WITHDRAWN
WRIGHT STATE UNIVERSITY LIBRARIES

D1521200

TISSUE ENGINEERING

ADVANCES IN EXPERIMENTAL MEDICINE AND BIOLOGY

Editorial Board:

NATHAN BACK, *State University of New York at Buffalo*
IRUN R. COHEN, *The Weizmann Institute of Science*
DAVID KRITCHEVSKY, *Wistar Institute*
ABEL LAJTHA, *N.S. Kline Institute for Psychiatric Research*
RODOLFO PAOLETTI, *University of Milan*

Recent Volumes in this Series

Volume 577
EARLY LIFE ORIGINS OF HEALTH AND DISEASE
Edited by E. Marelyn Wintour and Julie A. Owens

Volume 578
OXYGEN TRANSPORT TO TISSUE XXVII
Edited by Giuseppe Cicco, Duane Bruley, Marco Ferrari, and David K. Harrison

Volume 579
IMMUNE MECHANISMS IN INFLAMMATORY BOWEL DISEASE
Edited by Richard S. Blumberg

Volume 580
THE ARTERIAL CHEMORECEPTORS
Edited by Yoshiaki Hayashida, Constancio Gonzalez, and Hisatake Condo

Volume 581
THE NIDOVIRUSES: THE CONTROL OF SARS AND OTHER NIDOVIRUS DISEASES
Edited by Stanley Perlman and Kathryn Holmes

Volume 582
HOT TOPICS IN INFECTION AND IMMUNITY IN CHILDREN III
Edited by Andrew J. Pollard and Adam Finn

Volume 583
TAURINE 6: UPDATE 2005
Edited by Simo S. Oja and Pirjo Saransaari

Volume 584
LYMPHOCYTE SIGNAL TRANSDUCTION
Edited by Constantine Tsoukas

Volume 585
TISSUE ENGINEERING
Edited by John P. Fisher

Volume 586
CURRENT TOPICS IN COMPLEMENT
Edited by John D. Lambris

A Continuation Order Plan is available for this series. A continuation order will bring delivery of each new volume immediately upon publication. Volumes are billed only upon actual shipment. For further information please contact the publisher.

TISSUE ENGINEERING

Edited by

John P. Fisher
University of Maryland
College Park, Maryland

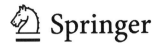 Springer

Editor:
John P. Fisher
University of Maryland
College Park, MD 20742
USA
jpfisher@umd.edu

Library of Congress Control Number: 2006925093

Printed on acid-free paper.

ISBN-10: 0-387-32664-2
ISBN-13: 978-0387-32664

Proceedings of the 2nd International Conference on Tissue Engineering, held in Crete, Greece, May 22–27 2005

© 2006 Springer Science+Business Media, LLC
All rights reserved. This work may not be translated or copied in whole or in part without the written permission of the publisher (Springer Science+Business Media, LLC, 233 Spring Street, New York, NY 10013, USA), except for brief excerpts in connection with reviews or scholarly analysis. Use in connection with any form of information storage and retrieval, electronic adaptation, computer software, or by similar or dissimilar methodology now known or hereafter developed is forbidden.
The use in this publication of trade names, trademarks, service marks and similar terms, even if they are not identified as such, is not to be taken as an expression of opinion as to whether or not they are subject to proprietary rights.

Printed in the United States of America.

9 8 7 6 5 4 3 2 1

springer.com

Preface

This special issue of Advances in Experimental Medicine and Biology includes much of the research presented at the recent Second International Tissue Engineering Conference. Held in Crete, Greece, as part of the Aegean Conference Series, the Second International Tissue Engineering Conference was organized by Dr. Kiki Hellman of the Hellman Group, Dr. John Jansen of the Nijmegen University Medical Center, and Dr. Antonios Mikos of Rice University. The conference brought over 150 researchers from around the world to the Knossos Royal Village Conference Center in Crete from May 22 to 27, 2005.

Following along the lines of the conference program, this volume is divided into seven sections, focusing on stem cells, signals, scaffolds, applied technologies, animal models, regulatory issues, as well as specific tissue engineering strategies. Both original research papers and review papers are presented. The chapters reflect a diverse group of authors, including both clinicians and academicians. Furthermore, the issue contains papers from Asia, Australia, Europe, and North America, demonstrating the international component of the conference.

The intended audience for this issue includes researchers, advanced students, and industrial investigators. This issue should be a useful reference for tissue engineering courses as well as for researchers developing engineered tissues for clinical applications.

Dr. John P. Fisher
University of Maryland
College Park, Maryland
jpfisher@umd.edu

Contents

List of Contributors xiii

Section 1: Stem Cells

Chapter 1

"Stem Cells into Liver" — Basic Research and Potential Clinical Applications.. 3
Agnieszka Banas, Gary Quinn, Yusuke Yamamoto, Takumi Teratani, and Takahiro Ochiya

Chapter 2

Mesenchymal Stem Cells Increase Self-Renewal of Small Intestinal Epithelium and Accelerate Structural Recovery after Radiation Injury 19
Alexandra Sémont, Sabine François, Moubarak Mouiseddine, Agnès François, Amandine Saché, Johanna Frick, Dominique Thierry, and Alain Chapel

Chapter 3

Optimizing Viral and Non-Viral Gene Transfer Methods for Genetic Modification of Porcine Mesenchymal Stem Cells................. 31
Maik Stiehler, Mogens Duch, Tina Mygind, Haisheng Li, Michael Ulrich-Vinther, Charlotte Modin, Anette Baatrup, Martin Lind, Finn S. Pedersen, and Cody E. Bünger

Chapter 4

Transplantation of Bone Marrow Stromal Cells for Treatment of Central Nervous System Diseases.. 49
Michael Chopp and Yi Li

Section 2: Soluble and Insoluble Signals

Chapter 5

Chondrocyte Signaling and Artificial Matrices for Articular Cartilage Engineering 67
Diana M. Yoon and John P. Fisher

Chapter 6

Osteoinduction with COLLOSS®, COLLOSS® E, and GFm 87
W.E. Huffer, J.J. Benedict, R. Rettenmaier, and A. Briest

Chapter 7

Biglycan Is a Positive Modulator of BMP-2-Induced Osteoblast Differentiation 101
Yoshiyuki Mochida, Duenpim Parisuthiman, and Mitsuo Yamauchi

Chapter 8

Use of Neopterin as a Bone Marrow Hematopoietic and Stromal Cell Growth Factor in Tissue-Engineered Devices 115
E. Zvetkova, Y. Gluhcheva, and D. Fuchs

Section 3: Scaffolds and Matrix Design

Chapter 9

Injectable Synthetic Extracellular Matrices for Tissue Engineering and Repair 125
Glenn D. Prestwich, Xiao Zheng Shu, Yanchun Liu, Shenshen Cai1, Jennifer F. Walsh, Casey W. Hughes, Shama Ahmad, Kelly R. Kirker, Bolan Yu, Richard R. Orlandi, Albert H. Park, Susan L. Thibeault, Suzy Duflo, and Marshall E. Smith

Chapter 10

Temporal Changes in PEG Hydrogel Structure Influence Human Mesenchymal Stem Cell Proliferation and Matrix Mineralization 135
Charles R. Nuttelman, April M. Kloxin, and Kristi S. Anseth

CONTENTS

Chapter 11

Novel Biophysical Techniques for Investigating Long-Term Cell Adhesion Dynamics on Biomaterial Surfaces 151
Z. Feng, N. Cai, V. Chan, P.S. Mhaisalka, K.S. Chian, B.D. Ratner, and K. Liao

Chapter 12

Evaluation of Various Types of Scaffold for Tissue-Engineered Intervertebral Disc 167
Soon Hee Kim, Sun Jung Yoon, Bangsil Choi, Hyun Jung Ha, John M. Rhee, Moon Suk Kim, Yoon Sun Yang, Hai Bang Lee, and Gilson Khang

Chapter 13

Physicochemical Characterization of Photopolymerizable PLGA Blends 183
Biancamaria Baroli

Chapter 14

Porous Tantalum Trabecular Metal Scaffolds in Combination with a Novel Marrow Processing Technique to Replace Autograft 197
Xuenong Zou, Haisheng Li, Lijin Zou, Tina Mygind, Martin Lind, and Cody Bünger

Chapter 15

Preparation of Sponge Using Porcine Small Intesinal Submucosa and Their Applications as a Scaffold and a Wound Dressing 209
Moon Suk Kim, Min Suk Lee, In Bum Song, Sang Jin Lee, Hai Bang Lee, Gilson Khang, and Il Woo Lee

Section 4: Bioreactor and Assessment Technologies

Chapter 16

Modulation of Cell Differentiation in Bone Tissue Engineering Constructs Cultured in a Bioreactor 225
Heidi L. Holtorf, John A. Jansen, and Antonios G. Mikos

Chapter 17

Bioreactors for Tissues of the Musculoskeletal System 243
Rita I. Abousleiman and Vassilios I. Sikavitsas

Chapter 18

Non-Invasive Monitoring of Tissue-Engineered Pancreatic Constructs by NMR Techniques... 261
Ioannis Constantinidis, Nicholas E. Simpson, Samuel C. Grant, Stephen J. Blackband, Robert C. Long Jr., and Athanassios Sambanis

Section 5: Animal Models and Clinical Strategies

Chapter 19

From Molecules to Matrix: Construction and Evaluation of Molecularly Defined Bioscaffolds 279
Paul J. Geutjes, Willeke F. Daamen, Pieter Buma, Wout F. Feitz, Kaeuis A. Faraj, and Toin H. van Kuppevelt

Chapter 20

Age-Related Differences in Articular Cartilage Wound Healing: A Potential Role for Transforming Growth Factor β1 in Adult Cartilage Repair 297
P.K. Bos, J.A.N. Verhaar, and G.J.V.M. van Osch

Chapter 21

Intrinsic versus Extrinsic Vascularization in Tissue Engineering........................... 311
Elias Polykandriotis, Raymund E. Horch, Andreas Arkudas, Apostolos Labanaris, Kay Brune, Peter Greil, Alexander D. Bach, Jürgen Kopp, Andreas Hess, and Ulrich Kneser

Chapter 22

Predictive Value of *in Vitro* and *in Vivo* Assays in Bone and Cartilage Repair — What Do They Really Tell Us about the Clinical Performance? 327
Pamela Habibovic, Tim Woodfield, Klaas de Groot, and Clemens van Blitterswijk

CONTENTS xi

Section 6: Science, Regulation, and the Public

Chapter 23

Engineered Tissues: The Regulatory Path from Concept to Market 363
Kiki B. Hellman

Section 7: Tissue Engineering Strategies

Chapter 24

Fibrin in Tissue Engineering 379
Daniela Eyrich, Achim Göpferich, and Torsten Blunk

Chapter 25

Ectopic Bone Induction by Equine Bone Protein Extract 393
*Haisheng Li, Marco Springer, Xuenong Zou, Arne Briest,
and Cody Bünger*

Chapter 26

Adipose Tissue Induction *in Vivo* 403
*Filip B.J.L. Stillaert, Phillip N. Blondeel, Keren Abberton,
Erik Thompson, and Wayne A. Morrison*

Chapter 27

Ocular Tissue Engineering 413
Florian Sommer, Ferdinand Brandl, and Achim Göpferich

Chapter 28

Molecular Mechanism of Osteochondroprogenitor Fate
Determination during Bone Formation 431
*Lijin Zou, Xuenong Zou, Haisheng Li, Tina Mygind,
Yuanlin Zeng, Nonghua Lü, and Cody Bünger*

Author Index 443

Subject Index 445

Contributors

Keren Abberton
Bernard O'Brien Institute of Microsurgery
University of Melbourne
Melbourne, Australia

Rita I. Abousleiman
Bioengineering Center
The University of Oklahoma
Norman, Oklahoma, USA

Shama Ahmad
Department of Bioengineering
The University of Utah
Salt Lake City, Utah, USA

Kristi S. Anseth
Department of Chemical & Biological
 Engineering
University of Colorado
Boulder, Colorado, USA

Andreas Arkudas
Department of Plastic & Hand Surgery
University of Erlangen
Erlangen, Germany

Anette Baatrup
Orthopaedic Research Laboratory
Department of Orthopaedic Surgery
Aarhus University Hospital
Aarhus, Denmark

Alexander D. Bach
Department of Plastic & Hand Surgery
University of Erlangen
Erlangen, Germany

Agnieszka Banas
Section for Studies on Metastasis
National Cancer Center Research Institute
Tokyo, Japan

Biancamaria Baroli
Dipartimento Farmaco Chimico
 Tecnologico
Università degli Studi di Cagliari
Facoltà di Farmacia
Cagliari, Sardinia, Italy

James J. Benedict
Arvada, Colorado

Stephen J. Blackband
Department of Medicine
University of Florida
Gainesville, Florida, USA

Phillip N. Blondeel
Department of Plastic & Reconstructive
 Surgery
University Hospital Ghent
Ghent, Belgium

Torsten Blunk
Department of Pharmaceutical Technology
University of Regensburg
Regensburg, Germany

P.K. Bos
Department of Orthopaedic Surgery
University Medical Center
Rotterdam, The Netherlands

Ferdinand Brandl
Department of Pharmaceutical Technology
University of Regensburg
Regensburg, Germany

Arne Briest
Research & Development
OSSACUR AG
Oberstenfeld, Denmark

Kay Brune
Institute of Pharmacology & Toxicology
University of Erlangen
Erlangen, Germany

Pieter Buma
Department of Orthopaedics
Radboud University Nijmegen
    Medical Centre
Nijmegen, The Netherlands

Cody E. Bünger
Orthopaedic Research Laboratory
Department of Orthopaedic
    Surgery
Aarhus University Hospital
Aarhus, Denmark

N. Cai
Department of Bioengineering
School of Chemical & Biomedical
    Engineering
Nanyang Technological University
Singapore

Shenshen Cai
Department of Medicinal Chemistry
The University of Utah
Salt Lake City, Utah, USA

V. Chan
Department of Chemical & Biomolecular
    Engineering
School of Chemical & Biomedical
    Engineering
Nanyang Technological University
Singapore

Alain Chapel
Laboratoire de Thérapie Cellulaire et de
    Radioprotection Accidentelle
Institut de Radioprotection et de
    Sûreté Nucléaire
Fontenay aux Roses, France

K.S. Chian
Tissue Engineering Laboratory
School of Mechanical & Aerospace
    Engineering
Nanyang Technological University
Singapore

Bangsil Choi
Department of Polymer/Nano Science
    & Technology
Chonbuk National University
Jeonju, Korea

Michael Chopp
Department of Neurology
Henry Ford Health Sciences Center
Detroit, Michigan, USA

Ioannis Constantinidis
Department of Medicine
University of Florida
Gainesville, Florida, USA

Willeke F. Daamen
Department of Orthopaedics
Nijmegen Centre for Molecular
    Life Sciences
Radboud University Nijmegen
    Medical Centre
Nijmegen, The Netherlands

Klaas de Groot
Institute for Biomedical Technology
University of Twente
Bilthoven, The Netherlands

Mogens Duch
Interdisciplinary Nanoscience Center
    (iNANO)
Department of Molecular Biology
University of Aarhus
Aarhus, Denmark

Suzy Duflo
Department of Surgery
The University of Utah
Salt Lake City, Utah, USA

Daniela Eyrich
Department of Pharmaceutical Technology
University of Regensburg
Regensburg, Germany

Kaeuis A. Faraj
Department of Biochemistry
Nijmegen Centre for Molecular
    Life Sciences
Radboud University Nijmegen
    Medical Centre
Nijmegen, The Netherlands

Wout F. Feitz
Department of Urology
Radboud University Nijmegen
    Medical Centre
Nijmegen, The Netherlands

Z. Feng
Biomedical Engineering Research Centre
Nanyang Technological University
Singapore

John P. Fisher
Department of Chemical & Biomolecular
    Engineering
University of Maryland
College Park, Maryland, USA

Agnès François
Laboratoire de Thérapie Cellulaire et
    de Radioprotection Accidentelle
Institut de Radioprotection et de
    Sûreté Nucléaire
Fontenay aux Roses, France

Sabine François
Laboratoire de Thérapie Cellulaire et
    de Radioprotection Accidentelle
Institut de Radioprotection et de
    Sûreté Nucléaire
Fontenay aux Roses, France

Johanna Frick
Laboratoire de Thérapie Cellulaire et
    de Radioprotection Accidentelle
Institut de Radioprotection et de
    Sûreté Nucléaire
Fontenay aux Roses, France

D. Fuchs
Division of Biological Chemistry
Innsbruck Medical University
Innsbruck, Austria

Paul J. Geutjes
Department of Biochemistry
Radboud University Nijmegen Medical
    Centre
Nijmegen, The Netherlands

Y. Gluhcheva
Institute of Experimental Morphology
    & Anthropology
Bulgarian Academy of Sciences
Sofia, Bulgaria

Achim Göpferich
Department of Pharmaceutical Technology
University of Regensburg
Regensburg, Germany

Samuel C. Grant
Department of Medicine
University of Florida
Gainesville, Florida, USA

Peter Greil
Department of Glass & Ceramics
Institute of Materials Sciences
University of Erlangen
Erlangen, Germany

Hyun Jung Ha
Department of Polymer/Nano Science
    & Technology
Chonbuk National University
Jeonju, Korea

Pamela Habibovic
Institute for Biomedical Technology
University of Twente
Bilthoven, The Netherlands

Moustapha Hamdi
Department of Plastic & Reconstructive
   Surgery
University Hospital Ghent
Ghent, Belgium

Kiki B. Hellman
The Hellman Group LLC
Clarksburg, Maryland, USA

Andreas Hess
Institute of Pharmacology & Toxicology
University of Erlangen
Erlangen, Germany

Heidi L. Holtorf
Division of Space Life Sciences
Universities Space Research Association
Houston, Texas, USA

Raymund.E. Horch
Department of Plastic & Hand Surgery
University of Erlangen
Erlangen, Germany

W.E. Huffer
Department of Pathology
University of Colorado Health Sciences
   Center
Denver, Colorado, USA

Casey W. Hughes
Department of Bioengineering
The University of Utah
Salt Lake City, Utah, USA

John A. Jansen
Department of Periodontology &
   Biomaterials
Radboud University Nijmegen
   Medical Centre
Nijmegen, The Netherlands

Gilson Khang
Department of Polymer/Nano Science
   & Technology
Chonbuk National University
Jeonju, Korea

Moon Suk Kim
Nanobiomaterials Laboratory
Korea Research Institutes of Chemical
   Technology
Daejeon, Korea

Soon Hee Kim
Department of Polymer/Nano Science &
   Technology
Chonbuk National University
Jeonju, Korea

L. Kin
School of Chemical & Biomedical
   Engineering
Nanyang Technological University
Singapore

Kelly R. Kirker
Department of Bioengineering
The University of Utah
Salt Lake City, Utah, USA

April M. Kloxin
Department of Chemical & Biological
   Engineering
University of Colorado
Boulder, Colorado, USA

Ulrich Kneser
Department of Plastic & Hand Surgery
University of Erlangen
Erlangen, Germany

Jürgen Kopp
Department of Plastic & Hand Surgery
University of Erlangen
Erlangen, Germany

Apostolos Labanaris
Department of Plastic & Hand Surgery
University of Erlangen
Erlangen, Germany

Hai Bang Lee
Nanobiomaterials Laboratory
Korea Research Institutes of
 Chemical Technology
Daejeon, Korea

Hye Ran Lee
Nanobiomaterials Laboratory
Korea Research Institutes of Chemical
 Technology
Daejeon, Korea

Il Woo Lee
Department of Neurosurgery
Catholic University of Korea
Daejeon, Korea

Min Suk Lee
Nanobiomaterials Laboratory
Korea Research Institutes of Chemical
 Technology
Daejeon, Korea

Sang Jin Lee
Nanobiomaterials Laboratory
Korea Research Institutes of Chemical
Technology
Daejeon, Korea

Haisheng Li
Orthopaedic Research Laboratory
Department of Orthopaedic Surgery
Aarhus University Hospital
Aarhus, Denmark

Yi Li
Department of Neurology
Henry Ford Health Sciences Center
Detroit, Michigan, USA

K. Liao
Department of Bioengineering
School of Chemical & Biomedical
 Engineering
Nanyang Technological University
Singapore

Martin Lind
Orthopaedic Research Laboratory
Department of Orthopaedic Surgery
Aarhus University Hospital
Aarhus, Denmark

Yanchun Liu
Department of Medicinal Chemistry
The University of Utah
Salt Lake City, Utah, USA

Robert C. Long Jr.
Department of Radiology
Emory University
Atlanta, Georgia, USA

Nonghua Lü
The First Affiliated Hospital of Nanchang
 University
Nanchang, China

P.S. Mhaisalka
Biomedical Engineering Research Centre
Nanyang Technological University
Singapore

Antonios G. Mikos
Department of Bioengineering
Rice University
Houston, Texas, USA

Yoshiyuki Mochida
Department of Pediatric Dentistry
Dental Research Center
University of North Carolina
Chapel Hill, North Carolina, USA

Charlotte Modin
Department of Molecular Biology
University of Aarhus
Aarhus, Denmark

Wayne A. Morrison
Bernard O'Brien Institute of Microsurgery
University of Melbourne
Melbourne, Australia

Moubarak Mouiseddine
Laboratoire de Thérapie Cellulaire et de Radioprotection Accidentelle
Institut de Radioprotection et de Sûreté Nucléaire
Fontenay aux Roses, France

Tina Mygind
Orthopaedic Research Laboratory
Department of Orthopaedic Surgery
Aarhus University Hospital
Aarhus, Denmark

Charles R. Nuttelman
Department of Chemical & Biological Engineering
University of Colorado
Boulder, Colorado, USA

Takahiro Ochiya
Section for Studies on Metastasis
National Cancer Center Research Institute
Tokyo, Japan

Richard R. Orlandi
Department of Surgery
The University of Utah
Salt Lake City, Utah, USA

Duenpim Parisuthiman
School of Dentistry
Thammasat University
Pathumthani, Thailand

Albert H. Park
Department of Surgery
The University of Utah
Salt Lake City, Utah, USA

Finn S. Pedersen
Department of Molecular Biology
University of Aarhus
Aarhus, Denmark

Elias Polykandriotis
Department of Plastic & Hand Surgery
University of Erlangen
Erlangen, Germany

Glenn D. Prestwich
Department of Medicinal Chemistry
The University of Utah
Salt Lake City, Utah, USA

Gary Quinn
Effector Cell Institute
Tokyo, Japan

B.D. Ratner
Departments of Bioengineering & Chemical Engineering
University of Washington
Seattle, Washington, USA

R. Rettenmaier
Veterinary Services
OSSACUR AG
Oberstenfeld, Denmark

John M. Rhee
Department of Polymer/Nano Science & Technology
Chonbuk National University
Jeonju, Korea

Amandine Saché
Laboratoire de Thérapie Cellulaire et de Radioprotection Accidentelle
Institut de Radioprotection et de Sûreté Nucléaire
Fontenay aux Roses, France

Athanassios Sambanis
School of Chemical and Biomolecular Engineering
Georgia Institute of Technology
Atlanta, Georgia, USA

Alexandra Sémont
Laboratoire de Thérapie Cellulaire et de Radioprotection Accidentelle
Institut de Radioprotection et de Sûreté Nucléaire
Fontenay aux Roses, France

Xiao Zheng Shu
Department of Medicinal Chemistry
The University of Utah
Salt Lake City, Utah, USA

Vassilios I. Sikavitsas
School of Chemical, Biological, & Materials
Engineering and Bioengineering Center
The University of Oklahoma
Norman, Oklahoma, USA

Nicholas E. Simpson
Department of Medicine
University of Florida
Gainesville, Florida, USA

Marshall E. Smith
Department of Surgery
The University of Utah
Salt Lake City, Utah, USA

Florian Sommer
Department of Pharmaceutical Technology
University of Regensburg
Regensburg, Germany

In Bum Song
Nanobiomaterials Laboratory
Korea Research Institutes of Chemical
    Technology
Daejeon, Korea

Marco Springer
OSSACUR AG
Oberstenfeld, Denmark

Maik Stiehler
Orthopaedic Research Laboratory
Department of Orthopaedic Surgery
Aarhus University Hospital
Aarhus, Denmark

Filip B.J.L. Stillaert
Department of Plastic & Reconstructive
    Surgery
University Hospital Ghent
Ghent, Belgium

Takumi Teratani
Section for Studies on Metastasis
National Cancer Center Research Institute
Tokyo, Japan

Susan L. Thibeault
Department of Surgery
The University of Utah
Salt Lake City, Utah, USA

Dominique Thierry
Laboratoire de Thérapie Cellulaire et de
    Radioprotection Accidentelle
Institut de Radioprotection et de Sûreté
    Nucléaire
Fontenay aux Roses, France

Erik Thompson
Bernard O'Brien Institute of Microsurgery
University of Melbourne
Melbourne, Australia

Michael Ulrich-Vinther
Orthopaedic Research Laboratory
Department of Orthopaedic Surgery
Aarhus University Hospital
Aarhus, Denmark

Clemens van Blitterswijk
Institute for Biomedical Technology
University of Twente
Bilthoven, The Netherlands

Toin H. van Kuppevelt
Department of Biochemistry
Nijmegen Centre for Molecular
    Life Sciences
Radboud University Nijmegen
    Medical Centre
Nijmegen, The Netherlands

G.J.V.M. van Osch
Departments of Orthopaedic Surgery &
    Otorhinolaryngology
University Medical Center
Rotterdam, The Netherlands

Jan Verhaar
Department of Orthopaedic Surgery
University Medical Center
Rotterdam, The Netherlands

Jennifer F. Walsh
Department of Bioengineering
The University of Utah
Salt Lake City, Utah, USA

Tim Woodfield
Centre for Bioengineering
University of Canterbury
Christchurch, New Zealand

Yusuke Yamamoto
Department of Biology
School of Education
Waseda University
Tokyo, Japan

Mitsuo Yamauchi
Dental Research Center
University of North Carolina
Chapel Hill, North Carolina, USA

Yoon Sun Yang
Asan Institute of Life Science
MEDIPOST Biomedical Research Institute
Seoul, Korea

Diana M. Yoon
Department of Chemical & Biomolecular
   Engineering
University of Maryland
College Park, Maryland, USA

Sun Jung Yoon
Department of Polymer/Nano Science
   & Technology
Chonbuk National University
Jeonju, Korea

Bolan Yu
Department of Medicinal Chemistry
The University of Utah
Salt Lake City, Utah, USA

Yuanlin Zeng
The First Affiliated Hospital of Nanchang
   University
Nanchang, China

Lijin Zou
Orthopaedic Research Laboratory
Aarhus University Hospital
Aarhus, Denmark

Xuenong Zou
Orthopaedic Research Laboratory
Aarhus University Hospital
Aarhus, Denmark

E. Zvetkova
Institute of Experimental Morphology
   & Anthropology
Bulgarian Academy of Sciences
Sofia, Bulgaria

SECTION 1
STEM CELLS

1

"STEM CELLS INTO LIVER"- BASIC RESEARCH AND POTENTIAL CLINICAL APPLICATIONS

Agnieszka Banas[1], Gary Quinn[1,2], Yusuke Yamamoto[1,3], Takumi Teratani[1] and Takahiro Ochiya[1]

1.1. INTRODUCTION

Regenerative medicine holds promise for the restoration of damaged tissues and organs. The concept of regenerative medicine radically changed when pluripotent human embryonic stem cells were isolated and cultured[1]. However, much more promising perspectives for clinical application are served by recently discovered multipotential adult stem cells, which may give rise to a large family of descendants, depending on the environments they are residing in[2,3,4]. Properties and plasticity of stem cells from different sources have been intensely investigated, regarding to their use in therapy. The liver is one target for which development of stem cell-based therapy is of great significance. Even though an injured liver is highly regenerative, many debilitating diseases lead to hepatocyte dysfunction and organ failure.

Liver transplantation is the only effective treatment for severe liver injuries. However, because of organ rejection and the limited number of donors, alternative therapeutic approaches are needed. Stem cell transplantation could offer a potentially unlimited and minimally invasive source of cells for hepatocyte replacement and regeneration and, therefore, might be superior to whole organ transplantation. A first step to establish such therapy is the development of a model where functional hepatocytes can be generated in vitro and the second step is the design of a microenvironment for long-term maintenance of cell and, finally, organ culture.

Many studies have been performed using stem cells to produce functional hepatocytes, but there are still many obstacles like teratoma formation, cell fusion or

---

[1] Section for Studies on Metastasis, National Cancer Center Research Institute, Tokyo, Japan
[2] Effector Cell Institute, Inc. Tokyo, Japan
[3] Department of Biology, School of Education, Waseda University, Tokyo, Japan

endless proliferative ability (potentially carcinogenic), which need to be overcome before clinical use. Nevertheless, investigations to establish a successful liver stem cell-based therapy are on the right track. With humbleness towards this difficult challenge, we will nevertheless attempt to resume achievements and discuss each of the potential stem cell-types (ES cells and adult stem cells) (Figure 1.1.) for use in liver therapy.

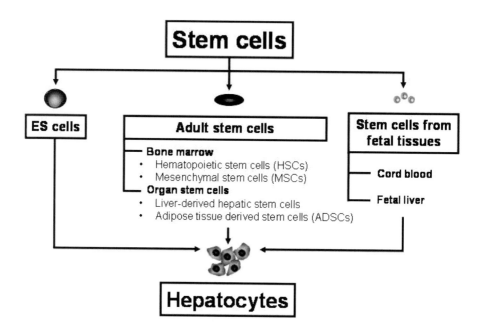

Figure 1.1. Generation of human hepatocytes from different stem cell sources. Embryonic stem (ES) cells, stem cells from fetal tissues (such as cord blood-derived mesenchymal stem cells) and adult stem cells (including bone marrow-derived mesenchymal stem cells (BM-MSCs) and adipose tissue-derived stem cells (ADSCs)) have potentiality to differentiate into hepatocytes in vitro and are promising candidates for hepatocyte production.

1.2. EMBRYONIC STEM CELLS

Pluripotent embryonic stem (ES) cells, isolated from the inner cell mass (ICM) of blastocysts are capable of giving rise to cells found in all three germ layers of the embryo. They are considered to have the greatest range of differentiation potential and are the cells that the majority of studies have used. In the context of serious ethical concerns, most of experiments are performed on animal ES cells. The pluripotency of ES cells was proven in vivo and in vitro. In vivo, injection of the ES cells generates teratomas harboring derivatives of all three embryonic germ layers. In vitro, after removal from the feeder layer or from LIF, ES cells aggregate in suspension to form spheroid clumps of cells called embryoid bodies (EBs).

1.2.1. Mouse ES Cells

Mouse ES cells can be maintained in their undifferentiated state for an indefinite continuous time, on mouse embryonic fibroblasts or by culture with a leukaemia inhibitory factor (LIF), which is a feeder-cell-derived molecule that plays a pivotal role in the maintenance of these cells.

Here we present a few systems of hepatic induction (in vitro and in vivo) from ES cells, utilized by different groups (Figure 1.2.). In vitro strategies include differentiation through EBs formation, co-culture and mono-culture systems, while in vivo strategies utilize animals with liver injury or liver regeneration.

In order to define hepatic differentiation, liver-specific markers, responsible for hepatocyte endodermal differentiation as well as hepatocyte functions need to be detected. The markers include hepatic transcription factors essential for endodermal development (hepatic nuclear factor (HNF)-3beta/forkhead box A2 (FOXA2) and HNF-4alpha), the carrier proteins (alpha-fetoprotein (AFP), responsible for fatty acids, copper and nickel transport, albumin (ALB), responsible for steroids, fatty acids and thyroid hormone transport, transthyretin (TTR), carrying retinol) as well as enzymes (tryptophan-2,3-dioxygenase (TDO2), catalyzing tryptophan oxidative degradation, glucose-6-phosphatase (G6P), involved in control of glucose homeostasis and cytochrom P450 (CYP) enzymes). The functional assays for hepatocytes are mainly albumin and urea synthesis, glucose production and glycogen storage ability.

1.2.1.1. In Vivo Differentiation

ES cells have a propensity to develop teratomas when implanted into animals. Teratomas form tumors and finally cause the death of the host animal, which introduces a handicap in respect to any naïve utilization of them clinically. However, ES cells have been used by Choi et al. in order to demonstrate their hepatic differentiation potential in vivo[5]. They injected ES cells into the spleen of immunosuppressed mice and, as a first, demonstrated that teratomas derived from injected ES cells revealed that some areas contained typical hepatocytes. Chinzei et al. demonstrated that cells isolated from EBs nine or more days after LIF removal have expressed a panel of hepatic markers and were capable of producing albumin and urea[6]. After transplantation into partial hepatectomy of female mice pretreated with 2-acetylaminofluorene, ES cell-derived cells survived and expressed ALB, whereas teratomas were found in mice transplanted with ES cells or EBs up to day six. They demonstrated that, while ES cells always developed teratomas in recipient mice, this incidence was decreased in case of implantation of EBs and depended on the culture period of EBs. In vivo differentiation of ES cells carrying green fluorescent protein (GFP) in the AFP locus was performed by Yin et al.[7] They selected a subpopulation of GFP positive and AFP expressing cells from differentiating in vitro ES cells. After transplantation into partially hepatectomized lacZ-positive ROSA26 mice,

GFP positive cells engrafted and differentiated into lacZ-negative and ALB-positive cells. In this case no teratomas were observed. Furthermore, using an animal with injured liver (regenerative condition), Yamamoto et al., reported that efficient differentiation of ES cells into transplantable hepatocytes with therapeutic properties has been successful[8].

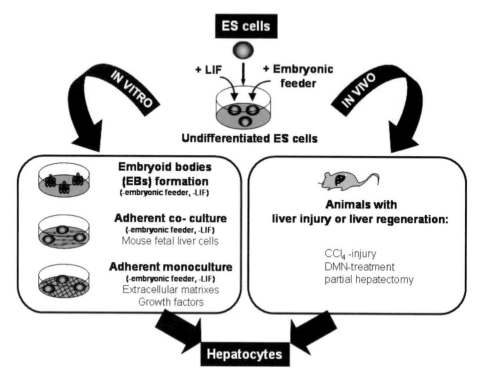

Figure 1.2. Strategies of hepatic induction from ES cells. In vivo strategies utilize factory on animals with liver injury or liver regeneration. In vitro hepatic differentiation strategies include: embryoid bodies (EBs) formation, co-culture and adherent monoculture systems.

1.2.1.2. In Vitro Differentiation

The EBs mature by the process of spontaneous differentiation and cavitations and the cells acquire markers for differentiated cell types. Dissociation of EBs and plating the differentiated cells as a monolayer reveal many cell lineages. Several growth factors and transcription factors have been shown to be capable of directing differentiation of mouse ES cells. Different matrix proteins may dramatically influence the generation and survival of the developed cells. Usually, collagen is used as the matrix for culturing the cells towards hepatic lineage since the liver bud proliferates and migrate into the septum transversum mesenchyme, which is composed of loose connective tissue containing collagen. Hamazaki et al. demonstrated that mouse EBs can be differentiated into hepatocyte-like cells when cultured on collagen-coated plates with early (fibroblast growth factors (FGFs)), middle (hepatocyte growth factor (HGF)) and late (oncostatin M

(OsM)), dexamethasone and insulin/transferrin/selenium) differentiation stage factors[9]. Jones et al. confirmed these observations, culturing ES cells carrying a gene trap vector insertion into an ankyrin-repeat-containing gene[10]. This modification induces beta-galactosidase expression when hepatocyte differentiation begins. Kuai et al. reported that beta-nerve growth factor (NGF) also promotes hepatic differentiation, which is increased in the presence of HGF and retinoic acid[11].

Miyashita et al. and Chinzei et al. also demonstrated in vitro hepatic differentiation through formation of EBs, without using hepatocyte-specific cytokines[12,6]. Yamada et al., by using an ES cell line carrying the enhanced green fluorescent protein (EGFP) gene, identified indocyanin-green (ICG) uptake by cells differentiated from mouse EBs and reported the presence of liver-specific markers using RT-PCR and immunocytochemistry[13]. Ishizaka et al. demonstrated that when transfected with HNF-3beta, mouse ES cells were able to differentiate into hepatocytes with liver-specific metabolic functions, after stimulation with FGF-2, dexamethasone, L-ascorbic-2-phosphate, and nicotinamide in a 3-dimensional culture system[14]. The same genetically modified ES cells were differentiated through EBs formation into hepatic-like cells by Kanda et al. on an attached culture system[15]. Importantly, later on they discovered that HNF-3beta transfected ES cell-derived hepatic-like cells have infinite proliferating potential, resulting in tumor formation and finally the death of the animals after transplantation.

EBs offer the advantage of providing a three-dimensional structure, which enhances cell-cell interactions that may be important for hepatocyte development. However, the complexity of the EBs is a problem, because of the cytokines and inducing factors generated within these structures which induce differentiation of other cell lineages as well. Until now, none of the hepatic differentiation systems based on EBs formation revealed an efficient induction of functional hepatocytes sufficient for experimental therapeutic study.

A co-culture strategy was used by Ishii et al[16]. They produced in vitro mature hepatocytes from ES cells (carrying GFP in AFP locus) entirely via isolation AFP-producing cells and subsequent maturation of these cells by co-culture with Thy1-positive (CD90) mouse fetal liver cells. The achieved hepatic-like cells produced and stored glycogen as well as revealed a capacity to clear ammonia. In a co-culture system differentiation takes place in contact with assisting cells (fetal liver cells or stromal cells), because of the presence of differentiation factors; however, undefined factors produced by these supportive cells may influence the differentiation of ES cells into undesired cell types. An additional disadvantage might be the difficulty with separation of the ES cell-derived hepatocytes from assisting cells.

Recently, Teratani et al. showed that ES cells can differentiate into functional hepatocytes without the requirement for EBs formation or in vivo transplantation or a co-culture system (Figure 1.2.)[17]. By comparison of genes between CCl_4-treated injured and untreated normal mouse liver, their group identified a hepatic induction factor cocktail (HIFC) (Figure 1.3.a.). ES cell-derived hepatocytes, after HIFC induction, expressed multiple liver specific makers: ALB, TDO2, TTR, G6P, cytochrome 450, as well as hepatocyte nuclear factors: HNF-3 beta and HNF-4 alpha. Additionally, AFP expression appeared in early and TDO2 at the late stage of differentiation, which means that ES cell-derived hepatocytes mimic normal liver development (Figure 1.3.b.). The functionality shown by glucose-producing ability, the capacity to clear ammonia and urea synthesis ability, display characteristics of mature hepatocytes. Also in this case no teratomas were observed and karyotyping analysis showed a normal chromosome number. Most importantly, transplantation of ES cell-derived hepatocytes in mice with cirrhosis generated by dimethylnitrosoamine (DMN) showed a significant therapeutic effect. This model could be easily adapted into human ES cells, allowing precise control of proliferation and differentiation during production of human hepatocytes. In support of this speculation, differentiation of hepatocytes from *Cynomolgus monkey* ES cells is achievable using the HIFC system (Teratani et al. unpublished data). In regard to utilizing human ES cells in liver therapy, knowledge of molecular mechanisms of hepatic differentiation is needed. Yamamoto et al., based on the HIFC differentiation system, compared the gene expression profile of ES cell-derived hepatocytes with adult mice liver and found significant similarities in gene expression profile[18]. Of 9172 analyzed genes in the HIFC treated ES cells; approximately 200 genes related to liver specific functions were radically altered in comparison with non treated ES cells. By using small interfering RNA (siRNA) technology, HNF-3beta has been found to be essential in in vitro hepatic differentiation, which indicates also that this system progresses via endoderm differentiation, imitating hepatic development in vivo: step 0-pluripotent ES cells, step 1-endoderm specification (HNF-3beta expression), step 2-immature hepatocytes (AFP, ALB), step 3: mature hepatocytes (ALB, TDO2) (Figure 1.3.b.).

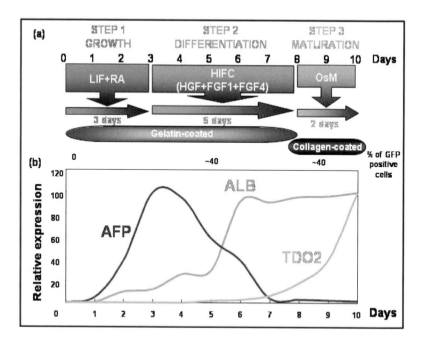

Figure 1.3. Hepatic induction system in adherent monoculture[17]. (a) Schematic representation of the differentiation protocol for the induction of the hepatocytes from ES cells by HIFC in monolayer culture. (b) Graph representation of AFP (alpha-fetoprotein), ALB (albumin) and TDO2 (tryptophan 2,3-dioxygenase) expression during HIFC treatment.

Experiments on human ES cells are limited because of obvious serious ethical concerns; however, there are strong speculations that after some modifications, experiments performed on animal models could be adapted into humans.

1.2.2. Human ES Cells

Schuldiner et al. showed the potential of human ES cells to differentiate into three embryonic germ layers after stimulation with different growth factors. EBs were dissociated and plated onto fibronectin-coated dishes and treated with growth factors, none of which induced the differentiation into any one specific cell type[19]. Rambhatla et al. used sodium butyrate to induce hepatocyte differentiation in human ES cells, through EBs formation[20]. Characteristics of hepatocyte morphology as well as ALB, alpha-1-antitripsin (AAT), cytokeratin (CK)-8 and CK-18, inducible cytochrome P450 expression and glycogen accumulation have been observed; however, sodium butyrate induced significant cell death. Levenberg et al. used biodegradable scaffolds of PLGA-poly(lactic-co-glycolic acid) and PLLA-poly(L-lactic acid) to induce tissue-like structures, after seeding ES cells or EBs and they found hepatocyte differentiation after stimulation with activin-A and insulin-like growth factor (IGF)[21]. 14 days after implantation of 2-week-old constructs into SCID mice; immunostaining analysis of cytokeratin and AFP indicated that the implanted constructs continued to express these human proteins.

ES cells have great potential, although they face limitations inherent in procurement from fetal tissues, problems related to histocompatibility and ethical concerns. Such handicaps might be sidestepped in the future by somatic cell nuclear transfer of a patient's own skin cells into donated oocytes. Further investigations concerning genomic stability, differentiation fidelity and cellular "reprogramming" need to be performed. Many controversies have emerged, but there are speculations that human ES cells might be investigated and used in regenerative medicine in the future without the need for embryos or oocytes.

1.3. ADULT STEM CELLS

Many adult tissues contain populations of multipotent stem cells, which have the capacity for renewal after trauma, disease, or ageing and indefinite proliferative potential, which makes them a very attractive and ethically non-controversial tool in stem cell therapy. In adults, there is a spectrum of stem cells with a different scale of potentiality (multipotent, unipotent) and quantity. They "are ready" to receive signals from circulating blood (also containing multipotential adult stem cells) to control homeostasis.

The liver, besides liver-derived bipotential cells[23], which can give rise to hepatocytes and biliary epithelial cells, is supported by stem cells deriving from bone marrow and blood[24]; however, the mechanism by which this balance is achieved is still enigmatic and controversial.

1.3.1. Bone Marrow

Bone marrow (BM) as a source of heterogeneous populations of stem cells (hematopoietic stem cells (HSC), mesenchymal stem cells (MSCs)), has been shown to contribute in liver regeneration.

1.3.1.1. Non-Fractioned BM

A huge focus on BM as a source of stem cells for regenerative medicine started when its contribution to liver regeneration in vivo was described. Petersen et al. showed that transplantation of unfractioned male BM into the livers of lethally irradiated female rats, whose livers were injured by 2-acetylaminofluorene and CCl_4, rescued the animals from radiation-induced BM ablation and simultaneously produced small numbers of BM-derived hepatic stem cells[25]. They demonstrated that host liver contained hepatocytes carrying genetic markers derived from implanted BM cells. Additional evidence of BM-derived hepatic stem cells was demonstrated by Theise et al., who also used the gender mismatch BM transplantation strategy and showed that over a six month period 1-2% of hepatocytes in mice liver may be derived from BM in the absence of any liver damage[26]. Further studies made by the same group demonstrated that also in humans, hepatocytes can derive from BM[27,28]. They examined the livers of female patients, who had received a BM transplant from male donors, and female livers transplanted into male recipients, which had to be removed for recurrent disease. In both cases Y-chromosome-positive hepatocytes were identified, but the degree of hepatic engraftment of HSCs into the human liver was highly variable. The most impressive generation of hepatocytes from BM cells has occurred after transplantation of BM into mice with lethal hepatic failure resulting from homozygous deletion of the fumaryl acetoacetate hydrolase (*Fah*) gene, corresponding to human tyrosinemia type 1[29]. Subsequent studies in the Fah-deficient model suggest that differentiation of HSCs to hepatocytes results from the fusion of HSCs descendant cells with Fah-negative hepatocytes, giving heterokaryotic cells[30,31]. The fusion might be observed as a result of the genetic alterations in the Fah-deficient mice; however, it remains unclear.

1.3.1.2. Purified BM-Derived Hematopoietic Stem Cells

Wang et al. did not observe cell fusion when transplanting purified human HSCs $CD34^+$ or $CD34^+$ $CD38^-$, $CD7^-$ from BM (and umbilical cord blood (UCB)) into non-obese diabetic immunodeficiency (NOD/SCID) mice and (NOD/SCID) beta-2-microglobulin–null mice[32]. They demonstrated after CCl_4 administration the presence of ALB in mice serum, and human ALB and CK19 mRNA in mice livers; however, they did not detect AFP. A recent report by Jang et al. showed as well that HSCs can differentiate without fusion into hepatocytes and that an injured liver's function was restored after transplantation[33]. They suggested that microenvironmental cues rather than fusion might be responsible for hepatocyte differentiation. Transdifferentiation is heavily debated topic and the mechanisms are not understood. It might be a rare and unphysiological event, occurring under special conditions only. Nevertheless, fusion of donor cells derived from BM or elsewhere with resident hepatocytes does not preclude stem cell-based therapies. It can bring as well a new opportunity for delivering new genetic material to cells for gene therapy.

There have also been reports that BM-derived HSCs can differentiate into mature hepatic phenotypes in vitro. Miyazaki et al. showed that BM-derived HSCs ($CD34^+$, Thy-1^+ (CD90) and c-kit$^+$ (CD117) express hepatic markers such as HGF receptor (c-Met) and AFP[34]. After culturing with growth factors (HGF, epidermal growth factor (EGF), BM stem cell-derived hepatic-like cells expressed ALB (protein) and TDO2 (mRNA). Fiegel et al. selected $CD34^+$ cells and cultured them on a collagen matrix with growth factors[35]. Unlike $CD34^-$ cells, $CD34^+$ derived cells expressed ALB and CK-19 mRNA. Similarly, Okumoto et al. used selected HSCs from rat BM and cultured them with mature hepatocytes or only with HGF[36]. The cells co-cultured with hepatocytes expressed HNF-1alpha, CK8, AFP and ALB mRNA, when cultured with HGF expressed HNF-1alpha and CK8.

In a co-culture system the cell fusion problem might be avoided; however, a proper separation protocol has to be developed.

1.3.1.3. Mesenchymal Stem Cells

Previously, a well-characterized BM stromal cell population[37] emerged as a focus for regenerative therapy. There is a little confusion in terminology with some authors suggesting[38] that subpopulations named colony forming units of fibroblasts (CFU-F), multipotent adult progenitor cells (MAPCs)[39], MSCs[37] or stromal cells are quite similar or highly related. Kucia et al. showed that human BM is composed of a heterogeneous nonhematopoietic (CXCR4+, CD34+, AC133+, lin-, CD45-) tissue-committed stem cell subpopulation[40]. They postulate that in BM there are stem cells with different levels of differentiation beginning from primitive pluripotent stem cells to tissue committed stem cells and so they suggest that the subpopulation of stem cells (e.g. HSCs, MSCs) taken into investigations should be carefully considered[40,41,42]. However, this subpopulation is different from MSCs (CXCR4-, CD34-). The predominant source for MSCs is the adult BM, but they can also be obtained from various tissues of the human body, including compact bone, peripheral blood, adipose tissue, cord blood, amniotic fluid and other fetal tissues. MSCs are capable of self renewal and multilineage differentiation (adipogenic, osteogenic, chondrogenic[37], myogenic[43], neurogenic[44]) and can be expanded in vitro, making it possible to engineer transplantable tissue in association with appropriate scaffolds. Schwartz et al. showed that rat, mouse and human BM-derived MAPCs, cultured with FGF-4 and HGF on Matrigel, can differentiate into cells expressing several liver-specific markers[39]. Sato et al. showed that human BM-MSCs xenografted into liver of the rat differentiate into human hepatocytes, which express liver-specific markers, without fusion.[45]. Zhao et al. have demonstrated a protective effect of MSCs isolated from rat BM on fibrosis caused by CCl_4 and DMN[46]. The HIFC system has been adapted by Teratani et al. to contribute to hepatic differentiation of human BM-derived MSCs[47].

Hepatocytes derived from human MSCs reveal morphological, biological, functional and therapeutic evidences.

Multipotential MSCs comprise a promising tool for cell therapy (Figure 1.4.). They can be obtained from the patient's own bone marrow (or other sources), expanded in vitro and implanted back into the liver as a native source for liver regeneration (this theory however needs to be confirmed) or after differentiating ex vivo (possibly with genetic modifications), maintained on a proper scaffold and implanted back into a diseased liver (without risk of rejection). There is high hope that in the future stem cell-derived hepatocytes might be used together with the advanced tissue engineering technology in entire liver system development.

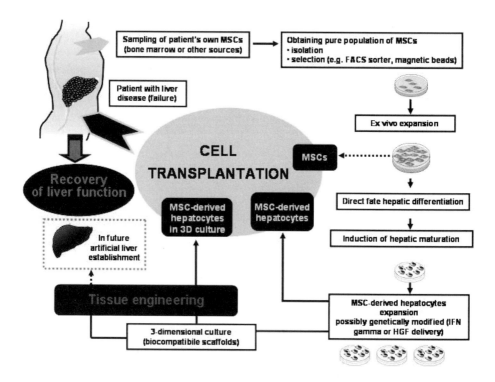

Figure 1.4 (see color insert, Figure 1.4). Schematic representation of mesenchymal stem cell (MSC)-based therapy and tissue engineering. MSCs can be obtained from patient's own tissue (bone marrow, adipose tissue), purified using MACS or FACS system and after expansion directly induced into hepatic lineage differentiation. Mature hepatocytes might be directly implanted or after genetic manipulations back into damaged liver of the patient or using tissue engineering technologies transplanted as small liver devices. Tissue engineering development holds promises for a future bioartificial liver establishment.

1.3.2. Adipose Tissue

Adipose tissue derived stem cells (ADSCs) are a heterogeneous population of cells similar to BM-derived MSCs[47] and are similarly able to differentiate into multiple lineages (adipocytes, osteoblasts, myoblasts, chondroblasts[48, 49], neuroblasts[50]). Their potentiality to differentiate into hepatocytes has been observed by Seo et al.[51]. Banas et al. has recently confirmed that the HIFC system allows hepatic induction from ADSCs (unpublished observations). ADSCs present an attractive tool for cell therapy, because they are easy to obtain, in large quantities and with minimal invasiveness.

1.4. STEM CELLS IN FETAL TISSUES

Lazaro et al. established a primary culture of human fetal liver hepatocytes, which retained hepatocyte morphology and gene expression patterns for several months[52]. After treatment with OsM, these fetal hepatocytes matured. Moreover, during culturing they formed a 3-dimensional structure, which after section revealed liver-like morphology. Importantly, the primary culture of mature hepatocytes either does not replicate sufficiently in vitro to produce the number of cells necessary for transplantation or does not maintain differentiated properties in vitro, and so fetal liver might be a better source of hepatocytes; however there are ethic concerns regarding utilization of fetal organs.

Human umbilical cord blood (UCB), placenta and amnion are normally discarded at birth and so they provide an easily accessible alternative source of stem cells. Human UCB, commonly used as part of clinical application for several hematopoietic diseases, besides HSCs, contains stem cells with properties similar to BM-derived MSCs. Lee et al. demonstrated a subpopulation of UCB-derived MSCs able to differentiate into hepatic-like cells, which were positive for immunofluorescence albumin staining and exhibited an ability to uptake low-density lipoprotein (LDL)[53]. Hong et al. reported differentiation of human UCB-derived stem cells into cells expressing hepatic markers (e.g. ALB, AFP, CK18)[54].

1.5. LONG-TERM MAINTENANCE OF HEPATIC FUNCTIONS BY BIOMATERIALS

Biomaterials with distinct properties are necessary to accommodate the growth and interactions of multiple cell lineages in composite tissue constructs[55]. The microenvironment for long-term culture with a possibility to maintain stem cell-derived hepatocyte functions is important in the context of stem cell-based liver therapy and tissue engineering[56]. The ideal scaffold is non-immunogenic, non-toxic, biocompatible, biodegradable and easy to manufacture. Scaffolds should permit easy diffusion of nutrients and cellular waste products and provide good mechanical support for cells during the repair process. Scaffolds currently used are natural or synthetic polymers. Liver tissue engineering started with maintaining a long-term culture of hepatocytes. Highly porous biocompatible polymers have been utilized, mainly poly (lactide-co-glycolide)[21], polyurethane, collagen, chitosan, alginate, hydrogel. In the three-dimensional (3D) culture system, using poly-N-para-vinylbenzyl-lactonamide (PVLA)-coated reticulated polyurethane Sato et al. maintained specific hepatocyte functions for up to 40 days in an in vitro culture. When transplanted into the peritoneal cavity of rats, the hepatocytes were able to survive and retain liver specific functions for more than one month[57]. Ohashi et al. successfully engrafted and maintained hepatocytes at extrahepatic sites, with extracellular matrix components for over 100 days[58]. For the first time, ES cell-derived hepatocytes were maintained for a long time by Teratani et al. in a three-dimensional culture with porous hyaluronic acid (HA) sponge (Figure 1.5.)[59].

In this study there is clear evidence that 3D HA sponge formed hepatocyte spheroids within the pores and sustained cell viability and liver functions, such as albumin secretion, ammonia detoxication and urea nitrogen synthesis for prolonged time (more than 20 days), when compared with a conventional monolayer culture and in collagen sponge cultures (17 days). Hepatocytes within HA sponge secreted a constant level of albumin up to 32 day.

The demonstrated results of 3-dimensional cultures along with advances in stem cell technology serve in the future as a basis for development of an artificial liver.

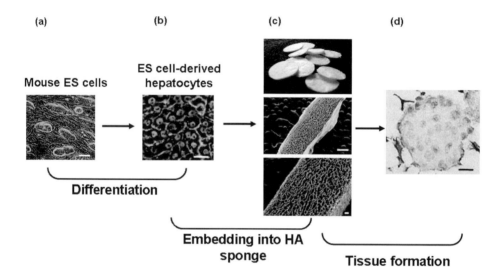

Figure 1.5. Liver tissue engineering[17,59].(a) Mouse ES cells (phase contrast microscopy) (scale bar represents 50μm) (b) Mouse ES cell-derived hepatocytes (phase contrast microscopy) (scale bar represents 20μm). (c) Hyaluronic acid (HA) sponge-discs and scanning electron microphotograph (scale bars represent 500μm). (d) ES cell-derived hepatocytes in HA sponge have formed multicellular spheroid in the reticulated pores (stained with May-Giemsa solution) (scale bar represents 5μm).

1.6. CONCLUSIONS AND FUTURE PERSPECTIVES

Excellent researchers with their in vitro and in vivo studies keep putting fresh items into the "stem cell puzzle", and it seems that liver devices or even the whole organ might be produced in the future by using tissue engineering advanced procedures. Until now the therapeutic potential of stem cells has been demonstrated and each stem cell (embryonic, fetal, and adult) has its advantages and disadvantages in the context of using it in therapy: the pluripotentiality of ES cells versus their uncontrolled differentiation and teratoma formation and the multipotentiality of adult stem cells versus their controlled differentiation and low risk of rejection or cancer formation. All groups should unify a view on adult stem cell isolation and characterization. It is essential to clarify the procedures as well as the similarities and the differences between the subpopulations of BM-derived stem cells to find answers for important questions: Which biological mechanism is predominant- fusion, transdifferentiation or independent proliferation? Which in vivo method of stem cell delivery is the best? How best to isolate and characterize a large number of highly pure stem cells? How to develop a stable ex vivo culture system of liver stem cells and adjust their differentiation? After a combined approach, composed of stem cell biology, gene therapy, immunology, bioengineering and transplant medicine, these questions will be answered and clinical applications will succeed.

We have to remember that Nature by itself was able to originate Life from "One Cell" (fertilized oocyte) and generate through many phenomena mechanisms such complex "Organ" as the human body. Moreover Nature by itself gave to this "Organ" an immunological system to fight against invasive factors. And so, our clinical applications and drug therapies should be very well considered, keeping in mind any dangerous consequences which might be generated by mistakes or an imprecise approach.

1.7. REFERENCES

1. J.A. Thomson, J. Itskovitz-Eldor, S.S. Shapiro, M.A. Waknitz, J.J. Swiergiel, V.S. Marshall, J.M. Jones, Embryonic stem cell lines derived from human blastocysts, *Science* **282**(5391), 1145-1147 (1998).
2. R.M. Lemoli, F. Bertolini, R. Cancedda, M. De Luca, A. Del Santo, G. Ferrari, S. Ferrari, G. Martino, F. Mavilio, S. Tura, Stem cell plasticity: time for a reappraisal?, *Haematologica* **90**(3), 360-381, (2005).
3. E. Fuchs, J. Segre, Stem cells: a new lease on life, *Cell* **100**(1), 143-155, (2000).
4. E.L. Herzog, L. Chai, D.S. Krause, Plasticity of marrow-derived stem cells, *Blood* **102**(10), 3483-3493, (2003).
5. D. Choi, H.J. Oh, U.J. Chang, S.K. Koo, J.X. Jiang, S.Y. Hwang, J.D. Lee, G.C. Yeoh, H.S. Shin, J.S. Lee, B. Oh, In vivo differentiation of mouse embryonic stem cells into hepatocytes, *Cell Transplant* **11**(4), 359-368, (2002).
6. R. Chinzei, Y. Tanaka, K. Shimizu-Saito, Y. Hara, S. Kakinuma, M. Watanabe, K. Teramoto, S. Arii, K. Takase, C. Sato, N. Terada, H. Teraoka, Embryoid-body cells derived from mouse embryonic stem cell line show differentiation into functional hepatocytes, *Hepatology* **36**(1), 22-29, (2002).
7. Y. Yin, Y.K. Lim, M. Salto-Tellez, S.C. Ng, C.S. Lin, S.K. Lim, AFP(+), ESC-derived cells engraft and differentiate into hepatocytes in vivo, *Stem Cells* **20**(4), 338-346, (2002).
8. H. Yamamoto, G. Quinn, A. Asari, H. Yamanokuchi, T. Teratani, M. Terada, T. Ochiya, Differentiation of embryonic stem cells into hepatocytes: biological functions and therapeutic application, *Hepatology* **37**(5), 983-993, (2003).
9. T. Hamazaki, Y. Iiboshi, M. Oka, P.J. Papst, A.M. Meacham, L.I. Zon, N. Terada, Hepatic maturation in differentiating embryonic stem cells in vitro, *FEBS Lett* **497**(1), 15-19, (2001).
10. E.A. Jones, D. Tosh, D.I. Wilson, S. Lindsay, L.M. Forrester, Hepatic differentiation of murine embryonic stem cells, *Exp Cell Res* **272**(1), 15-22, (2002).
11. X.L. Kuai, X.Q. Cong, X.L. Li, S.D. Xiao, Generation of hepatocytes from cultured mouse embryonic stem cells, *Liver Transplant* **9**(10), 1094-1099, (2003).
12. H. Miyashita, A. Suzuki, K. Fukao, H. Nakauchi, H. Taniguchi, Evidence for hepatocyte differentiation from embryonic stem cells in vitro, *Cell Transplant* **11**(5), 429-434, (2002).
13. T. Yamada, M. Yoshikawa, S. Kanda, Y. Kato, Y. Nakajima, S. Ishizaka, Y. Tsunoda, In vitro differentiation of embryonic stem cells into hepatocyte-like cells identified by cellular uptake of indocyanine green, *Stem Cells* **20**(2), 146-154, (2002).
14. S. Ishizaka, A. Shiroi, S. Kanda, M. Yoshikawa, H. Tsujinoue, S. Kuriyama, T. Hasuma, K. Nakatani, K. Takahashi, Development of hepatocytes from ES cells after transfection with the HNF-3beta gene, *FASEB J.* **16**(11), 1444-1446, (2002).

15. S. Kanda, A. Shiroi, Y. Ouji, J. Birumachi, S. Ueda, H. Fukui, K. Tatsumi, S. Ishizaka, Y. Takahashi, M. Yoshikawa, In vitro differentiation of hepatocyte-like cells from embryonic stem cells promoted by gene transfer of hepatocytes nuclear factor 3 beta, *Hepatol Res* **26**(3), 225-231, (2003).
16. T. Ishii, K. Yasuchika, H. Fujii, H. Toshitaka, B. Shinji, M. Naito, T. Machimoto, N. Kamo, H. Suemori, N. Nakatsuji, I. Ikai, In vitro differentiation and maturation of mouse embryonic stem cells into hepatocytes. *Exp Cell Res*, (2005) (in press).
17. T. Teratani, H. Yamamoto, K. Aoyagi, H. Sasaki, A. Asari, G. Quinn, H. Sasaki, M. Terada, T. Ochiya, Direct hepatic fate specification from mouse embryonic stem cells, *Hepatology* **41**(4), 836-846, (2005).
18. Y. Yamamoto, T. Teratani, H. Yamamoto, G. Quinn, S. Murata, R. Ikeda, K. Kinoshita, K. Matsubara, T. Kato, T. Ochiya, Recapitulation of in vivo gene expression during hepatic differentiation from embryonic stem cells, *Hepatology* **42**(3), 558-567, (2005).
19. M. Schuldiner, O. Yanuka, J. Itskovitz-Eldor, D.A. Melton, N. Benvenisty, Effects of eight growths factors on the differentiation of cells derived from human embryonic stem cells, *Proc Natl Acad Sci USA* **97**(21), 11307-11312, (2000).
20. L. Rambhatla, C.P. Chiu, P. Kundu, Y. Peng, M.K. Carpenter, Generation of hepatocyte-like cells from human embryonic stem cells, *Cell Transplant* **12**(1), 1-11, (2003).
21. S. Levenberg, N.F. Huang, E. Lavik, A.B. Rogers, J. Itskovitz-Eldor, R. Langer, Differentiation of human embryonic stem cells on three-dimensional polymer scaffolds, *Proc Natl Acad Sci USA* **100**(22), 12741-12746, (2003).
23. X. Wang, M. Foster, M. Al-Dhalimy, E. Lagasse, M. Finegold, M. Grompe, The origin and liver repopulating capacity of murine oval cells, *Proc Natl Acad Sci USA* **100**(Supplement1), 11881-11888, (2003).
24. J. Laurson, C. Selden, H.J.F. Hodgson, Hepatocytes progenitors in man and in rodents-multiple pathways, multiple candidates, *Int J Exp Pathol* **86**(1), 1-18, (2005).
25. B.E. Petersen, W.C. Bowen, K.D. Patrene, W.M. Mars, A.K. Sullivan, N. Murase, S.S. Boggs, J.S. Greenberger, J.P. Goff, Bone marrow as a potential source of hepatic oval cells, *Science* **284**(5417), 1168-1170, (1999).
26. N.D. Theise, S. Badve, R. Saxena, O. Henegariu, S. Sell, J.M. Crawford, D.S. Krause, Derivation of hepatocytes from bone marrow cells in mice after radiation-induced myeloablation, *Hepatology* **31**(1), 235-240, (2000).
27. M.R. Alison, R. Poulsom, R. Jaffery, A.P. Dhillon, A. Quaglia, J. Jacob, M. Novelli, G. Prentice, J. Williamson, N.A. Wright, Hepatocytes from non-hepatic adult stem cells, *Nature* **406**(6793), 257, (2000).
28. N.D. Theise, M. Nimmakayalu, R. Gardner, P.B. Illei, G. Morgan, L. Teperman, O. Henegariu, D.S. Krause, Liver from bone marrow in humans, *Hepatology* **32**(1), 11-16, (2000).
29. E. Lagasse, H. Connors, M. Al-Dhalimy, M. Reitsma, M. Dohse, L. Osborne, X. Wang, M. Finegold, I.L. Weissman, M. Grompe, Purified hematopoietic stem cells can differentiate into hepatocytes in vivo, *Nat Med* **6**(11), 1229-1234, (2000).
30. G. Vassilopoulos, P.R. Wang, D.W. Russell, Transplanted bone marrow regenerates liver by cell fusion, *Nature* **422**(6934), 901-904, (2003).
31. X. Wang, H. Willenbring, Y. Akkari, Y. Torimaru, M. Foster, M. Al-Dhalimy, E. Lagasse, M. Finegold, S. Olson, M. Grompe, Cell fusion in the principal source of bone marrow-derived hepatocytes, *Nature* **422**(6934), 897-901, (2003).
32. X. Wang, S. Ge, G. McNanara, Q.L. Hao, G.M. Crooks, J.M. Nolta, Albumin-expressing hepatocyte-like cells develop in the livers of immune-deficient mice that received transplants of highly purified human hematopoietic stem cells, *Blood* **101**(10), 4201-4208, (2003).
33. Y.Y. Jang, M.I. Collector, S.B. Baylin, A. Mae Diehl, S.J. Sharkis, Hematopoietic stem cells convert into liver cells within days without fusion, *Nat Cell Biol* **6**(6), 532-539, (2004).
34. M. Miyazaki, I. Akiyama, M. Sakaguchi, E. Nakashima, M. Okada, K. Kataoka, N.H. Huh, Improved conditions to induce hepatocytes from rat bone marrow cells in culture, *Biochem Bioph Res Co* **298**(1), 24-30, (2002).
35. H.C. Fiegel, M.V. Lioznov, L. Cortes-Dericks, C. Lange, D. Kluth, B. Fehse, A.R. Zander, Liver-specific gene expression in cultured human hematopoietic stem cells, *Stem Cells* **21**(1), 98-104, (2003).
36. K. Okumoto, T. Saito, E. Hattori, J.I. Ito, T. Adachi, T. Takeda, K. Sugahara, H. Watanabe, K. Saito, H. Togashi, S. Kawata, Differentiation of bone marrow cells into cells that express liver-specific genes in vitro: implication of the Notch signals in differentiation, *Biochem Bioph Res Co* **304**(4), 691-695, (2003).
37. M.F. Pittenger, A.M. Mackay, S.C. Beck, R.K. Jaiswal, R. Douglas, J.D. Mosca, M.A. Moorman, D.W. Simonetti, S. Craig, D.R. Marshak, Multilineage potential of adult human mesenchymal stem cells, *Science* **284**(5411), 143-147, (1999).
38. M.H. Dahlke, F.C. Popp, S. Larsen, H.J. Schlitt, J.E.J. Rasko, Stem cell therapy of the liver-fusion or fiction?, *Liver Transplant* **10**(4), 471-479, (2004).

39. R.E. Schwartz, M. Reyes, L. Koodie, Y. Jiang, M. Blackstad, T. Lund, T. Lenvic, S. Johnson, W.S. Hu, C.M. Verfaillie, Multipotent adult progenitor cells from bone marrow differentiate into functional hepatocyte-like cells, *J Clin Invest* **109**(10), 1291-1302, (2002).
40. M. Kucia, R. Reca, V.R. Jala, B. Dawn, J. Ratajczak, M.Z. Ratajczak, Bone marrow as a home of heterogenous populations of nonhematopoietic stem cells, *Leukemia* **19**(7), 1118-1127, (2005).
41. M. Kucia, J. Ratajczak, M.Z. Ratajczak, Are bone marrow stem cells plastic or heterogenous- that is the question, *Exp Hematol* **33**(6), 613-623, (2005).
42. M. Majka, M. Kucia, M.Z. Ratajczak, Stem cell biology-never ending quest for understanding, *Acta Biochim Pol* **52**(2), 353-358, (2005).
43. G. Ferrari, G. Cusella-De Angelis, M. Coletta, E. Paolucci, A. Stornaiuolo, G. Cossu, F. Mavilio, Muscle regeneration by bone-marrow-derived myogenic progenitors, *Science* **279**(5356), 1528-1530, (1998).
44. D. Woodbury, B. Reynoldsk, I.B. Black, Adult bone marrow stromal stem cells express germline, ectodermal, endodermal and mesodermal genes prior to neurogenesis, *J Neurosci Res* **69**(6), 908-917, (2002).
45. Y. Sato, H. Araki, J. Kato, K. Nakamura, Y. Kawano, M. Kobune, T. Sato, K. Miyanishi, T. Takayama, M. Takahashi, R. Takimoto, S. Iyama, T. Matsunaga, S. Ohtani, A. Matsuura, H. Hamada, Y. Niitsu, Human mesenchymal stem cells xenografted directly to rat liver are differentiated into human hepatocytes without fusion, *Blood* **106**(2), 756-763, (2005).
46. D.C. Zhao, J.X. Lei, R. Chen, W.H. Yu, X.M. Zhang, S.N. Li, P. Xiang, Bone marrow-derived mesenchymal stem cells protect against experimental liver fibrosis in rats, *World J Gastroentero* **11**(22), 3431-3440, (2005).
47. T. Teratani, T. Ochiya, Stem cells, ES cells and Mesenchymal stem cells: Induction of mature hepatocytes from human mesenchymal stem cells (in Japanese), *Regenerative medicine* **3**(4), 126-133, (2005).
48. R.H. Lee, B.C. Kim, I.S. Choi, H. Kim, H.S. Choi, K.T. Suh, Y.C. Bae, J.S. Jung, Characterization and expression analysis of mesenchymal stem cells from human bone marrow and adipose tissue, *Cell Physiol Biochem* **14**(4-6), 311-324, (2004).
49. P.A. Zuk, M. Zhu, H. Mizuno, J. Huang, J.W. Futrell, A.J. Katz, P. Benheim, H.P. Lorenz, M.H. Hedrick, Multilineage cells from human adipose tissue: implications for cell-based therapies, *Tissue Eng* **7**(2), 211-228, (2001).
50. K.M. Safford, K.C. Hicok, S.D. Safford, Y.D. Halvorsen, W.O. Wilkinson, J.M. Gimble, H.E. Rice, Neurogenic differentiation of murine and human adipose-derived stromal cells, *Biochem Bioph Res Co* **294**(2), 371-379, (2002).
51. M.J. Seo, S.Y. Suh, Y.C. Bae, J.S. Jung, Differentiation of human adipose stromal cells into hepatic lineage in vitro and in vivo, *Biochem Bioph Res Co* **328**(1), 258-264, (2005).
52. C.A. Lazaro, E.J. Croager, C. Mitchell, J.S. Campbell, C. Yu, J. Foraker, J.A. Rhim, G.C.T. Yeoh, N. Fausto, Establishment, characterization, and long-term maintenance of cultures of human fetal hepatocytes, *Hepatology* **38**(5), 1095-1106 (2003).
53. O.K. Lee, T.K. Kuo, W.M. Chen, K.D. Lee, S.L. Hsieh, T.H. Chen, Isolation of multipotent mesenchymal stem cells from umbilical cord blood, *Blood* **103**(5), 1669-1675, (2004).
54. S.H. Hong, E.J. Gang, J.A. Jeong, C. Ahn, S.H. Hwang, I.H. Yang, H.K. Park, H. Han, H. Kim, In vitro differentiation of human umbilical cord blood-derived mesenchymal stem cells into hepatocyte-like cells, *Biochem Bioph Res Co* **330**(4), 1153-1161, (2005).
55. L.G. Griffith, G. Naughton, Tissue engineering-current challenges and expanding opportunities, *Science* **295**(5557), 1009-1014, (2002).
56. B.C. Heng, H. Yu, Y. Yin, S.G. Lim, T. Cao, Factors influencing stem cell differentiation into the hepatic lineage in vitro, *J Gastroen Hepatol* **20**(7), 975-987, (2005).
57. Y. Sato, T. Ochiya, Y. Yasuda, K. Matsubara, A new three-dimensional culture system for hepatocytes using reticulated polyurethane, *Hepatology* **19**(4), 1023-1028, (1994).
58. K. Ohashi, J.M. Waugh, M.D. Dake, T. Yokoyama, H. Kuge, Y. Nakajima, M. Yamanouchi, H. Naka, A. Yoshioka, M.A. Kay, Liver tissue engineering at extrahepatic sites in mice as a potential new therapy for genetic liver diseases, *Hepatology* **41**(4), 132-140, (2005).
59. T. Teratani, G. Quinn, Y. Yamamoto, T. Sato, H. Yamanokuchi, A. Asari, T. Ochiya, Long-term maintenance of liver-specific functions in cultured ES-derived hepatocytes with hyaluronic acid sponge, *Cell Trasplant*, **14**(9), (2005).

2

MESENCHYMAL STEM CELLS INCREASE SELF-RENEWAL OF SMALL INTESTINAL EPITHELIUM AND ACCELERATE STRUCTURAL RECOVERY AFTER RADIATION INJURY

Alexandra Sémont[1], Sabine François[1], Moubarak Mouiseddine[1], Agnès François[1], Amandine Saché[1], Johanna Frick[1], Dominique Thierry[1] and Alain Chapel[1]

2.1. ABSTRACT

Patients who undergo pelvic or abdominal radiotherapy may develop side effects that can be life threatening. Tissue complications caused by radiation-induced stem cell depletion may result in structural and functional alterations of the gastrointestinal (GI) tract. Stem cell therapy using mesenchymal stem cells (MSC) is a promising approach for replenishment of the depleted stem cell compartment during radiotherapy. There is little information on the therapeutic potential of MSC in injured-GI tract following radiation exposure. In this study, we addressed the ability of MSC to support the structural regeneration of the small intestine after abdominal irradiation.

We isolated MSC from human bone marrow and human mesenchymal stem cells (hMSC) were transplanted into immunotolerent NOD/SCID mice with a dose of 5.10^6 cells via the systemic route. Using a model of radiation-induced intestinal injury, we studied the link between damage, hMSC engraftment and the capacity of hMSC to sustain structural recovery. Tissue injury was assessed by histological analysis. hMSC engraftment in tissues was quantified by PCR assay.

Following abdominal irradiation, the histological analysis of small intestinal structure confirms the presence of partial and transient (three days) mucosal atrophy. PCR analysis evidences a low but significant hMSC implantation in small intestine (0.17%) but also at all the sites of local irradiation (kidney, stomach and spleen). Finally, in presence of hMSC, the small intestinal structure is already recovered at three days after abdominal radiation exposure. We show a structural recovery accompanied by an increase of small intestinal villus height, three and fifteen days following abdominal radiation exposure.

---

[1] UPRES 1638, IRSN, Fontenay aux Roses, France

In this study, we show that radiation-induced small intestinal injury may play a role in the recruitment of MSC for the improvement of tissue recovery. This work supports, the use of MSC infusion to repair damaged GI tract in patients subjected to radiotherapy. MSC therapy to avoid extended intestinal crypt sterilization is a promising approach to diminish healthy tissue alterations during the course of pelvic radiotherapy.

2.2. INTRODUCTION

Radiotherapy efficacy is governed by an optimal compromise between tumour control and normal tissue damage, i.e the risk/benefit ratio (Denham and Hauer-Jensen, 2002). Intestinal tissue injury after abdominal or pelvic radiotherapy may lead to acute and/or chronic gastrointestinal (GI) complications that can affect patient's quality of life and/or may be life threatening (Allgood et al 1996, Francois et al 2005). Limitation of GI tract damage by radiotherapy would reduce side effects and would enhance the control of tumours in so far as the radiation dose delivered could be increased.

The bordering epithelium of the intestine is composed of epithelial cells, which come from the intestinal stem cell residing in the base of the crypts of Lieberkühn. The intestinal stem cells give rise to four main lineages of differentiated cells, namely, absorptive cells, goblet cells, enteroendocrine cells and Paneth cells (Marshman et al 2002, Leedham et al 2005). Differentiated intestinal epithelial cells are involved in lineage specific functions such as the transport of intestinal nutrients, water and electrolyte movements, mucus secretion, neuropeptide production and immune defense. The epithelium is quickly and continuously renewed and its structural and functional integrity is governed by the proliferating capacity of stem cells. Intestinal radiation injury is characterized by crypt stem cell loss and subsequent impaired epithelial renewing, leading to mucosal disruption and intestinal structural and functional abnormalities (Francois et al 2005). Ionizing radiations have been postulated to target and deplete epithelial stem cells within the crypt of healthy intestine initiating GI complications (Potten CS 2004). So far, there is a need for the development of new treatments of GI complications after radiotheraphy.

In this regard, stem cell therapy using MSC is a promising approach. MSC have the capacity to differentiate *in vivo* and *in vitro* into several mesenchymal tissues including bone, cartilage tendon, muscle, adipose tissue and bone marrow stroma (Pittenger et al 1999, Deans and Moseley 2000). We also showed that MSC were able to migrate and to home at the site of injury in small intestine (Chapel et al 2003). Moreover, studies indicate a possible therapeutic effect of MSC in human osteogenesis imperfecta (Horwitz et al 2001) and in animal models with myocardial infarction (Shake et al 2002, Kinnaird et al 2004, Tang et al 2004). MSC multipotential property, their easy isolation and high *ex vivo* proliferating capacity as well as their use in various clinical settings make these cells good candidates for replenishment of the depleted stem cell compartment during radiotherapy.

In this study, we addressed the question of the therapeutic potential of MSC in the context of radiation-induced GI injury. We tested the regenerative capacity of hMSC on structural alterations in small intestine after radiation exposure in a NOD/SCID mouse model.

2.3. MATERIAL AND METHODS

2.3.1. Culture of Human MSC

Bone marrow (BM) cells were obtained from iliac crest aspirates of healthy volunteers after informed consent and were used in accordance with the procedures approved by the human experimentation and ethic committees of Hôpital St Antoine. As previously described (Bensidhoum et al 2004), 50 ml of BM were taken from different donors in the presence of heparin (Sanofi-synthélabo, France). Low-density mononuclear cells were separated on Ficoll Hypaque density gradient (d 1.077). Mononuclear cells (MNC) were plated at a density of $1.33 \; 10^6$ cells / cm^2 corresponding to a concentration of 10^7 cells/10 ml of McCoy's 5A medium supplemented with 12.5% fetal calf serum, 12.5% horse serum, 1% sodium bicarbonate, 1% sodium pyruvate, 0.4% MEM non essential amino acids, 0.8% MEM essential amino acids, 1% MEM vitamin solution, 1% L-glutamine (200 mM), 1% penicillin-streptomycin solution (all from Invitrogen, Groningen, The Netherland), 10^{-6} M hydrocortisone (Stem Cell Technologies®), 2 ng/ml human basic recombinant fibroblast growth factor (R&D System, Abington, UK) in T-75 cm^2 tissue culture flasks and incubated at 37°C in humidified, 5% CO_2 atmosphere. After three days, non-adherent cells were washed with PBS and complete fresh medium (without Hydrocortisone) was added. Samples of hMSC of different donors were collected at passage 2 for transplantation. At the time of infusion, hMSC were characterized by expression of CD73 (SH3) and CD105 (SH2) and lack of expression of CD45 using FACS analysis (data not shown).

2.3.2. NOD/SCID Mouse Model

All experiments and procedures were performed in accordance with the French Ministry of Agriculture regulations for animal experimentation (Act n°87-847 October 19th, 1987, modified May, 2001) and were approved by the animal care committee of the Institut de Radioprotection et de Sûreté Nucléaire (IRSN). NOD-LtSz-*scid/scid* (NOD-SCID) mice, from breeding pairs originally purchased from Jackson Laboratory (Bar Harbor, ME, USA) were bred in our pathogen-free unit and maintained in sterile micro isolator cages. A total of 60 eight-week-old mice divided into 6 groups were used for this study. Three groups were transplanted with a dose of 5.10^6 hMSC via the systemic route. Group 1 was not irradiated before receiving MSC infusion. Groups 2 received total body irradiation (TBI) at a sublethal dose of 3.5 Grays 24 hours before MSC infusion. Group 3 received 24 hours before MSC infusion 3.5 Grays TBI followed by local irradiation to the abdomen at a dose of 4.5 Grays for a total of 8 Grays to the abdominal region. Group 4 received only TBI and Group 5 abdominal irradiation immediately after TBI. Group 6 was a non-irradiated control group that did not receive hMSC.

The animals were sacrificed three and fifteen days after irradiation. Peripheral blood, bone marrow (femur), lung, liver, kidney, spleen, stomach and small intestine, were collected and the quantitative distribution of the hMSC was defined by PCR experiments on day fifteen after irradiation. Intestinal alterations were studied by histological analysis on days three and fifteen.

2.3.3. DNA Extraction and PCR Analysis

Genomic DNA for PCR analysis was prepared from tissues using the QIAamp DNA Mini Kit (Qiagen, Courtaboeuf, France). Amplifications were performed following the standard recommended amplification conditions (Applied Biosytems, Foster City, CA) as previously described by Heid et al (1996). One hundred nanograms of purified DNA from various tissues were amplified using TaqMan universal PCR master mix (Applied Biosytems). The primers and probe for human β-GLOBIN were forward primer 5'GTGCACCTGACTCCTGAGGAGA3' and reverse primer 5'CCTTGATACCAACCTGCCCAGG3'. The probe labeled with fluorescent reporter and quencher was:5'FALM-AAGGTGAACGTGGATGAAGTTGGTGG-TAMRA-3. Endogenous mouse RAPSYN gene (Receptor-Associated Protein at the Synapse) was also amplified, as an internal control. The primers and probe for mouse RAPSYN gene were forward primer 5'ACCCACCCATCCTGCAAAT3' and reverse primer 5'ACCTGTCCGTGCTGCAGAA3'. After 10 min at 95°C, amplification was performed by 40 cycles of 15s at 95°C and 1 min at 60°C. In order to determine the efficiency of amplification and the assay precision, calibration curves for human β-GLOBIN and mouse RAPSYN were constructed with a 0,99 correlation coefficient and an efficiency superior to 98%. Mouse DNA was isolated from the identical tissues of non-transplanted NOD/SCID mice and used as a negative control. As well, human DNA was isolated from human MSC culture and used as a positive control. Evaluation of specificity of human β-GLOBIN amplification was demonstrated using tenfold dilution for 100 ng to 0.05 ng of human MSC DNA with mouse DNA, without cross reactivity. Since the number of cells is directly related to the copies numbers of human β-GLOBIN and mouse RAPSYN, the results were expressed as number of human cells per 100 mouse cells in each tissue.

2.3.4. Histology

Formalin-fixed, paraffin-embedded small intestine from NOD/SCID mice were cut at 5 μm on a rotary microtome (Leica Microsystems AG, Wetzlar Germany) and mounted on polysine slides. Sections were deparaffinized in xylene and rehydrated with ethanol and PBS. Sections were stained with hematoxylin, eosin and safran (HES). Villus height was measured in μm using an image analysis software (Visiolab, Biocom, France)

2.3.5. Statistical Analysis

All values were expressed as the mean and SEM (standard error of the mean). To compare results between groups, we have used a T test or a one-way ANOVA followed by Tukey's test with Sigmastat software (Systat Software Incorporation). Significance for all analyses was set at $p<0.001$

2.4. RESULTS

2.4.1. Human MSC Implantation 15 Days after Irradiation of NOD/SCID Mice

We previously have reported no significant hMSC engraftment in small intestine of non-irradiated NOD/SCID mice (Francois et al in press in Stem Cells). In this study, we investigated the engraftment of hMSC following radiation exposure. Figure 2.1 indicates the levels of hMSC engraftment in animals receiving only TBI in comparison with animals receiving both TBI and localized irradiation to the abdomen. Fifteen days after TBI, we observed low hMSC engraftment in all organs tested. The level of hMSC engraftment significantly increased to reach 0.17% in small intestine and 0.12% in stomach in mice receiving abdominal irradiation in addition to TBI. Moreover, abdominal irradiation in addition to TBI also gave rise to a significant hMSC engraftment in the kidney (0.10%), and spleen (0.94%). Our results suggested an engraftment of hMSC in injured organs located in areas of the body having received the highest irradiation dose. We also observed an engraftment in filtering organs located outside of the abdominal irradiation field, such as liver (0.44%) and lung (0.82%). By contrast, no difference in the percentage of implanted hMSC was observed in the bone marrow according to the radiation schedule. Moreover, no circulating hMSC were observed in blood of mice receiving TBI or both TBI and abdominal irradiation (data not shown).

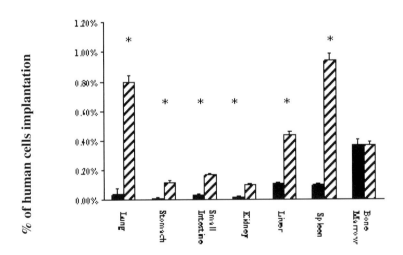

Figure 2.1. Implantation of hMSC in NOD/SCID mice 15 days after TBI with or without abdominal irradiation. Histogram represents the percentage of hMSC detected by PCR in various tissues following TBI (dark histogram) or TBI with abdominal radiation exposure (hatched histogram). Results are the mean ± SEM of 10 animals per group. *$p<0.001$ versus the TBI (T-test).

2.4.2. Effects of Human MSC Infusion on Non-Irradiated NOD/SCID Mice Small Intestine

Histological analysis of the small intestine (jejunum) were carried out. The thickness of the intestinal epithelium is criterion of the structure intestine integrity. The thickness of the intestinal epithelium is characterized by villus height and/or crypt of Lieberkühn depth. Figure 2.2Aa and 2.3Aa show control NOD/SCID mouse jejunum with long finger-like villi (230.3 ± 5.3 µm) and crypts (82.6 ± 1.3 µm). To analysis small intestine alteration or regeneration, we have focused on the quantification of villus height. In non-irradiated mice, two days after hMSC infusion, we observed a significant increase (1.4 fold, p< 0.001) of small intestine villus height (Figures 2.2Ac and 2.2B). This effect was enhanced fourteen days after hMSC infusion (Figures 2.3Ac and 2.3B).

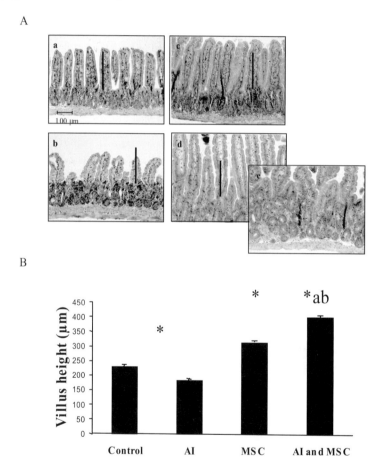

Figure 2.2. Effects of hMSC infusion on NOD/SCID mice small intestine alterations 3 days after abdominal irradiation (AI) at a dose of 8 Grays. A) Histologic sections of jejunum stained with hematoxylin, eosin and safran (HES). a. unirradiated and hMSC uninjected, control animals b. AI with TBI and hMSC uninjected animals, c. unirradiated and hMSC injected animals, d,e. AI with TBI and hMSC injected animals. B) Histogram represents the villus height (µm) with 3 to 5 animals per group. Each value represents the average of 20 to 30 independent measurements of villus height per slice and per mice. * p < 0.001 versus the control, [a]p < 0.001 versus the AI, [b]p < 0.001 versus the MSC (one way ANOVA followed by Tuchey's test). Original magnitude, x100

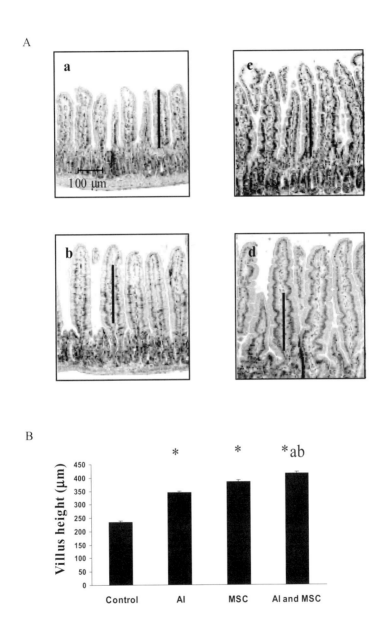

Figure 2.3. Effects of hMSC infusion on NOD/SCID mice small intestine alterations 15 days after abdominal irradiation (AI) at a dose of 8 Grays. A) Histologic sections of jejunum stained with hematoxylin, eosin and safran (HES). a. unirradiated and hMSC uninjected as control animals b. AI with TBI and hMSC uninjected animals, c. unirradiated and hMSC injected animals, d. AI with TBI and hMSC injected animals. B) Histogram represents the villus height (μm) with 3 to 5 animals per group. Each value represents the average of 20 to 30 independent measurements of villus height per slice and per mice. *p< 0.001 versus the control, [a]p< 0.001 versus the AI, [b]p< 0.001 versus the Sham (one way ANOVA followed by Tuchey's test). Original magnitude, x100.

2.4.3. Abdominal Irradiation Induces Small Intestinal Injury in Non-Transplanted NOD/SCID Mice

Abdominal irradiation in addition to TBI resulted in partial atrophy of small intestinal mucosa with villus height reduction (1.25 fold decrease versus control group, $p < 0.001$) and apex dilatation three days post-exposure (Figures 2.2Ab and 2.2B). At fifteen days, intestinal structure recovered its integrity (Figures 2.3Ab and 2.3B). At this time, we observed an increase of the villi height (1.5 fold increase, $p < 0.001$) as compared to the control group suggesting a compensatory hyperplasia of NOD/SCID mice small intestine.

2.4.4. Human MSC Infusion Improves the Regeneration of Small Intestinal Mucosa in NOD/SCID Mice Receiving Abdominal Irradiation

We then tested the capacity of hMSC to improve structural small intestinal recovery. Three days after abdominal irradiation, the integrity of small intestine was already regained in hMSC injected mice. The villus height was significantly increased (1.7 fold compared with control, $p < 0.001$) to reach 399.6 ± 7.4 μm (Figures 2Ad and 2B). We also observed many regenerating crypt zones (Figure 2.2Ae). Fifteen days after irradiation, the villus height remained elevated (426 ± 6.6 μm) and was significantly increased in comparison with control group (Figures 2.3Ad and 2.3B). This demonstrated that hMSC could accelerate small intestinal mucosa regeneration following radiation exposure.

2.5. DISCUSSION

In this study, we addressed the question of the therapeutic potential of MSC in the context of radiation-induced intestinal damages. This study was realized in a preclinical model in which hMSC were intravenously injected to NOD/SCID mice following sublethal TBI at 3.5 Grays. We previously demonstrated in this model that TBI at 3.5 Grays causes minor damages to the gut (Francois et al in press in Stem Cells). In this study, to induce additional intestinal lesions, NOD/SCID mice were subjected to an abdominal irradiation of 4.5 Grays in addition to 3.5 Grays TBI leading to a total dose received to the abdomen of 8 Grays.

With this radiation dose, we have observed a rapid (three days after irradiation) structural damage of small intestine (jejunum) with partial mucosal atrophy. These mucosal alterations have completely disappeared at fifteen days. The small intestinal epithelium has thus a high potential to repair mucosal damage and to recover from radiation injury. That remarkable property of the intestinal epithelium has already been described in rodent models (Lesher et al 1975, Bisht et al 2000, Potten et al 2003, Dublineau et al 2004, Brittan et al 2005) along the entire GI tract. These authors have shown that intestinal recover is a very rapid process already achieved at seven days.

The well-known properties of MSC, namely, easy expansion in culture and ability to differentiate *in vitro* and *in vivo* into multiple tissue lineages, make this cell population a very attractive option for a wide range of clinical applications (Gregory et al 2005). Relevant Le Blanc's work (2004) showed strikingly clinical improvement of GI dysfunction after MSC transplantation in a patient with severe treatment-resistant graft-versus-host diseases of the gut and liver. Nevertheless, although healing effects on the damaged gut epithelium are suggested by these authors, as yet there is no evidence of structural and fully-functioning intestinal organ rescues with purified MSC population transplantation.

In this study, we present novel findings, concerning MSC contribution to spontaneous renewal and damage repair of the small intestinal mucosa. These aspects are discussed in the following sections. First, we have reported that MSC can increase the self-renewal potential of small intestinal mucosa. This process is persistent over time. Indeed, a significant high increase of small intestinal villus height was found at two days after systemic injection of hMSC in NOD/SCID mice and this increase was enhanced at forteen days post-infusion. In contrast with other works (Devine et al 2003, Anjos-Alfonso 2004) we did not detect any hMSC engraftment in small intestine, in the absence of substantial injury (Francois et al in press in Stem Cells). This might be due to the sensitivity of PCR, which could not detect low levels of hMSC engraftment. We secondly have shown that in our model, hMSC engraft into small intestine after irradiation and contribute to structural recovery acceleration. At three days in presence of hMSC, the structure of NOD/SCID mouse small intestine has regained its integrity. Human MSC implantation at the site of injury could be triggered by inflammatory chemokines released following irradiation (Grimm et al 2001, Van der Meeren et al 2004, Lüttichau et al 2005). Implantation of hMSC in organs receiving lesser irradiation dose such as liver or lung could be related to the role of physiological filter of these organs or might be caused by circulating cytokines and chemokines consequent to the small intestine inflammatory response (Van der Meeren et al 2005). The MSC contribution to tissue repair has broadly been reported for many different organs such as kidney (Herrera et al 2004), lung (Ortiz et al 2003), heart (Mangi et al 2003, Pittenger and Martin 2004), muscles (Ferrari et al 1998, Santa Maria et al 2004), skin (Deng et al 2005), spinal cord (Chopp et al 2000) and liver (Peterson et al 1999, Wang et al 2002). It as been previously reported that, following irradiation, transplanted MSC were found at the site of small intestinal injury in non-human primate models (Chapel et al 2003, Devine et al 2003). Hori's experiment (2002) on tissue engineering of small intestine by MSC seeding onto collagen scaffold, has shown a partial regenerating potential at the site of the scaffold graft. However, our results evidence for the first time the effect of MSC on structural regeneration of the small intestine. The rescue of intestine is joined by an increase of regenerating crypt zones and villus height (approximately two folds) indicating that MSC could sustain crypt cell proliferation and newly differentiated intestinal epithelial cell turnover and replacement. Such an enhancement of villus height might result in an improvement of several functions of intestinal mucosa such as mechanical barrier, nutrient absorption and production. Future examination of MSC-induced functional regeneration following radiation exposure could be of interest.

The mechanisms involved in MSC improvement of structural recover of the small intestine have not been yet clarified. It has been previously shown that bone marrow-derived cells could reside in the small intestine as late transit cells with limited dividing potential (Marshman et al 2002) and in turn could give rise to differentiated cells within an extremely short period. To restore small intestinal structure, bone marrow-derived cells could also transdifferentiate to form specific epithelial cell lineages (Okamato et al 2002, Okamato et al 2003, Matsumoto et al 2005). However, a more simple assumption would be that MSC implant in pericryptal and lamina proprial meshwork to form mesenchymal cell lineages as regulator of epithelial cell proliferation and differentiation via mesenchymal-epithelial paracrine interactions (Brittan et al 2002, Direkze et al 2003, Brittan et al 2005). The precise histological localization of implanted hMSC would help to choose between these two assumptions.

Our results support the use of hMSC infusion to repair injured small intestine. Human MSC therapy to avoid extended intestinal crypt sterilization is a promising approach to diminish healthy tissue alterations during the course of pelvic radiotherapy.

2.6. ACKNOWLEDGMENTS

We wish to thank Patrice Richard and Noelle Mathieu for their help concerning the present work and Jean-Marc Bertho for revising the manuscript. This work was supported by grants from EDF (électricité de France) and EEC (FIRST: contract number 503436).

2.7. REFERENCES

Allgood J.W., Langberg C.W., Sung C.C., and Hauer-Jensen M., 1996, Timing of concomitant boost irradiation affects incidence and severity of intestinal complications, *Int. J. Radiat. Oncology boil. Phys.* 34(2):381-387.

Anjos-Afonso F., Siapati E.K., and Bonnet D., 2004, In vivo contribution of murine mesenchymal stem cells into multiple cell-types under minimal damage conditions, *J. Cell Sci.* 117:5655-5664.

Bensidhoum M., Chapel A., Francois S., Demarquay C., Mazurier C., Fouillard L., Bouchet S., Bertho JM., Gourmelon P., Aigueperse J., Charbord P., Gorin N.C., Thierry D., and Lopez M., 2004, Homing of in vitro expanded Stro-1⁻ or stro-1⁺ human mesenchymal stem cells into the NOD/SCID mouse and their role in supporting human CD34 cell engraftment, *Blood* 103(9): 3313-3319.

Bisht K.S., Prabhu S., and Devi P.U., 2000, Modification of radiation induced damage in mouse intestine by WR-2721. *Indian J. Exp. Biol.* 38(7):669-674.

Brittan M., Hunt T., Jeffery R., Poulsom R., Forbes S.J., Hodivala-Dilke K., Goldman J., Alison M.R., and Wright N.A., 2002, Bone marrow derivation of pericryptal myofibroblasts in the mouse and human small intestine and colon, *Gut* 50:752-757.

Brittan M., Chance V., Elia G., Poulsom R;, Alison M.R., MacDonald T.T., Wright N.A., 2005, A regenerative role for bone marrow following experimental colitis: contribution to neovasculogenesis and Myofibroblasts, *Gastroenterology* 128:1984-1995.

Chapel A., Bertho J.M., Bensidhoum M., Fouillard L., Young R.G., Frick J., Demarquay C., Cuvelier F., Mathieu E., Trompier F., Dudoignon N., Germain C., Mazurier C., Aigueperse J., Borneman J., Gorin N.C., Gourmelon P., and Thierry D., 2003, Mesenchymal stem cells home to injured tissues when co-infused with hematopoeitic cells to treat a radiation-induced multi-organ failure syndrome. *J. Gene Med.* 5(12):1028-1038.

Chopp M., Zhang X.H., Li Y., Wang L., Chen J., Lu D., Lu M., and Rosenblum M., 2000, Spinal cord injury in rat: treatment with bone marrow stromal cell transplantation, *Neuroreport* 11(13):3001-3005.

Deans R.J., and Moseley A.B., 2000, Mesenchymal stem cells: biology and potential clinical uses. *Exp. Hematol.* 28(8):875-884.

Deng W., Han Q., Liao L., Li C., Ge W., Zhao Z., You S., Deng H., Murad F., and Zhao R.C.H., 2005, Engrafted bone marrow-derived FlK-1⁺ mesenchymal stem cells regenerate skin tissue. *Tissue Eng.* 11(1/2): 110-119.

Denham J.W., and Hauer-Jensen M., 2002, The radiotherapeuthic injury-a complex wound, *Radiother. Oncol.* 63:129-145.

Devine S.M., Cobbs C., Jennings M., Bartholomew A., and Hoffman R;, 2003, Mesenchymal stem cells distribute to a wide range of tissues following systemic infusion into nonhuman primates, *Blood* 101(8): 2999-3001.

Direkze N.C., Forbes S.J., Brittan M., Hunt T., Jeffery R., Preston S.L., Poulsom R., Hodivala-Dilke K., Alison M.R., and Wright N.A., 2003, Multiple organ engraftment by bone marrow-derived myofibroblasts and fibroblasts in bone marrow-transplanted mic,. *Stem cells* 21:514-520.

Dublineau I., Lebrun F., Grison S., and Griffiths N.M., 2004, Functional and structural alterations of epithelial barrier properties of rat ileum following X-irradiation, *Can. J. Physiol. Pharmacol.* 82(2):84-93.

Ferrari G., Cusella-De Angelis G., Coletta M., Paolucci E., Sornaiuolo A., Cossu G., andMavilio F., 1998, Muscle regeneration by bone marrow-derived myogenic progenitors, *Science* 279(5356):1528-1530.

Francois A., Milliat F., and Vozenin-Brotons M.C., 2005, Bowel injury associated with pelvic radiotherapy, *Radiat. Phys. Chemistry* 72:399-407.

Gregory C.A., Prockop D.J., and Spees J.L., 2005, Non-hemotopoietic bone marrow stem cells: Molecular control of expansion and differentiation, *Exp. Cell Res.* 306:330-335.

Grimm P.C., Nickerson P., Jeffery J., Savani R.C., Gough J., McKenna R.M., Stern E., and Rush D.N., 2001 Neointimal and tubulointerstitial infiltration by recipient mesenchymal cells in chronic renal-allograft rejection, *N. Engl. J. Med.* 345(2):93-97.

Heid C.A., Stevens J., Livak K.J., and Williams P.M., 1996, Real time quantitative PCR, *Genome Res.* 6 (10): 986-994.

Herrera M.B., Bussolati B., Bruno S., Fonsato V., Romanazzi G.M., and Camussi G., 2004, Mesenchymal stem cells contribute to renal repair of acute tubular epithelial injury, *Int. J. Mol. Med.* 14:1035-1041.

Hori Y., Nakamura T., Kimura D., Kaino K., Kurokawa Y., Satomi S., and Shimizu Y., 2002, Experimental study on tissue engineering of the small intestine by mesenchymal stem cell seeding, *J. Surg. Res.* 102:156-160

Horwitz E.M., Prockop D.J., Gordon P.L., Koo W.W., Fitzpatrick L.A., Neel M.D., McCarville M.E., Orchard P.J., Pyeritz R.E., and Brenner M.K., 2001, Clinical responses to bone marrow transplantation in children with severe osteogenesis imperfecta. *Blood* 97:1227-1231.

Kinnaird T., Stabile E., Burnett M.S., Shou M., Lee C.W., Barr S., Fuchs S., and Epstein S.E., 2004, Local delivery of marrow-derived stromal cells augments collateral perfusion through paracrine mechanisms, *Circulation* 109(12):1543-1549.

Le Blanc K., Rasmusson I., Sundberg B., Götherström C., Hassan M., Uzunel M., and Ringden O., 2004 Treatment of severe acute graft-versus-host disease with third party haploidentical mesenchymal stem cells, *Lancet* 363:1439-1441.

Leedham S.J., Brittan M., McDonald A.S.C., and Wright N.A., 2005, Intestinal stem cells, *J. Cell Mol. Med.* 9(1):11-24.

Lesher S., Cooper J., Hagemann R., and Lesher J., 1975, Proliferative patterns in the mouse jejunal epithelium after fractionated abdominal X-irradiation, *Curr. Top. Radiat. Res. Q.* 10(3):229-261.

Lüttichau I.V., Notohamiprodjo M., Wechselberger A., Peters C., Henger A., Seliger C., Djafarzadeh R., Huss R., and Nelson P.J., 2005, Human Adult CD34(-) progenitor cells functionally express the chemokine receptors CCR1, CCR4, CCR7, CXCR5 and CCR10 but not CXCR4, *Stem Cells Dev.* 14:329-336.

Mangi A.A., Noiseux N., Kong D., He H., Rezvani M., Ingwall J.S., and Dzau V.J., 2003, Mesenchymal stem cells modified with Akt prevent remodeling and restore performance of infracted hearts, *Nat. Med.* 9:1195-1201.

Marshman E., Booth C., Potten C.S., 2002, The intestinal epithelial stem cell, *Bioessays* 24:91-98.

Matsumoto T., Okamoto R., Yajima T., Mori T., Okamato S., Ikeda Y., Mukai M., Yamazaki M., Oshima S., Tsuchiya K., Nakamura T., Kanai T., Okano H., Inazawa J., Hibi J., and Watanabe M., 2005, Increase of bone marrow-derived secretory lineage epithelial cells during regeneration in the human intestine, *Gastroenterology* 128:1851-1867.

Okamoto R., Yajima T., Yamazaki M., Kanai T., Mukai M., Okamoto S., Ikeda Y., Hibi T., Inazawa J., and Watanabe M., 2002, Damaged epithelia regenerated by bone marrow-derived cells in the human gastrointestinal tract, *Nat. Med.* 8:1011-1017.

Okamoto R., and Watanabe M., 2003, Prospects for regeneration of gastrointestinal epithelia using bone marrow cells, *Trends Mol. Med.* 9:286-290.

Ortiz L.A, Gambelli F., McBride C., Gaupp D., Maddoo M., Kaminski N., and Phinney D.G., 2003, Mesenchymal stem cell engraftment in lung is enhanced in response to bleomycin exposure and ameliorates its fibrotic effects. *Proc. Natl. Acad. Sci. U.S.A.* 100:8407-8411.

Petersen B.E., Bowen W.C., Patrene K.D., Mars W.M., Sullivan A.K., Murase N., Boggs S.S., Greenberger J.S., and Goff J.P., 1999, Bone marrow as a potential source of hepatic oval cells, *Science* 284(5417):1168-1170.

Pittenger M.F., Mackay A.M., Beck S.C., Jaiswal R.K., Douglas R., Mosca J.D., Moorman M.A., Simonetti D.W., Craig S., and Marshak D.R., 1999, Multilineage potential of adult human mesenchymal Stem Cells, *Science* 284(5411):143-147.

Pittenger M.F., Martin B.J., 2004, Mesenchymal stem cells and their potential as cardiac therapeutic, *Circ. Res.* 95(1):9-20.

Potten C.S., Booth C, Tudor G.L., Booth D., Brady G., Hurley P., Ashton G., Clarke R., Sakakibara S., Okano H., 2003, Identification of a putative intestinal stem cell and early lineage marker; musashi-1, *Differentiation* 71:28-41.

Potten C.S., 2004, Radiation, the ideal cytotoxic agent for studying the cell biology of tissues such as the small intestine, *Radiat. Res.* 161:123-136.

Santa Maria L., Rojas C.V., and Minguell J.J., 2004, Signals from damaged but not undamaged skeletal muscle induce myogenic differentiation of rat bone marrow-derived mesenchymal stem cells, *Exp. Cell Res.* 300(2):418-426.

Shake J.G., Gruber P.J., Baumgartner W.A., Senechal G., Meyers J., Redmond J.M., Pittenger M.F., and Martin B.J., 2002, Mesenchymal stem cell implantation in a swine myocardial infarct model: engraftment and functional effects, *Ann. Thorac. Surg.* 73(6):1919-1925; discussion 1926.

Tang Y.L., Zhao Q., Zhang Y.C., Cheng L., Liu M., Shi J., Yang Y.Z;, Pan C., Ge J., and Phillips M.I., 2004, Autologous mesenchymal stem cell transplantation induce VEGF and neovascularization in ischemic myocardium, *Regul. Pept.* 117:3-10.

Van der Meeren A., Mouthon M.A., Vandamme A., Squiban C., and Aigueperse J., 2004, Combinations of cytokines promote survival of mice and limit acute radiation damage in concert with amelioration of vascular damage, *Radiat. Res.* 161(5):549-559.

Van der Meeren A., Monti P., Vandamme M., Squiban C., Wysocki J., and Griffiths N., 2005, Abdominal radiation exposure elicits inflammatory responses and abscopal effects in the lungs of mice, *Radiat. Res.* 163:144-152.

Wang X., Montini E., Al-Dhalimy M., Lagasse E., Finegold M., and Grompe M., 2002, Kinetics of liver repopulation after bone marrow transplantation, *Am. J. Pathol.* 161(2):349-350.

3

OPTIMIZING VIRAL AND NON-VIRAL GENE TRANSFER METHODS FOR GENETIC MODIFICATION OF PORCINE MESENCHYMAL STEM CELLS

Maik Stiehler[1,2], Mogens Duch[2], Tina Mygind[1], Haisheng Li[1], Michael Ulrich-Vinther[1], Charlotte Modin[2], Anette Baatrup[1], Martin Lind[1], Finn S. Pedersen[2], and Cody E. Bünger[1]

3.1. ABSTRACT

INTRODUCTION: Mesenchymal stem cells (MSCs) provide an excellent source of pluripotent progenitor cells for tissue-engineering applications due to their proliferation capacity and differentiation potential. Genetic modification of MSCs with genes encoding tissue-specific growth factors and cytokines can induce and maintain lineage-specific differentiation. Due to anatomical and physiological similarities to humans, porcine research models have been proven valuable for the preclinical testing of tissue engineering protocols in large animals. The aim of this study was to evaluate optimized viral and non-viral *ex vivo* gene delivery systems with respect to gene transfer efficiency, maintenance of transgene expression, and safety issues using primary porcine MSCs as target cells.

MATERIALS AND METHODS: MSCs were purified from bone marrow aspirates from the proximal tibiae of four 3-month-old Danish landrace pigs by Ficoll step gradient separation and polystyrene adherence technique. Vectors expressing enhanced green fluorescent protein (eGFP) and human bone morphogenetic protein-2 (BMP-2) were

---

[1] Orthopaedic Research Laboratory, Department of Orthopaedic Surgery E, Aarhus University Hospital, Aarhus, Denmark
[2] Interdisciplinary Nanoscience Center (iNANO) and Department of Molecular Biology, University of Aarhus, Aarhus, Denmark
Address correspondence to: Maik Stiehler, MD; Orthopaedic Research Laboratory; Aarhus University Hospital; Norrebrogade 44, building 1A; 8000 Aarhus C, Denmark; *Tel.:* +45.8949.4162; *Fax:* +45.8949.4150; *Email:* maik.stiehler@ki.au.dk

transferred to the cells by different non-viral methods and by use of recombinant adeno-associated virus (rAAV)-mediated and retroviral gene delivery. Each method for gene delivery was optimized. Gene transfer efficiency was compared on the basis of eGFP expression as assessed by fluorescence microscopy and fluorescence-activated flow cytometry. BMP-2 gene expression and osteogenic differentiation were evaluated by real-time quantitative RT-PCR and histochemical detection of alkaline phosphatase activity, respectively.

RESULTS: Non-viral gene delivery methods resulted in transient eGFP expression by less than 2% of the cells. Using high titer rAAV-based vector up to 90% of the cells were transiently transduced. The efficiency of rAAV-mediated gene delivery was proportional to the rAAV vector titer applied. Retroviral gene delivery resulted in long-term transgene expression of porcine MSCs. A 26-fold increase in percentage of eGFP expressing cells (1.7% ±0.2% versus 44.1% ±5.0%, mean ±SD) and a 68-fold increase in mean fluorescence intensity (327.4 ±56.6 versus 4.8 ±1.3) was observed by centrifugation of retroviral particles onto the target cell layer. Porcine MSCs that were BMP-2 transduced by optimized retroviral gene delivery demonstrated a significant increase in BMP-2 gene expression and showed increased osteogenic differentiation. Retrovirally transduced porcine MSCs were furthermore tested free of replication-competent viruses.

DISCUSSION: The non-viral gene transfer methods applied were significantly less efficient compared to the viral methods tested. However, due to advantages with respect to safety issues and ease of handling, improvement of non-viral gene delivery to primary MSCs deserves further attention. The high efficiency of rAAV-mediated gene delivery observed at high titers can be explained by the ability of rAAV vector to transduce nondividing cells and by its tropism towards porcine MSCs. rAAV-mediated gene delivery resulted in transient transgene expression due to lack of stable AAV genome integration. MLV-mediated retroviral gene delivery can be considered a safe method for long-term transgene expression by porcine MSCs, and is therefore particularly attractive for advanced tissue engineering strategies requiring extended transgene expression.

3.2. INTRODUCTION

Mesenchymal stem cells (MSCs) are adult non-haematopoietic stem cells providing an excellent source of pluripotent progenitor cells. The utility of MSCs consists of their relative ease of isolation from bone-marrow aspirates, their proliferative capacity, and their potential to differentiate into distinct mesenchymal tissues, i.e., bone, cartilage, adipose, muscle, tendon, and haematopoiesis-supporting stroma [1-5]. This lineage-specific differentiation of MSCs is controlled by specific growth factors and cytokines. Bone morphogenetic protein-2 (BMP-2), for example, stimulates osteogenic differentiation of MSCs [6]. Gene delivery methods enable the intracellular transfer of one or more genes of interest, resulting in an expression of the corresponding foreign protein by the target cell. Genetically modified MSCs, (over)expressing tissue-specific growth factors or cytokines, provide both autocrine and paracrine stimuli to induce and maintain tissue-specific differentiation, and are therefore promising cellular components for advanced tissue engineering applications [7].

Gene delivery methods can be divided into systems using non-viral techniques and those using viral vectors. The basic principle of all non-viral methods is to transfer foreign deoxyribonucleic acid (DNA) constructs into recipient cells without the help of viral gene transfer machinery. This can be achieved by chemical (e.g., calcium phosphate co-precipitation, cationic liposome-mediated transfection), physical (e.g., electro–poration), and mechanical methods (e.g., microinjection, gene gun therapy), as well as by use of magnetic force (e.g., Magnetofection^{TM}).

The most promising viral gene transfer methods include systems using recombinant adeno-associated virus (rAAV)-based vectors and murine leukemia virus (MLV)-based retroviral vectors. AAV is a non-pathogenic, replication-defective, small (20 nm), nonenveloped single-stranded DNA parvovirus that has been known since 1965 [8]. The viral genome contains two open reading frames encoding four replication and three capsid proteins and is flanked by the inverse terminal repeats (ITR), which are the only *cis*-acting elements that are essential for replication, packaging, and integration [9]. Recent studies indicate that the ITR also possess weak transcriptional promoter activity [10]. Thus, the entire AAV genome, except for the ITR, can be replaced by a transgene cassette of interest to form a biologically active recombinant AAV vector [9]. AAV vector DNA primarily persists as episomal molecules without chromosomal integration [11]. AAV vectors have several properties that make them attractive for gene therapy including a broad cellular tropism, the ability to infect both proliferating and non-dividing cells [12-15], and the production of high titer by a simple, helper virus-free ultra high grade purification [16].

Retroviruses are 100 nm large, enveloped, plus-strand ribonucleic acid (RNA) viruses. The retroviral genome encoding the various viral proteins needed for replication is approximately 7,000-10,000 nucleotides in length and is flanked by the long terminal repeats (LTR) that harbour control elements for transcription, reverse transcription, and integration [17]. Retroviral gene transfer systems consist of two components: the packaging cell and the retroviral transfer vector. The packaging cell harbors engineered packaging constructs that direct the synthesis of proteins needed for production of retroviral particles. In advanced packaging cells, the coding regions are split into two constructs and the viral control elements are replaced by heterologous signals. The transfer vector consists of virus-derived elements necessary for encapsidation of the RNA into the retroviral particle, reverse transcription of RNA into DNA and integration of the vector into the host DNA. Furthermore, the transfer vector contains the necessary signals to secure transcription of the full-length vector RNA in the packaging cell and transcription and translation of its genes by the host machinery in the target cell. RNA transcribed from the introduced transfer vector DNA will form viral particles together with the viral proteins of the packaging cell. Retroviral vectors developed from MLVs were the first to be taken into clinical trials. By 2005, 1076 clinical gene therapy and gene marking trials had been approved and about one-fourth of these use retroviral vectors (www.wiley.com/wileychi/genmed/clinical).

Ex vivo gene delivery to specific target cells isolated from the patient limits undesired transduction to nontarget cells and allows for re-implantation of selected genetically modified tissue-engineered cells. Gene delivery to primary MSCs of porcine origin is of special interest as porcine research models have proven valuable for the preclinical testing of tissue engineering protocols in large animals.

The aim of this study was to evaluate optimized viral and non-viral *ex vivo* gene delivery systems with respect to gene transfer efficiency, maintenance of transgene expression, and safety issues using primary porcine MSCs as recipient cells.

3.3. MATERIALS AND METHODS

3.3.1. Cell Culture

Dulbeccos Modified Eagles Medium + 4500 mg/L glucose + GlutaMAX™ I + pyruvate supplemented with 10% fetal calf serum (Gibco Invitrogen) was used as complete cell culture medium. If not stated otherwise, cell cultures were maintained in a humidified atmosphere of 95% air and 5% CO_2 at 37°C. Cells were trypsinized according to a standardized protocol. Briefly, following two washes with phosphate buffered saline solution (PBS), 4 mL trypsin ethylenediaminetetraacetic acid (EDTA)-solution (0,125% trypsin, 5 mM EDTA in PBS) was added to a subconfluent T75-cm^2 cell culture dish. Following 5 min incubation at 37°C, 6 mL complete medium was added. The cell suspension was centrifuged at 300 x g for 10 min and resuspended in complete medium. The cells were counted using a Bürker-Türk hematocytometer. Frozen stocks of cells were prepared in complete medium supplemented with 10% dimethyl sulfoxide and kept at -140°C until use.

3.3.2. MSC Isolation

MSCs were isolated from bone marrow samples by density gradient separation and polystyrene adherence. Briefly, bone marrow was aspirated from the proximal tibiae of 4 different 3-month-old Danish landrace pigs under general anesthesia. Fifty milliliters of bone marrow were mixed with 10 mL PBS including 300 IU Heparin in order to prevent blood coagulation. A low-density cell fraction was obtained by centrifugation of the cell suspension over a density gradient (1.077 g/mL; Ficoll-Paque Plus, Amersham) at 400 x g for 30 min. Cells were collected from the interface, diluted with two volumes of PBS, centrifuged at 200 x g for 10 min and finally resuspended in complete medium supplemented with penicillin and streptomycin (50 IU/mL and 50 µg/mL, respectively; Sigma-Aldrich), then counted and plated for primary culture at a concentration of 1.5 x 10^6 cells/cm^2. Complete medium was renewed twice weekly to remove non-adherent cells. Following culture expansion for 48 h, usually a fraction of about 0.05% of the cells was adherent to polystyrene. Subconfluency of the cell layer was reached after 10 to 14 days of culture. For all experiments, only early passage (less than 4) MSCs were used.

3.3.3. Non-Viral Gene Delivery Methods

3.3.3.1. Calcium Phosphate Co-Precipitation

One day prior to transfection, 5 x 10^5 - 5 x 10^6 porcine MSCs were plated in a 75-cm^2 cell culture dish in complete medium. Culture medium was renewed 1 h prior to transfection. Ten micrograms of total DNA consisting of 1 µg (2 µg, 4 µg, and 8 µg, respectively) vector DNA (pLXSN-eGFP, Figure 3.1.a) supplemented with 9 µg (8 µg, 6 µg, and 2 µg, respectively) pUC19 carrier DNA were dissolved in 450 µL dd$H_2$0 and 50 µL 2.5 M $CaCl_2$ was added. The DNA/$CaCl_2$ solution was mixed and incubated for 10 min at room temperature. The precipitated DNA/$CaCl_2$ complexes were then added dropwise to 500 µL 2x HEPES buffer while constantly mixing the buffer by air insufflation. One day post transfection, the culture medium was renewed. The following day, the cells were evaluated for expression of enhanced green fluorescence protein (eGFP) by fluorescence microscopy.

3.3.3.2. Cationic Liposome-Mediated Transfection

Different cationic liposome-based transfection reagents (jetPEI^{TM}, Qbiogene; GenePORTER^{TM}, Genlantis; GeneJammer$^®$, Stratagene; TransIT^{TM}, Mirus; Lipofect–AMINE^{TM}, Invitrogen; Fugene^{TM}, Roche) were tested under varying combinations of cell seeding densities and transfection reagent/DNA ratios. Following assessment of gene transfer efficiency and cytotoxicity by use of fluorescence-activated flow cytometric analysis and light microscopy, the following optimized protocol including LipofectAMINE^{TM} transfection reagent was selected for cationic lipid mediated transfection. One day prior to transfection, 1.6 x 10^6 porcine MSCs were plated per 75-cm^2 cell culture dish in complete medium. Forty micrograms of vector DNA (pLXSN-eGFP, Figure 3.1.a) were dissolved in 1 mL serum-free medium. Four hundred microliters Plus reagent were added, mixed, and incubated for 15 min at room temperature. One hundred µl of LipofectAMINE^{TM} reagent were dissolved in 1 mL serum-free medium. Finally, the DNA solution was mixed with the solution containing LipofectAMINE^{TM} and incubated for 15 min at room temperature. Culture medium was removed and 7.5 mL fresh complete medium was added to the target cells. The DNA/liposome complexes were added drop-wise to the cell layer. Four hours post transfection, 20 mL complete medium were added to the cells. The following day, the culture medium was renewed.

3.3.3.3. Electroporation

Two micrograms vector DNA (pLXSN-eGFP, Figure 3.1.a) were added to 5 x 10^5 cells suspended in 100 µL Human MSC Nucleofector^{TM} solution (AMAXA Biosystems). Electroporation was performed using Nucleofector^{TM} programs U-23 and C-17 for high transfection efficiency and high cell survival, respectively, as described in the protocol provided by the manufacturer. Following electroporation, the cells were cultured in complete culture medium in 6-well tissue culture plates.

3.3.3.4. Magnetofection^{TM}

After optimizing the ratio of PolyMag (OZ Biosciences)/DNA and the nucleic acid dose according to the manufacturer's recommendation, the following protocol was applied. One day prior to Magnetofection^{TM}, 3 x 10^4 porcine MSCs were plated onto 12-well plates. Three micrograms of plasmid DNA (pLXSN-eGFP, Figure 3.1.a) were added to a total of 100 µL serum-free culture medium, mixed with 4.5 µg PolyMag material, and incubated for 20 min at room temperature. The DNA/PolyMag complexes were added to the target cell layer drop-wise and the cells were exposed to a magnetic field for 15 min at 37°C and 5% CO_2. The following day, culture medium was renewed.

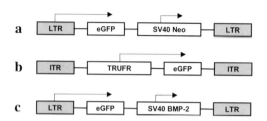

Figure 3.1. Schematic representation of the transfer vectors used for MLV-based retroviral gene transfer (**a, c**) and rAAV-mediated gene transfer (**b**). The arrows indicate direction of transgene transcription. *LTR*, long terminal repeats; *eGFP*, enhanced green fluorescence protein gene; *SV40*, simian virus 40 promoter; *Neo*, neomycin phosphotransferase gene; *ITR*, inverted terminal repeats; *TRUFR*, TRUFR promoter; *BMP-2*, human bone morphogenetic protein-2 gene.

3.3.4. Viral Gene Delivery Methods

3.3.4.1. Recombinant Adeno-Associated Virus (rAAV) System

The eGFP gene under transcriptional control of a *TRUFR* promoter was cloned into the rAAV-vector backbone (Figure 3.1.b) [18]. rAAV-eGFP virus was prepared by the Gene Core Facility, University of North Carolina at Chapel Hill, NC, USA using an adenovirus-free system cotransfecting the transfer vector with pXX2 and pXX6 plasmid into 293T cells, as described previously [16]. The concentration of infectious rAAV-eGFP particles was approximately 2.1×10^{10} mL^{-1} determined by titration on human embryonic kidney cells. rAAV-eGFP was added to the cultures at different multiplicities of infection (MOIs). Non-transduced porcine MSCs (MOI 0) served as negative controls. After the observation periods, intra-cellular eGFP expression was determined by flow cytometry as described below.

3.3.4.2. Murine leukemia Virus (MLV)-Based Retroviral System

The gene encoding eGFP was cloned into the MLV-based retroviral transfer vector pLXSN generating pLXSN-eGFP (Figure 3.1.a) [19]. If not otherwise stated, this vector was used for retroviral gene transfer. The gene encoding human BMP-2 protein was cloned into pLXSN-eGFP replacing Neo by BlnI-RsrII digestion generating pLXSBMP2-eGFP. In that way, transcription of the genes encoding eGFP and BMP-2 is directed by the LTR promoter and by the heterologous SV40 promoter, respectively (Figure 3.1.c). The transfer vector of interest was transfected into the xenotropic packaging cell line ProPak-X.36 (LGC Promochem, Boras, Sweden) by calcium phosphate co-precipitation. Briefly, 3.75×10^6 packaging cells were plated per 75-cm^2 cell culture flask in 10 ml complete medium at 37°C. Each flask was transfected as described above. One day after transfection the medium was replaced by 10 mL of fresh complete medium per flask and porcine primary MSCs were seeded in cell culture flasks or well-plates at a concentration of 5-10 x 10^3/cm^2. Forty-eight hours after transfection the retroviral vector-containing supernatants were cleared from cellular debris by filtration through 0.45 μm nitrocellulose filters (Minisart®, Sartorius) and supplemented with 6 µg Polybrene® (Sigma-Aldrich)/mL. One milliliter of the retroviral vector supernatant was added per 10^3 seeded target cells. Only fresh vector supernatants were used for this study, as thawed stocks resulted in a titer drop in the range of 10^1 (data not shown). After defined incubation periods, the genetically modified porcine MSCs were evaluated for eGFP expression as described below.

The following four optimization strategies were applied. First, the infectious supernatant was concentrated to yield an increase in vector titer using centrifugal filters (Centricon® Plus-20, Millipore) according to the manufacturer's instructions. Second, the Magnetofection™ method (OZ Biosciences) was applied. Briefly, one day prior to Magnetofection™, 3×10^4 porcine MSCs were plated per 12-wells. The following day, 1.5 µL, 3 µL, and 6 µL CombiMag were added to 1.5 mL infectious supernatant each, which was produced and harvested as described above. Polybrene® was avoided. After 20 min incubation at room temperature, the magnetic particle/vector-solution was added to the porcine MSCs. The cells were then exposed to a magnetic field for 15 min at 37°C and 5% CO_2. On the third day, culture medium was renewed. Third and fourth, as described by Kotani et al. [20], the packaging cells were incubated at 32°C during expansion and vector production and the infectious supernatant was centrifuged onto the target cell layer for 90 min at 1000 x g and 32°C. All optimization methods were tested in triplicate per experimental unit in at least two independent experiments.

3.3.5. Bioassay for Detection of Replication-Competent Viruses (RCVs)

Human 293 cells (LGC Promochem, CRL-1573), primary porcine MSCs, and murine NIH3T3 cells (LGC Promochem, CRL-1658) were cultured in triplicate for 4 days in supernatants from MLV-transduced porcine MSCs that were harvested 2 days and 7 days after retroviral transduction. The experiment was repeated four times using supernatants from 4 different MLV-transduced porcine MSC populations. Supernatants from pLXSN-eGFP transfected packaging cells served as positive controls. The test cells were assessed for expression of eGFP by fluorescence microscopy as described below.

3.3.6. Evaluation of Transgene Expression

If not otherwise stated, eGFP expression was assessed by flow cytometric analysis. Briefly, the cells were washed with PBS, trypsinized, resuspended in complete medium, counted and centrifuged at 200 x g for 10 min 2 d post gene transfer. The pellet was dissolved in PBS supplemented with 1% paraformaldehyde at a final cell concentration of approximately 10^6 cells per milliliter. The cells were fixated for 48 h at 4°C. Mock-transduced cells were used as negative controls. Fluorescence-activated cytometry was performed using a FACSCalibur™ machine (Becton Dickinson) counting a minimum of 3×10^4 cells per acquisition. Both percentage of viable eGFP expressing cells and mean fluorescence intensity (MFI) were evaluated for each population using CellQuest™ (Becton Dickinson) and FlowJo™ (Tree Star) software. A maximum level of 1% was set as the background auto-fluorescence in viable control cells. Figure 3.2. shows an example of three rAAV-eGFP transduced primary porcine MSC populations and two non-transduced baseline population.

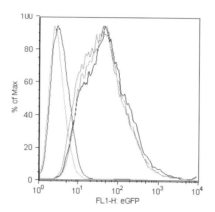

Figure 3.2. Flow cytometric analysis demonstrating three right-shifted rAAV-eGFP transduced porcine MSC populations (MOI 1000) and two non-transduced baseline populations. Percentages of maximum number of events are plotted as a function of logarithmic green fluorescence intensity.

For optimization of non-viral gene transfer methods, porcine MSCs expressing eGFP were counted using fluorescence microscopy (Olympus IX70) and normalized to the total number of cells counted 2 days post gene transfer. A minimum of 3 x 100 cells were counted for each experimental unit. Moreover, fluorescence microscopy was used for detection of replication-competent viruses as described above.

Osteogenic differentiation of retrovirally BMP-2 transduced porcine MSCs was assessed by histochemical detection of alkaline phosphatase activity. Briefly, 7×10^5 cells were plated in triplicate in 6-well cell culture plates. Porcine MSCs transduced with pLXSN-eGFP vector (Figure 3.1.a) served as controls. After 7 d culturing, the confluent cell layer was washed in PBS, fixed in 3.5% paraformaldehyde in PBS for 30 min, and washed again in PBS. The cells were then equilibrated in NTMT buffer (0.1 M NaCl, 50 mM MgCl, 0.1% Tween-20, 0.1 M Tris-HCl pH 9.5, in ddH$_2$O) and stained with 2% NBT/BCIP solution (Roche) overnight. A positive reaction gave an insoluble blue-black precipitate with nitroblue tetrazolium salt substrate as evaluated by light microscopy.

Transcription of the transgene encoding BMP-2 was assessed by real-time quantitative reverse transcription polymerase chain reaction (RT-PCR). Briefly, 4 d post retroviral transduction, total RNA was isolated by Trizol® method according to the manufacturer's directions. Following DNase-treatment (TURBO DNA-free™, Ambion) the amount and purity of the RNA samples were determined by optical densitometry at 260 nm and 280 nm. RNA integrity was confirmed by agarose gel electrophoresis. Using the High Capacity cDNA Archive Kit (Applied Biosystems, cat. no. 4322171) RNA was converted into complementary DNA (cDNA). Real-time quantitative RT-PCR was performed on a 7500 Fast Real-Time PCR system (Applied Biosystems) using TaqMan® Gene Expression Assays Hs00154192_m1 and Hs99999901_s1 for BMP-2 and 18S rRNA with standard enzymes and cycling conditions for the 7500 Fast System. Template cDNA corresponding to 40 ng of RNA was added to each PCR reaction and each sample was run in triplicate. The experiment was repeated three times. Data analysis was performed using 7500 Fast System Sequence Detection Software version 1.3 (Applied Biosystems). Expression levels of the BMP-2 gene were normalized to 18S rRNA gene expression according to the equation:

relative BMP-2 expression = $2^{\,Ct\,(BMP-2)\,-\,Ct\,(18S)}$, where Ct is the threshold cycle.

3.3.7. Statistical Analyses

The data were tested for normal distribution and homogeneity of variances and when these conditions were fulfilled, parametric analyses were performed (*t*-test for comparison of two groups, One Way Analysis of Variance for multiple comparisons), otherwise non-parametric analyses were applied (Mann-Whitney rank sum test, Kruskal-Wallis rank test). Statistical significance was determined as $p < 0.05$ (two-tailed). Data are presented as mean and standard deviation of the mean.

3.4. RESULTS

3.4.1. Non-Viral Gene Transfer

No transduced porcine MSCs could be detected following calcium phosphate co-precipitation method, even after optimization by varying cell density and amount of vector DNA used. Optimized cationic liposome-mediated transfection, electroporation, and Magnetofection™ resulted in eGFP expression by not more than 2% of the cells. Figure 3.3. shows the maximum achievable percentage of eGFP expressing cells by the non-viral methods tested compared to rAAV-based and MLV-based retroviral gene delivery method. Following all non-viral methods tested higher percentages of non-viable cells were observed compared to the viral methods applied as assessed by light microscopy (data not shown).

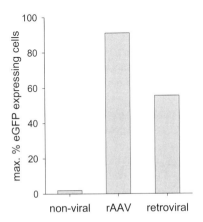

Figure 3.3. Maximum achievable percentages of eGFP-expression by primary porcine mesenchymal stem cells using non-viral, rAAV-mediated, and retroviral gene delivery. Flow cytometric analysis was performed within 7 d post transduction.

3.4.2. rAAV-Mediated Gene Transfer

To assess the inter-individual variation of rAAV-mediated gene transfer efficiency and the effect of MOI on rAAV-mediated gene transfer efficiency, primary porcine MSC populations from four different pigs were transduced in quadruplicate with rAAV-eGFP vector at MOI 10, MOI 100, and MOI 1000. Four days post transduction, the cells were prepared for flow cytometric analysis and the percentages of eGFP expressing cells and MFIs were determined. The results are visualized in Figure 3.4.. We were able to demonstrate percentages of eGFP expressing cells of 8.1% (inter-individual SD, ±4.9%), 48.0% (±9.8%), and 73.4% (±7.8%), corresponding to MOIs of 10, 100, and 1000, respectively (Figure 3.4.a). The MFIs were 8.0 (±3.6), 86.0 (±50.4), and 671.9 (±652.4) for the corresponding MOIs of 10, 100, and 1000, respectively (Figure 3.4.b).

To evaluate temporal rAAV-mediated transgene expression, one porcine MSC population was transduced with rAAV-eGFP in quadruplicate at MOI 100 and MOI 1000 and the percentages of eGFP-expressing cells and MFIs were assessed at 2 d, 7 d, 14 d, and 21 d post transduction (Figure 3.5.). Porcine MSCs transduced at the highest titer (MOI 1000) showed a higher percentage of eGFP expression and an increased MFI compared to those transduced at MOI 100 at all time points. Maximum transgene expression was reached 7 d post rAAV-eGFP transduction at MOI 1000 (% eGFP-expressing cells, 90.3% ±0.7%; MFI, 214.8 ±28.8) and 2 d post transduction at MOI 100 (% eGFP-expressing cells, 61.3% ±6.1%; MFI, 58.0% ±19.7%), respectively. These peaks were followed by a continuous decrease in transgene expression. After 14 d 16.8% ±1.5% (MOI 1000) and 7.2% ±2.4% (MOI 100) of the cells were eGFP-positive. Twenty one days post transduction, about 6% of the cells were still transduced for both titers used.

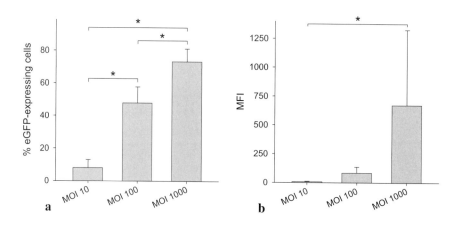

Figure 3.4. Effect of rAAV titer on gene transfer efficiency. MSC populations (N=4) were rAAV-eGFP transduced in quadruplicate at MOI 10, MOI 100, and MOI 1000. Percentages of eGFP-expressing cells (**a**) and

mean fluorescence intensities (MFIs, **b**) were assessed by flow cytometric analysis 4 d post transduction. Data are presented as mean ±SD. * P<0.05.

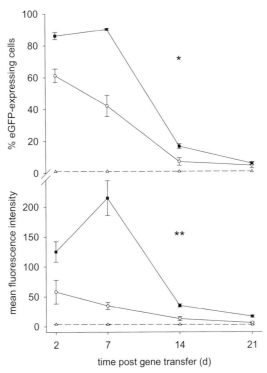

Figure 3.5. Temporal rAAV transgene expression in porcine MSCs. One porcine MSC population was rAAV-eGFP transduced in triplicate at MOI 100 (—○—) and MOI 1000 (—■—). Non-transduced cells (– △ –) served as controls. Percentages of eGFP-expressing cells (upper graph) and mean fluorescence intensities (MFIs, lower graph) were assessed by flow cytometric analysis. Data are presented as mean ±SD. * P<0.05 within and between MOI 1000 and MOI 100 groups for all time points. ** P<0.05 for MOI 1000 (7 d) versus MOI 100 (21 d).

3.4.3. MLV-Based Retroviral Gene Transfer

Using a protocol including centrifugation of retroviral vector onto porcine MSCs, we were able to show eGFP expression in 44.1% ±5.0% (mean ±SD) of the cells and MFIs of 327.4 ±56.6. This denotes a 26-fold increase in percentage of transduction and a 68-fold increase in MFI compared to the standard protocol not including centrifugation (% eGFP-expressing cells, 1.7% ±0.2%; MFI, 4.8% ±1.3%). None of the other optimization methods could increase MLV-based retroviral gene transfer efficiency compared to the conventional protocol. Figure 3.6. summarizes the results from the optimization of retroviral gene transfer.

To confirm transcription of the BMP-2 transgene, a porcine MSC population was retrovirally transduced in triplicate with pLXSBMP2-eGFP vector (Figure 3.1.c) using the optimized retroviral gene delivery protocol described above. Cells from the same population transduced with pLXSN-eGFP vector (Figure 3.1.a) served as controls. Using real-time quantitative RT-PCR we observed a 220-fold increase in BMP-2 gene expression by the BMP-2 transduced cells compared to the control cells (Figure 3.7.a). The BMP-2 transduced porcine MSCs demonstrated furthermore increased osteogenic differentiation as determined by histochemical detection of alkaline phosphatase activity (Figure 3.7.b).

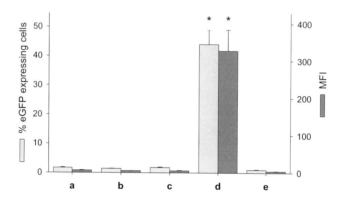

Figure 3.6. Optimization of MLV-based retroviral gene transfer to porcine MSCs. (a) 32°C incubation of packaging cells during expansion and vector production. (b) Concentration of infectious supernatant using Centricon® Plus-20 centrifugal filters. (c) Magnetofection™ method. (d) Centrifugation of infectious supernatant onto the target cells. (e) Conventional transduction protocol (control). Percentages of eGFP-expressing cells and mean fluorescence intensities (MFIs) were assessed by flow cytometric analysis 4 d post transduction (N=8). Data are presented as mean ±SD. * P < 0.05 versus control.

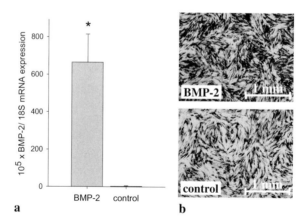

Figure 3.7. Genetic modification of porcine MSCs by optimized MLV-based retroviral gene delivery using pLXSBMP2-eGFP vector. Cells transduced with pLXSN-eGFP served as controls. (a) BMP-2 gene expression was increased by 220-fold compared to the control cells as assessed by real-time quantitative RT-PCR. Data are presented as mean ±SD (N=3). * P<0.05 versus control. (b) Representative micrographs demonstrating increased osteogenic differentiation of BMP-2 transduced cells by histochemical determination of alkaline phosphatase activity (**b**).

3.5. DISCUSSION

3.5.1. Non-Viral Gene Transfer

Due to safety concerns in relation to viral gene transfer systems non-viral, synthetic vectors and physical DNA-delivery methods have gained increasing interest. The advantages of non-viral gene transfer include low immunogenicity, low acute toxicity, simplicity, few restrictions on the size of the gene of interest, and feasibility to be produced on a large scale. There are, however, drawbacks concerning non-viral gene delivery including lower gene transfer efficiency than in viral systems and only transient gene expression in the host cells [21]. In this study, primary porcine MSCs transfected by calcium phosphate co-precipitation, cationic liposome-mediated transfection, electroporation, and Magnetofection™ did not show acceptable transgene expression levels, even when optimization protocols were applied. However, due to advantages with respect to safety issues and ease of handling, the improvement of existing non-viral methods and the development of new strategies for non-viral gene delivery to primary porcine MSCs deserve further attention.

3.5.2. rAAV-Mediated Gene Transfer

3.5.2.1. Gene Transfer Efficiency and Effect of Viral Load

In contrast to the moderate inter-individual variation percentage of eGFP-expressing cells (Figure 3.4.a), we observed high inter-individual variation in MFI using rAAV-mediated gene transfer, in particular at the highest titers used (Figure 3.4.b). High-titer rAAV-mediated transduction of porcine MSCs resulted in maximum percentages of eGFP-expressing cells of 90.3% ±0.7% (Figure 3.5.). A prerequisite for this high efficiency is a high tropism of rAAV vector system towards porcine MSCs. In addition, rAAV vectors are characterized by the ability to transduce cells that are not actively undergoing cell division, as opposed to, e.g., MLV vectors, that are dependent on the breakdown of the nuclear membrane during cell division for the vector DNA to gain access to the chromosomal DNA of the host cell.

Porcine MSCs transduced at higher rAAV-eGFP titers showed increased percentage of eGFP-expressing cells and MFIs compared to those transduced at lower MOIs at all time points (Figure 3.5.) and in all four porcine MSC populations investigated (Figure 3.4.). The increase in percentage of eGFP-expressing cells with increasing MOI can be explained by the fact that more target cells are transduced due to a higher vector density around the target cells. The increase in MFI at higher titers is likely to result from multiple rAAV-infections per target cell. This leads to a higher translation of transgenic proteins per cell. We conclude that there is a positive correlation between viral rAAV vector load and gene transfer efficiency in porcine MSCs.

3.5.2.2. Temporal Transgene Expression

Transduction of porcine MSCs at MOI 100 resulted in a decrease in transgene expression already during the first week post transduction, whereas cells transduced at MOI 1000 showed a delayed decrease in transgene expression with maximum eGFP expression 7 d post transduction. Following infection, the single-stranded DNA rAAV genome rapidly translocates to the nucleus [22,23], where it remains in an inert state until the second strand is synthesized to generate the transducing episomal molecule. This rAAV episome does not integrate into the host cell's genome [11,24]. The second-strand synthesis is the rate-limiting step in rAAV transduction [25,26]. During high-titer transduction each target cell is infected by multiple rAAV vectors as mentioned above. The delayed maximum transgene expression observed at rAAV transduction using the highest titer can therefore be explained by intracellular accumulation of rAAV genome prior to second-strand synthesis.

Unlike retroviral vectors, AAV does not require active cell division or integration for expression to occur. Compared to slowly proliferating cells, e.g., neurons, chondrocytes, or muscle cells the porcine MSCs used in this study are characterized by a high cellular turnover. The observed decrease in transgene expression (Figure 3.5.) can be explained by a "dilution effect", i.e., each nuclear episomal vector DNA is passed down to only one daughter cell during cell division thereby reducing the percentage of transduced cells ("dilution"). The duration of rAAV-mediated transgene expression is therefore largely dependent on the proliferation rate of the target cell. However, two weeks post high-titer rAAV-mediated transduction, 16.8% ±1.5% of porcine MSCs were still expressing the transgenic reporter protein.

3.5.2.3. Safety Issues

To address concerns of the potential for adenoviral contamination of the AAV vector stocks, and the presence of adenoviral denatured proteins, which is unacceptable for clinical use, a three plasmid co-transfection procedure was used for production of viral AAV vectors [16]. The three plasmids are: (1) the genes required for capsid and replication are provided by a pAAV packaging construct, pXX2, containing only the AAV cap and rep genes — this plasmid increases the rAAV yield by 15-fold compared to the conventional packaging plasmid pAAV/Ad [16]; (2) the adenovirus helper functions are delivered from a plasmid, pXX6, which contains the essential helper genes but lacks the adenoviral structural and replication genes; (3) the cloned plasmid encoding the transgene of interest flanked by the AAV ITR (Figure 3.1.b). The combination of these plasmids ensures a vector production method providing high titer AAV vector preparations that are completely free of adenovirus and wild type AAV. To ensure the absence of RCVs a bioassay as described for the retroviral vectors can be applied for the safety assessment of rAAV-based gene delivery systems.

3.5.2.4. Application

Ex vivo genetic modification of porcine MSCs by rAAV-mediated gene delivery is of special interest for tissue engineering systems requiring transient expression of one or more genes of interest. The intensity and duration of transgene expression can be controlled by the MOI applied.

3.5.3. MLV-Based Retroviral Gene Transfer

3.5.3.1. Optimization of Gene Transfer Efficiency

Retroviral infection begins by interaction of the viral envelope surface protein with a specific receptor protein on the cytoplasmic membrane of a target cell. MLVs can form infectious particles with various envelope surface proteins that allow entry via different receptors. Since receptor abundance varies among cell types, the choice of envelope protein may influence the efficacy of gene delivery [17]. Mosca et al. demonstrated the dependence on retroviral envelope for transduction of MSCs isolated from pigs and other species [27]. This also reflects our experience as we did not achieve acceptable retroviral gene transfer efficiencies using amphotropic compared to xenotropic envelope vectors (data not shown). For this reason, a packaging cell line producing xenotropic envelope vectors was used in this study.

Incubation of packaging cells at 32°C, which has been shown to improve retroviral vector production [20], vector particle concentration, and Magnetofection^{TM} method did not enhance retroviral transduction efficiency of porcine MSCs compared to the conventional transduction protocol. We solved the problem of inefficient retroviral gene transfer by including a simple centrifugation step, which resulted in a 26-fold increase in percentage of eGFP-expressing cells and a 68-fold increase in MFI compared to the standard transduction protocol (Figure 3.6.). We conclude that centrifugation facilitated the approximation of viral vector to the target cell layer which is a crucial prerequisite for the early steps of retroviral infection.

In concordance with the eGFP reporter gene study, optimized retroviral transduction of porcine MSCs with a vector containing the gene encoding the osteogenic growth factor BMP-2 in addition to the reporter gene resulted in a dramatic increase in BMP-2 gene transcription. BMP-2 activity was not measured directly. However, we were able to demonstrate an increased osteogenic differentiation of the BMP-2 transduced porcine MSCs as assessed by histochemical determination of alkaline phosphatase activity (Figure 3.7.). We interpret this finding as an effect of transgenic BMP-2.

3.5.3.2. Safety Issues

Specific safety concerns are associated with the handling and clinical use of retroviral vectors.

The contribution of retrovirally mediated gene transfer to the induction of leukaemia in two children with X-linked SCID after transplantation of retrovirally corrected haematopoietic stem cells in a gene therapy trial has recently raised concerns about the potential risk of insertional mutagenesis resulting from random retroviral integration [28]. However, an extended clinical follow-up and molecular analysis in nonhuman primates and dogs that received retrovirally transduced haematopoietic stem cells did not provide evidence for the induction of leukaemia by retroviral vectors *in vivo* [29]. It is therefore most likely that patient- or transgene-specific factors contributed to the occurrence of leukemia in the above mentioned X-SCID gene therapy trial. Retroviral transfer vectors containing the weak transcriptional Akv enhancer sustained acceptable transgene expression levels [30]. In this context, the application of such low- or non-leukaemogenic murine retroviral vectors can be advantageous for gene therapy protocols.

The risk of generating replication-competent viruses (RCVs) denotes another key issue in safety assessment of retroviral vector systems. RCVs may spread beyond the target cells and lead to multiple cycles of vector transfer, raising concerns of (1) transgene expression in non-target cells, (2) spread of the transfer vector to other individuals, (3) damage caused by an immune reaction against virus-infected cells, and (4) excessive mutations of the host genome caused by provirus insertions during multiple rounds of replication. However, a three-component retroviral gene transfer system requires 3 crossover events between transfer vector and packaging construct RNAs for generation of RCVs [17]. Importantly, the packaging cells' RNAs that direct translation of viral proteins are devoid of signals for incorporation into virions. Accordingly, the resulting retroviral particles deliver transfer vectors but not viral protein encoding genes to the target cells. Such transduced target cells without viral proteins will not give rise to infectious particles. Using this scheme of single cycle replication-defective retroviral vector propagation, we did not detect any RCVs by bioassay including human, porcine, and murine recipient cells. In clinical trials using *ex vivo* retrovirally mediated gene therapy absence of RCVs should be confirmed by such assays before re-implantation of the genetically modified material. Furthermore, transfer and recombination of endogenous viruses can be prevented by screening the recipients' genome for endogenous retroviral sequences potentially interacting with the MLV-based gene transfer machinery.

3.5.3.3. Application

Unlike AAV-based and non-viral gene transfer, retroviral gene delivery resulted in long-term transgene expression by porcine MSCs. This can be explained by the retroviral replication via a DNA intermediate which becomes stably integrated into the chromosomal DNA of the host cell. *Ex vivo* genetic modification of porcine MSCs by optimized MLV-based retroviral gene transfer is in particular attractive for the preclinical testing of advanced tissue engineering strategies requiring long-term transgene expression.

3.6. SUMMARY

Ex vivo genetic modification of autologous MSCs with genes encoding specific growth factors and cytokines is an attractive strategy to induce and maintain differentiation towards the tissue of interest. Gene transfer to primary MSCs of porcine origin is of special interest as porcine research models have proven valuable for the preclinical testing of tissue engineering protocols in large animals. In this context, the choice of gene delivery method denotes a crucial step.

The low efficiency of non-viral gene transfer methods observed in this study requires further improvement of existing non-viral methods and the development of new strategies for non-viral gene delivery to primary porcine MSCs.

High-titer rAAV-mediated gene transfer resulted in highly efficient, though transient, genetic modification of porcine MSCs with maximum percentages of eGFP-expressing cells in the range of 90%, due to a sufficient tropism of rAAV vectors towards porcine MSCs and their ability to infect nondividing cells. *Ex vivo* genetic modification of porcine MSCs by rAAV-mediated gene delivery is therefore interesting for tissue engineering systems requiring transient expression of one or more genes of interest. The intensity and duration of transgene expression can be controlled by the MOI applied.

Using a protocol including xenotropic envelopes and centrifugation of retroviral particles onto the target cell layer we observed stable transduction of porcine MSCs by retroviral vectors with maximum percentages of eGFP-expressing cells of about 45%. Porcine MSCs that were BMP-2 transduced by optimized retroviral gene transfer method demonstrated a significant increase in BMP-2 gene expression and showed increased osteogenic differentiation compared to mock-transduced control cells. By use of bioassays including human, porcine, and murine target cells we did not detect formation of RCVs. *Ex vivo* genetic modification of porcine MSCs by optimized retroviral gene delivery is in particular attractive for the preclinical testing of advanced tissue engineering strategies requiring long-term transgene expression.

3.7. ACKNOWLEDGMENTS

This work was financially supported by the Interdisciplinary Research Group "Nanoscience and Biocompatibility", grant no. 2052-01-0049, Danish Research Agency, and by the Family Hede Nielsen Foundation. Dieter Klein, DVM, University of Veterinary Medicine, Vienna generously provided the transfer vector pLXSN-eGFP. We would like to thank Ane Kjeldsen for excellent technical assistance in cell culture and Alexander Schmitz, MSc, PhD, Xuenong Zou, MD, PhD and Jeannette Justesen, MSc, PhD for initiating flow cytometric analysis, cell purification method and RCV bioassay, respectively.

3.8. REFERENCES

1. S.E. Haynesworth, J. Goshima, V.M. Goldberg, and A.I. Caplan, Characterization of cells with osteogenic potential from human marrow, *Bone* **13**(1), 81-88 (1992).
2. M.F. Pittenger, A.M. Mackay, S.C. Beck, R.K. Jaiswal, R. Douglas, J.D. Mosca, M.A. Moorman, D.W. Simonetti, S. Craig, and D.R. Marshak, Multilineage potential of adult human mesenchymal stem cells, *Science* **284**(5411), 143-147 (1999).
3. H.A. Awad, D.L. Butler, G.P. Boivin, F.N. Smith, P. Malaviya, B. Huibregtse, and A.I. Caplan, Autologous mesenchymal stem cell-mediated repair of tendon, *Tissue Eng.* **5**(3), 267-277 (1999).
4. G. Ferrari, G. Cusella-De Angelis, M. Coletta, E. Paolucci, A. Stornaiuolo, G. Cossu, and F. Mavilio, Muscle regeneration by bone marrow-derived myogenic progenitors, *Science* **279**(5356), 1528-1530 (1998).
5. P. Bianco and P.G. Robey, Stem cells in tissue engineering, *Nature* **414**(6859), 118-121 (2001).
6. F. Gori, T. Thomas, K.C. Hicok, T.C. Spelsberg, and B.L. Riggs, Differentiation of human marrow stromal precursor cells: bone morphogenetic protein-2 increases OSF2/CBFA1, enhances osteoblast commitment, and inhibits late adipocyte maturation, *J. Bone Miner. Res.* **14**(9), 1522-1535 (1999).
7. A.I. Caplan, Mesenchymal stem cells and gene therapy, *Clin. Orthop.* **379**, S67-S70 (2000).
8. K.W. Culver and R.M. Blaese, Gene therapy for cancer, *Trends Genet.* **10**(5), 174-178 (1994).
9. V. Cottard, D. Mulleman, P. Bouille, M. Mezzina, M.C. Boissier, and N. Bessis, Adeno-associated virus-mediated delivery of IL-4 prevents collagen-induced arthritis, *Gene Ther.* **7**(22), 1930-1939 (2000).
10. K.R. Clark, T.J. Sferra, and P.R. Johnson, Recombinant adeno-associated viral vectors mediate long-term transgene expression in muscle, *Hum. Gene Ther.* **8**(6), 659-669 (1997).
11. D. Duan, P. Sharma, J. Yang, Y. Yue, L. Dudus, Y. Zhang, K.J. Fisher, and J.F. Engelhardt, Circular intermediates of recombinant adeno-associated virus have defined structural characteristics responsible for long-term episomal persistence in muscle tissue, *J. Virol.* **72**(11), 8568-8577 (1998).

12. M.G. Kaplitt, P. Leone, R.J. Samulski, X. Xiao, D.W. Pfaff, K.L. O'Malley, and M.J. During, Long-term gene expression and phenotypic correction using adeno-associated virus vectors in the mammalian brain, *Nat. Genet.* **8**(2), 148-154 (1994).
13. T. Ikeda, T. Kubo, Y. Arai, T. Nakanishi, K. Kobayashi, K. Takahashi, J. Imanishi, M. Takigawa, and Y.Hirasawa, Adenovirus mediated gene delivery to the joints of guinea pigs, *J. Rheumatol.* **25**(9), 1666-1673 (1998).
14. A.M. Douar, K. Poulard, D. Stockholm, and O. Danos, Intracellular trafficking of adeno-associated virus vectors: routing to the late endosomal compartment and proteasome degradation, *J. Virol.* **75**(4), 1824-1833 (2001).
15. J. Goater, R. Muller, G. Kollias, G.S. Firestein, I. Sanz, R.J. O'Keefe, and E.M. Schwarz, Empirical advantages of adeno associated viral vectors in vivo gene therapy for arthritis, *J. Rheumatol.* **27**(4): 983-989 (2000).
16. X. Xiao, J. Li, and R.J. Samulski, Production of high-titer recombinant adeno-associated virus vectors in the absence of helper adenovirus, *J. Virol.* **72**(3), 2224-2232 (1998).
17. F. S. Pedersen and M. Duch, Retroviruses in human gene therapy, *Encyclopedia of Life Sciences* (2003); http://els.wiley.com.
18. M. Ulrich-Vinther, M.D. Maloney, J.J. Goater, K. Soballe, M.B. Goldring, R.J. O'Keefe, and E.M. Schwarz, Light-activated gene transduction enhances adeno-associated virus vector-mediated gene expression in human articular chondrocytes, *Arthritis Rheum.* **46**(8), 2095-2104 (2002).
19. D. Klein, S. Indraccolo, K. von Rombs, A. Amadori, B. Salmons, and W.H. Gunzburg, Rapid identification of viable retrovirus-transduced cells using the green fluorescent protein as a marker, *Gene Ther.* **4**(11), 1256-1260 (1997).
20. H. Kotani, P.B. Newton 3rd, S. Zhang, Y.L. Chiang, E. Otto, L. Weaver, R.M. Blaese, W.F.Anderson, and G.J.McGarrity, Improved methods of retroviral vector transduction and production for gene therapy, *Hum. Gene Ther.* **5**(1), 19-28 (1994).
21. K.A. Partridge and R.O. Oreffo, Gene delivery in bone tissue engineering: progress and prospects using viral and nonviral strategies, *Tissue Eng.* **10**(1-2), 295-307 (2004).
22. A.M. Douar, K. Poulard, D. Stockholm, and O. Danos, Intracellular trafficking of adeno-associated virus vectors: routing to the late endosomal compartment and proteasome degradation, *J Virol* **75**(4):1824-1833 (2001).
23. G. Seisenberger, M.U. Ried, T. Endress, H. Buning, M. Hallek, and C. Brauchle, Real-time single-molecule imaging of the infection pathway of an adeno-associated virus." Science 2001.Nov.30.;294.(5548.):1929.-32. 294,(November 2001):1929-32.
24. T.R. Flotte, S.A. Afione, and P.L. Zeitlin, Adeno-associated virus vector gene expression occurs in nondividing cells in the absence of vector DNA integration, *Am. J. Respir. Cell Mol. Biol.* **11**(5), 517-521 (1994).
25. G. Seisenberger, M.U. Ried, T. Endress, H. Buning, M. Hallek, and C. Brauchle, Real-time single-molecule imaging of the infection pathway of an adeno-associated virus, *Science* **294**(5548), 1929-1932 (2001).
26. K.J. Fisher, G.P. Gao, M.D. Weitzman, R. DeMatteo, J.F. Burda, and J.M. Wilson, Transduction with recombinant adeno-associated virus for gene therapy is limited by leading-strand synthesis, *J. Virol.* **70**(1), 520-532 (1996).
27. J.D. Mosca, J.K. Hendricks, D. Buyaner, J. Davis-Sproul, L.C. Chuang, M.K. Majumdar, R. Chopra, F. Barry, M. Murphy, M.A. Thiede, U. Junker, R.J. Rigg, S.P. Forestell, E. Bohnlein, R. Storb, and B.M. Sandmaier, Mesenchymal stem cells as vehicles for gene delivery, *Clin. Orthop.* **379**, S71-S90 (2000).
28. S. Hacein-Bey-Abina, C. von Kalle, M. Schmidt, M.P. McCormack, N. Wulffraat, P. Leboulch, A. Lim, C.S.Osborne, R.Pawliuk, E.Morillon, R.Sorensen, A.Forster, P.Fraser, J.I.Cohen, B.G.de Saint, I. Alexander, U. Wintergerst, T. Frebourg, A. Aurias, D. Stoppa-Lyonnet, S. Romana, I. Radford-Weiss, F. Gross, F. Valensi, E. Delabesse, E. Macintyre, F. Sigaux, J. Soulier, L.E. Leiva, M. issler, C. Prinz, T.H. Rabbitts, F. Le Deist, A. Fischer, and M. Cavazzana-Calvo, LMO2-associated clonal T cell proliferation in two patients after gene therapy for SCID-X1, *Science* **302**(5644), 415-419 (2003).
29. H.P. Kiem, S. Sellers, B. Thomasson, J.C. Morris, J.F. Tisdale, P.A. Horn, P. Hematti, R. Adler, K. Kuramoto, B. Calmels, A. Bonifacino, J. Hu, C. von Kalle, M. Schmidt, B. Sorrentino, A. Nienhuis, C.A. Blau, R.G. Andrews, R.E. Donahue, and C.E. Dunbar, Long-term clinical and molecular follow-up of large animals receiving retrovirally transduced stem and progenitor cells: no progression to clonal hematopoiesis or leukemia, *Mol. Ther.* **9**(3), 389-395 (2004).
30. M. Duch, K. Paludan, J. Lovmand, M.S. Sorensen, P. Jorgensen, and F.S. Pedersen, The effect of selection for high-level vector expression on the genetic and functional stability of a single transcript vector derived from a low-leukemogenic murine retrovirus, *Hum. Gene Ther.* **6**(3), 289-296 (1995).

4

TRANSPLANTATION OF BONE MARROW STROMAL CELLS FOR TREATMENT OF CENTRAL NERVOUS SYSTEM DISEASES

Michael Chopp[1] and Yi Li[2]

4.1. INTRODUCTION

In this review article, we primarily focus on data generated in our laboratory using bone marrow stromal cells (BMSCs) for the treatment of stroke, and other central nervous system (CNS) disorders, such as traumatic brain injury, intracerebral hemorrhage, spinal cord injury, Parkinson's disease, multiple sclerosis and brain tumor in rodents. BMSCs obtained from donor rats, mice or humans have been transplanted into the CNS via local and systemic routes. BMSCs selectively target damaged tissue, promote neurological functional recovery, and remodel brain architecture. Although some BMSCs express proteins phenotypic of neural cells, it is highly unlikely that benefit is derived by replacement of damaged tissues and rewiring brain with transdifferentiated BMSCs. The far more reasonable explanation is that BMSCs secrete and induce within parenchymal cells expression of growth or trophic factors that activate endogenous restorative processes, e.g., angiogenesis, synaptogenesis, gliogenesis and neurogenesis (Figure 4.1).

Brain after stroke or neural injury responds by necrotic and apoptotic cell death in the lesion areas, and reverts to a quasi-developmental state in peri-lesion areas.[1] This developmental state is recognized at the molecular level. Embryonic and developmental proteins and genes are expressed in adult damaged brains. Proteins such as nestin,[2,3] growth-associated protein 43 (GAP-43),[4,5] cyclin D1,[5] synaptophysin,[5] vascular endothelial growth factor (VEGF)[6] that promote neurogenesis, synaptogenesis and angiogenesis are profusely expressed in the region of tissue adjacent to the ischemic lesion. Within the ischemic boundary tissue having quasi-developmental characteristics, we hypothesized that stem and progenitor cells in the subventricular zone (SVZ) respond to and affect this developmental microenvironment. These molecular alterations of the ischemic boundary zones occur at a time at which there is enhanced neurogenesis in the SVZ.[7,8] These two remodeling events may act syner-

---

[1] Department of Neurology, Henry Ford Health Sciences Center, Detroit, Michigan, USA, Department of Physics, Oakland University, Rochester, Michigan, USA.
[2] Department of Neurology, Henry Ford Health Sciences Center, Detroit, Michigan, USA

gistically to promote repair of brain and recovery of neurological function. Adult brain is a highly dynamic structure.[9] The adult brain has the ability to repair itself with its endogenous pool of parenchymal cells; however, the supply of cells is limited. Novel strategies for the treatment of stroke and other CNS disorders are needed in order to enhance the recovery processes.

Bone marrow is composed of non-adherent hematopoetic and adherent stromal cell compartments. BMSCs provide a stromal microenvironment for hematopoiesis, including, stem-cell factor (SCF), granulocyte colony stimulating factors (G-CSF), macrophage colony stimulating factors (M-CSF), granulocyte-macrophage colony-stimulating factor (GM-CSF), tumor necrosis factors, interferon-gamma (IFN-gamma) and interleukins (IL) -6, IL-7.[10, 11] Some of the cytokines have been reported to exert influence on proliferation and differentiation of cells. These data indicate that BMSCs supply autocrine, paracrine, and juxtacrine factors that influence the cells of the marrow microenvironment itself.[10] In addition to cytokines, BMSCs express factors associated with bone formation such as bone morphogenetic proteins (BMPs),[11] which define patterning and morphogenesis, play a regulatory role during differentiation of embryonic cells, by modifying mesodermal and neuroectodermal pathways.[12] BMSCs also secrete neurotrophins that are target-derived soluble factors required for neuronal survival, including nerve growth factor (NGF) and brain-derived neurotrophic factor (BDNF).[11] Given the robust therapeutic benefit of BMSCs in experimental models with neural diseases, and the fact that BMSCs have been employed in the treatment of human diseases, additional investigations leading to clinical studies for the treatment of CNS diseases are warranted.

4.2. TREATMENT OF CNS DISEASES WITH BMSCs

We have performed therapeutic interventions with bone marrow cells for experimental stroke,[7, 13-20] traumatic brain injury,[21-28] intracerebral hemorrhage,[29] spinal cord injury,[30] Parkinson's disease,[31] multiple sclerosis[32] and brain tumor[33] in more than 6,000 rodents. Our data reveal an obvious reduction of neurological deficits with effective doses of the BMSCs for all studies. Those effective doses are different upon various experimental therapeutic regimens: the strain of animal, cell origin, cell preparation and purification, route of administration, therapeutic window, as well as short-term or long-term observations.

The principal hypothesis to be tested was that these bone marrow cells promote functional recovery. A complete neurological examination was employed in our studies for stroke and traumatic brain injury (Figure 4.1, Functional Tests), referred to as, the modified neurological severity score (mNSS).[13] This test provides an index of motor, sensory, balance and reflex. Additional tests were performed for stroke and other CNS disorders: Adhesive-removal somatosensory test,[34] Corner test,[35] Footfault test,[36] Rotarod test,[31] Water maze test,[37] and grading 0-5 multiple sclerosis score.[32] A sophisticated integrated outcome analysis, call the "global test", was performed to measure the BMSC effect on functional recovery.[38]

4.2.1. Stroke

Stroke is characterized by extensive tissue injury in the territory of an affected vessel. For example, occlusion of the middle cerebral artery (MCAo), the major cause of stroke, induces a sudden attack of weakness and other symptoms affecting the opposite side of the body to the MCA. We have induced stroke by insertion of a nylon suture[13] or an embolus[39] into the internal carotid artery to block the middle cerebral artery in the male and female[7] young adult (2-3 m),[13] and retired breeder (10-12 m) rats,[18] as well as mice.[40] After onset of a severe cerebral ischemia, brain cells died by necrosis or apoptosis.[41-43] The ischemic boundary zone (the penumbra of infarct) is a metabolically, biochemically, and molecularly active region where a variety of mutagens, trophic factors, adhesion molecules, intra- and extra- cellular matrix molecules, among others, are uniquely elaborated in the stroke brain.[44-48]

Relying on the hypothesis that BMSCs promote functional recovery after stroke, we were confronted with an array of options of implementing preclinical cellular therapy protocols. Among questions to address were, when and where to implant the cells? We initially elected to treat the rodent at one day after MCAo.[14, 20] This time point is clinically reasonable. If deficits persist for one day after a stroke, then the event is classified as a stroke and not as a transient ischemic attack (TIA). We expanded the time window to 7 days[13] and till one month. The most direct route of placement of cells into damaged brain is intracerebral surgical transplantation[14, 20] and intracisternal cell injection[49] (Figure 4.1, Routes of Injections). The success of the direct implantation of BMSCs into brain prompted experiments to test a less invasive vascular route of administration. The carotid artery ipsilateral to the ischemic hemisphere was cannulated for injection of BMSCs,[15] and then, a more clinically relevant venous route was used for BMSC administration.[13] As described above, rats were subjected to a battery of neurological outcome measures, and exhibited a significant functional improvement with treatment of BMSCs. However, dead BMSCs,[21] and liver fibroblasts[16] showed no therapeutic benefit above that of phosphate buffered saline (PBS) treated control animals.

One question addressed with histological analysis was, whether BMSCs differentiate into brain parenchymal cells? It is necessary to mark the injected BMSCs, so that they can be identified in tissue. BMSCs pre-labeled with bromodeoxyuridine (BrdU, a thymidine analog, which is incorporated into newly formed DNA)[14, 20] or male derived BMSCs injected into female rats and the sex Y-chromosome identified by in situ hybridization[7] or human cells were injected into rats and specific anti human antibodies (e.g., MAB1281) were employed.[16] BMSCs selectively target injured tissue. In all the studies, therapeutic benefit became evident within days of transplantation. Yet, the numbers of BMSCs transplanted are miniscule compared to the approximately 35-39% of the hemispheric brain tissue infarcted after induction of MCAo. For example, at 14 days after MCAo in rats with 3×10^6 BMSC intravenous (IV) administration, $\sim 3.2 \times 10^4 \pm 0.8 \times 10^4$ BMSCs survive (~12% of transplanted BMSCs),[14] of which a small percentage of cells express neural proteins (~1% neuronal nuclear marker, NeuN; ~2% neuronal cytoplasm marker, MAP-2; and ~5% astrocytic marker, GFAP) in the injured brain, far too few to even potentially replace the infarcted tissue. Very few (~0.01%-0.5%) injected BMSCs were also found in the host bone marrow, muscle, spleen, kidney, lung, and liver. Most BMSCs encircle vessels in these organs, with few cells located in parenchyma. Injected BMSCs expressed of brain cell phenotypic proteins do not indicate true differentiation and neuronal or glial cell function. It is also highly unlikely that after such a short time period, these BMSCs truly integrate into tissue and form complex connections, which enhance function. The issue of the mechanisms of action will be discussed in the next section when interwoven events are considered.

4.2.2. Traumatic Brain Injury

Traumatic brain injury is defined as brain damage caused by externally inflicted trauma to the head. Rats were subjected to controlled cortical impact in male [21, 22] and female[23] rats. The cumulative data from our laboratory indicate that both rats[21, 27, 28] and human[26] BMSC therapy show substantial promise in the treatment of traumatic brain injury. Intracerebral transplantation of BMSCs improves neurological outcome.[23, 25] Although BMSCs enter brain using the carotid route, functional benefit was not present, likely because the route of administration required ligation of the internal carotid artery, causing an imposed hypoperfusion exacerbating brain injury.[22] To measure the effect of BMSCs administered IV on rats subjected to traumatic brain injury,[26, 27, 50] we injected BMSCs into the tail vein. The cells preferentially entered and migrated into the parenchyma of the injured brain. BMSCs were also found in other organs and were primarily localized to the vascular structures, without any obvious adverse effects. BMSC treatment via both intracerebral and intravenous reroutes, significantly increased neurological benefit. BMSC treatment enhanced endogenous brain repair in the SVZ, the sub granular zone (SGZ) of the hippocampus and the contusion boundary zone, which may contribute to the functional improvement observed in these rats.

4.2.3. Intracerebral Hemorrhage

Intracerebral hemorrhage is bleeding from a cerebral artery into the tissue of the brain. To investigate whether BMSCs administered by IV injection have a beneficial effect on the outcome after intracerebral hemorrhage in rats, intracerebral hemorrhage was induced in rats by stereotactic injection of autologous blood into the right striatum.[29] IV infusion of the BMSCs was performed 1 day after intracerebral hemorrhage. After 7 and 14 days, the rats that received the BMSC administration showed significant improvement in functional scores compared to the control rats. This improvement in the treated animals is associated with reduced tissue loss and increased local presence of the BMSCs, synaptogenesis and neural remodeling.

4.2.4. Spinal Cord Injury

We tested the hypothesis that transplantation of BMSCs into the spinal cord after a contusion injury promotes functional outcome.[30] Rats were subjected to a weight driven implant injury. BMSCs or PBS was implanted adjacent to a contusion spinal cord lesion 7 days after injury. Functional outcome measurements using the Basso-Beattie-Bresnehan score were performed weekly to 5 weeks post-injury. Sections of tissue were analyzed by double-labeled immunohistochemistry for BMSC identification. Significant improvement was detected in functional outcome in animals treated with BMSC transplantation compared to control animals. Scattered cells derived from BMSCs expressed neural protein markers. These data suggest that transplantation of BMSCs may have a therapeutic role after spinal cord injury.

4.2.5. Parkinson's Disease

Parkinson's Disease is a disorder characterized by tremor, rigidity and poverty of spontaneous movements and is affecting the basal ganglia and track of stratum-

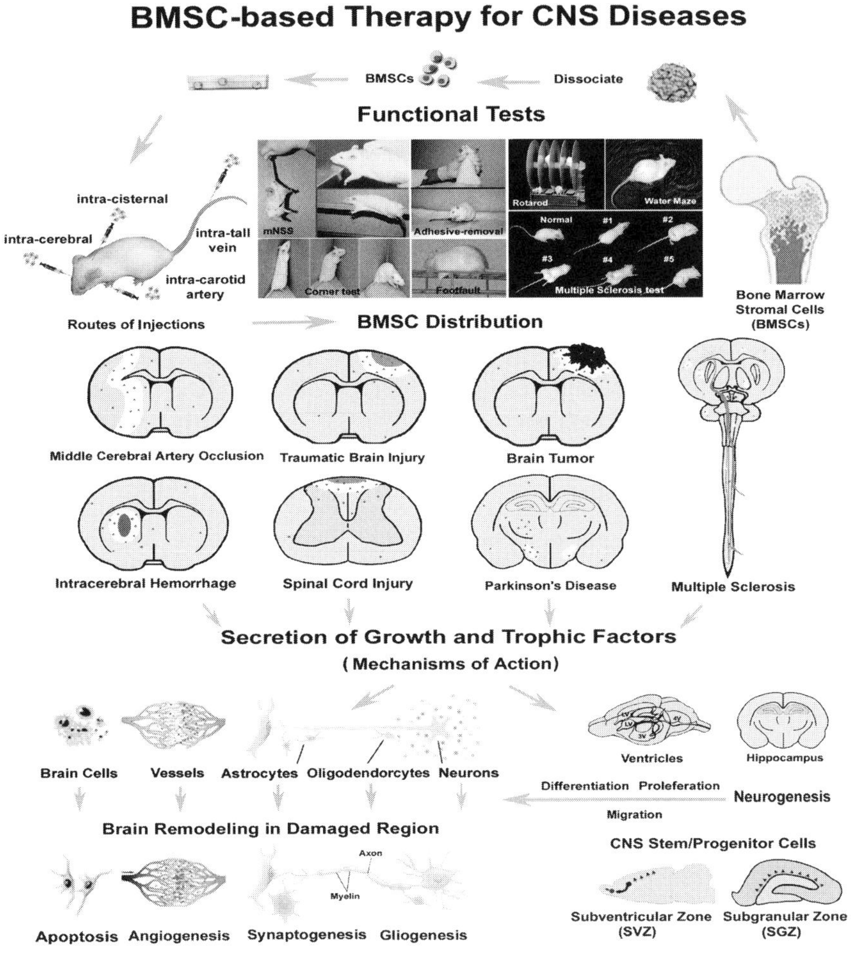

Figure 4.1. Illustration of our experimental studies supporting the potential treatment of CNS disorders with bone marrow stromal cells (BMSCs). BMSCs are extracted, separated and cultured. They are then injected via different local or systemic routes into the animal with CNS diseases. A battery of neurological functional tests are performed, such as the modified neurological severity score (mNSS, e.g., raising the rat tail shows forepaw flexes for motor test, closing the rat to an object shows no vision for sensory test, and beam balance test), Adhesive-removal test (A-R test, time of removal of a sticky tab from the paw), Corner test (turning in one versus the other direction while the vibrissae are stimulated), Footfault test (the foot falls while walking on a grid), Rotarod test (the duration of persisting on an accelerating treadmill), Water Maze test (learning and memory), and specific grading 0-5 score for multiple sclerosis test. BMSCs selectively migrate and survive in the damaged tissue and the peri-lesion areas in the animals with stroke, traumatic brain injury, intracerebral hemorrhage, spinal cord injury, brain tumor and multiple sclerosis. An array of restorative events are mediated by BMSC and possibly by parenchymal-cell secretion of cytokines, growth and trophic factors, e.g., NGF, BDNF, bFGF, VEGF, and IGF. These factors may decrease apoptosis, increase angiogenesis, gliogenesis, synaptogenesis and neurogenesis for brain remodeling and may enhance neuroprotective and neurorestorative mechanisms to improve functional recovery.

substantia nigra system of the brain. 1-methyl-4-phenyl-1,2,3,6- tetrahydropyridine (MPTP) can induce bilateral Parkinson's disease (PD) – like lesion. A study of intraparenchymal transplantation of BMSCs into one side of the striatum of MPTP-PD mice was demonstrated significant recovery of motor function.[31] Intrastriatal transplantation of BMSCs was performed 7 days after MPTP administration. MPTP-PD mice with BMSC intrastriatal transplantation exhibit significant improvement on the Rotarod test at day 35 compared with PBS controls. Immunohistochemistry shows that BrdU reactive cells survive in the transplanted areas in the MPTP-PD striatum at 4 weeks after administration. Scattered BMSCs express tyrosine hydroxylase (TH) immunoreactivity, which reduced by the MPTP administration. Our findings suggest that BMSCs injected intrastriatally survive, express dopaminergic protein TH immunoreactivity, and promote functional recovery.

4.2.6. Multiple Sclerosis

Multiple sclerosis is a chronic disease affecting the myelin sheaths surrounding nerves in the multi-regions of brain and spinal cord which affects the function of the nerves involved. The course of the illness is characterized by recurrent relapse followed by remission. Incomplete remyelination from oligodendrocyes is one the main reasons for multiple sclerosis. We investigated the treatment of remitting-relapsing experimental autoimmune encephalomyelitis (EAE) in mice with BMSCs.[32] EAE was induced in female SJL/J mice by subcutaneous injection with myelin proteolipid protein (PLP). BMSCs were injected IV into EAE mice upon onset of paresis. Neurological functional tests were scored daily by grading clinical signs (Figure 4.1, score 0-5, multiple sclerosis test). The maximum clinical score and the average clinical scores were significantly decreased in the BMSC transplanted mice compared to the PBS treated EAE controls. Immunohistochemistry was performed to measure the transplanted BMSCs, cell proliferation (BrdU), oligodendrocyte progenitor cells (NG2), immature and mature oligodendrocytes (RIP), and BDNF. Demyelination significantly decreased, and BrdU+ and BDNF+ cells significantly increased in the BMSC treated mice compared to controls. Some BrdU+ cells were colocalized with NG2+ and RIP+ immunostaining. These data indicate that BMSC treatment improved functional recovery after EAE in mice, possibly, via reducing demyelination areas, stimulating oligodendrogenesis, and by elevating BDNF expression.

4.2.7. Brain Tumor

In our studies, we employed a 9L-gliosarcoma, which grows rapidly spreading through the otherwise normal brain tissue and causes progressive neurological disability. The effects of grafted BMSCs on 9L-gliosarcoma of the rat were tested using magnetic resonance imaging (MRI), a method which permits noninvasive tracking of injected cells.[33] The BMSCs were labeled with lipophilic dye-coated superparamagnetic particles. The labeled BMSCs were transplanted to rats via a tail vein at 7 days after 9L-gliosarcoma cell implantation on the cortex. Three-dimensional (3D) gradient echo and contrast agent images revealed dynamic migration of BMSCs detected by loss of MRI signals towards tumor mass and infiltrated tumor cells. Fluorescent microscope analysis showed that grafted cells targeted tumor cells, and the areas with grafted cells corresponded to the areas with loss of MRI signals. These results demonstrate that BMSCs can target tumor sults demonstrate that BMSCs can target tumor aggregates in the brain and that the MRI technique provides a sensitive method for in vivo assessment of grafted cells targeting tumor mass and infiltrated tumor cells. BMSCs as vehicles target tumor and interfere tumor growth with novel treatment strategies may alter brain function and life quality.

4.3. MECHANISMS OF ACTION

BMSCs administered to animals with various CNS diseases provide significant functional benefit. There are multiple basic questions to address, including why the BMSCs survive in the injured brain? What mechanisms target these cells specifically to sites of injury? How do BMSCs provide their benefit? Is there any significance to the lesion-site localization of these BMSCs and to the distance-site of the germinal areas – the SVZ and SGZ? How do the BMSCs affect brain and thereby promote restorative processes? The most interesting question is, however, how these effects translate into therapeutic benefit?

4.3.1. Immune Priority of Both Brain and BMSCs

For any new treatment, safety issues must be first addressed. The immune reaction of syngeneic and allogeneic rat (r)BMSCs in rodents were investigated in stroke rats. Wistar rats were IV injected with allogeneic ACI- or syngeneic Wistar-rBMSCs at 24 hrs after MCAo and sacrificed at 28 days. Significant functional recovery was found in both cell-treated groups compared to PBS controls, but no difference was detected between allogeneic and syngeneic cell treated rats. T cells from mesenteric and cervical lymph nodes of syn-rBMSC or allo-rBMSC-treated rats were evaluated by T cell activation to antigens by the one-way mixed lymphocyte reaction (MLR) assay. Rats were bled at sacrifice, and their sera were evaluated for antibodies specific for rBMSCs by flow cytometry. There was no significant difference between the two treatment groups compared with the control PBS group, indicating that syn- and allo-rBMSCs did not elicit immune response. Our findings of allogeneic "immune privilege" of BMSCs in the rat model suggest that the animals may have been tolerized to ACI alloantigens by the rBMSC injection. No evidence of T cell priming or humoral antibody production to rBMSCs was found in recipient rats after treatment with allogeneic cells. Human (h)BMSCs were also injected IV into rats one day after MCAo.[16, 17] Effective functional improvement was found after hBMSC treatment in stroke rats. T lymphocytes are implicated as an initiator of graft-versus-host fatal iatrogenic disease. Graft-versus-host T cell response was measured using a 51Cr assay to determine the lytic effect.[16] We neither observe any indication of immunorejection nor any obvious increase in inflammatory response to hBMSCs. Additional support for the absence of rejection was obtained from evaluation of splenic cell proliferation and cytotoxic T lymphocyte (CTL) responses of exposed splenic cells. These data indicate that although hBMSCs are capable of inducing a primary proliferative response in the rat splenic lymphocytes, the administration of hBMSCs to the rats fails to sensitize lymphocytes in vivo for a secondary in vitro proliferative response. In addition, hBMSCs failed to induce a cytotoxic T lymphocyte response in the rat spleen cells.

Immune monitoring studies demonstrated that syn- and allo-rBMSC or hBMSC treatment after stroke in rats improved neurological recovery with no indication of T cell sensitization or antibody production in immunocompetent recipients. These findings are in agreement with previous reports showing that BMSCs do not stimulate divison of allogeneic T cells in vitro, probably due to active suppressive mechanisms.[51, 52] hBMSCs have been employed to treat patients with cancer,[53, 54] multiple sclerosis[55] and stroke.[56] Thus, safety data in humans are available. It is possible that, allogeneic cells, and not autologous cells may be used to treat patients.

4.3.2. Targeting BMSCs to Sites of Cerebral Damage

Where do the injected cells go, especially after the more clinically relevant IV injection? Damaged brain appears to attract BMSCs (Figure 4.1, BMSC Distribution), with the majority of these cells congregating in the perilesional areas,[13] and many cells present adjacent to or within vessels. Signals which target inflammatory cells to injured tissue likely direct BMSCs to injury sites. Using a microchemotaxis Boyden chamber, an in vitro assay, was performed for cell migration between an upper and a lower chambers separated by a permeable membrane.[57, 58] BMSCs are placed in the upper chamber. Chemotactic molecules MIP-1, MCP-1, IL-8, or adhesion molecules, such as ICAM-1, which attract inflammatory cells into brain tissue were placed into the lower chamber. A dose-dependent effect of chemotactic molecules on BMSC migration into the lower chamber was found. The enhanced migration was effectively blocked by placement of antibodies to these molecules into the lower chamber. This suggests, that BMSCs respond to chemotactic factors as do inflammatory cells. Instead of specific chemotactic or adhesion agents, brain tissue from injured and stroke brain placed in the lower chambers, also significantly increased BMSC migration.[57, 58] These data provide insight into how the cells assume an inflammatory-like cell identity, and how they "know" to target specifically injured tissue. Thus, any brain damage, which may have an inflammatory response, including neurodegenerative processes, such as multiple sclerosis, may guide BMSCs to the affected sites. The dependence of guidance on the degree of injury also provides a form of titration of "effective" dose of BMSCs. The more severe the injury and concomitant inflammatory response, the greater the numbers of BMSCs are recruited to the site.

4.3.3. Secretion of Trophic Factors and Brain Remodeling

Secretion by BMSCs of an array of cytokines and trophic factors from BMSCs may activate restorative mechanisms (Figure 4.1, Secretion of Growth and Trophic Factors, Mechanisms of Action – Interwoven Events). BMSCs behave as small molecular "factories". We and others have demonstrated that BMSCs induce significant increases in injured brain of various trophic and growth factors, such as HGF, NGF, BDNF, VEGF, basic fibroblast growth factor (bFGF), and insulin-like growth factor 1 (IGF-1), among many others in animals.[9, 27, 59] In addition, BMSCs secrete many of these factors in vitro.[60, 61] A very important observation is that BMSCs when cultured under different ionic microenvironments, e.g. calcium, respond to the cues of the ionic microenvironment by adjusting growth factor expression.[62] Thus, the degree of tissue injury and the corresponding disruption of the ionic environment may dictate the secretion levels of trophic factors. It is the dynamic effect of this variety of factors secreted by BMSCs and not the single bullet of a particular growth factor that facilitates the beneficial effect. Given the assumption that BMSCs selectively enter injured brain and secrete growth and trophic factors in a tissue feedback loop, the question remains how these factors possibly alter brain to promote therapeutic benefit? We speculate that the process that promotes restoration of function is not a single modification of tissue. Therapeutic benefit is induced by a set of events associated with brain plasticity. This includes but is not restricted to a reduction of apoptosis and glial scarring, and an increase in angiogenesis, synaptogenesis, gliogenesis, reconstruct glial-axonal architectures; and within the germinal SVZ and SGZ, an increase in neurogenesis followed by cell proliferation, migration and differentiation.

4.3.4. Apoptosis versus Cell Survival

Apoptosis is an ongoing process that persists for months after stroke[42, 43] or brain trauma. The peri-lesioned area is highly susceptible to apoptotic cell death.[42, 43] Cell death or survival is mediated by the production of growth factors, such as NGF within the injured brain.[63] The reduction of apoptosis within this region may sustain cerebral rewiring. We demonstrated that treatment of stroke with BMSCs significantly reduces apoptosis within the perilesioned area after MCAo in the rat.[7] Apoptosis is present in many cells in brain, including neurons, astrocytes, endothelial cells, after stroke.[43] Astrocytes are the most numerous cells in brain, and astrocytes are known to provide structural, trophic and metabolic support for neurons. Thus, astrocytes are critical for neural survival post-ischemia. In our in vitro studies,[64] we investigated the influence of BMSCs on rat astrocytic apoptosis and survival post-ischemia employing an anaerobic chamber. Our data indicate that BMSCs reduce apoptotic cell death, and increase the DNA proliferation rate in astrocytes post-ischemia. MEK/Erk and PI3K/Akt pathways are involved in cell survival. Western blot showed that BMSCs activate these two pathways in astrocytes post-ischemia, and upregulate total Erk 1/2 and Akt. BMSCs increase astrocyte survival via upregulation of PI3K/Akt and MEK/Erk pathways and stimulate astrocyte trophic factor gene expression after anaerobic insult. Since astrocytes produce various neurotrophic factors, we performed RT-PCR to investigate BMSC effect on astrocyte growth factor gene expression post-ischemia. We observed that BDNF, VEGF and bFGF gene expression was enhanced by BMSC coculture. These data suggest that BMSCs increase astrocytic survival post-ischemic injury, which may involve the activation of MEK/Erk and PI3K/Akt pathways and upregulation of BDNF, VEGF and bFGF.

4.3.5. Angiogenesis and Brain Repair

We tested the effect of BMSCs or supernatant from BMSCs on the induction of angiogenesis both in vitro[61] and in vivo.[65] Rats were subjected to MCAo and were injected IV with BMSCs at 24 hrs later. To examine cerebral microvessels, rats were injected IV with FITC-dextran 5 min before sacrifice. Vascular structure was measured in three dimensions using quantitative laser scanning confocal microscopy. VEGF and bFGF are potent angiogenic agents.[66, 67] Immunohistochemistry was used to identify BrdU and VEGF expression. The BMSC treatment group revealed a significant increase in total surface area of vessels in the ipsilateral hemisphere compared with PBS treated animals. Microvessels were enlarged and exhibited a significant increase in BrdU+ endothelial cells compared with PBS treated rats. BMSC treatment promoted VEGF expression in the ischemic boundary zone. In vitro, the secretion of VEGF by BMSCs was measured using ELISA. BMSC-conditioned medium was tested by measuring formation of capillary-like tubes from brain microvascular endothelial cells. BMSC supernatant significantly induced capillary-like tube formation compared with regular medium. BMSCs secrete and induce expression of VEGF in vitro and in vivo, respectively, and promote endothelial cell proliferation and angiogenesis after stroke. The classic vascular corneal assay was also employed as an additional in vivo assay.[68] A surgical incision forms a pocket in the cornea, into which a collagen wafer coated with BMSC supernatant is placed, or alternatively BMSCs are directly placed within the pocket.[69] Our data demonstrated rapid and robust corneal angiogenesis in the wafer loaded with BMSC supernatant. The induction of angiogenesis is more robust with the BMSC supernatant than with the direct use of VEGF, suggesting that the supernatant is a highly effective source of angiogenic factors. Although the induction of angiogenesis does not directly translate into promotion of function, we have previously demonstrated that treatment of stroke with VEGF one or more days after stroke significantly enhances functional recovery and enhances angiogenesis.[70, 71]

4.3.6. Synaptogenesis and Synaptic Modification

Though neurotrophins were initially characterized for their roles in promoting neuronal survival and differentiation, they also participate in many aspects of synapse function.[72] Growth factors, such as BDNF and NGF play an important role in synaptogenesis in the developing brain.[73] A current hypothesis proposed that plasticity, and therefore, learning new skills, is based on changes in synaptic function. Synapse formation and stabilization in the CNS is a dynamic process, requiring bi-directional communication between pre- and postsynaptic partners. It is necessary for mature neurons to sprout and establish new synaptic connections in the CNS during adult life because of changes in circuitry resulting from environmental changes or cell death[73]. Astrocytes and possibly oligodendrocytes, contribute to activity-dependent structural plasticity in the adult brain.[74] The powerful transport function of astrocytes helps terminate the postsynaptic action of neurotransmitters released presynaptically and the replenishment of the neurotransmitter pool. An alteration of these two processes could cause severe neuronal dysfunction and neuronal death. A significant increase of the synapse maker synaptophysin immunoreactivity was detected in rats subjected to MCAo with BMSC treatment compared with non-treated animals. The BMSC mediated increased synapse activity may enhance functional benefit of the treatment of CNS diseases with BMSCs. This effect is mediated directly by BMSC secretion of neurotrophins or indirectly through astrocyte-related microenvironment plasticity.

4.3.7. Gliogenesis and Glial-Axonal Remodeling

Communication between neurons and glia is essential for axonal conduction, synaptic transmission and information processing, and is required for normal functioning of the nervous system during development and throughout adult life.[75] There are two types of neuronal degeneration, anterograde and retrograde degeneration[76] with both types of degeneration affecting the synapse. Axonal sprouting is supported by astrocytes; however, it is inhibited under some conditions by the astrocytic scar.[77]

The white matter contains large amounts of the insulating material, myelin. After stroke, myelin repair is evident in the brain.[78] Microglia release compounds that affect the inflammatory and immune reactions of the CNS[79]. Investigation of glial-axonal remodeling after CNS damage may provide insight into restorative processes after stroke. Retired breeder rats were subjected to MCAo and injected IV with BMSCs at 7 days, and sacrificed at 4 months.[18] Concomitant with neurological benefit, BMSC treatment significantly decreased the thickness of the scar wall and reduced the numbers of microglia/macrophages within the scar wall. Double staining showed increased expression of an axonal marker (GAP-43), among reactive astrocytes in the scar boundary zone and in the SVZ in the treated rats. BrdU in cells preferentially colocalized with markers of astrocytes (GFAP) and oligodendrocytes (RIP) in the ipsilateral hemisphere, and gliogenesis was enhanced in the SVZ of the rats treated with BMSCs. BrdU in cells colocalized with NG-2 (oligodendrocyte precursors and/or new NG-2+ glia), and RIP (early oligodendrocyte differentiation), in the SVZ and in the striatum, corpus callosum, cingulum of the white matter. This study demonstrates that brain tissue repair is an ongoing chronic process with reactive glial-axonal remodeling.

4.3.8. Neurogenesis with Proliferation, Migration and Differentiation

The CNS can partially self-repair from injury.[80-83] A significant increase in new cell numbers identified by $BrdU^+$ and $Ki67^+$ immunoreactivity was measured in the SVZ after stroke.[84-87] Many of these cells expressed progenitor like molecular markers, such as nestin, TUJ-1, and NG2, indicative of the activation of adult cerebral tissue into a quasi-developmental state after brain injury.[3, 19] BMSCs amplify neurogenesis within the SVZ after MCAo. Our traumatic brain injury data confirm BMSC administration promotes endogenous cellular proliferation in rats. Newly generating cells were mainly present in the SVZ, SGZ, and boundary zone of contusion.[28] Induction of cell proliferation and differentiation by means of BMSCs may contribute to functional improvement after brain injury.

The presence of factors secreted from BMSCs appears to promote the rapid induction and migration of new cells from a primary source within the SVZ into the injured brain. For example, we tested the hypothesis that IV injection of BMSCs promotes bFGF secretion and SVZ cell migration in vitro and in vivo after stroke in rats subjected to 2 hrs MCAo and sacrificed at 14 days.[7] Immunohistochemistry staining of bFGF and doublecortin (DCX, a neuronal migration marker) was employed. To test whether BMSCs increase bFGF which promote neuronal migration, SVZ explants were extracted from rats 7 days after MCAo and cultured with supernatant of BMSCs or bFGF. The lengths of SVZ cell migration from the explant were measured in vitro. Morphological analyses revealed significant increases in the density of bFGF+ cells in the ischemic boundary zone in rats with BMSC treatment compared with control. In addition, treatment with BMSCs after stroke significantly increased DCX. In vitro, SVZ explant migration was significantly enhanced by BMSC supernatant and bFGF alone compared with normal control medium. The neutralizing antibody to bFGF significantly inhibited BMSC supernatant induced SVZ explant migration. Thus, bFGF plays an important role in neuronal migration induced by BMSC treatment after stroke. The migration of these new cells into the damaged cerebral tissue may be guided by astrocytic-like projections emanating from the SVZ,[18] resembling morphogenesis within the developing brain.

4.4. FROM BENCH TO BED

We seek to fully develop BMSC-based therapies in experimental models of CNS diseases in animals to prepare the groundwork for cell administration to the patient. As we look back at the discoveries made in the animals, one finding that stands out is that the transplanted BMSCs enhance functional recovery. Thus, the application of BMSC transplantation appears to be a strong candidate for cell-based neurorestorative therapy. The basic biologic profiles for BMSC transplantation remain to be demonstrated, and the dynamics of affected growth factor and corresponding receptors also need to be measured. The subsequent events induced by secretions of BMSCs require further investigation. Studies using transgenic animals are useful to tease out the role for specific growth factors. BMSCs have been employed for patients with cancer patients,[53, 54] multiple sclerosis[55] and stroke with autologous cells.[56] The basic and preclinical studies described in this review indicate that treatment of CNS diseases with BMSCs may provide a viable and highly effective restorative therapy. Thus, clinical studies to bring this therapeutic procedure to the patients are warranted.

4.5. CONCLUSIONS

We have demonstrated a remarkable improvement in functional outcome after stroke and various CNS disorders with the BMSC treatment. Mechanisms that enhance the recovery from neurological deficits have been widely studied at cellular and molecular levels. BMSC therapy can enhance the endogenous restorative mechanisms of the injured brain, assisting the tissue as it returns to a "developmental" state and supporting the process of angiogenesis, synaptogenesis, gliogenesis and neurogenesis, and the interwoven events, neural reorganization. It is anticipated that cellular therapy, in combination with standard rehabilitation therapy and neural retraining, can improve functional outcomes following CNS diseases.

4.6. REFERENCES

1. S. C. Cramer and M. Chopp, Recovery recapitulates ontogeny, *Trends Neurosci* 23(6), 265-271 (2000).
2. N. Duggal, R. Schmidt-Kastner and A. M. Hakim, Nestin expression in reactive astrocytes following focal cerebral ischemia in rats, *Brain Res* 768, 1-9 (1997).
3. Y. Li and M. Chopp, Temporal profile of nestin expression after focal cerebral ischemia in adult rat, *Brain Res* 838, 1-10 (1999).
4. R. P. Stroemer, T. A. Kent and C. E. Hulsebosch, Neocortical neural sprouting, synaptogenesis, and behavioral recovery after neocortical infarction in rats, *Stroke* 26(11), 2135-2144 (1995).
5. Y. Li, N. Jiang, C. Powers and M. Chopp, Neuronal damage and plasticity identified by microtubule-associated protein 2, growth-associated protein 43, and cyclin d1 immunoreactivity after focal cerebral ischemia in rats, *Stroke* 29(9), 1972-1980 (1998).
6. Z. Zhang and M. Chopp, Vascular endothelial growth factor and angiopoietins in focal cerebral ischemia, *Trends Cardiovasc Med* 12(2), 62-66 (2002).
7. J. Chen, Y. Li, M. Katakowski, X. Chen, L. Wang, D. Lu, M. Lu, S. C. Gautam and M. Chopp, Intravenous bone marrow stromal cell therapy reduces apoptosis and promotes endogenous cell proliferation after stroke in female rat, *J Neurosci Res* 73(6), 778-786 (2003).
8. R. Zhang, Z. Zhang, L. Wang, Y. Wang, A. Gousev, L. Zhang, K. L. Ho, C. Morshead and M. Chopp, Activated neural stem cells contribute to stroke-induced neurogenesis and neuroblast migration toward the infarct boundary in adult rats, *J Cereb Blood Flow Metab* 24(4), 441-448 (2004).

9. G. Kempermann, H. van Praag and F. H. Gage, Activity-dependent regulation of neuronal plasticity and self repair, *Prog Brain Res* 127, 35-48 (2000).
10. S. E. Haynesworth, M. A. Baber and A. I. Caplan, Cytokine expression by human marrow-derived mesenchymal progenitor cells in vitro: Effects of dexamethasone and il-1 alpha, *J Cell Physiol* 166(3), 585-592 (1996).
11. S. P. Dormady, O. Bashayan, R. Dougherty, X. M. Zhang and R. S. Basch, Immortalized multipotential mesenchymal cells and the hematopoietic microenvironment, *J Hematother Stem Cell Res* 10(1), 125-140 (2001).
12. J. Rohwedel, K. Guan, W. Zuschratter, S. Jin, G. Ahnert-Hilger, D. Furst, R. Fassler and A. M. Wobus, Loss of beta1 integrin function results in a retardation of myogenic, but an acceleration of neuronal, differentiation of embryonic stem cells in vitro, *Dev Biol* 201(2), 167-184 (1998).
13. J. Chen, Y. Li, L. Wang, Z. Zhang, D. Lu, M. Lu and M. Chopp, Therapeutic benefit of intravenous administration of bone marrow stromal cells after cerebral ischemia in rats, *Stroke* 32(4), 1005-1011 (2001).
14. J. Chen, Y. Li, L. Wang, M. Lu, X. Zhang and M. Chopp, Therapeutic benefit of intracerebral transplantation of bone marrow stromal cells after cerebral ischemia in rats, *J Neurol Sci* 189, 49-57 (2001).
15. Y. Li, J. Chen, L. Wang, M. Lu and M. Chopp, Treatment of stroke in rat with intracarotid administration of marrow stromal cells, *Neurology* 56(12), 1666-1672 (2001).
16. Y. Li, J. Chen, X. G. Chen, L. Wang, S. C. Gautam, Y. X. Xu, M. Katakowski, L. J. Zhang, M. Lu, N. Janakiraman and M. Chopp, Human marrow stromal cell therapy for stroke in rat: Neurotrophins and functional recovery, *Neurology* 59(4), 514-523 (2002).
17. J. Chen, Y. Li, R. Zhang, M. Katakowski, S. C. Gautam, Y. Xu, M. Lu, Z. Zhang and M. Chopp, Combination therapy of stroke in rats with a nitric oxide donor and human bone marrow stromal cells enhances angiogenesis and neurogenesis, *Brain Res* 1005, 21-28 (2004).
18. Y. Li, J. Chen, C. L. Zhang, L. Wang, D. Lu, M. Katakowski, Q. Gao, L. H. Shen, J. Zhang, M. Lu and M. Chopp, Gliosis and brain remodeling after treatment of stroke in rats with marrow stromal cells, *Glia* 49(3), 407-417 (2005).
19. Y. Li, J. Chen and M. Chopp, Adult bone marrow transplantation after stroke in adult rats, *Cell Transplant* 10(1), 31-40 (2001).
20. Y. Li, M. Chopp, J. Chen, L. Wang, S. C. Gautam, Y. X. Xu and Z. Zhang, Intrastriatal transplantation of bone marrow nonhematopoietic cells improves functional recovery after stroke in adult mice, *J Cereb Blood Flow Metab* 20(9), 1311-1319 (2000).
21. D. Lu, A. Mahmood, L. Wang, Y. Li, M. Lu and M. Chopp, Adult bone marrow stromal cells administered intravenously to rats after traumatic brain injury migrate into brain and improve neurological outcome, *Neuroreport* 12(3), 559-563 (2001).
22. D. Lu, Y. Li, L. Wang, J. Chen, A. Mahmood and M. Chopp, Intraarterial administration of marrow stromal cells in a rat model of traumatic brain injury, *J Neurotrauma* 18 (8), 813-819 (2001).
23. A. Mahmood, D. Lu, L. Yi, J. L. Chen and M. Chopp, Intracranial bone marrow transplantation after traumatic brain injury improving functional outcome in adult rats, *J Neurosurg* 94(4), 589-595 (2001).
24. A. Mahmood, D. Lu, L. Wang, Y. Li, M. Lu and M. Chopp, Treatment of traumatic brain injury in female rats with intravenous administration of bone marrow stromal cells, *Neurosurgery* 49(5), 1196-1203 (2001).
25. A. Mahmood, D. Lu, L. Wang and M. Chopp, Intracerebral transplantation of marrow stromal cells cultured with neurotrophic factors promotes functional recovery in adult rats subjected to traumatic brain injury, *J Neurotrauma* 19(12), 1609-1617 (2002).
26. A. Mahmood, D. Lu, M. Lu and M. Chopp, Treatment of traumatic brain injury in adult rats with intravenous administration of human bone marrow stromal cells, *Neurosurgery* 53(3), 697-702 (2003).
27. A. Mahmood, D. Lu and M. Chopp, Intravenous administration of marrow stromal cells (MSCs) increases the expression of growth factors in rat brain after traumatic brain injury, *J Neurotrauma* 21(1), 33-39 (2004).
28. ---, Marrow stromal cell transplantation after traumatic brain injury promotes cellular proliferation within the brain, *Neurosurgery* 55(5), 1185-1193 (2004).
29. D. Seyfried, J. Ding, Y. Han, Y. Li, J. Chen and M. Chopp, Intravenous administration of human bone marrow stromal cells improves recovery and reduces neural tissue loss after intracerebral hemorrhage in rats, *J Neurosurg* 104:1–6 (2006).
30. M. Chopp, X. H. Zhang, Y. Li, L. Wang, J. Chen, D. Lu, M. Lu and M. Rosenblum, Spinal cord injury in rat: Treatment with bone marrow stromal cell transplantation, *Neuroreport* 11(13), 3001-3005 (2000).
31. Y. Li, J. Chen, L. Wang, L. Zhang, M. Lu and M. Chopp, Intracerebral transplantation of bone marrow stromal cells in a 1- methyl-4-phenyl-1,2,3,6-tetrahydropyridine mouse model of parkinson's disease, *Neurosci Lett* 316(2), 67-70 (2001).

32. J. Zhang, Y. Li, J. Chen, Y. Cui, M. Lu, S. B. Elias, J. B. Mitchell, L. Hammill, P. Vanguri and M. Chopp, Human bone marrow stromal cell treatment improves neurological functional recovery in EAE mice, *Exp Neurol* (in press) (2005).
33. Z. Zhang, Q. Jiang, F. Jiang, G. Ding, R. Zhang, L. Wang, L. Zhang, A. M. Robin, M. Katakowski and M. Chopp, In vivo magnetic resonance imaging tracks adult neural progenitor cell targeting of brain tumor, *Neuroimage* 23(1), 281-287 (2004).
34. T. Schallert, M. Upchurch, N. Lobaugh, S. B. Farrar, W. W. Spirduso, P. Gilliam, D. Vaughn and R. E. Wilcox, Tactile extinction: Distinguishing between sensorimotor and motor asymmetries in rats with unilateral nigrostriatal damage, *Pharmacol Biochem Behav* 16(3), 455-462 (1982).
35. L. Zhang, T. Schallert, Z. G. Zhang, Q. Jiang, P. Arniego, Q. Li, M. Lu and M. Chopp, A test for detecting long-term sensorimotor dysfunction in the mouse after focal cerebral ischemia, *J Neurosci Methods* 117(2), 207-214 (2002).
36. J. Chen, C. Zhang, H. Jiang, Y. Li, L. Zhang, A. Robin, M. Katakowski, M. Lu and M. Chopp, Atorvastatin induction of vegf and bdnf promotes brain plasticity after stroke in mice, *J Cereb Blood Flow Metab* 25(2), 281-290 (2005).
37. D. Lu, A. Mahmood, A. Goussev, T. Schallert, C. Qu, Z. G. Zhang, Y. Li, M. Lu and M. Chopp, Atorvastatin reduction of intravascular thrombosis, increase in cerebral microvascular patency and integrity, and enhancement of spatial learning in rats subjected to traumatic brain injury, *J Neurosurg* 101(5), 813-821 (2004).
38. M. Lu, J. Chen, D. Lu, L. Yi, A. Mahmood and M. Chopp, Global test statistics for treatment effect of stroke and traumatic brain injury in rats with administration of bone marrow stromal cells, *J Neurosci Methods* 128, 183-190 (2003).
39. R. L. Zhang, M. Chopp, Z. G. Zhang, Q. Jiang and J. R. Ewing, A rat model of focal embolic cerebral ischemia, *Brain Res* 766, 83-92 (1997).
40. Z. Zhang, M. Chopp, R. L. Zhang and A. Goussev, A mouse model of embolic focal cerebral ischemia, *J Cereb Blood Flow Metab* 17(10), 1081-1088 (1997).
41. J. H. Garcia, Y. Yoshida, H. Chen, Y. Li, Z. G. Zhang, J. Lian, S. Chen and M. Chopp, Progression from ischemic injury to infarct following middle cerebral artery occlusion in the rat, *Am J Pathol* 142(2), 623-635 (1993).
42. Y. Li, V. G. Sharov, N. Jiang, C. Zaloga, H. N. Sabbah and M. Chopp, Ultrastructural and light microscopic evidence of apoptosis after middle cerebral artery occlusion in the rat, *Am J Pathol* 146(5), 1045-1051 (1995).
43. Y. Li, M. Chopp, N. Jiang, F. Yao and C. Zaloga, Temporal profile of in situ DNA fragmentation after transient middle cerebral artery occlusion in the rat, *J Cereb Blood Flow Metab* 15(3), 389-397 (1995).
44. Y. Li, M. Chopp, J. H. Garcia, Y. Yoshida, Z. G. Zhang and S. R. Levine, Distribution of the 72-kd heat-shock protein as a function of transient focal cerebral ischemia in rats, *Stroke* 23(9), 1292-1298 (1992).
45. Y. Li, M. Chopp, Z. G. Zhang, C. Zaloga, L. Niewenhuis and S. Gautam, P53-immunoreactive protein and p53 mrna expression after transient middle cerebral artery occlusion in rats, *Stroke* 25(4), 849-855 (1994).
46. Y. Li, M. Chopp, C. Powers and N. Jiang, Immunoreactivity of cyclin d1/cdk4 in neurons and oligodendrocytes after focal cerebral ischemia in rat, *J Cereb Blood Flow Metab* 17(8), 846-856 (1997).
47. R. L. Zhang, M. Chopp, Y. Li, C. Zaloga, N. Jiang, M. L. Jones, M. Miyasaka and P. A. Ward, Anti-icam-1 antibody reduces ischemic cell damage after transient middle cerebral artery occlusion in the rat, *Neurology* 44(9), 1747-1751 (1994).
48. Z. G. Zhang, M. Chopp, F. Bailey and T. Malinski, Nitric oxide changes in the rat brain after transient middle cerebral artery occlusion, *J Neurol Sci* 128(1), 22-27 (1995).
49. Z. G. Zhang, L. Zhang, Q. Jiang and M. Chopp, Bone marrow-derived endothelial progenitor cells participate in cerebral neovascularization after focal cerebral ischemia in the adult mouse, *Circ Res* 90(3), 284-288 (2002).
50. D. Lu, P. R. Sanberg, A. Mahmood, Y. Li, L. Wang, J. Sanchez-Ramos and M. Chopp, Intravenous administration of human umbilical cord blood reduces neurological deficit in the rat after traumatic brain injury, *Cell Transplant* 11(3), 275-281 (2002).
51. K. R. McIntosh, K. Beggs, R. Dodds, A. Lyubimov, A. Bartholomew, C. Cobbs, A. Smith and A. Moseley, High dose administration of allogeneic mesenchymal stem cells to immunocompetent baboons. *Supplement of the Bone Marrow Transplantation* 29, S38. (Abstract) (2002).
52. W. T. Tse, J. D. Pendleton, W. M. Beyer, M. C. Egalka and E. C. Guinan, Suppression of allogeneic t-cell proliferation by human marrow stromal cells: Implications in transplantation, *Transplantation* 75(3), 389-397 (2003).
53. O. N. Koc, S. L. Gerson, B. W. Cooper, S. M. Dyhouse, S. E. Haynesworth, A. I. Caplan and H. M. Lazarus, Rapid hematopoietic recovery after coinfusion of autologous-blood stem cells and culture-expanded marrow mesenchymal stem cells in advanced breast cancer patients receiving high-dose chemotherapy, *J Clin Oncol* 18(2), 307-316 (2000).

54. O. N. Koc and H. M. Lazarus, Mesenchymal stem cells: Heading into the clinic, *Bone Marrow Transplant* 27(3), 235-239 (2001).
55. P. Mandalfino, G. Rice, A. Smith, J. L. Klein, L. Rystedt and G. C. Ebers, Bone marrow transplantation in multiple sclerosis, *J Neurol* 247(9), 691-695 (2000).
56. O. Y. Bang, J. S. Lee, P. H. Lee and G. Lee, Autologous mesenchymal stem cell transplantation in stroke patients, *Ann Neurol* 57(6), 874-882 (2005).
57. L. Wang, Y. Li, J. Chen, S. C. Gautam, Z. Zhang, M. Lu and M. Chopp, Ischemic cerebral tissue and mcp-1 enhance rat bone marrow stromal cell migration in interface culture, *Exp Hematol* 30(7), 831-836 (2002).
58. L. Wang, Y. Li, X. Chen, J. Chen, S. C. Gautam, Y. Xu and M. Chopp, Mcp-1, mip-1, il-8 and ischemic cerebral tissue enhance human bone marrow stromal cell migration in interface culture, *Hematology* 7(2), 113-117 (2002).
59. J. Zhang, Y. Li, J. Chen, M. Yang, M. Katakowski, M. Lu and M. Chopp, Expression of insulin-like growth factor 1 and receptor in ischemic rats treated with human marrow stromal cells, *Brain Res* 1030(1), 19-27 (2004).
60. X. Chen, Y. Li, L. Wang, M. Katakowski, L. Zhang, J. Chen, Y. Xu, S. C. Gautam and M. Chopp, Ischemic rat brain extracts induce human marrow stromal cell growth factor production, *Neuropathology* 22(4), 275-279 (2002).
61. X. Chen, M. Katakowski, Y. Li, D. Lu, L. Wang, L. Zhang, J. Chen, Y. Xu, S. Gautam, A. Mahmood and M. Chopp, Human bone marrow stromal cell cultures conditioned by traumatic brain tissue extracts: Growth factor production, *J Neurosci Res* 69(5), 687-691 (2002).
62. X. G. Chen, Li Y, Wang L, Katakowski M, Zhang L.J, Chen J, Xu Y.X, Gautam S.C, Chopp M, Calcium promotes secretion of growth factors from human bone marrow stromal cells (hMSCs) and tube formation of human brain microvessel endothelial cells, *Stroke* 33(1), 401 (Abstract) (2002).
63. C. Guegan, B. Onteniente, Y. Makiura, M. Merad-Boudia, I. Ceballos-Picot and B. Sola, Reduction of cortical infarction and impairment of apoptosis in ngf- transgenic mice subjected to permanent focal ischemia, *Brain Res Mol Brain Res* 55(1), 133-140 (1998).
64. Q. Gao, Y. Li and M. Chopp, Bone marrow stromal cells increase astrocyte survival via upregulation of pi3k/akt and mek/erk pathways and stimulate astrocyte trophic factor gene expression after anaerobic insult., *Neuroscience*, (in press) (2005).
65. J. Chen, Z. G. Zhang, Y. Li, L. Wang, Y. X. Xu, S. C. Gautam, M. Lu, Z. Zhu and M. Chopp, Intravenous administration of human bone marrow stromal cells induces angiogenesis in the ischemic boundary zone after stroke in rats, *Circ Res* 92(6), 692-699 (2003).
66. Y. Tamada, C. Fukiage, D. L. Boyle, M. Azuma and T. R. Shearer, Involvement of cysteine proteases in bfgf-induced angiogenesis in guinea pig and rat cornea, *J Ocul Pharmacol Ther* 16(3), 271-283 (2000).
67. K. Hamano, T. S. Li, T. Kobayashi, S. Kobayashi, M. Matsuzaki and K. Esato, Angiogenesis induced by the implantation of self-bone marrow cells: A new material for therapeutic angiogenesis, *Cell Transplant* 9(3), 439-443 (2000).
68. G. A. Fournier, G. A. Lutty, S. Watt, A. Fenselau and A. Patz, A corneal micropocket assay for angiogenesis in the rat eye, *Invest Ophthalmol Vis Sci* 21(2), 351-354 (1981).
69. M. Chopp and Y. Li, Treatment of neural injury with marrow stromal cells, *Lancet Neurol* 1(2), 92-100 (2002).
70. Z. G. Zhang, L. Zhang, W. Tsang, H. Soltanian-Zadeh, D. Morris, R. Zhang, A. Goussev, C. Powers, T. Yeich and M. Chopp, Correlation of vegf and angiopoietin expression with disruption of blood-brain barrier and angiogenesis after focal cerebral ischemia, *J Cereb Blood Flow Metab* 22(4), 379-392 (2002).
71. Z. G. Zhang, W. Tsang, L. Zhang, C. Powers and M. Chopp, Up-regulation of neuropilin-1 in neovasculature after focal cerebral ischemia in the adult rat, *J Cereb Blood Flow Metab* 21(5), 541-549 (2001).
72. M. M. Poo, Neurotrophins as synaptic modulators, *Nat Rev Neurosci* 2(1), 24-32 (2001).
73. S. Cohen-Cory, The developing synapse: Construction and modulation of synaptic structures and circuits, *Science* 298(5594), 770-776 (2002).
74. D. T. Theodosis and D. A. Poulain, *Contribution of astrocytes to activity-dependent structural plasticity in the adult brain*, pp175-182 Kluwer Academic / Plenum Publishers, New York, (1999).
75. R. D. Fields and B. Stevens-Graham, New insights into neuron-glia communication, *Science* 298(5593), 556-562 (2002).
76. J. P. Kelly, *Principles of neural science*, Elsevier, Nw York, (1985).
77. R. J. McKeon, A. Hoke and J. Silver, Injury-induced proteoglycans inhibit the potential for laminin-mediated axon growth on astrocytic scars, *Exp Neurol* 136(1), 32-43 (1995).
78. J. Fok-Seang, N. A. DiProspero, S. Meiners, E. Muir and J. W. Fawcett, Cytokine-induced changes in the ability of astrocytes to support migration of oligodendrocyte precursors and axon growth, *Eur J Neurosci* 10(7), 2400-2415 (1998).

79. N. G. Gourmala, S. Limonta, D. Bochelen, A. Sauter and H. W. Boddeke, Localization of macrophage inflammatory protein: Macrophage inflammatory protein-1 expression in rat brain after peripheral administration of lipopolysaccharide and focal cerebral ischemia, *Neuroscience* 88(4), 1255-1266 (1999).
80. V. Darsalia, U. Heldmann, O. Lindvall and Z. Kokaia, Stroke-induced neurogenesis in aged brain, *Stroke* 36(8): 1790-1795 (2005).
81. R. J. Lichtenwalner and J. M. Parent, Adult neurogenesis and the ischemic forebrain, *J Cereb Blood Flow Metab* Advance online publication 15 June (2005).
82. P. M. Rossini and G. Dal Forno, Neuronal post-stroke plasticity in the adult, *Restor Neurol Neurosci* 22(3-5), 193-206 (2004).
83. S. B. Frost, S. Barbay, K. M. Friel, E. J. Plautz and R. J. Nudo, Reorganization of remote cortical regions after ischemic brain injury: A potential substrate for stroke recovery, *J Neurophysiol* 89(6), 3205-3214 (2003).
84. Y. Li, J. Chen and M. Chopp, Cell proliferation and differentiation from ependymal, subependymal and choroid plexus cells in response to stroke in rats, *J Neurol Sci* 193(2), 137-146 (2002).
85. R. L. Zhang, Z. G. Zhang, L. Zhang and M. Chopp, Proliferation and differentiation of progenitor cells in the cortex and the subventricular zone in the adult rat after focal cerebral ischemia, *Neuroscience* 105(1), 33-41 (2001).
86. R. L. Zhang, L. Zhang, Z. G. Zhang, D. Morris, Q. Jiang, L. Wang, L. J. Zhang and M. Chopp, Migration and differentiation of adult rat subventricular zone progenitor cells transplanted into the adult rat striatum, *Neuroscience* 116(2), 373-382 (2003).
87. R. Zhang, Z. Zhang, C. Zhang, L. Zhang, A. Robin, Y. Wang, M. Lu and M. Chopp, Stroke transiently increases subventricular zone cell division from asymmetric to symmetric and increases neuronal differentiation in the adult rat, *J Neurosci* 24(25), 5810-5815 (2004).

SECTION 2

SOLUBLE AND INSOLUBLE SIGNALS

5

CHONDROCYTE SIGNALING AND ARTIFICIAL MATRICES FOR ARTICULAR CARTILAGE ENGINEERING

Diana M. Yoon[1] and John P. Fisher[1,2]

5.1. INTRODUCTION

The proper functionality of healthy tissue requires maintenance. Even after tissue has undergone trauma, it attempts to repair itself. However, there are tissues within the body that are unable to completely regenerate when inflicted with severe stress, such as articular cartilage. The field of tissue engineering can alleviate this problem by providing cells, biological molecules and scaffolding materials to facilitate regeneration of healthy tissue. In order to achieve this task, fundamental mechanisms of cartilage tissue function needs to be understood. Cartilage is composed of components, such as cells, proteins and macromolecules, which all play a role in maintaining the well-being of the tissue. There has been considerable evidence that the interaction of chondrocytes with proteins and extracellular matrix play an important role in the homeostasis of cartilage. This is a continuously evolving area of study as biologists are intensely discovering new details of the cellular signaling pathways involved in the communication of chondrocytes. Recent studies have implicated that alterations in the signaling pathways of chondrocytes can lead to osteoarthritis, a degenerative condition of articular cartilage. We propose that the success of tissue engineers involves understanding the intricacy of chondrocytes signaling mechanisms in order to maintain their proper function while in contact with biomaterial scaffolds. To this end, we first discuss the basic biology of articular cartilage. Then we will explore the activation of signaling pathways that occur by chondrocytes due to the interaction with proteins (growth factors and cytokines) and extracellular matrix components (type II collagen, glycosaminoglycans and proteoglycans). Finally, we discuss the effects polymeric biomaterials may have on chondrocyte signaling.

---

[1] Department of Chemical and Biomolecular Engineering, University of Maryland, College Park, MD, USA
[2] Bioengineering Graduate Program, University of Maryland, College Park, MD, USA

Table 5.1: Abbreviations for Proteins Involved in Chondrocyte Signaling

ACTR	activin receptor
ALK	activin-like receptor
AP1	activating protein 1
BMP	bone morphogenic protein
c-met	hepatocyte growth factor receptor
COX2	cyclooxygenase-2
DAN	differential screening-selected gene aberrative in neuroblastoma
ECM	extracellular matrix
EGF	epithelial growth factor
ERK	extracellular signal-regulated kinase
FADD	fas-activated death domain protein
FAK	focal adhesion kinase
FGF	fibroblastic growth factor
FGFR	fibroblastic growth factor receptor
Flt-1	fms-like tyrosine kinase
GAG	glycosaminoglycan
Grb2	growth factor receptor-binding protein 2
IGF	insulin-like growth factor
IGF-1R	insulin-like growth factor-1 receptor
IGFBP	insulin-like growth factor binding protein
IKK	inhibitor of NF-κB kinase
IL	interleukin
IL-1ra	interleukin-1 receptor antagonist
IL-1RacP	interleukin-1 receptor associated protein
IL-R	interleukin receptor
IRAK	interleukin-1 receptor activate kinase
IRS	insulin receptor substrate
I-κB	inhibitor of kappa B
JNK	c-jun N-terminal protein kinase
KDR	kinase insert domain-containing receptor
MAPK	mitogen-activated protein kinase
MEK	mitogen-activated protein kinase kinase
MH2	mad homology 2
MMP	metallanoproteinases
MyD88	adaptor protein
NF-κB	nuclear transcription factor-kappa B
NIK	NF-κB-inducing kinase
NRP-1	neutropilin-1
PDGF	platelet-derived growth factor
PDK	phosphatidylinositol 3-kinase-dependent kinases
PGE_2	prostaglandin E_2
PI3K	phosphatidylinositol 3-kinase
PKC	protein kinase C
Ras	rat sarcoma guanine triphosphatase
SH2	src homology 2
Shc	src homology 2 domain containing transforming protein 1

SOS	son-of-sevenless
Sox9	sex-determining region Y-related gene
Src	sarcoma
STAT	signal transducer and activator of transcription
TACE	tumor necrosis factor-converting enzyme
TGF	transforming growth factor
TNF	tumor necrosis factor
TNF-R	tumor necrosis factor receptor
TRADD	tumor necrosis factor receptor-associated death domain protein
TRAF	tumor necrosis factor receptor-associated factor
VEGF	vascular endothelial growth factor

5.2. BIOLOGY OF ARTICULAR CARTILAGE

Articular cartilage is an avascular, alymphatic tissue that is predominately found on the surface of articulating joints[1,2]. Its function is to provide protection and enable articulation of subchondronal bone, allowing the joint to undergo compressive forces as well as smooth movement[3,4]. This functionality may be attributed to the zonal architectural composition of articular cartilage, which is composed of extracellular matrix (ECM) components and chondrocytes. (All proteins, and their abbreviations, involved in chondrocyte signaling are listed in Table 5.1.) There are four subsections of articular cartilage known as the superficial, middle, deep and calcified zones[1,4-6].

The main ECM components in articular cartilage are collagen, glycosaminoglycans (GAGs) and proteoglycans. Structural integrity of articular cartilage is sustained partially by the relationship of all the ECM components. The predominant collagen found in articular cartilage is type II collagen, which provides an interconnected network of support through the mobile restriction of GAGs and proteoglycans[2,4,6-8]. Articular cartilage has two main types of GAGs: chondroitin sulfate and keratin sulfate[2,9]. Proteoglycans are large protein core molecules that have numerous amounts of GAGs attached to it, comprising up to 95% of their composition[9]. Aggrecan and hyaluronic acid are the most prevalent proteoglycans in articular cartilage and are partially responsible for maintaining the integrity of articular cartilage under compressive forces[6,9,10]. Other smaller proteoglycans in articular cartilage include decorin, biglycan and perlecan[1,2,5,11]. Glycosaminoglycans and proteoglycans are both negatively charged, allowing for continuous hydration of the tissue[4]. Thus, the water content in articular cartilage can comprise about 75% of the total weight[2,4,12]. This high water content, as well as a lack of vascularization of articular cartilage necessitates diffusion the leading mechanism for nutrient and waste exchange between chondrocytes and the synovial fluid.

The extracellular matrix is the structural component of articular cartilage that provides a framework for cell viability and function. Chondrocytes, which are the primary cell in articular cartilage, comprise only 5% of cartilage volume[2,4,13]. They have a unique physical appearance in that they maintain a spherical morphology. Chondrocytes also provide the necessary homeostasis for healthy articular cartilage by communicating with both the ECM and soluble proteins within and surrounding the tissue[4]. These interactions are controlled by protein receptors, which are located within the plasma membrane of chondrocytes. Each receptor has specific affinity for their respective ligand, which is crucial to cellular signaling.

Like most tissue, articular cartilage can become diseased or damaged. One of the most common articular cartilage diseases is known as osteoarthritis. In this state, articular cartilage is more fibrous and contain higher levels of type I collagen and type X collagen versus type II collagen[8,12,14,15]. Additionally, the appearance of chondrocytes seems to be more fibroblastic in shape rather than spherical[14]. In order to repair osteoarthritic cartilage it is vital to understand how chondrocytes maintain the balance of growth factors necessary to create a healthy extracellular matrix. Finally, it is critical to understand how chondrocytes interact with the extracellular matrix itself.

5.3. BASIC PRINCIPLES OF CELLULAR SIGNALING

The functions of chondrocytes are stimulated during their attachment to the extracellular matrix or specifically when an extracellular signaling molecule binds to a receptor. These extracellular interactions start a cascade of steps that eventually leads to cellular effects of the cytoskeleton, gene expression and metabolism. A general outline of a signal cascade starts with an extracellular signal that attaches to a receptor protein within the plasma membrane of the cell[16-18]. Cell surface receptors are proteins located within the plasma membrane. Their basic structural makeup is an amino terminus, transmembrane domain and carboxyl tail. The attachment of extracellular signaling molecules to the amino terminus of the receptor results in the release or activation of intracellular signaling molecules by the cytoplasmic side of the receptor[19]. The intracellular signaling molecules then interact with target proteins to further relay its signal. There are multitudes of signaling pathways that can be activated to result in several different outcomes[20]. Furthermore, these pathways can be integrated with one another[16]. Additionally, there are a variety of regulatory proteins present in the extracellular matrix and cytoplasm of the cell.

5.4. NATIVE EFFECTORS ON CHONDROCYTE SIGNALING

5.4.1. Extracellular Matrix

The structural integrity and properties of articular cartilage is partially due to the extracellular matrix. Chondrocytes are responsible for maintaining compounds in the ECM, such as type II collagen and aggrecan. Conversely, chondrocytes need the ECM to function. This is mediated by integrin receptors within the cell membrane of chondrocytes that become activated when bound to the ECM[10,11,21-23]. Additionally, integrin signaling can affect growth factor and cytokine receptors[22,24].

Integrins are glycoproteins that contain α and β subunits that have an influence in signal transduction and cell shape[18,25,26]. The response of the integrin is controlled by both the extracellular and cytoplasmic domains. However, the β subunits interact with cytoskeletal proteins to activate various signaling cascades (Figure 5.1). Signaling through integrins depends on the formation of focal adhesions, where cytoskeletal and other proteins are concentrated at the surface of the plasma membrane. Aggregation of these focal adhesions activates the FAK and Shc pathways. Intracellular activation of FAK involves phosphorylation by the β subunit of the integrin. This activation allows FAK to attach to the Src homology 2 (SH2) domains of the Src proteins[22]. FAK has been found to affect the JNK, MAPK, p38 and PI3K pathways[22]. The activation of the Shc pathway is initiated by the phosphorylation of the Shc protein when in contact with an integrin attached to the extracellular matrix. This results in the recruitment of Grb2 and SOS proteins that eventually attach to a Ras protein, responsible for activating the MAPK pathway.

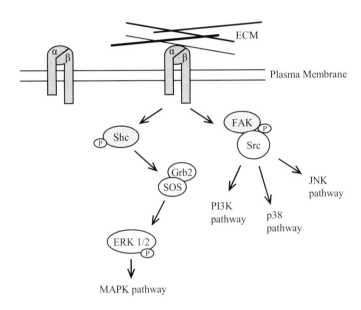

Figure 5.1. Integrin signaling pathway of chondrocytes. Integrins interact with ECM proteins to phosphorylate Shc and/or FAK proteins. These molecules lead to the activation of the MAPK, PI3K, p38 and/or JNK pathways.

The most predominant integrin expressed by chondrocytes is the α5β1, which is known to be a fibronectin receptor[24,25,27,28]. However, α5β1 has also been found to interact with type II collagen[27]. Other integrins that interact with type II collagen are α1β1, α2β1 and α10β1[24,28]. β1 integrins have a vital role in the relationship of chondrocytes to the ECM and have been identified in cartilage[11,23,28,29]. Chondrocyte attachment to type II collagen through integrins α1β1, α2β1 and α3β1 has recently been identified and is critical to chondrocyte survival[24,27,30]. Others have stated that α1 and β3 integrins are not expressed by chondrocytes and α2 expression is low in the presence of type II collagen[23]. Another well known integrin receptor is CD44, which interacts with hyaluronan and has been found to be highly expressed in cartilage[10,11]. The interaction of chondrocytes with fibronectin resulted in higher phosphorylation levels of FAK and ERK 1/2 protein compared to when the cells were in suspension[24]. When chondrocytes are in contact with insulin-like growth factor-1 protein and type II collagen, the production of the Shc, Grb2 and ERK 1/2 proteins increased[31]. However, the presence of these respective proteins was less apparent when chondrocytes were attached to type I collagen surfaces in the presence of IGF-1. These results indicate that there is an interactive merging of the integrin and growth factor signaling pathways.

5.5. SIGNALING MOLECULES OF CHONDROCYTES

An initiator for cellular signaling is an extracellular signaling molecule, allowing cells to communicate amongst one another. There are several different signaling transportation mechanisms: autocrine, paracrine and endocrine. A cell that releases signaling molecules that bind to receptors from the same cell is known as autocrine signaling. When a signal acts as a local mediator to neighboring cells it is referred to as paracrine signaling. Finally, endocrine signaling involves ligands being distributed throughout the body. Extracellular signaling molecules function is mediated by its binding to its receptor, which is located within the cell's plasma membrane. However, the extracellular signaling molecules are inhibited by antagonists, binding proteins that block the signaling protein's ability to bind a cell surface receptor. Most ligands have extracellular antagonists that can inhibit their function. A balance must exist between the signal concentration, antagonist concentration and their affinities for one another. Additionally, extracellular signaling molecules can become degraded by enzymes as well as immobilized within the ECM.

Chondrocytes synthesize and express various proteins referred to as growth factors, which affect their function. The two main types of growth factors are anabolic and catabolic. Anabolic growth factors enable chondrocytes to produce the necessary proteins to maintain its environment. Catabolic growth factors do the opposite in that they degrade molecules within the extracellular matrix. The interplay between these two types of growth factors is necessary in order to maintain homeostasis for articular cartilage through the initiation of appropriate signaling pathways.

5.5.1. Growth Factors

5.5.1.1. Insulin-Like Growth Factor-1

In articular cartilage, insulin-like growth factor-1 (IGF-1) is a dominant growth factor that leads to type II collagen, hyaluronan and aggrecan synthesis[2,14,32-35]. Additionally, IGF-2 has also been found to affect the proteoglycan synthesis[36]. Insulin-like growth factor is a protein that has similar homology to insulin[37]. More specifically, IGF-1 is a small soluble protein with a molecular weight of 7.5 kDa[38-40]. Normal versus reparative cartilage show a lower response to IGF[41]. In the extracellular part of chondrocytes, IGF-1 is bound to an antagonist that maintains its stability. There are 6 known IGF binding proteins (IGFBP) in cartilage, which can bind to extracellular matrix proteins[34,42,43]. The most predominant is IGFBP-3, which has a high affinity for IGF-1[39,40,43,44]. IGFBP-3 has been found in both normal and osteoarthritic cartilage[36,45]. However, its degradation is more apparent in cartilage that is damaged. It has been found that IGFBP-3 has a higher affinity for IGF-1 than its receptor, IGF-1R. These binding proteins regulate the availability of the IGF-1. In order for IGF-1 to bind to IGF-1R, the binding protein must undergo proteolytic cleavage[38,43]. IGF-1R is a heterodimeric protein, containing two α and two β subunits that are attached by disulfide bonds[37,39,40].

The binding of IGF-1 to the α subunits activates the β subunits to initiate several intracellular signaling pathways (Figure 5.2)[39,40]. The tyrosine kinases of insulin receptor substrates (IRS) can become activated as well as Shc proteins by phosphorylation. Insulin receptor substrates lead to the activation of PI3K and MAPK pathways by binding to

Grb2/SOS proteins. When the Ras attaches to a Raf protein this initiates the MEK 1/2 and then ERK 1/2 intracellular protein. Both IRS and Shc lead to the same pathway. Besides the MAPK pathway it can go through the JNK and p38 pathway. Conversely, IGF-1 has been observed not to activate JNK or p38 proteins[46]. For the PI3K pathway, the p85 and p110 subunits of PI3 kinase activate PDK1 and PDK2 to move and phosphorylate an Akt protein located within the membrane. Through the activation of the PI3K pathway by IGF-1, chondrocytes have been found to express type II collagen and proteoglycans[39,40]. Additionally, this has shown to inhibit nitric oxide production, which is stimulated through the p38, ERK1/2 and PKC pathways[39,40]. The inhibition of nitric oxide is implicated in the reduction of apoptosis.

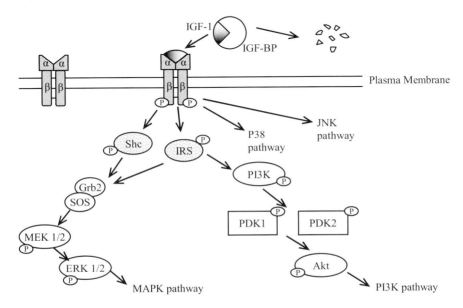

Figure 5.2. Signaling cascade of IGF-1. IGF-1 growth factors activate the β subunits of IGF-1R, which translocates proteins to the integrin to active the MAPK, PI3K, p38 and/or JNK pathway.

5.5.1.2. Transforming Growth Factor-β Superfamily

There are several ligands within the class of the transforming growth factor-β (TGF-β) superfamily. In chondrocytes, the two major types are TGF-β1 and bone morphogenic proteins (BMPs). Both of these ligands interact with two receptors, type I and type II, which are both required to transduce an intracellular signaling response[47]. When a ligand adheres to the dimeric type II receptor, it causes the formation of a heterotetrameric complex with the dimeric type I receptor. The activation of the type I receptor through phosphorylation of its serine/threonine kinase domains in the intracellular domain initiates the signaling cascade[48]. Since the type II receptor is constantly in an active state, the type I receptor recruits the specific proteins (Figure 5.3).

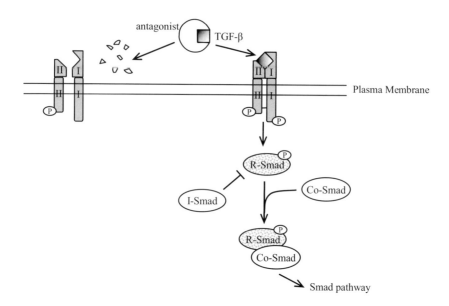

Figure 5.3. Scheme of the TGF-β superfamily activation pathway. Type I and II receptors integrate together after the adherence to TGF-β proteins. This results in the phosphorylation of R-Smads. I-Smads act as intracellular antagonists to regulate the Smad signaling pathway. Co-Smads aid in the translocation of R-Smads into the nucleus, which affects chondrocyte gene expression.

Most commonly in this pathway, the first intracellular proteins involved are Smad proteins. There are three types of Smad proteins, which are referred to as regulator Smads (R-Smads), common Smads (Co-Smads) and inhibitory Smads (I-Smads)[49-52]. All Smads except for I-Smads contain two important domains, an amino terminal (MH1) and carboxyl terminal (MH2), which have been found to be inactive when linked. I-Smads have been found not to contain MH1 domains. When R-Smads become phosphorylated by type II receptors, the interaction between MH1 and MH2 domains is terminated. This enables the MH2 domains of R-Smads to interact with Co-Smads, whose role is to aid in transporting this complex to the nucleus and affect gene transcription[47]. I-Smads regulate and inhibit the activation of R-Smads by adhering to type I receptors. In general I-Smads have a higher affinity for type I receptors than R-Smads, which dissociate after time[53,54]. Another regulation mechanism in the cytoplasm of chondrocytes is the proteolytic degradation of Smads. There is also competition between the TGF-β and BMP signaling pathway for R-Smads (e.g., Smad-4), since they share a common pathway[53,54].

5.5.1.2.a. Transforming Growth Factor- β1

Transforming growth factor-β1 (TGF-β1) is a protein that is part of the TGF-β superfamily that stimulates ECM synthesis[47,53-56]. TGF-β1 has been found to affect the production and prevent degradation of proteoglycans in cartilage. More specifically, TGF-β1 increases aggrecan mRNA expression[14,57]. A higher level of total proteoglycan synthesis was observed in the presence of type II collagen and TGF-β1[14,57]. The stability and activation of TGF-β1 is regulated by the extracellular matrix, with a strong affinity for proteoglycan decorin[10,58].

Three TGF-β isoforms, TGF-β1, TGF-β2 and TGF-β3, are present in cartilage. However, the most prominent form in chondrocytes is TGF-β1, which is a 100 kDa peptide that contains two subunits, active (25 kDa) and inactive (75 kDa)[15,59-61]. In order for TGF-β1 to bind to its receptor, TGF-βI (ALK5) or TGF-βII (ALK1), TGF-β1 must first remove the inactive peptide[48,49].

The specific Smad proteins that are part of the TGF-β1 pathway are Smad-2, -3, -4, -6 and -7[48,50]. The two R-Smad proteins are Smad-2 and -3. The Co-Smad protein is Smad-4. Finally, Smad-6 and -7 are considered I-Smads, which prevent complex formation of R-Smads to Co-Smads[48,49]. The amino terminal of Smad-7 has been found to affect the MH2 domain of R-Smads to inhibit TGF-β1 signaling[47]. The TGF-β1 signaling pathway includes Smad, ERK, JNK and p38 kinases as well as the JAK/STAT pathways[47,48,53,54]. In the MAP kinase pathway, ERK prevents the transport of R-Smads and their Co-Smads into the nucleus. This is true for both TGF-β1 and BMP[54].

It has been shown that tumor necrosis-α, a cytokine, prevents the activation of the TGF-β signaling through Smad-7, which can be produced by NF-κB[62]. Another cytokine, interleukin-1 has been found to increases the degradation of proteoglycans within articular cartilage. When TGF-β1 was introduced to cartilage, it was found to overwhelm the tissue and prevent the effects of interleukin-1[56]. This could be a result of Smad-7, which is responsible for inducing other signaling pathways, such as interleukin-1[54]. The expression of aggrecan has been found to occur when Smad-2 is phosphorylated by TGF-β. By expressing Smad-7 at high levels, it has been found to prevent the effects of TGF-β1 on the proteoglycan synthesis[55]. The intracellular signaling proteins Smad-2 and Smad-3 both became phosphorylated when human chondrocytes are stimulated by TGF-β1, type II collagen or both simultaneously[63]. This indicates a possible interaction of the integrin and TGF-β signaling pathways.

5.5.1.2.b. Bone Morphogenic Protein

Bone morphogenic proteins (BMP), also referred to as osteogenic proteins (OP), are part of the TGF-β superfamily. BMPs are dimeric proteins that are approximately 32-36 kDa. Several BMPs have been found to affect chondrocyte function, including BMP-2, -4, -6 and -7[12,51,64,65]. However, the most notable effects have been found with BMP-7[13]. Initially, BMPs are synthesized with an amino terminal region. The removal of this region allows BMPs to become activated. When BMPs bind to type I and type II receptors (e.g., BMPR-IA, BMPR-IB, ACTR-I, BMPRII, ACTRII and/or ACTR-IIB), the serine/threonine kinases become phosphorylated. Additionally, the interaction between type I and type II receptors lead to the initiation of R-Smads (Smad-1, -5 or -8)[50,51,55]. The Co-Smad (Smad-4) aids in the translocation of the R-Smads to the nucleus allowing for gene transcription to occur.

The BMP signaling pathway can be controlled both in the extracellular and intracellular part of the cell. A few extracellular antagonists for BMP are noggin, chordin, follistan and DAN[66]. BMP-2, -4 and -7 bind to noggin and chordin with a higher affinity than to BMP receptors[48,50,51,66,67]. DAN has been found to bind to BMP-2.[50] The interaction of BMPs to their binding proteins can be broken down by BMP-1, a metalloprotease[51,66]. Additionally, BMPs can adhere to extracellular matrix components such as collagen and heparin derivatives to prevent receptor activation[11,66]. Soluble inhibitory intracellular proteins are present in chondrocytes, commonly referred to as Smad-6 and -7. They both reside in the nucleus and travel into the cytoplasm after R-Smad activation. I-Smads adhere to the type I receptor and prevent the receptor interaction with the appropriate R-Smads. There are a few regulatory elements in the BMP Smad signaling pathway. For instance, Smad-6 can form a complex with Smad-1, therefore, preventing Smad-4 from binding.

Several BMPs have been found to affect chondrocyte production of type II collagen, such as BMP-2, -4, -6 and -7[12]. BMP-2 has been shown to promote the expression of type II collagen, aggrecan and not type X collagen[13,15]. However, it does cause matrix degradation as well as induce the formation of proteases[13,68]. BMP-7 was found to maintain type II collagen and produce extracellular matrix components[13,15,69-71]. In comparison to basal medium, chondrocytes incubated with BMP-7 showed an increase in proteoglycan synthesis, with 95% being chondroitin sulfate[71]. Additionally, when chondrocytes were induced with BMP-7 an increase in the expression of the intracellular protein FAK, as well as other focal adhesion proteins, occurred[70]. In the presence of interleukin-1, BMP-7 allowed chondrocytes to maintain and continue synthesizing proteoglycans[15].

5.5.1.3. Platelet-Derived Growth Factor

Platelet-derived growth factor (PDGF) is a 30 kDa glycoprotein found at platelet migration sites, such as injured tissue[12]. PDGF is a disulfide-linked heterodimer with four types of isoforms (PDGF-A, -B, -C and –D)[72]. There are two receptors for PDGF (-α, -β), which are both tyrosine kinase enzymes. Individually, the two receptors have specificity for the different PDGF isoforms. PDGF-α and PDGF-β can also bind together, which results in an increase in enzymatic activity compared to when they are alone[72,73]. The MAPK, PI3K and PKC signaling pathways have been found to become activated by PDGF in various cell lines[72]. PDGF has been shown to be produced locally in cartilage by chondrocytes[12,15,73]. PDGF can induce proteoglycan synthesis and aggrecan without inducing chondrocyte proliferation[15,74,75]. By inducing chondrocytes with PDGF, an increase in interleukin-1 receptor gene expression was observed[75]. When PDGF and interleukin-1 were incubated together, there was noticeably more proteoglycan and aggrecan degradation. This also correlated with an increase in mRNA of proteases, such as metalloproteinases. However, the extracellular matrix was maintained with PDGF and interleukin-1 combined compared to just interleukin-1 alone.

5.5.1.4. Fibroblastic Growth Factor

Fibroblast growth factor (FGF) is a polypeptide that is 14-16 kDa in molecular weight that binds to heparin proteoglycans, present in articular cartilage[11,12]. It is known to be in a basic and acidic form. FGF regulation of chondrocyte function is important to articular cartilage homeostasis by aiding in the synthesis and degradation of proteoglycans and type II collagen[76]. FGF determines its functionality as either an anabolic or catabolic growth factor by its concentration within articular cartilage. The interaction of FGF with chondrocytes and its effect on the signaling pathway is still trying to be understood. It has been found that FGF-18, a specific type of fibroblastic growth factor, attaches to the FGF receptor-3 (FGFR-3). The activation of the FGFR-3 increased the gene expression of α1 integrin, which has been found to adhere to type II collagen. Additionally, when FGF and interleukin-1 are exogenously added to chondrocytes, the expression of the interleukin-1 receptor increases, leading to an increase in matrix degradation attributed to interleukin-1[77].

5.5.1.5. Epithelial Growth Factor, Vascular Endothelial Growth Factor, Hepatocyte Growth Factor

Endothelial growth factor (EGF) is a very small protein, approximately 1.6 kDa[12]. It has been found to degenerate articular cartilage by breaking down proteoglycans. The expression of type II collagen and aggrecan decreases in the presence of EGF[12,78]. Some inflammatory responses that occur due to EGF have been a higher expression of cyclooxygenase-2 (COX2) and production of prostaglandin E_2 (PGE$_2$)[79]. EGF has been found to activate the ERK 1/2 pathway but not effect Sox9, which aids in the transcription of type II collagen and aggrecan[78]. However, a correlation between EGF and these inflammatory proteins can be seen by the activation of two pathways, primarily the ERK 1/2 and p38 kinase pathway[79].

Vascular endothelial growth factor (VEGF) is a 23-kDa protein, commonly associated with angiogenic activity[12,80]. Several different isoforms of VEGF (VEGF$_{121}$, VEGF$_{165}$ and VEGR$_{189}$) that have been found in normal and osteoarthritic cartilage[80,81]. These VEGF proteins adhere to two different types of receptors, VEGF-R1 (Flt-1) and VEGF-RII (KDR). Additionally, the co-receptor neutropilin-1 (NRP-1) increases the ability of VEGF to bind to VEGF-R[80,82]. This co-receptor is activated in osteoarthritic cartilage at higher amounts compared to healthy cartilage[80]. VEGF has been found to adhere to heparin and heparin-sulfate proteoglycans. Additionally, the adhesion of VEGF to the ECM can loosen the binding of basic FGF[82]. VEGF receptor gene expression is present in osteoarthritic cartilage with an increase in metalloproteinases (MMP) synthesis, specifically MMP1 and MMP3[80]. When chondrocytes are induced with interleukin-1β, VEGF protein synthesis decreases. However, VEGF production increases when chondrocytes are incubated with both interleukin-1β and TGF-β[83].

Hepatocyte growth factor (HGF) is a heterodimeric glycoprotein with an α and β subunit with molecular weights of 69 and 32 kDa, respectively[84]. It has been found to bind collagen, chondroitin sulfate and hyaluronic acid. When chondrocytes are introduced to HGF, there is an increase in proteoglycan synthesis compared to basal levels. HGF attaches to a transmembrane receptor, *c-met*, which is a tyrosine kinase. The mRNA for HGF and *c-met* have both been observed in normal and arthritic cartilage. However, HGF protein and *c-met* have are present at higher levels in damaged cartilage[15,84]. This correlates to other data, indicating that HGF expression increased in the presence of interleukin-1[15].

5.5.2. Catabolic Growth Factors/Cytokines

5.5.2.1. Interleukin-1

Interleukins (ILs) are cytokines present in articular cartilage that have been associated with degenerative cartilage. There are many different forms of interleukins (IL-1, -4, -6, -8, -10, -11,-17 and -18)[12,46,85]. IL-1β has been found to strongly associate with damaged cartilage, increasing the expression of MMPs and decreasing the expression of ECM components, such as type II collagen and aggrecan[12,21,70,84,86-88]. IL-1β is synthesized with two components to maintain it at an inactive state at a molecular weight of 31 kDa[46]. An enzyme breaks down the IL-1β protein into a smaller active 17-kDa fragment[21,46].

There are two antagonists that control the extracellular IL-1s (Figure 5.4). The interleukin-1 receptor I (IL-1RI) can attach to IL-1ra to inhibit signal transduction. Additionally, interleukin-1 receptor II (IL-1RII) binds to IL-1β[21,35]. When IL-1β attaches to IL-1RI, an intracellular protein is recruited and becomes attached to the receptor. This protein is known as the IL-1 associating protein (IL-1RAcP). This enables an adaptor protein, MyD88, to procure kinases IRAK-1 and -2 to activate further intracellular proteins. IRAK-1 and -2 stimulate the response of the NF-κB inducing kinase (NIK) to activate the IKKαβ complex, which finally induces the NF-κB protein to effect gene transcription. Other signaling pathways that can become activated by IL-1 are the MAPK and PI3K pathway[21,46,89]. It has been found that IL-1 activates the expression of MMPs through JNK and p38 kinases[46]. Other interleukins, such as IL-6, activate the JAK/STAT pathway[89,90]. IL-6 as well as IL-1 negatively affects the mRNA and protein amounts of Sox9, a protein that has been attributed to enable the gene expression of type II collagen and aggrecan[21,78,90].

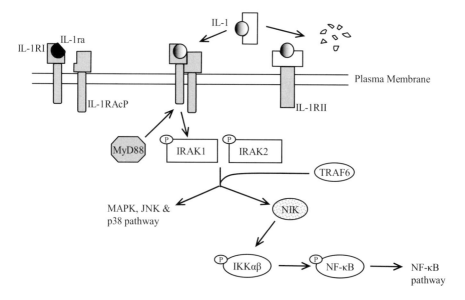

Figure 5.4. The transduction of the IL-1 pathway by chondrocytes. IL-1 can be bound to the IL-1RII antagonist, which is present within the plasma membrane and in soluble form. Additionally, IL-1ra prevents IL-1 from adhering to its respective receptor, IL-1RI. The activation of IL-1RI results in either the activation of MAPK, JNK, p38 and/or NF-κB pathways.

In order for ILs to have an effect on gene expression by chondrocytes, they adhere to their respective receptors (IL-1R). Low levels of ILs are maintained in healthy cartilage. Additionally, this lessens the extent of MMP production as well as its gene expression[46]. However, in the presence of TGF-β, osteoarthritic cartilage was found to increase the expression of IL-6[46,85]. Additionally, IL-1β was found to increase the expression of TGF-β. When chondrocytes are incubated with exogenous IGF-1, there is an upregulation of IL-1RII[35].

Other forms of IL have shown to effect chondrocytes function. In the presence of IL-17 and IL-18, chondrocytes induce the expression and synthesis of several MMPs as well as produce nitric oxide, which causes apoptosis[21,46,91]. Therefore, this decreases the normal level of proteoglycan synthesis. In arthritic cartilage, the mRNA of IL-6 and -8 has been found to be present more often compared to healthy cartilage[46,86]. The mRNA of several ILs show a trend of higher expression in damaged versus healthy cartilage, such as IL-6, IL-8 and IL-18[86]. Chondrocytes expression of IL-18 increases in the presence of IL-1β. When IL-1β and IL-18 are incubated with chondrocytes together, the results indicate that nitric oxide is produced concurrently with a decrease in proteoglycan synthesis[92].

5.5.2.2. Tumor Necrosis Factor-α

Tumor necrosis factor-α (TNF-α) is another cytokine that acts similarly to ILs on chondrocytes[93]. TNF-α has been found to increase gene expression of MMPs and decrease the expression of extracellular matrix components[12,78,93]. TNF-α gene expression and their respective receptors are more present in damaged cartilage compared to normal cartilage[86,94]. It has an initial molecular weight of 51 kDa and reduces down to 17 kDa[12,95]. It is synthesized as a membrane bound protein, but after it is cleaved off the membrane by a metalloproteinase known as TACE, it becomes activated and can adhere to its appropriate receptor, TNF-R1 or TNF-R2[94-96]. This enables the receptors to attach to either two cytoplasmic proteins, TRAF2/5 and FADD, through an adaptor protein, TRADD (TNF-R1 associated death domain protein)[95,96]. The TRAF protein activates two main signaling pathways, MAPK and NF-κB. The MAPK signaling pathway includes transcriptional factors such as AP1[96]. It has been recently discovered that chondrocytes activate the MEK pathways with minimal detection of the p38 and JNK pathways[93,97]. The activation of the NF-κB transcriptional protein is initiated by the TRAF protein. NF-κB can be further controlled by I-κB proteins through the IKK complex, which is also recruited by TRAF proteins[95,96]. Through the activation of the NF-κB signaling pathway, TNF-α, similar to IL-1β, affects type II collagen expression[78,93].

Chondrocytes incubated with exogenous TNF-α resulted in the expression of IL-6[85]. The synthesis of IGFBPs by chondrocytes was shown to be greater in the presence of TNF-α, which could limit the availability of IGF-1[98]. Other studies have shown that chondrocytes induced with EGF and TNF-α affects the mRNA of type II collagen and aggrecan more significantly compared to their individual effects[78,93].

5.6. TISSUE ENGINEERING APPROACHES TO REGULATE SIGNALING

The interactions of environmental cues and chondrocytes have been proven to be important in determining cell function. In the field of tissue engineering, it is vital to fully understand these underlying principles to create an appropriate biomaterial scaffold that can integrate and eventually heal the tissue. Therefore, many researchers have looked into biomaterials. Both natural and synthetic polymers have been utilized to aid in chondrocyte encapsulation. Natural polymers are typically polysaccharides or polypeptide chains isolated from natural plants or organisms. While synthetic polymers are fabricated and their properties can be altered more readily compared to natural polymers. These polymers can be shaped into various three dimensional forms, such as meshes, foams and gels. However, a common form that mimics the articular cartilage environment is a hydrogel. The primary reason for interest in hydrogels as artificial matrices for chondrocytes is that they are water-laden polymer networks that have the ability to retain up to 99% water volume[99-101]. This attribute enables the encapsulation of chondrocytes as well as proteins within the bulk of the network. Hydrogels have been shown to maintain the spherical morphology and gene expression of chondrocytes[102].

Alginate is common natural polymer that has been used to encapsulate chondrocytes. A unique property of alginate is that there is limited cellular adhesion due to the lack of cellular recognition proteins. It has been found that chondrocytes encapsulated in alginate are able to express their phenotypic type II collagen expression[103-105]. Adult human chondrocytes were found to express aggrecan, metalloproteinases-3 and -8 for as long as eight months after their encapsulation in alginate beads[106]. The expression of BMP-2 was also apparent for chondrocytes in alginate[105]. A recent study has shown that when chondrocytes in alginate were incubated with exogenous IGF-1, there was an activation of both the PI3K and MAPK pathway, as demonstrated by phosphorylation of the Akt and ERK proteins respectively[107]. Inhibitors of Akt promoted a decrease in proteoglycan synthesis at a greater extent than compared to MEK inhibitors. Thus, indicating the importance in the PI3K pathway with production of extracellular matrix components. The effects of catabolic growth factor, IL-1β activated ERK, p38 and JNK proteins, but not Akt proteins[107].

Arginine-glycine-aspartic acid (RGD) sequences, which are commonly found in the ECM, have been covalently bound to alginate, forming a natural and synthetic hybrid. These constructs have allowed chondrocytes to express type II collagen at a far greater extent than when cultured in unmodified alginate[104]. Alternatively, cyclic RGD incubated with chondrocytes inside alginate decreased proteoglycan synthesis[23]. This work indicates that chondrocyte adhesion is critical to extracellular matrix production. Alginate gels that were embedded with fibrin gels allowed chondrocyte production of type II collagen and proteoglycans, such as aggrecan[108,109]. Alginate and type II collagen constructs promoted an increase in chondroitin-6 sulfate production by chondrocyte[110]. When stimulated with TGF-β1, an increase in keratin sulfate synthesis by chondrocytes was observed but also a decrease in the expression of chondroitin-6-sulfate was noted[57,110]. The expression of type II collagen of chondrocytes within alginate beads was negatively effected by IL-1 while TGF-β1 and BMP-2 individually showed an enhancement[13,105,106]. BMP-2 also showed an greater aggrecan expression of chondrocytes in alginate[105]. When cultured in alginate, BMP-7 was found to effect the synthesis of type II collagen and proteoglycans greater than with just serum[111].

In terms of integrin expression, chondrocytes encapsulated in type II collagen and alginate were found to express $\alpha 5\beta 1$[23]. When these chondrocytes were incubated with an antibody that attached to β1 integrins with exogenous TGF-β1 there was a significant decrease in proteoglycan synthesis[23]. However, there was no effect when β1 integrins were blocked without TGF-β1. This indicates that there is a possible interaction of TGF-β1 to integrin signaling activation. Further studies also show the effects of integrin signaling on chondrocytes. When fibronectin beads are in contact with chondrocytes, the activation of the α5β1 integrin occurs[112]. This resulted in the phosphorylation of focal adhesion kinases, indicating the role of integrin signaling. A higher level of proteoglycan synthesis is observed when FGF and IGF-1 are incubated with chondrocytes and fibronectin beads, further suggesting that integrin activation can be enhanced or aided by growth factors.

Hyaluronic acid is a component in the extracellular matrix and therefore has been of interest for tissue engineers to encapsulate chondrocytes. For instance, TGF-β mRNA expression increased when chondrocytes adhered to hyaluronic acid through the CD44 integrin[10]. A modification of hyaluronic acid has been made with benzyl alcohol. In these constructs, chondrocytes expression of type II collagen and Sox9 increased while maintaining their low level of type I collagen expression and high level of aggrecan[113]. Hyaluronic acid has also been incorporated with other types of polymers, including alginate. Chondrocytes are able to produce type II collagen and proteoglycans in both alginate beads and sponges that contain hyaluronic acid. Investigations additionally indicated that the ECM protein levels were stabilized in the alginate beads versus alginate sponge structures[114].

Synthetic scaffolds have also been researched in determining the effect of chondrocyte signaling. On poly(glycolic acid) meshes, it was found that chondrocytes produce type II collagen[8]. Further studies have been done with chondrocytes on a poly(glycolic acid) scaffold with incorporation of various growth factors[33]. IGF-1 increased the GAG fraction compared to constructs with low protein supplemented media. TGF-β resulted in high type II collagen expression. IL-4 prevented a decrease in GAG compared to other growth factors and PDGF was found to decrease GAG concentration. Chondrocytes were encapsulated in photopolymerized poly(ethylene oxide) hydrogels with TGF-β1 and IGF-1 growth factors within poly(lactic-glycolic) acid microspheres[115]. There was an increase in the glycosaminoglycans concentrations with IGF-1 individually and with a combination of IGF-1 and TGF-β1. Poly(ethylene glycol) has also been co-polymerized with various other synthetic polymers. A poly(propylene fumarate-co-ethylene glycol) was shown to maintain the viability of chondrocytes encapsulated within this construct[116]. Proteoglycan synthesis occurred in these constructs, but was found to be lower when compared to alginate and agarose hydrogels by producing 25% of type II collagen. Recently, different armed-poly(ethylene glycol) polymers have been altered with MMP sensitive peptides[117]. This polymeric construct encapsulated chondrocytes and showed that the mRNA expression for type II collagen and aggrecan was the highest for poly(ethylene glycol) polymers that contained the MMP sensitive peptides versus without the peptides. Additionally, in these scaffolds, the expression of MMP-13 was the lowest compared to the scaffolds without MMP sensitive peptides.

The effect of biomaterials on chondrocyte function is vital for creating a proper scaffolding environment to recreate articular cartilage. It is important to investigate the effect of biomaterial properties on controlling molecular signaling of chondrocytes and therefore chondrocyte function. We propose that fully understanding the interactions of chondrocytes amongst the extracellular matrix proteins and the cells to one another will enhance our ability to engineer a viable construct for articular cartilage.

5.7. SUMMARY

Chondrocytes depend on their environment to aid in their expression of appropriate proteins. It has been found that the interaction of integrin receptors with chondrocytes effects the production of extracellular molecules such as type II collagen and aggrecan.

Additionally, the presence of growth factors such as IGF-1, TGF-β1 and BMP-7 induce various signaling pathways that also aid in transducing phenotypic expressions by chondrocytes. Natural and synthetic polymers have been used to act as a scaffold for chondrocytes. The production of extracellular matrix proteins by chondrocytes has been studied. As tissue engineers, it is advantageous to explore the possibility of how altering biomaterial properties affect the signaling cascades by activation of receptors and transduction through the cytoplasm. This vital information will be able to aid in the future of engineering an appropriate biomaterial that can incorporate chondrocytes to act as a scaffold for articular cartilage.

5.8. ACKNOWLEDGMENTS

This work was supported by the National Science Foundation (0448684), Minta Martin Foundation, and University of Maryland, College Park.

5.9. REFERENCES

1. Poole, A.R. et al. Composition and structure of articular cartilage: a template for tissue repair. *Clin Orthop Relat Res*, S26-33 (2001).
2. Ulrich-Vinther, M., Maloney, M.D., Schwarz, E.M., Rosier, R. & O'Keefe, R.J. Articular cartilage biology. *J Am Acad Orthop Surg* **11**, 421-30 (2003).
3. Randolph, M.A., Anseth, K. & Yaremchuk, M.J. Tissue engineering of cartilage. *Clin Plast Surg* **30**, 519-37 (2003).
4. Newman, A.P. Articular cartilage repair. *Am J Sports Med* **26**, 309-24 (1998).
5. Almarza, A.J. & Athanasiou, K.A. Design characteristics for the tissue engineering of cartilaginous tissues. *Ann Biomed Eng* **32**, 2-17 (2004).
6. Woodfield, T.B., Bezemer, J.M., Pieper, J.S., van Blitterswijk, C.A. & Riesle, J. Scaffolds for tissue engineering of cartilage. *Crit Rev Eukaryot Gene Expr* **12**, 209-36 (2002).
7. Goessler, U.R., Hormann, K. & Riedel, F. Tissue engineering with chondrocytes and function of the extracellular matrix (Review). *Int J Mol Med* **13**, 505-13 (2004).
8. Riesle, J., Hollander, A.P., Langer, R., Freed, L.E. & Vunjak-Novakovic, G. Collagen in tissue-engineered cartilage: types, structure, and crosslinks. *J Cell Biochem* **71**, 313-27 (1998).
9. Temenoff, J.S. & Mikos, A.G. Review: tissue engineering for regeneration of articular cartilage. *Biomaterials* **21**, 431-40 (2000).
10. Ishida, O., Tanaka, Y., Morimoto, I., Takigawa, M. & Eto, S. Chondrocytes are regulated by cellular adhesion through CD44 and hyaluronic acid pathway. *J Bone Miner Res* **12**, 1657-63 (1997).
11. van der Kraan, P.M., Buma, P., van Kuppevelt, T. & van den Berg, W.B. Interaction of chondrocytes, extracellular matrix and growth factors: relevance for articular cartilage tissue engineering. *Osteoarthritis Cartilage* **10**, 631-7 (2002).
12. Holland, T.A. & Mikos, A.G. Advances in drug delivery for articular cartilage. *J Control Release* **86**, 1-14 (2003).
13. Chubinskaya, S. & Kuettner, K.E. Regulation of osteogenic proteins by chondrocytes. *Int J Biochem Cell Biol* **35**, 1323-40 (2003).
14. Darling, E.M. & Athanasiou, K.A. Growth factor impact on articular cartilage subpopulations. *Cell Tissue Res*, 1-11 (2005).
15. Hickey, D.G., Frenkel, S.R. & Di Cesare, P.E. Clinical applications of growth factors for articular cartilage repair. *Am J Orthop* **32**, 70-6 (2003).
16. Hunter, T. Signaling--2000 and beyond. *Cell* **100**, 113-27 (2000).
17. Martin, G.S. Cell signaling and cancer. *Cancer Cell* **4**, 167-74 (2003).
18. Dhanasekaran, N. Cell signaling: an overview. *Oncogene* **17**, 1329-30 (1998).
19. Brumley, L.M. & Marchase, R.B. Receptor synthesis and routing to the plasma membrane. *Am J Med Sci* **302**, 238-43 (1991).

20. Geiger, B., Bershadsky, A., Pankov, R. & Yamada, K.M. Transmembrane crosstalk between the extracellular matrix--cytoskeleton crosstalk. *Nat Rev Mol Cell Biol* **2**, 793-805 (2001).
21. Lotz, M. Cytokines in cartilage injury and repair. *Clin Orthop Relat Res*, S108-15 (2001).
22. Hering, T.M. Regulation of chondrocyte gene expression. *Front Biosci* **4**, D743-61 (1999).
23. Lee, J.W., Qi, W.N. & Scully, S.P. The involvement of beta1 integrin in the modulation by collagen of chondrocyte-response to transforming growth factor-beta1. *J Orthop Res* **20**, 66-75 (2002).
24. Loeser, R.F. Integrins and cell signaling in chondrocytes. *Biorheology* **39**, 119-24 (2002).
25. Loeser, R.F., Carlson, C.S. & McGee, M.P. Expression of beta 1 integrins by cultured articular chondrocytes and in osteoarthritic cartilage. *Exp Cell Res* **217**, 248-57 (1995).
26. Glowacki, J., Trepman, E. & Folkman, J. Cell shape and phenotypic expression in chondrocytes. *Proc Soc Exp Biol Med* **172**, 93-8 (1983).
27. Salter, D.M., Hughes, D.E., Simpson, R. & Gardner, D.L. Integrin expression by human articular chondrocytes. *Br J Rheumatol* **31**, 231-4 (1992).
28. Enomoto, M., Leboy, P.S., Menko, A.S. & Boettiger, D. Beta 1 integrins mediate chondrocyte interaction with type I collagen, type II collagen, and fibronectin. *Exp Cell Res* **205**, 276-85 (1993).
29. Kurtis, M.S. et al. Mechanisms of chondrocyte adhesion to cartilage: role of beta1-integrins, CD44, and annexin V. *J Orthop Res* **19**, 1122-30 (2001).
30. Cao, L. et al. beta-Integrin-collagen interaction reduces chondrocyte apoptosis. *Matrix Biol* **18**, 343-55 (1999).
31. Shakibaei, M., John, T., De Souza, P., Rahmanzadeh, R. & Merker, H.J. Signal transduction by beta1 integrin receptors in human chondrocytes in vitro: collaboration with the insulin-like growth factor-I receptor. *Biochem J* **342 Pt 3**, 615-23 (1999).
32. Curtis, A.J., Ng, C.K., Handley, C.J. & Robinson, H.C. Effect of insulin-like growth factor-I on the synthesis and distribution of link protein and hyaluronan in explant cultures of articular cartilage. *Biochim Biophys Acta* **1135**, 309-17 (1992).
33. Blunk, T. et al. Differential effects of growth factors on tissue-engineered cartilage. *Tissue Eng* **8**, 73-84 (2002).
34. Bhakta, N.R., Garcia, A.M., Frank, E.H., Grodzinsky, A.J. & Morales, T.I. The insulin-like growth factors (IGFs) I and II bind to articular cartilage via the IGF-binding proteins. *J Biol Chem* **275**, 5860-6 (2000).
35. Wang, J., Elewaut, D., Veys, E.M. & Verbruggen, G. Insulin-like growth factor 1-induced interleukin-1 receptor II overrides the activity of interleukin-1 and controls the homeostasis of the extracellular matrix of cartilage. *Arthritis Rheum* **48**, 1281-91 (2003).
36. Morales, T.I. The role and content of endogenous insulin-like growth factor-binding proteins in bovine articular cartilage. *Arch Biochem Biophys* **343**, 164-72 (1997).
37. Claeys, I. et al. Insulin-related peptides and their conserved signal transduction pathway. *Peptides* **23**, 807-16 (2002).
38. Bunn, R.C. & Fowlkes, J.L. Insulin-like growth factor binding protein proteolysis. *Trends Endocrinol Metab* **14**, 176-81 (2003).
39. Dupont, J., Dunn, S.E., Barrett, J.C. & LeRoith, D. Microarray analysis and identification of novel molecules involved in insulin-like growth factor-1 receptor signaling and gene expression. *Recent Prog Horm Res* **58**, 325-42 (2003).
40. Dupont, J. & Holzenberger, M. Biology of insulin-like growth factors in development. *Birth Defects Res C Embryo Today* **69**, 257-71 (2003).
41. Nakajima, H., Goto, T., Horikawa, O., Kikuchi, T. & Shinmei, M. Characterization of the cells in the repair tissue of full-thickness articular cartilage defects. *Histochem Cell Biol* **109**, 331-8 (1998).
42. Jones, J.I. & Clemmons, D.R. Insulin-like growth factors and their binding proteins: biological actions. *Endocr Rev* **16**, 3-34 (1995).
43. Matsumoto, T., Gargosky, S.E., Iwasaki, K. & Rosenfeld, R.G. Identification and characterization of insulin-like growth factors (IGFs), IGF-binding proteins (IGFBPs), and IGFBP proteases in human synovial fluid. *J Clin Endocrinol Metab* **81**, 150-5 (1996).
44. Clemmons, D.R. IGF binding proteins: regulation of cellular actions. *Growth Regul* **2**, 80-7 (1992).
45. Morales, T.I. The insulin-like growth factor binding proteins in uncultured human cartilage: increases in insulin-like growth factor binding protein 3 during osteoarthritis. *Arthritis Rheum* **46**, 2358-67 (2002).
46. Malemud, C.J. Cytokines as therapeutic targets for osteoarthritis. *BioDrugs* **18**, 23-35 (2004).
47. Miyazawa, K., Shinozaki, M., Hara, T., Furuya, T. & Miyazono, K. Two major Smad pathways in TGF-beta superfamily signalling. *Genes Cells* **7**, 1191-204 (2002).
48. Zimmerman, C.M. & Padgett, R.W. Transforming growth factor beta signaling mediators and modulators. *Gene* **249**, 17-30 (2000).
49. Heldin, C.H., Miyazono, K. & ten Dijke, P. TGF-beta signalling from cell membrane to nucleus through SMAD proteins. *Nature* **390**, 465-71 (1997).

50. Balemans, W. & Van Hul, W. Extracellular regulation of BMP signaling in vertebrates: a cocktail of modulators. *Dev Biol* **250**, 231-50 (2002).
51. Reddi, A.H. Bone morphogenetic proteins: from basic science to clinical applications. *J Bone Joint Surg Am* **83-A Suppl 1**, S1-6 (2001).
52. Reddi, A.H. Interplay between bone morphogenetic proteins and cognate binding proteins in bone and cartilage development: noggin, chordin and DAN. *Arthritis Res* **3**, 1-5 (2001).
53. Miyazono, K. Positive and negative regulation of TGF-beta signaling. *J Cell Sci* **113 (Pt 7)**, 1101-9 (2000).
54. Miyazono, K., Kusanagi, K. & Inoue, H. Divergence and convergence of TGF-beta/BMP signaling. *J Cell Physiol* **187**, 265-76 (2001).
55. Li, T.F., O'Keefe, R.J. & Chen, D. TGF-beta signaling in chondrocytes. *Front Biosci* **10**, 681-8 (2005).
56. van Beuningen, H.M., van der Kraan, P.M., Arntz, O.J. & van den Berg, W.B. Protection from interleukin 1 induced destruction of articular cartilage by transforming growth factor beta: studies in anatomically intact cartilage in vitro and in vivo. *Ann Rheum Dis* **52**, 185-91 (1993).
57. Qi, W.N. & Scully, S.P. Effect of type II collagen in chondrocyte response to TGF-beta 1 regulation. *Exp Cell Res* **241**, 142-50 (1998).
58. Pedrozo, H.A. et al. Growth plate chondrocytes store latent transforming growth factor (TGF)-beta 1 in their matrix through latent TGF-beta 1 binding protein-1. *J Cell Physiol* **177**, 343-54 (1998).
59. Hynes, R.O. Cell adhesion: old and new questions. *Trends Cell Biol* **9**, M33-7 (1999).
60. Morales, T.I. Transforming growth factor-beta 1 stimulates synthesis of proteoglycan aggregates in calf articular cartilage organ cultures. *Arch Biochem Biophys* **286**, 99-106 (1991).
61. Guerne, P.A., Sublet, A. & Lotz, M. Growth factor responsiveness of human articular chondrocytes: distinct profiles in primary chondrocytes, subcultured chondrocytes, and fibroblasts. *J Cell Physiol* **158**, 476-84 (1994).
62. Bitzer, M. et al. A mechanism of suppression of TGF-beta/SMAD signaling by NF-kappa B/RelA. *Genes Dev* **14**, 187-97 (2000).
63. Schneiderbauer, M.M., Dutton, C.M. & Scully, S.P. Signaling "cross-talk" between TGF-beta1 and ECM signals in chondrocytic cells. *Cell Signal* **16**, 1133-40 (2004).
64. Cook, S.D., Barrack, R.L., Patron, L.P. & Salkeld, S.L. Osteogenic protein-1 in knee arthritis and arthroplasty. *Clin Orthop Relat Res*, 140-5 (2004).
65. Luyten, F.P. et al. Natural bovine osteogenin and recombinant human bone morphogenetic protein-2B are equipotent in the maintenance of proteoglycans in bovine articular cartilage explant cultures. *J Biol Chem* **267**, 3691-5 (1992).
66. Reddi, A.H. Morphogenesis and tissue engineering of bone and cartilage: inductive signals, stem cells, and biomimetic biomaterials. *Tissue Eng* **6**, 351-9 (2000).
67. Brunet, L.J., McMahon, J.A., McMahon, A.P. & Harland, R.M. Noggin, cartilage morphogenesis, and joint formation in the mammalian skeleton. *Science* **280**, 1455-7 (1998).
68. Frenkel, S.R. et al. Transforming growth factor beta superfamily members: role in cartilage modeling. *Plast Reconstr Surg* **105**, 980-90 (2000).
69. Nishida, Y., Knudson, C.B., Kuettner, K.E. & Knudson, W. Osteogenic protein-1 promotes the synthesis and retention of extracellular matrix within bovine articular cartilage and chondrocyte cultures. *Osteoarthritis Cartilage* **8**, 127-36 (2000).
70. Vinall, R.L., Lo, S.H. & Reddi, A.H. Regulation of articular chondrocyte phenotype by bone morphogenetic protein 7, interleukin 1, and cellular context is dependent on the cytoskeleton. *Exp Cell Res* **272**, 32-44 (2002).
71. Lietman, S.A., Yanagishita, M., Sampath, T.K. & Reddi, A.H. Stimulation of proteoglycan synthesis in explants of porcine articular cartilage by recombinant osteogenic protein-1 (bone morphogenetic protein-7). *J Bone Joint Surg Am* **79**, 1132-7 (1997).
72. Heldin, C.H. Platelet-derived growth factor--an introduction. *Cytokine Growth Factor Rev* **15**, 195-6 (2004).
73. Betsholtz, C. Biology of platelet-derived growth factors in development. *Birth Defects Res C Embryo Today* **69**, 272-85 (2003).
74. Schafer, S.J., Luyten, F.P., Yanagishita, M. & Reddi, A.H. Proteoglycan metabolism is age related and modulated by isoforms of platelet-derived growth factor in bovine articular cartilage explant cultures. *Arch Biochem Biophys* **302**, 431-8 (1993).
75. Harvey, A.K., Stack, S.T. & Chandrasekhar, S. Differential modulation of degradative and repair responses of interleukin-1-treated chondrocytes by platelet-derived growth factor. *Biochem J* **292 (Pt 1)**, 129-36 (1993).
76. Sah, R.L., Chen, A.C., Grodzinsky, A.J. & Trippel, S.B. Differential effects of bFGF and IGF-I on matrix metabolism in calf and adult bovine cartilage explants. *Arch Biochem Biophys* **308**, 137-47 (1994).

77. Chin, J.E., Hatfield, C.A., Krzesicki, R.F. & Herblin, W.F. Interactions between interleukin-1 and basic fibroblast growth factor on articular chondrocytes. Effects on cell growth, prostanoid production, and receptor modulation. *Arthritis Rheum* **34**, 314-24 (1991).
78. Klooster, A.R. & Bernier, S.M. Tumor necrosis factor alpha and epidermal growth factor act additively to inhibit matrix gene expression by chondrocyte. *Arthritis Res Ther* **7**, R127-38 (2005).
79. Huh, Y.H., Kim, S.H., Kim, S.J. & Chun, J.S. Differentiation status-dependent regulation of cyclooxygenase-2 expression and prostaglandin E2 production by epidermal growth factor via mitogen-activated protein kinase in articular chondrocytes. *J Biol Chem* **278**, 9691-7 (2003).
80. Enomoto, H. et al. Vascular endothelial growth factor isoforms and their receptors are expressed in human osteoarthritic cartilage. *Am J Pathol* **162**, 171-81 (2003).
81. Pufe, T., Petersen, W., Tillmann, B. & Mentlein, R. The splice variants VEGF121 and VEGF189 of the angiogenic peptide vascular endothelial growth factor are expressed in osteoarthritic cartilage. *Arthritis Rheum* **44**, 1082-8 (2001).
82. Neufeld, G., Cohen, T., Gengrinovitch, S. & Poltorak, Z. Vascular endothelial growth factor (VEGF) and its receptors. *Faseb J* **13**, 9-22 (1999).
83. Pulsatelli, L. et al. Vascular endothelial growth factor activities on osteoarthritic chondrocytes. *Clin Exp Rheumatol* **23**, 487-93 (2005).
84. Pfander, D. et al. Hepatocyte growth factor in human osteoarthritic cartilage. *Osteoarthritis Cartilage* **7**, 548-59 (1999).
85. Moo, V., Sieper, J., Herzog, V. & Muller, B.M. Regulation of expression of cytokines and growth factors in osteoarthritic cartilage explants. *Clin Rheumatol* **20**, 353-8 (2001).
86. Attur, M.G., Dave, M., Akamatsu, M., Katoh, M. & Amin, A.R. Osteoarthritis or osteoarthrosis: the definition of inflammation becomes a semantic issue in the genomic era of molecular medicine. *Osteoarthritis Cartilage* **10**, 1-4 (2002).
87. Pfander, D., Heinz, N., Rothe, P., Carl, H.D. & Swoboda, B. Tenascin and aggrecan expression by articular chondrocytes is influenced by interleukin 1beta: a possible explanation for the changes in matrix synthesis during osteoarthritis. *Ann Rheum Dis* **63**, 240-4 (2004).
88. Stabellini, G. et al. Effects of interleukin-1beta on chondroblast viability and extracellular matrix changes in bovine articular cartilage explants. *Biomed Pharmacother* **57**, 314-9 (2003).
89. Vosshenrich, C.A. & Di Santo, J.P. Interleukin signaling. *Curr Biol* **12**, R760-3 (2002).
90. Legendre, F., Dudhia, J., Pujol, J.P. & Bogdanowicz, P. JAK/STAT but not ERK1/ERK2 pathway mediates interleukin (IL)-6/soluble IL-6R down-regulation of Type II collagen, aggrecan core, and link protein transcription in articular chondrocytes. Association with a down-regulation of SOX9 expression. *J Biol Chem* **278**, 2903-12 (2003).
91. Blanco, F.J., Ochs, R.L., Schwarz, H. & Lotz, M. Chondrocyte apoptosis induced by nitric oxide. *Am J Pathol* **146**, 75-85 (1995).
92. Olee, T., Hashimoto, S., Quach, J. & Lotz, M. IL-18 is produced by articular chondrocytes and induces proinflammatory and catabolic responses. *J Immunol* **162**, 1096-100 (1999).
93. Seguin, C.A. & Bernier, S.M. TNFalpha suppresses link protein and type II collagen expression in chondrocytes: Role of MEK1/2 and NF-kappaB signaling pathways. *J Cell Physiol* **197**, 356-69 (2003).
94. Malemud, C.J. Fundamental pathways in osteoarthritis: an overview. *Front Biosci* **4**, D659-61 (1999).
95. Wajant, H., Pfizenmaier, K. & Scheurich, P. Tumor necrosis factor signaling. *Cell Death Differ* **10**, 45-65 (2003).
96. Baud, V. & Karin, M. Signal transduction by tumor necrosis factor and its relatives. *Trends Cell Biol* **11**, 372-7 (2001).
97. Scherle, P.A., Pratta, M.A., Feeser, W.S., Tancula, E.J. & Arner, E.C. The effects of IL-1 on mitogen-activated protein kinases in rabbit articular chondrocytes. *Biochem Biophys Res Commun* **230**, 573-7 (1997).
98. Olney, R.C., Wilson, D.M., Mohtai, M., Fielder, P.J. & Smith, R.L. Interleukin-1 and tumor necrosis factor-alpha increase insulin-like growth factor-binding protein-3 (IGFBP-3) production and IGFBP-3 protease activity in human articular chondrocytes. *J Endocrinol* **146**, 279-86 (1995).
99. Hoffman, A.S. Hydrogels for biomedical applications. *Adv Drug Deliv Rev* **54**, 3-12 (2002).
100. Lee, K.Y. & Mooney, D.J. Hydrogels for tissue engineering. *Chem Rev* **101**, 1869-79 (2001).
101. Gutowska, A., Jeong, B. & Jasionowski, M. Injectable gels for tissue engineering. *Anat Rec* **263**, 342-9 (2001).
102. Benya, P.D. & Shaffer, J.D. Dedifferentiated chondrocytes reexpress the differentiated collagen phenotype when cultured in agarose gels. *Cell* **30**, 215-24 (1982).
103. Elisseeff, J.H., Lee, A., Kleinman, H.K. & Yamada, Y. Biological response of chondrocytes to hydrogels. *Ann N Y Acad Sci* **961**, 118-22 (2002).

104. Alsberg, E., Anderson, K.W., Albeiruti, A., Rowley, J.A. & Mooney, D.J. Engineering growing tissues. *Proc Natl Acad Sci U S A* **99**, 12025-30 (2002).
105. Grunder, T. et al. Bone morphogenetic protein (BMP)-2 enhances the expression of type II collagen and aggrecan in chondrocytes embedded in alginate beads. *Osteoarthritis Cartilage* **12**, 559-67 (2004).
106. Chubinskaya, S. et al. Gene expression by human articular chondrocytes cultured in alginate beads. *J Histochem Cytochem* **49**, 1211-20 (2001).
107. Starkman, B.G., Cravero, J.D., Delcarlo, M. & Loeser, R.F. IGF-I stimulation of proteoglycan synthesis by chondrocytes requires activation of the PI 3-kinase pathway but not ERK MAPK. *Biochem J* **389**, 723-9 (2005).
108. Almqvist, K.F. et al. Culture of chondrocytes in alginate surrounded by fibrin gel: characteristics of the cells over a period of eight weeks. *Ann Rheum Dis* **60**, 781-90 (2001).
109. Perka, C., Spitzer, R.S., Lindenhayn, K., Sittinger, M. & Schultz, O. Matrix-mixed culture: new methodology for chondrocyte culture and preparation of cartilage transplants. *J Biomed Mater Res* **49**, 305-11 (2000).
110. Qi, W.N. & Scully, S.P. Type II collagen modulates the composition of extracellular matrix synthesized by articular chondrocytes. *J Orthop Res* **21**, 282-9 (2003).
111. Flechtenmacher, J. et al. Recombinant human osteogenic protein 1 is a potent stimulator of the synthesis of cartilage proteoglycans and collagens by human articular chondrocytes. *Arthritis Rheum* **39**, 1896-904 (1996).
112. Clancy, R.M. et al. Outside-in signaling in the chondrocyte. Nitric oxide disrupts fibronectin-induced assembly of a subplasmalemmal actin/rho A/focal adhesion kinase signaling complex. *J Clin Invest* **100**, 1789-96 (1997).
113. Girotto, D. et al. Tissue-specific gene expression in chondrocytes grown on three-dimensional hyaluronic acid scaffolds. *Biomaterials* **24**, 3265-75 (2003).
114. Miralles, G. et al. Sodium alginate sponges with or without sodium hyaluronate: in vitro engineering of cartilage. *J Biomed Mater Res* **57**, 268-78 (2001).
115. Elisseeff, J., McIntosh, W., Fu, K., Blunk, B.T. & Langer, R. Controlled-release of IGF-I and TGF-beta1 in a photopolymerizing hydrogel for cartilage tissue engineering. *J Orthop Res* **19**, 1098-104 (2001).
116. Fisher, J.P., Jo, S., Mikos, A.G. & Reddi, A.H. Thermoreversible hydrogel scaffolds for articular cartilage engineering. *J Biomed Mater Res A* **71**, 268-74 (2004).
117. Park, Y., Lutolf, M.P., Hubbell, J.A., Hunziker, E.B. & Wong, M. Bovine primary chondrocyte culture in synthetic matrix metalloproteinase-sensitive poly(ethylene glycol)-based hydrogels as a scaffold for cartilage repair. *Tissue Eng* **10**, 515-22 (2004).

6

OSTEOINDUCTION WITH COLLOSS®, COLLOSS® E, AND GFm

WE Huffer[1], JJ Benedict[2], R Rettenmaier[3], and A Briest[3]

6.1. INTRODUCTION

COLLOSS® and COLLOSS® E are bone void fillers consisting of lyophilized type I collagen and non-collagenous proteins extracted with chaotropic solvents from acid demineralized bovine and equine bone, respectively. The protein extracts are precipitated and further purified by methods similar to those used for isolating bone morphogenetic proteins[1]. COLLOSS® achieved the same rate and percentage of new bone formation as autologous bone graft in a porcine anterior spinal fusion model[2] and both COLLOSS® and COLLOSS® E were equal osteoinductive than autograft bone in a sheep cortical bone defect model[3]. This osteoinductive activity was thought to be most likely mediated by BMPs, because an earlier study had shown that COLLOSS® enclosed in titanium mesh and implanted subcutaneously in rats, induced bone formation[4]. In this study we used histology and histomorphometry to confirm those results and to better define the osteoinductive potency and the phenotypic diversity of ectopic skeletal tissues induced in weanling Long Evans rats by COLLOSS® and COLLOSS® E. Osteoinduction in response to those materials was compared with induction of bone in response to known amounts of a purified mixture of bovine bone BMPs, GFm.

6.2. MATERIALS AND METHODS

COLLOSS®, and COLLOSS® E obtained from OSSACUR AG, Oberstenfeld, Germany are cotton-like lyophilisates in which the bone type I collagen is thought to act

---

[1] Department of Pathology, University of Colorado Health Sciences Center, Denver, CO
[2] Arvada, CO
[3] OSSACUR AG, Oberstenfeld, DE

as a carrier matrix for putative BMPs. Twenty and 60 mg samples were compressed into 10 mm discs and implanted in ventral and dorsal SC implants in ten 100-300 g female Long Evans rats. Immunodeficient rats were not used in order to better mimic physiologic processes of bone formation as immunologic processes are shown to be important in initial bone healing. Ten and 35 µg aliquots of GFm obtained from Sulzer Biologics, Wheat Ridge CO. were dissolved in 10 mM HCl, applied to 6.5 mg discs (8x3 mm) capsules of type I bovine tendon collagen (Regen Biologics, Redwood, CA), re-lyophilized, and similarly implanted into the same group of 10 animals. Extensive experience with this technique has shown us that significant differences between means and medians of experimental treatment groups can be achieved with groups of N=5. In these experiments we wanted to compare effects of 2 doses of COLLOSS®, COLLOSS E®, and GFm on formation of ectopic bone (6 experimental conditions using groups of N=5 or greater). Each animal in a group of 10 received 4 non-randomly allocated implants to form 6 treatment groups of the following sizes: GFm, 10 µg, N=5; GFm, 35 µg, N=5; COLLOSS®, 20 mg, N= 10; COLLOSS E®, 20 mg, N=10; COLLOSS®, 60 mg N=5; and COLLOSS E®, 60 mg, N=5. COLLOSS® and COLLOSS E® were overrepresented at 20mg because prior studies had indicated that those were the optimal doses for those materials. Death of 1 animal following surgery reduced the size of the 35 µg GFm and 60 mg COLLOSS E® groups to 4, and the 20 mg COLLOSS E® group to 8. Development of an abscess in one of the 35 µg GFm sites further reduced the size of that group to 3.

Animals received 2 mg/g of Tylenol in their drinking water 48 hours prior to and 24 hours after surgery, and were anesthetized with 80 mg/g Ketamine and 16 mg/g Xylazine, IP. Each animal had 4 implants sterilely inserted with forceps into subcutaneous muscle pouches through two 1 cm ventral incisions on either side of the sternum and 2 similar dorsal thoracic incisions on either side of the spinal column. Incisions were closed with 2-3 sutures. Animals were humanely sacrificed and the implants recovered 26 days after implantation. All animal procedures were approved by UCHSC Animal Care Committee Protocol # 38003602(05)1E.

Implants were photographed, X-rayed, fixed 24 hours in 10 % neutral buffered formalin, decalcified and embedded in paraffin. Five µm sections from the center of the implants cut parallel to their longest axes were stained with hematoxylin and eosin. This technique provided a standardized biopsy comparable from one sample to another demonstrating maximal implant area with a representative sampling of induced skeletal tissues which were known from prior experience to be distributed non-randomly around the center of the implant. Areas occupied by fibrous and fibrovascular tissue, hyaline and fibrocartilage, hematopoietic marrow, and bone were traced and measured in 40X and 100X digital images obtained via an Optronics VI-470 television camera attached to a Leitz Laborlux K microscope using software of the Bioquant Nova Image Analysis System.

Mean values for each implant group were compared by ANOVA with post-hoc comparisons by the Tukey-Kramer method using software of the NCSS Statistical System, Kayesville, UT. This methodology combines the variance for all the experimental groups in the study taking into account differences in sample size among the different groups and avoids errors due to multiple comparisons of groups of different sizes. The relative incidence of different types of skeletal tissues among different treatment groups was compared by Chi square analysis of a contingency table using the NCSS program.

6.3. ECTOPIC BONE FORMATION INDUCED BY GFm

GFm formed smooth oval ossicles of cortical and cancellous bone around a central fibrovascular core (Figure 6.1).

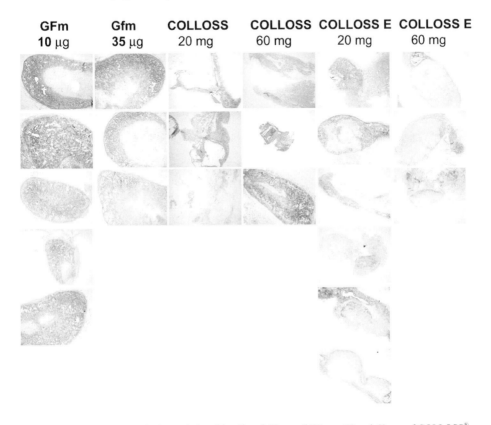

Figure 6.1. Overview of ectopic tissues induced by 10 and 35 µg of GFm or 20 and 60 mg of COLLOSS® or COLLOSS® E. 25X Digital images of Hematoxylin and eosin-stained sections.

The ossicles continued to form new bone and marrow by three closely related, but distinctive mechanisms, membranous, endochondral, and accelerated endochondral bone growth. In each case osteoclasts, osteoblasts, blood vessels, and hematopoietic cells arising from cancellous bone and marrow formed during early stages of the osteoinductive process grew centripetally into the remaining fibrovascular core by resorbing and replacing one of three types of calcified tissues in the outer perimeter of that core (Figures. 6.2-4).

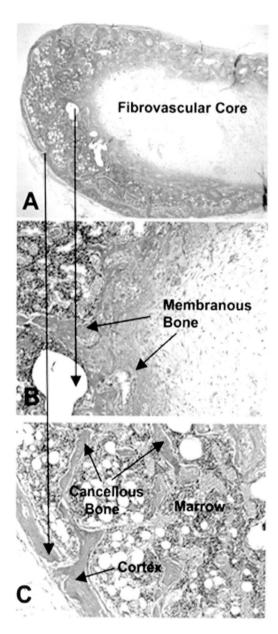

Figure 6.2. Cancellous bone and marrow and cortical bone formed by remodeling of membranous bone differentiating in the fibrovascular core of a 10μg GFm implantation site. Hematoxylin and eosin-stained sections. A. 25X view of one end of the implant. Arrows point to corresponding locations in (B) and (C). B. 100X view of membranous bone differentiating around the outer perimeter of the fibrovascular core and being remodeled by osteoclasts, osteoblasts, and other cells derived from cancellous bone and marrow. C. 100X view of cortical bone formed by remodeling of cancellous bone and marrow. The cortex has an osteoblastic bone-forming endosteal, and an osteoclastic bone-resorbing periosteal surface.

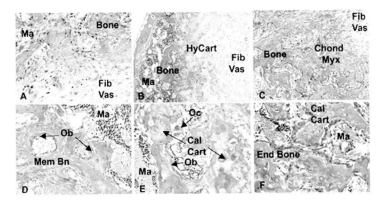

Figure 6.3. Membranous bone formation (A,D), Endochondral bone formation (B,E), and Acelerated Endochondral bone formation (C,F) in GFm implants. 100X (A), 40X (B,-C), and 250X (D-F) Hematoxylin and eosin-stained sections. A. Membranous bone formed by osteoblasts differentiating in the outer perimeter of the fibrovascular core (FibVas) (right lower) is being invaded and remodeled by osteoclasts and osteoblasts invading from the marrow (Ma) (upper left). B. Hyaline cartilage (HyCart) formed by chondrocytes differentiating in the outer perimeter of the fibrovascular core is being invaded and resorbed by chondroclasts and blood vessels, and having bone formed on its surface by osteoblasts arising in cancellous bone and marrow. C. Chondromxyoid (ChondMyx) stroma formed by chondrocytes and spindled and stellate fibroblasts rather than typical hyaline cartilage in the outer perimeter of the fibrovascular core is being resorbed and replaced by bone by cells similar to those in B. In other studies we have shown that such endochondral bone is formed more rapidly than that formed from hyaline cartilage. D. More mature membranous bone (MemBn) trabeculae around the outer perimeter of the implant have no remnants of calcified cartilage and are being enlarged by layers of osteoblasts (Ob) arising from marrow stromal cells. E. Endochondral bone trabeculae with remnants of calcified cartilage in their cores are being enlarged by osteoblasts arising from marrow stromal cells. Osteoclasts (Oc) are initiating trabecular remodeling by resorbing calcified cartilage remnants (CalCart) in the trabecular core. F. Osteoblasts are enlarging and osteoclasts remodeling endochondral bone trabeculae containing remnants of calcified chondromyxoid tissue (Cal Cart) which differs from calcified hyaline cartilage because chondrocyte lacunae are smaller and less prominent and the matrix is composed of basophilic fibrillar material rather than homogenous pale staining cartilage.

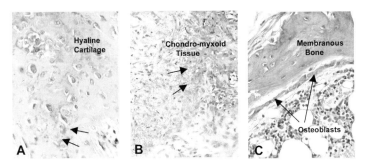

Figure 6.4. Different histologic characteristics of hyaline cartilage, chondromyxoid tissue, and membranous bone forming in the outer perimeter of the fibrovascular core of GFm implants. Hematoxylin and eosin-stained sections, 400X. A. Hyaline cartilage has homogeneous pale blue to pink matrix containing round chondrocytes of varying size in well defined lacunae. Arrows point to a region where hypertrophic chondrocytes have released large irregular clumps of calcifying matrix vesicles into the surrounding matrix. B .Chondromyxoid tissue is basophilic, fibrillar, and contains a mixture of small rounded chondrocytes in indistinct lacunae, and elongated and stellate fibroblasts. The tissue is more vascular than hyaline cartilage and contains large numbers of small uniform calcifying matrix vesicles (arrows). C. Membranous bone is undergoing resorption by mononuclear osteoclasts (upper surface) and bone formation by osteoblasts (lower surface). The marrow consists of adipocytes and hematopoietic cells.

The three types of calcified tissues were membranous bone, calcified hyaline cartilage, and calcified chondromyxoid tissue. In regions in which cells in the outer perimeter of the fibrous core were differentiating into osteoblasts they formed membranous bone. The cancellous bone in those regions lacked calcified cartilage cores, and contained no calcifying matrix granules (Figures 6.2B, 6.3A, and 6.3D). In other regions, cells in the fibrovascular core differentiated into chondrocytes, formed cartilage matrix, hypertrophied, and released calcifying matrix vesicles into the surrounding cartilage matrix. In these regions remodeling cells from the bone and marrow excavated the calcified cartilage and deposited endochondral bone on the walls of the excavation site. Bone trabeculae formed in this way had cores of calcified cartilage with lacunar chondrocytes (Figures 6.3B, 6.3E, and 6.4A).

Finally, in regions of accelerated endochondral bone growth, the substrate for the remodeling cells was chondro-myxoid tissue formed by small, round, spindle-shaped, or stellate fibrovascular vascular core cells and consisting of a loose, fibrillar basophilic matrix with occasional small lacunae, and large numbers of small calcifying matrix vesicles (Figures. 6.3C, 6.3F, and 6.4B). Bone trabeculae in these regions had cores of calcified chondro-myxoid tissue.

In GFm implants cancellous bone and marrow grew centripetally, and matured centrifugally to form a thin layer of cortical bone around the outer perimeter of the implants (Figures 6.2C, 6.3B and 6.4C). The cortex also moved centripetally as a result of osteoblastic bone formation on its endosteal surface, and osteoclastic bone resorption on its outer periosteal surface (Figure 6.4C).

6.4. ECTOPIC BONE FORMATION INDUCED BY COLLOSS® AND COLLOSS E®

COLLOSS® and COLLOSS E® implants were more irregular in size and shape and had a different distribution of bone and cartilage than that in GFm implants (Figure 6.1). With both COLLOSS® and COLLOSS E®, the major cellular mechanism of bone formation was membranous, and the bone was arranged in plates rather than spherical ossicles (Figures 6.5 and 6.6).

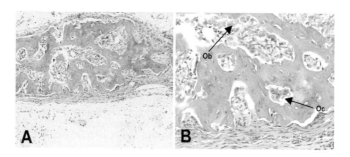

Figure 6.5. Membranous bone formation in response in a 20 mg COLLOSS E® implantation site. Hematoxylin and eosin stained sections, 40X (A) and 100X (B). Irregular trabeculae of woven bone lying within a fibrous membrane are undergoing remodeling by osteoblasts and osteoclasts.

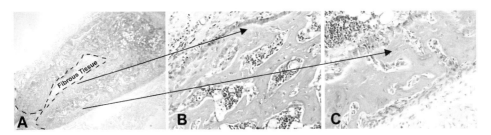

Figure 6.6. Formation of cortical dipoles in membranous bone of a 60 mg COLLOSS® implantation site. Hematoxylin and eosin-stained sections. 25X (A) and 250 X (B,C). A. Two plates of membranous bone (left) protrude from a much thicker plate (right) composed of cancellous bone and marrow separating an upper and lower cortical surface. The protrusion on the lower right (arrows) also has a dipolar structure with developing cancellous bone and marrow continuous with the main central marrow cavity on the right. B. The developing upper cortical dipole has an osteoblastic periosteal surface and no clearly defined endosteal surface. C. The better-developed lower cortical dipole has a clearly demarcated osteoblastic bone forming endosteal surface and a resorptive osteoclastic periosteal surface.

Bone formation (Figure 6.5) was similar to embryonic development of the calvarium, and remodeled to form a dipole of compact cortical bone separated by cancellous bone and hematopoietic marrow (Figure 6.6). The cortical bone formed in response to COLLOSS® and COLLOSS E® had coupled bone modeling surfaces with osteoblasts forming bone on one side, and osteoclasts resorbing bone on the opposite side. Cortical endosteal and periosteal surfaces in COLLOSS® and COLLOSS E® implants could be either both osteoblastic and osteoclastic, but the opposite surface was always coupled to the opposite functional activity (Figure 6.6).

In three of six 20 mg COLLOSS® E implants the cancellous bone and marrow space between the cortical dipoles was focally interrupted by islands of fibrous tissue and cartilage (Figure 6.7A). Cartilage in such foci was more abundant than that seen in GFm implants, had a higher ratio of matrix to chondrocytes, and showed only focal hypertrophy, mineralization and replacement by endochondral bone (Figures 6.7B and 6.7C). Junctions between cartilage and fibrovascular tissue were populated by chondrocyte precursors, and the outer surface of the cartilage underwent only focal replacement by endochondral bone and marrow. Thus the fibro-cartilaginous foci were analogous to the fibrovascular cores of GFm implants, but formed a morphologically different type of cartilage which was much less active in stimulating endochondral bone formation.

Sixty milligrams implants of COLLOSS® E showed only small foci of immature membranous bone adjacent to much larger masses of hyaline cartilage and fibrocartilage (Figure 6.8).

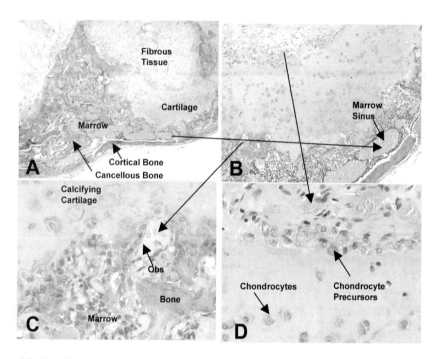

Figure 6.7. Focal fibro-cartilaginous nodule within the membranous cortical dipole of a 20 mg COLLOSS® E implantation site. Hematoxylin and eosin-stained sections. 25X (A), 40X (B), and 250X (C, D). A. A large fibrous and cartilaginous nodule is partially enclosed by and expands, and displaces cancellous bone and marrow in the center of membranous bone otherwise forming a cortical dipole. B. The cartilaginous portion of the nodule has a small focus of endochondral bone formation (arrow to C) but is directly apposed to marrow sinuses and has no endochondral bone forming on most of its lower surface. Its upper surface (arrow to D) is in contact with fibrous tissue. C. Osteoblasts and chondroclasts from the marrow are focally invading and replacing the cartilage with new bone and marrow, but there is no chondrocyte hypertrophy or formation of calcifying matrix vesicles. D. At the junction between fibrous tissue and cartilage, precursor cells with fibroblasts morphology in the fibrous tissue are differentiating into rounded chondrocytes. The fibrous tissue is therefore analogous to the fibrovascular core of a GFm implant.

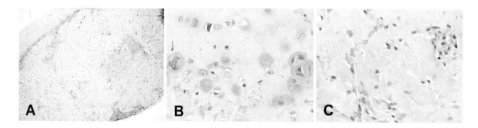

Figure 6.8. Hyaline cartilage and fibrocartilage formation in a 60 mg COLLOSS® E implant site. Hematoxylin and eosin-stained sections. 25X (A), 250X (B,C). A. A rounded nodule of cartilage and fibrocartilage is surrounded by fibrous tissue with no evidence of membranous bone formation. B. Multiple foci within the nodule had rounded chondrocytes in lacunae but there was no chondrocyte hypertrophy or formation of calcifying matrix vesicles. C. Much of the nodule consisted of homogeneous cartilage-like matrix containing a few small rounded chondrocytes in lacunae and penetrated by bands of fibrovascular tissue with elongated cells with fibroblast morphology.

The hyaline cartilage contained clusters of small and large chondrocytes, but no hypertrophic chondrocytes or calcifying matrix vesicles (Figure 6.8B). Cartilage merged with fibrocartilage consisting of small round chondrocytes and elongated cells with fibroblasts morphology (Figure 6.8C).

6.5. INCIDENCE AND AMOUNTS OF DIFFERENT TYPES OF SKELETAL TISSUES

Ectopic tissue of any type was present in 8/9 of GFm, 9/12 of COLLOSS E®, and 6/15 of the COLLOSS® implantation sites (Figure 6.9, Table 6.1).

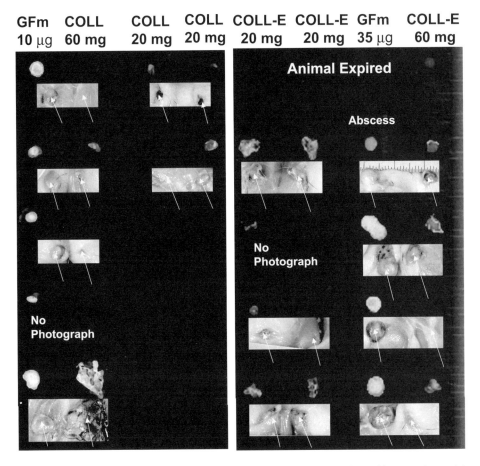

Figure 6.9. Composite of in situ photographs and X-rays of all implantation sites (white arrows) containing ectopic tissues of any type. Completely empty squares in the grid used for holding specimens for X-rays correspond to sites where no ectopic tissues were found. Circles within the squares for the expired animal were small drops of water in advertently placed in the squares. The radio-opaque circle and the yellow nodule under the word abscess were an abscess composed entirely of polymorphonuclear leucocytes.

Table 6.1. Incidence of Tissues and Types of Bone Formation Induced by GFm, COLLOSS®, and COLLOSS®E.

Tissue	GFm	COLLOSS®	COLLOSS E®	Chi-Square	P<0.05
Any Tissue	8/9	6/15	9/12	9.7	+
Hyaline Cartilage*	1/8	0/6	4/9	4.8	-
Fibro-Cartilage*	0/8	0/6	3/6	5.4	-
Cancellous Bone	8/8	1/6	8/9	14.1	+
Cortical Bone	6/8	1/6	4/9	4.7	-
Marrow	8/8	1/6	4/9	10.6	+
Bone Formation					
Endochondral					
Hyaline^	6/8	0/6	3/9	8.3	+
Chondromyxoid	5/8	0/6	0/9	12.0	+
Membranous Bone	4/8	3/6	7/9	1.8	-

*Foci of hyaline or fibrocartilage at least 1 mm^2
^ Foci of hyaline cartilage less than 1 mm^2 containing 1 to 20 chondrocytes surrounded by cartilage matrix.

One 35 µg GFm site without ectopic skeletal tissue was an abscess (Figure 6.9). The low incidence of ectopic tissues in the COLLOSS® group was significant ($P < 0.05$) by Chi-square analysis (Table 6.1).

X-rays showed heavy uniform mineralization of all GFm sites (Figure 6.9). COLLOSS® sites contained only small foci of mineralization with the exception of one heavily mineralized 60 mg site. COLLOSS E® sites had less mineral than GFm sites. The mineral deposits were linear, consistent with the histologic pattern of membranous bone formation described above.

Although 6/8 of GFm implants had multiple small foci of hyaline cartilage contributing to endochondral bone formation, only 1 implant site had a focus of hyaline cartilage 1 mm^2. Foci of hyaline cartilage 1 mm^2 or larger were present in 4/9 of COLLOSS® E implants and absent from COLLOSS® implants (Table 6.1). Foci of fibrocartilage 1 mm^2 or larger were present in 3/6 COLLOSS® E implants and absent from GFm and COLLOSS® implants (Table 6.1). Differences in the incidences of these larger foci of hyaline cartilage or fibrocartilage among GFm, COLLOSS®, or COLLOSS® E groups were not significant by Chi-square analysis. Low incidences of cancellous bone, hematopoietic marrow, and endochondral bone formation in the COLLOSS® group, and limitation of accelerated endochondral bone formation to the GFm group were also significant by Chi-square analyses (Table 6.1).

Analysis of mean tissue areas by one-way ANOVA and post-hoc comparisons by the Tukey-Kramer method showed that the mean bone area in the 35 µg GFm group was significantly greater than those of all but the 10 µg GFm group. The mean fibrovascular core area in the 35 µg GFm group was significantly greater than those of all other groups (Figure 6.10).

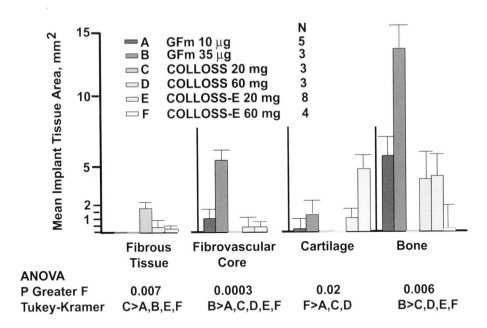

Figure 6.10. Bar Graphs with standard deviations of the mean areas (mm^2) occupied by fibrous tissue, the fibrovascular core or its equivalent, combined hyaline cartilage and fibrocartilage, and bone in implant sites containing 2 doses of GFm COLLOSS®, or COLLOSS® E. Results of one-way ANOVA and post-hoc analysis by the Tukey-Kramer method are given below each tissue panel.

The mean combined hyaline and fibrocartilage area (Cartilage in Figure 6.10) was higher in the 60 mg COLLOSS® E group than those of the 10 μg GFm, or the 20 mg and 60 mg COLLOSS® groups. The mean fibrous tissue area was higher in the 20 mg COLLOSS® group than those in all but the 60 mg COLLOSS® group.

6.6. DISCUSSION

One objective of this study was to confirm that COLLOSS® and COLLOSS® E had osteoinductive BMP activity. BMPs were originally defined by their ability to induce bone in non-skeletal tissues in rodents[5,6]. Subsequently they have been defined molecularly and found to be the largest sub-group within the transforming growth factor beta (TGFß) superfamily[7] with multiple functions other than cartilage and bone induction that make them essential for development and maintenance of many organ systems in addition to the skeleton[8,9]. Individual members of the BMP family vary in their ability to induce cartilage and bone, and some induce other types of skeletal tissues such as tendons and ligaments. For example, BMP-3 does not stimulate ectopic bone in rats and inhibits ectopic bone formation in response to BMP-2[10]. BMP 13 induces mainly ectopic tendon and ligament and only small amounts of cartilage and bone[11]. However, induction of ectopic cartilage and bone in rats is still accepted as evidence that a mixture of proteins contains BMPs[12]. Therefore, this study confirmed that COLLOSS® and COLLOSS® E contain osteo- and chondro-inductive BMPs.

Another objective of the study was to better define the osteoinductive potency of COLLOSS® and COLLOSS® E in comparison to GFm. GFm was used as a reference material since its composition is known. COLLOSS® and COLLOSS® E were assumed to contain qualitatively similar growth and differentiation factors, since all three substances were prepared from similar starting materials[13]. GFm consists of a core osteoinductive protein fraction containing BMPs 2, and 4-8, TGFβ-1, and -3, and FGF-1, each comprising less than 1 % of the total protein, and another major fraction comprising 65 % of the weight whose 2 major components are BMP-3 and TGFβ-2[14]. For maximal osteoinductive activity, the inductive proteins must be delivered on carrier systems that retain them in the osteoinductive site, promote movement of inducible cells into the site, and provide space for new bone formation to occur[15]. With GFm the osteoinductive activity was delivered on 6.5 mg of type I tendon collagen, and with COLLOSS® E and COLLOSS® on 20 and 60 mg, respectively, of bone type I collagen and other non-osteoinductive bone proteins. Thus, per mg of carrier COLLOSS® E was 0.3, and COLLOSS® 0.1 times as potent as 10 μg of GFm.

The analyses above were complicated by a lower incidence of osteoinduction in response to COLLOSS® (Figure 6.9, Table 6.1), and a non-linear dose response to COLLOSS® E (Figure 6.10). These discrepancies may have been due in part to inhibition of osteogenic responses to COLLOSS® and COLLOSS® E by immunogenic components. Studies in the 1980s showed that 4M guanidine-HCl extracts of rat bone restored osteoinductive activity of demineralized rat bone extracted with the same solvent[16]. Similar extracts of bovine, monkey, and human bone gave reduced (bovine) or no (human and monkey) osteoinduction, but reconstitution with 4 M guanidine-HCl extract fractions containing proteins 50,000 Daltons or less gave equivalent osteoinduction for all species[17]. Those studies were interpreted as indicating that xenograft bone extracts contained immunogenic inhibitory substances that reduced osteoinduction. Thus it is possible that the low incidence of osteoinductive responses to COLLOSS®, and decreased osteoinduction with higher doses of COLLOSS® E may have been due to similar inhibitory substances. Such effects would have been maximized in this study by applying the materials subcutaneously, and using immunocompetent Long Evans, rather than athymic rats. On the other hand studies showing that COLLOSS® and COLLOSS® E are more osteoinductive than autologous bone in sheep cortical bone defects[3] and lack of evidence for xenogenic rejection following use of COLLOSS® as a bone filler in rabbits, pigs, or humans[2,18-23] suggest that these putative immunogenic effects may be less important in species other than rats, and in skeletal tissues.

A third purpose of this study was to determine what types of skeletal tissues and mechanisms of bone formation COLLOSS® and COLLOSS® E induce. Previous studies have shown that those parameters vary depending on the composition of BMPs and other growth and differentiation factors present in the induction mixture[24]. For example, complete GFm typically induces an ossicle of cancellous bone and marrow surrounded by a thin rim of cortical bone by endochondral mechanisms as described in this study. Formation of cancellous bone and marrow by remodeling of membranous bone formation as described in this study is unusual with GFm, but was the major osteoinductive response to COLLOSS® and lower doses of COLLOSS® E. These observations were consistent with the actions of these materials in sheep cortical bone defects where they elicited extensive membranous bone formation[3]. This may be related to the characteristics of the carrier proteins. Previous studies have described independent foci of membranous and endochondral bone formation in response to implantation of partially purified bovine BMPs on a bovine fibrous membrane carrier[25] or of rBMP2 on type I collagen carriers[26,27]. This suggests that the type I collagen in COLLOSS® and COLLOSS® E may promote membranous bone formation. Others have described membranous bone formation in response to implantation of BMP 4/7 heterodimers on pure collagen carriers[28]. Such dimers are known to occur in GFm (unpublished observations, JJ Benedict). Whether they are present in COLLOSS® or COLLOSS® E is not known. Formation of ectopic membranous bone in response to rhBMP2 has also been ascribed to differences in pore size in hydroxyapatite, collagen membrane, and bioglass carriers[29]. With the bioglass carrier system addition of increasing amounts of an angiogenic inhibitor progressively reduced the formation of membranous bone but not cartilage[30]. Those results were consistent with observations in this and other studies of GFm-induced bone formation that membranous bone formation occurred in implants with heavily vascularized central cores, and endochondral bone formation persisted if central core failed to vascularize. It is thus possible that membranous bone formation with COLLOSS® and COLLOSS® E is related to better penetration of those materials by blood vessels. Conversely, chondrogenic responses to COLLOSS® E may have been related to local compression of the carrier proteins impairing vascularization. Whatever the causes, induction of membranous bone formation appears to be the most characteristic response to COLLOSS® and COLLOSS® E.

6.7. SUMMARY

This study provided data relevant to three major goals. It confirmed that both COLLOSS® and COLLOSS® E contain osteo- and chondro-inductive BMPs as shown by their ability to produce new bone in an ectopic location in rats. Second, based on the area of bone produced in standardized implant sections by osteoinductive growth factors in GFm, COLLOSS®, and COLLOSS® E and their respective collagenous carrier matrices, the study showed that COLLOSS® was 0.1, and COLLOSS® E 0.3 time as potent as 10 µg of GFm. Finally, the study showed that ordinary and accelerated endochondral bone formation were more frequent in response to GFm than to COLLOSS® and COLLOSS® E, whereas membranous bone formation was more frequent in response to COLLOSS® E than to COLLOSS® or GFm.

6.8. REFERENCES

1. Urist MR. Bone Morphogenetic Protein Composition. patent 4,619,989. 1986.
2. Li H, Zou X, Woo C, Ding M, Lind M, Bunger C. Experimental anterior lumbar interbody fusion with an osteoinductive bovine bone collagen extract. Spine 2005; 30(8):890-896.
3. Huffer WE, Benedict JJ, Turner AS, Laib.A., Briest A, Rettenmaier R. Repair of sheep long bone cortical defects filled with COLLOSS, COLLOSS E, OSSAPLAST, and fresh iliac autografts. Biomaterials (submitted).

4. Walboomers XF, Jansen JA. Bone tissue induction, using a COLLOSS-filled titanium fiber mesh-scaffolding material. Biomaterials 2005; 26(23):4779-4785.
5. Urist MR. Bone formation by autoinduction. Science 1965; 150:893-899.
6. Wozney JM, Rosen V, Celeste AJ, Mitsock LM, Whitters MJ, Kriz RW et al. Novel regulators of bone formation: molecular clones and activities. Science 1988, 242(4885).1528-1534.
7. Wozney JM. The bone morphogenetic protein family: multifunctional cellular regulators in the embryo and adult. [Review] [44 refs]. European Journal of Oral Sciences 1998; 106 Suppl 1:160-166.
8. Hoffmann A, Weich HA, Gross G, Hillmann G. Perspectives in the biological function, the technical and therapeutic application of bone morphogenetic proteins. Appl Microbiol Biotechnol 2001; 57(3):294-308.
9. Hogan LM. Bone morphogenetic proteins: multifunctional regulators of vertebrate development. Genes & Development 10, 1580-1594. 1996. Ref Type: Generic
10. Bahamonde ME, Lyons KM. BMP3: to be or not to be a BMP. J Bone Joint Surg Am 2001; 83-A Suppl 1(Pt 1):S56-S62.
11. Helm GA, Li JZ, Alden TD, Hudson SB, Beres EJ, Cunningham M et al. A light and electron microscopic study of ectopic tendon and ligament formation induced by bone morphogenetic protein-13 adenoviral gene therapy. J Neurosurg 2001; 95(2):298-307.
12. Wozney JM. Overview of bone morphogenetic proteins. Spine 2002; 27(16 Suppl 1):S2-S8.
13. Poser JW, Benedict JJ. Intermedics Orthopedics/Denver Inc.Wheat Ridge C, editor. Osteoinducitve protein mixture and purification processes. patent 5290763. 1994.
14. Roethy W, Fiehn E, Suehiro K, Gu A, Yi GH, Shimizu J et al. A growth factor mixture that significantly enhances angiogenesis in vivo. J Pharmacol Exp Ther 2001; 299(2):494-500.
15. Seeherman H, Wozney J, Li R. Bone morphogenetic protein delivery systems. Spine 2002; 27(16 Suppl 1):S16-S23.
16. Sampath TK, Reddi AH. Dissociative extraction and reconstitution of extracellular matrix components involved in local bone differentiaton. Proc Natl Acad Sci USA 1981; 78:7599-7602.
17. Sampath T.K., Reddi AH. Homology of bone-inductive proteins from human, monkey, bovine, and rat extracellular matrix. Proc Natl Acad Sci USA 1983; 80(21):6591-6595.
18. Bertagnoli R. Osteoinductive bone regeneration substance Colloss in spinal fusion. European Spine Journal 11, 189-190. 2002. Ref Type: Generic
19. Cornell CN. Initial clinical experience with the use of Collagraft as a bone graft substitute. Techniques Orth 1992; 7(2):55-63.
20. Feifel H. [Bone regeneration in Pro Osteon 500 alone and in combination with Colloss in the patellar gliding model of the rabbit]. Mund Kiefer Gesichtschir 2000; 4 Suppl 2:S527-S530.
21. Kloss FR, Schlegel KA, Felszeghy E, Falk S, Wiltfang J. [Applying an osteoinductive protein complex for regeneration of osseous defects]. Mund Kiefer Gesichtschir 2004; 8(1):12-17.
22. Schlegel KA, Kloss FR, Kessler P, Schultze-Mosgau S, Nkenke E, Wiltfang J. Bone conditioning to enhance implant osseointegration: an experimental study in pigs. Int J Oral Maxillofac Implants 2003; 18(4):505-511.
23. Wiltfang J, Kloss FR, Kessler P, Nkenke E, Schultze-Mosgau S, Zimmermann R et al. Effects of platelet-rich plasma on bone healing in combination with autogenous bone and bone substitutes in critical-size defects. An animal experiment. Clin Oral Implants Res 2004; 15(2):187-193.
24. Huffer WE, Lewis M, Barnes T, Benedict JJ. Strategies for tailoring bone and connective tissue regeneration using bone protein. In: Davies JE, editor. Bone Engineering: An International Workshop. Toronto: University of Toronto Press, 2001: 408-420.
25. Sasano Y, Ohtani E, Narita K, Kagayama M, Murata M, Saito T et al. BMPs induce direct bone formation in ectopic sites independent of the endochondral ossification in vivo. Anat Rec 1993; 236(2):373-380.
26. Stoeger T, Proetzel GE, Welzel H, Papadimitriou A, Dony C, Balling R et al. In situ gene expression analysis during BMP2-induced ectopic bone formation in mice shows simultaneous endochondral and intramembranous ossification. Growth Factors 2002; 20(4):197-210.
27. Nakagawa T, Tagawa T. Ultrastructural study of direct bone formation induced by BMPs-collagen complex implanted into an ectopic site. Oral Dis 2000; 6(3):172-179.
28. Aono A, Hazama M, Notoya K, Taketomi S, Yamasaki H, Tsukuda R et al. Potent ectopic bone-inducing activity of bone morphogenetic protein-4/7 heterodimer. Biochem Biophys Res Commun 1995; 210(3):670-677.
29. Kuboki Y, Jin Q, Kikuchi M, Mamood J, Takita H. Geometry of artificial ECM: sizes of pores controlling phenotype expression in BMP-induced osteogenesis and chondrogenesis. Connect Tissue Res 2002; 43(2-3):529-534.
30. Takita H, Kikuchi M, Sato Y, Kuboki Y. Inhibition of BMP-induced ectopic bone formation by an antiangiogenic agent (epigallocatechin 3-gallate). Connect Tissue Res 2002; 43(2-3):520-523.

7

BIGLYCAN IS A POSITIVE MODULATOR OF BMP-2 INDUCED OSTEOBLAST DIFFERENTIATION

Yoshiyuki Mochida[1], Duenpim Parisuthiman[1], and Mitsuo Yamauchi[1,2]

7.1. INTRODUCTION

Development of the vertebrate skeleton is a complex process involving genes that control a series of cellular events such as proliferation, migration, mesenchymal condensations and eventually differentiation into osteoblasts and chondrocytes[1]. For osteoblast differentiation, an intricate and highly regulated interplay of growth factors, receptors/co-receptors, specific extracellular milieu and transcription factors is required[2]. Bone morphogenetic proteins (BMPs), members of the transforming growth factor-beta (TGF-β) superfamily, are multifunctional growth factors critically involved in osteoblast differentiation. The BMP functions are exerted through their interaction with specific cell surface receptors, BMP type I and II receptors, leading to the regulation of specific BMP target genes. The signaling is regulated at numerous steps at extracellular, cell surface and intracellular levels[3,4].

The extracellular matrix is a complex three dimensional network composed of heterogeneous macromolecules, including a number of small leucine-rich proteoglycans (SLRPs)[5,6]. Biglycan (BGN), a member of SLRP family, is highly expressed in the areas of growth of skeletal tissues and on the cell surface of both chondroblasts and osteoblasts[7]. Due to its location, BGN has been speculated to have roles in cell differentiation/function distinct from the closely related molecule decorin (DCN) that is mainly localized in the extracellular matrix[7].

It has been reported that mice with targeted disruption of *bgn* gene develop an age-dependent osteoporosis-like phenotype[8]. The absence of BGN may in part cause an insufficient modulation of growth factors such as TGF-β resulting in the reduced number of osteoprogenitor cells, subsequently, impaired bone formation[9,10]. Indeed several studies have demonstrated that BGN binds a number of growth factors including TGF-β superfamily[11], TGF-α[12], and tumor necrosis factor-alpha (TNF-α)[13],

---

[1] CB#7455 Dental Research Center, University of North Carolina at Chapel Hill, NC, USA.
[2] Corresponding author. Tel. 1-919-966-3441. E-mail address: mitsuo_yamauchi@dentistry.unc.edu

indicating that BGN modulates various signaling pathways. In support of this notion, BGN deficient cells responded poorly to TGF-β and BMP-4 in vitro[9, 14]. BGN also appears to modulate BMP-4 signaling in concert with chordin and twisted gastrulation, the well known BMP antagonist/agonist[15].

The multifunctionality of BGN may be associated with its ability to bind multiple molecules, thereby, inducing diverse roles depending on cell/tissue types and developmental stages. Most recently, by over- and underexpressing *bgn*, we have demonstrated that BGN promotes osteoblast differentiation[16]. In order to obtain insights into the BGN modulation of osteoblast differentiation, here we report the binding specificity of BGN to BMPs (BMP-2, -4, -6 and -7) and 8 known TGF-β/BMP receptors, and the effects of BGN on BMP-induced signaling and osteoblast differentiation.

7.2. MATERIALS AND METHODS

7.2.1. Cell Culture

Human embryonic kidney 293 cells were purchased from Clontech and maintained in Dulbecco's modified Eagle's medium (DMEM, Invitrogen) containing a high concentration of glucose (4.5 mg/ml), supplemented with 10% fetal bovine serum (FBS, Sigma). The mouse C2C12 myoblastic cells were obtained from American Type Culture Collection (ATCC; CRL-1772) and maintained in DMEM containing 15% FBS. The mouse calvaria-derived MC3T3-E1 cells (subclone 4, ATCC; CRL-2593) were maintained in α-minimum essential medium (α-MEM, Invitrogen) containing 10% FBS. Every growth medium was supplemented with 100 units/ml penicillin and 100μg/ml streptomycin. The medium was changed twice a week.

7.2.2. cDNA Construct

Mouse BMP-2, -4, -6 and -7 cDNA were isolated from MC3T3-E1 cells by reverse transcription-polymerase chain reaction (RT-PCR) employing Hotstar *Taq* polymerase (Qiagen). The sequences of the primers were designed based on the public database and they were as follows: BMP-2 forward primer, 5' ACCATGGTGGCCGGGACCCGCTG 3' and reverse primer, 5' ACGACACCCGC AGCCCTCCACAAC 3', BMP-4 forward primer, 5' ACCATGATTCCTGGTAAC CGAATGCTG 3' and reverse primer, 5' GCGGCATCCACACCCCTCTACCAC 3', BMP-6 forward primer 5' GCGATG CCCGGGCTGGGGCG 3' and reverse primer, 5' ATGGCAACCACAAGCTTCAC 3', BMP-7 forward primer, 5' GCGATGCACG TGCGCTCGCTGCGC 3' and reverse primer, 5' GTGGCAGCCACAGGCC CGGACCAC 3'. The PCR products of each BMP were ligated into pcDNA3.1-V5/His-TOPO mammalian expression vector (Invitrogen), sequenced at the UNC-CH DNA Sequencing Facility (University of North Carolina, Chapel Hill, NC), and the plasmids harboring V5/His-tagged BMP cDNAs (pcDNA3.1-BMPs -V5/His vectors) were obtained. The BGN cDNA cloned previously[16] was ligated into pcDNA3 vector (Invitrogen) with hemagglutinin (HA) tag (kindly provided by Dr. H. Ichijo, University of Tokyo, Japan), and the construct (pcDNA3-BGN-HA) was obtained and sequenced.

The HA-tagged vectors harboring TGF-β/BMP type I receptors, i.e. activin receptor-like kinase 1-6 (ALK1-6), TGF-β/BMP type II receptors (TGFβRII and BMPRII)[17-19] were generous gifts from Drs. K. Miyazono (University of Tokyo, Japan) and T. Imamura (The JFCR Cancer Institute, Japan).

7.2.3. Immunoprecipitation-Western Blot Analyses

293 cells were transfected with a combination of a pcDNA3-BGN-HA vector and each of the pcDNA3.1-BMP (2, 4, 6, 7)-V5/His vectors using FuGENE6 transfection reagent (Roche Diagnostics) according to the manufacturer's instructions. After 72 hours, the cultured medium was collected and immunoprecipitated (IP) with either anti-V5 antibody (Invitrogen) or anti-HA antibody (clone 12CA5, Roche Diagnostics). After addition of protein A-sepharose 4B conjugate (Zymed Laboratories), the samples were incubated for additional 15 min, and the beads were washed once with RIPA buffer containing 150mM NaCl, 50mM Tris-HCl pH8.0, 1% NP-40, 0.1% sodium dodecyl sulfate (SDS), 0.5% deoxycholate, 1.5% aprotinin and 1mM phenylmethylsulfonyl fluoride (PMSF), and twice with lysis buffer containing 150mM NaCl, 20mM Tris-HCl pH7.5, 10mM EDTA, 1% Triton X-100, 1% deoxycholate, 1.5% aprotinin and 1mM PMSF. Proteins bound to the beads were dissolved in SDS sample buffer (100mM Tris-HCl pH8.8, 0.01% bromophenol blue, 36% glycerol, 4% SDS) in the presence of 10mM dithiothreitol (DTT), applied to 4-12% gradient SDS-polyacrylamide gel electrophoresis (PAGE), transferred onto a polyvinylidene fluoride (PVDF) membrane (Immobilon-P, Millipore), and Western blot (WB) analysis was performed with either anti-V5 antibody or anti-HA antibody (clone 3F10, Roche Diagnostics). The immunoreactive bands were visualized with an Alkaline Phosphatase Conjugate Substrate Kit (Bio-rad).

To investigate the binding between BGN and TGF-β/BMP receptors, 293 cells were cotransfected with a combination of a pcDNA3.1-BGN-V5/His vector and each of the HA-tagged TGF-β/BMP receptor (ALK1-6, TGF-βRII, BMPRII) containing vectors in a similar manner as described. After the transfection, the expression of BGN was confirmed by analyzing the cultured media by IP-WB with anti-V5 antibody. The cells were then lysed with lysis buffer, and the supernatants obtained by the centrifugation were further immunoprecipitated with anti-HA antibody. IP-WB analyses were performed and the binding of BGN to the receptors was examined using anti-V5 antibody. Aliquots of the supernatants were subjected to WB analysis to confirm the expression of the receptors. After the binding of BGN to ALK6 was determined using 293 cells, the binding was further confirmed by the use of MC3T3-E1 osteoblastic cells. In this set of experiment, various amounts of pcDNA3.1-BGN-V5/His vector (0.45, 0.75, and 1.5 µg) were transfected together with 2.0 µg of HA-tagged ALK6 vector, the cells were lysed in the same manner as described above, and the supernatants were immunoprecipitated using anti-V5 antibody. Proteins bound to the beads were dissolved in SDS sample buffer, applied to 10% SDS-PAGE, and WB analysis was performed in the same manner as described.

7.2.4. Generation of Recombinant Glutathione-S-Transferase (GST)-BGN Fusion Protein

In order to examine the direct binding of BGN to BMPs, recombinant BGN fused with GST protein (GST-BGN) was generated. The primer sequences of BGN cDNA corresponding to its mature core protein (amino acids 38-369; Asp^{38}-Lys^{369}) were designed as follows: forward primer, 5' GCGGATCCGATGAGGAGGCTTCAGGT 3' and reverse primer, 5' GCCTCGAGCTACTTCTTATAATTTCC 3'. The PCR products amplified were then ligated into a pGEX4T-1 vector (Amersham Biosciences), sequenced, and the plasmid harboring the mature BGN cDNA (pGEX4T-1-BGN) was obtained. pGEX4T-1-BGN or pGEX4T-1 empty vector was transformed into BL21-CodonPlus bacterial strain (Stratagene), cultured, and the synthesis of GST-BGN fusion protein or GST protein alone was induced by isopropylthio-β-galactosidase (IPTG, Fisher). The bacteria were further cultured at 20 °C overnight. The cultures were then centrifuged and lysed in phosphate buffered saline (PBS) containing 1% Triton X-100. After the centrifugation, the supernatants were incubated with glutathione-sepharose beads (Amersham Biosciences) overnight and the beads were extensively washed with PBS. The beads were then treated with the elution buffer (10mM glutathione, 50mM Tris-HCl pH8.0) to release the conjugated proteins. The eluted proteins were pooled, dialyzed against distilled water, lyophilized and resuspended in distilled water. The protein concentration of each GST protein was measured by a plate reader using a DC protein assay kit (Bio-rad). Aliquots of each GST protein were mixed with SDS sample buffer, applied to 4-12 % SDS-PAGE, and stained with Coomassie Brilliant Blue R-250 (CBB) (Bio-rad). An aliquot of the GST-BGN protein generated was subjected to WB analysis with polyclonal antibody against mouse BGN core protein (LF-159, generous gift from Dr. Fisher L.W., NIDCR, MD) and the immunoreactivity of the protein was confirmed.

7.2.5. GST Pull Down Assay

In order to investigate the direct interaction between BGN and BMPs, GST protein or GST-BGN protein was incubated with 500 ng of each recombinant human BMP (rhBMP-2, -4, -6, and -7, R&D systems) at 4 °C overnight. After addition of glutathione-sepharose beads, the samples were washed with lysis buffer twice, mixed with SDS sample buffer, applied to 4-12 % SDS-PAGE and stained using a Silver stain plus kit (Bio-rad). The consistency of the amounts of rhBMPs mixed with GST proteins were also verified by 4-12% SDS-PAGE followed by CBB staining.

7.2.6. Smad Phosphorylation Assay

C2C12 cells were treated with 50 ng/ml of rhBMP-2 in combination with GST protein or GST-BGN protein, and incubated up to 4 hours. At four time points (0, 1, 2, and 4 hours), cells were washed with PBS twice, and cell extracts were prepared with RIPA buffer. After the centrifugation, the supernatants were collected, dissolved in SDS sample buffer, and applied to 4-12% SDS-PAGE. WB analyses were performed with anti-phospho-Smad1/5/8 antibody (Cell Signaling), or anti-Smad1 antibody (clone A-4, Santa Cruz). Signals were detected by the immunoreactivity and were analyzed by Scion Image Software (Scion corporation).

7.2.7. Alkaline Phosphatase (ALP) Activity

C2C12 cells were plated onto 35 mm plastic dishes in duplicate at a density of 2 $X10^5$ cells/well. On the following day, the concentration of FBS was reduced to 5%, and cells were treated with varied concentrations (0, 50, 100ng/ml) of rhBMP-2 in combination with GST protein or GST-BGN protein. After 4 days, cell cultures were washed with PBS twice and ALP activity was analyzed using an alkaline phosphatase kit (Sigma Diagnostics) according to the manufacturer's instructions. Three independent experiments were performed to confirm the results.

7.2.8. Quantitative Real Time RT-PCR

C2C12 cells were plated onto 35 mm plastic dishes in duplicate at a density of 2 $\times 10^5$ cells/well, and were treated with or without 100 ng/ml of rhBMP-2 in combination with GST protein or GST-BGN protein in the same manner as described above. After 4 days, total RNA was extracted by means of the TRIzol REAGENT (Invitrogen) solution. Two µg of total RNA extract was used for RT using an Omniscript RT Kit (Qiagen) according to the manufacturer's protocol. Real time PCR primers-probes of myogenic and osteogenic markers used in this study were as follows; myogenic differentiation 1 (Myod1, ABI assay number: Mm00440387_m1); core binding factor 1/runt-related transcription factor 2 (Cbfa1/Runx2, Mm00501578_m1); alkaline phosphatase 2, liver (Akp2, Mm00475831_m1); type I collagen alpha 2 chain (Col1A2, Mm00483888_m1); bone sialoprotein (BSP, Mm00492555_m1); osterix (Osx, Mm00504574_m1). Real time PCR was performed in triplicate using the ABI Prism 7000 Sequence detection system (Applied Biosystems). The mean fold changes in the expression of each myogenic and osteogenic marker relative to that of glyceraldehyde-3-phosphate dehydrogenase (GAPDH, ABI assay number: 4308313) were calculated using the values of cDNA derived from the cell culture treated with GST protein alone as a calibrator by means of $2^{-\Delta\Delta C_T}$ method as described previously[20].

7.3. RESULTS

7.3.1. BGN Directly Binds to BMP-2

In order to determine the binding of BGN to several BMP members that are known to be expressed in osteoblastic cells[2], we first examined the binding by cotransfecting 293 cells with BGN- and BMP-containing vectors followed by IP-WB. As shown in Figure 7.1.a, BGN appeared as a smear band (lower panel, lanes 2-6) indicating that BGN was synthesized as a proteoglycan. The BMP expression levels are relatively consistent (middle panel). The binding of BGN to BMPs is shown in the upper panel of Figure 7.1.a. The results demonstrated that the binding of BGN to BMP-2 (lane 2), -4 (lane 3) and -6 (lane 4) occurred in a cell culture system. No binding was observed between BGN and BMP-7 (lane 5). In order to determine whether or not the binding observed is direct (i.e. without the presence of other molecules), we next examined the binding by incubating the recombinant BMP (rhBMP)-2, -4, -6, or -7 with recombinant GST-BGN fusion protein *in vitro* followed by GST pull down assay (Figure 7.1.b). The amounts of rhBMPs, GST and GST-BGN used for the pull down are shown in the lower panels of the figure, and the binding in the upper panel. GST alone did not bind to any rhBMPs tested (upper panel). When incubated with GST-BGN, only BMP-2, but not -4, -6 and -7, showed the binding (upper panel). These results suggest that BMP-2 is a direct binding partner of BGN.

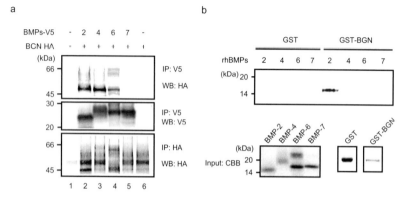

Figure 7.1. BGN directly binds to BMP-2. (a) Binding assay in a cell culture system. 293 cells were transiently cotransfected with BGN-HA and BMPs-V5 containing expression vectors. The cultured medium was collected, incubated with either anti-V5 antibody or anti-HA antibody. BGN bound to BMPs was analyzed by Western blotting (WB) using anti-HA antibody (upper panel). The comparable expression levels of several BMPs or BGN in each lane were verified by WB using anti-V5 antibody (middle panel) or anti-HA antibody (lower panel), respectively. Positions of molecular weight standards (kDa) are indicated on each panel. Note the significant binding of BGN to BMP-2 and, to a lesser extent to BMP-4 and -6 (upper panel). (b) Binding assay by GST pull down. The recombinant BMPs were incubated with either GST protein alone or GST-BGN protein and coupled to glutathione beads. After washing the beads, the bound proteins were visualized by Silver staining (upper panel). The amounts of recombinant BMPs, GST proteins and GST-BGN protein were assessed by Coomassie Brilliant Blue (CBB) staining to ensure the comparable amounts of BMPs, GST, and GST-BGN proteins used (lower panels). Positions of molecular weight standards (kDa) are indicated. Note that GST protein alone does not bind to any BMPs but GST-BGN binds only to BMP-2 (upper panel).

7.3.2. Effects of BGN on BMP-2-induced Smad Phosphorylation in C2C12 Cells

It has been generally accepted that upon BMP stimulation, specific downstream signaling molecules Smad 1/5/8 are phosphorylated via the hetero-oligomeric association of BMP type I and II receptors[21]. The phosphorylated Smad proteins are then translocated into the nucleus to regulate the expression of several osteogenic markers[4]. Thus, we next investigated the effect of BGN on the Smad 1/5/8 phosphorylation using C2C12 cells. This cell line has been well characterized and widely used to investigate the BMP-2 induced transdifferentiation from myoblast to osteoblastic cells[22]. When BMP-2 together with GST protein was added to C2C12 cells, the phosphorylation of Smad1/5/8 was observed at 1 hour, and decreased thereafter (Figure 7.2.a), showing a similar pattern to that induced by BMP-4 reported previously[23]. However, when combined with GST-BGN, the phosphorylation was enhanced at 1 hr, and the high level was sustained after this time point up to 4 hrs (Figure 7.2.a). These results strongly indicate that BGN enhances BMP-2 induced signaling.

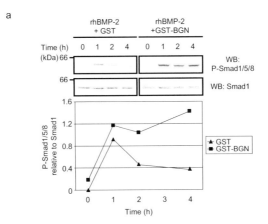
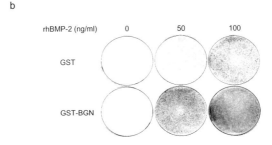

Figure 7.2. BGN enhances BMP-2-induced-Smad phosphorylation and -ALP activity in C2C12 cells. (a) Effects of BGN on BMP-2-induced Smad phosphorylation. C2C12 cells were treated with 50 ng/ml of BMP-2 (rhBMP-2) together with GST protein or GST-BGN protein, and were incubated for the indicated time periods. The cell lysates were analyzed by WB using anti-phospho Smad1/5/8 antibody (P-Smad1/5/8) and anti-Smad1 antibody, respectively. The level of phosphorylated Smad proteins was normalized to that of Smad1 protein in the same lysates using Scion Image Software. Note that GST-BGN significantly enhances and sustains the Smad phosphorylation. (b) Effects of BGN on BMP-2-induced ALP activity. C2C12 cells were treated with varied concentration of BMP-2 together with GST protein or GST-BGN protein and incubated for 4 days. ALP activity was analyzed as described in Methods. Three independent experiments were performed and similar results were obtained.

7.3.3. Effects of BGN on BMP-2-induced ALP Activity in C2C12 Cells

The effect of BGN on BMP-2 induced osteoblast differentiation was then investigated by the use of C2C12 cells. The cells were treated with various concentrations of rhBMP-2 together with GST protein or GST-BGN protein, cultured for 4 days, and the activities of alkaline phosphatase (ALP), an early osteogenic marker, were determined (Figure 7.2.b). The results demonstrated that rhBMP-2 in the presence of GST protein increased the ALP activity in a dose dependent manner as reported previously[22]. When rhBMP-2 was combined with GST-BGN protein, the ALP activities were synergistically increased in the cell cultures in comparison to those treated with rhBMP-2 and GST protein. No ALP activity was observed in the cell cultures treated with GST protein or GST-BGN alone. These results clearly demonstrate that BGN enhances the BMP-2-induced ALP activity, thus osteoblast differentiation, likely through its direct interaction with BMP-2.

7.3.4. Effects of BGN on the Expression of Myogenic and Osteogenic Markers in C2C12 Cells Stimulated by BMP-2

When differentiated into osteoblasts by BMP-2, C2C12 cells are known to suppress myogenic makers and upregulate several osteogenic markers[24]. Thus, the effects of BGN on the expression of those markers in this process were assessed by quantitative real time PCR (Figure 7.3.). The expression level of Myod1, a myogenic marker[25], was downregulated with the treatment of GST-BGN protein or rhBMP-2 alone. When treated with both rhBMP-2 and GST-BGN protein combined, the expression level was further decreased in comparison to the treatment with GST-BGN protein or rhBMP-2 alone.

For osteogenic markers, when treated with BMP-2 and GST-BGN protein combined, the expression levels of Cbfa1/Runx2 and Col1A2 were significantly upregulated in the cell culture in comparison to those treated with GST-BGN protein or rhBMP-2 alone. The expression of other osteogenic markers such as Akp2, BSP, and Osx was synergistically upregulated upon the treatment of both GST-BGN protein and BMP-2 in comparison with that of GST-BGN protein or BMP-2 alone.

7.3.5. BGN Specifically Binds to ALK6, a BMP-2 Receptor

It has been demonstrated that BGN is localized on the cell surface[7], thereby, assisting BMP binding to the cells[14]. Thus, in order to gain insights into the BGN-assisted BMP-2 function, we further examined a potential binding of BGN to the known TGF- /BMP cell surface receptors. 293 cells were cotransfected with vectors containing BGN-V5 and each of the TGF-β/BMP type I and II receptors (ALK1-6, TGFβRII or BMPRII)-HA, and IP-WB analyses were performed in the same manner as described above. As shown in Figure 7.4.a, among the receptors tested, ALK6 showed a specific binding to BGN (upper panel of Figure 7.4.a, lane 7). A slight binding of BGN to ALK5, a TGF-β type I receptor, was also detected (upper panel of Figure 7.4.a, lane 6). In order to confirm the specific binding of BGN to ALK6 in osteoblasts, MC3T3-E1 cells were cotransfected with vectors containing ALK6-HA and various amounts of BGN-V5, and the cell lysate was immunoprecipitated using anti-V5 antibody. As shown in Figure 7.4.b, the specific binding between BGN and ALK6 was also confirmed in MC3T3-E1 osteoblastic cells and the binding indeed occurred in a dose dependent manner.

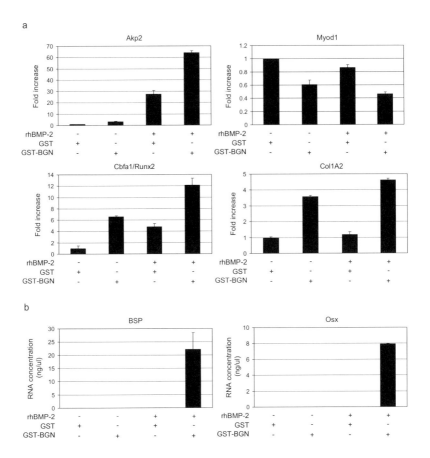

Figure 7.3. Effects of BGN on BMP-2 induced osteoblast differentiation in C2C12 cells. Quantitative real time RT-PCR was performed using specific primers-probes for a myogenic marker (Myod1) and several osteogenic markers (Akp2, Cbfa1/Runx2, Col1A2, BSP, and Osx). The mean fold changes in the expression of each marker relative to that of GAPDH were calculated using the expression value of the samples treated with GST protein alone as a calibrator, and are shown in (a). Since the expression of BSP and Osx was detected only when cells were treated with BMP-2 in the presence of GST-BGN protein, the expression levels were calculated based on their own standard curves, and are shown as RNA concentrations in (b). The values are shown as mean ± S.D. based on triplicate measurements.

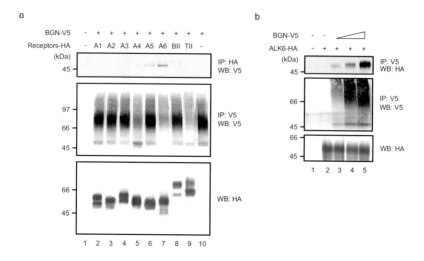

Figure 7.4. BGN binds to ALK6. (a) 293 cells were transiently cotransfected with BGN-V5 and TGF-β/BMP receptor-HA expression vectors (A1-A6; ALK1-6, B II; BMP type II receptor, T II; TGF-β type II receptor) and IP-WB analyses were performed as described in Methods. Positions of molecular weight standards (kDa) are shown on the left of each panel. Note, though a very slight binding to ALK5 was detected, BGN binds most specifically to ALK6 among all the receptors tested. (b) BGN-ALK6 binding using MC3T3-E1 osteoblasts. MC3T3-E1 cells were cotransfected with BGN-V5 and ALK6-HA expression vectors. To verify the binding of BGN to ALK6, various doses of BGN were used for transfection together with ALK6, and the binding was detected by IP-WB analysis as described in Methods. The binding between BGN and ALK6 was observed in a dose dependent manner. Positions of molecular weight standards (kDa) are shown on the left of each panel.

7.4. DISCUSSION

BMPs were originally identified by their abilities to induce ectopic bone formation[26]. Of more than 20 BMP members, it has been reported that BMP-2, -4 and -7 are expressed in MC3T3-E1 osteoblastic cells[2] and the expression of BMP-6 in this cell line was confirmed in the present study. Recent studies have indicated that the BMP functions are partially modulated by an extracellular matrix proteoglycan, BGN[14-16]. Though an interaction between BGN and BMP-4 was indicated in these studies, the binding of BGN to other BMPs is not well understood. In the present study, we investigated the binding specificity of BGN to BMPs and their receptors, and the effect of BGN on BMP-2 induced osteoblast differentiation.

The results of our binding assay in a cell culture system indicated that BGN binds to BMP-2, -4 and -6, but not to -7 (Figure 7.1.a). However, when GST pull down assay was performed using recombinant GST-BGN and rhBMPs, the binding of GST-BGN was seen only to BMP-2, but not other BMPs including BMP-4 and -6. It is not clear as to why GST-BGN protein failed to bind to BMP-4 and -6 *in vitro* (Figure 7.1.b). The possible explanations include; 1) the binding sites of BGN to BMP-4 or -6 might be associated with glycosaminoglycan (GAG) chains, propeptide, and/or the N-glycosylated regions of BGN, since GST-BGN was produced in bacteria as a mature form (i.e. no propeptide) without any posttranslational modifications, 2) the binding between BGN and BMP-4 or -6 might involve other molecules, thus not direct. The involvement of GAG chains is less likely since BGN after treatment with chondroitinase ABC still binds at least to BMP-2 and -4[15]. In any case, it is clear that of the four BMPs tested, BMP-2 is a direct and preferential binding partner of BGN. This preferential binding is rather surprising considering the high level of sequence identity between BMP-2 and -4 (85% identical among the mature forms). A possible explanation may be the difference in the number of N-glycosylation sites that are present near the receptor binding regions of those BMPs[27]. Based on the NetNGlyc 1.0 Server program (http://www.cbs.dtu.dk/services/NetNGlyc/), it is predicted that BMP-2 has only one N-glycosylation site, while BMP-4 has two. The slower migration position of BMP-4 than BMP-2 on SDS-PAGE may reflect this difference (Figure 7.1.a; middle panel, lanes 2 and 3, and 7.1.b; lower panel). Recently, it has been demonstrated that BGN can form a multi binding complex together with BMP-4 and chordin[15], a well known BMP-4 antagonist. The failure of recombinant GST-BGN to bind BMP-4 or BMP-6 may also be due to the absence of such other BMP binding molecules in vitro.

There are a number of extracellular BMP antagonists identified[28], however, little is known about the positive extracellular modulators. It has been reported that loss of glycosylphosphatidylinositol (GPI)-anchoring heparin sulfate large proteoglycan, glypican-3 (GPC3) abrogated the effects of BMP-2-Smad signaling, suggesting GPC3 modulates BMP-2 signaling pathway[29]. Very recently, it has been demonstrated that DRAGON, another GPI-anchoring protein, enhances BMP-specific signaling via the direct interaction with BMP-2 and -4, but not with BMP-7 or TGF-β[30]. BGN lacks any transmembrane regions or C-terminal GPI attachment site based on the PSORT II prediction program (http://psort.nibb.ac.jp/ form2.html) and the detection/prediction of GPI cleavage site (GPI-anchor) in a protein program (http://129.194.185.165/dgpi/ DGPI_demo_en.html) *in silico*. Thus, BGN acts as a positive modulator of BMP-2 signaling through a mechanism distinct from those GPI-anchoring molecules. Our novel finding on the ability of BGN to bind both BMP-2 and its receptor, ALK6 (Figures 7.1. and 7.4.), may imply a potential mechanism. ALK6 has been demonstrated as a type I receptor for BMP-2[31] and shown to be expressed in MC3T3-E1 osteoblastic cells[32]. A BGN-BMP-2 complex may be a more efficient ligand for the BMP-2 receptor, thus, enhancing its signaling. Or BGN may stabilize the interaction of BMP-2 with ALK6 by binding both molecules, thus, help sustain the BMP-2/ALK6 binding and the subsequent phosphorylation/signaling as shown in Figure 7.2.a. The binding may lead to ALK6 involved specific gene expression and promote osteoblast differentiation.

The positive regulation of BMP-2 signaling by BGN is also apparent by its effects on BMP-2 induced osteoblast differentiation of C2C12 cells. The addition of GST-BGN to BMP-2 further suppressed the myogenic marker, Myod1, and synergistically upregulated the expression of osteogenic markers, Akp2, BSP and Osx. The effects on the Cbfa1/Runx2 and Col1A2 expression were rather additional. The synergistic effect of BGN was also seen on the ALP activity (Figure 7.2.b). Interestingly, our recent study has shown that in the clones underexpressing BGN, the expression of Cbfa1/Runx2, Col1A2, BSP, and Osx was downregulated at day 7 in culture, but at day 14 the expression of the first two markers; i.e. Cbfa1/Runx2 and Col1A2 became comparable to that of the control cells while that of BSP and Osx still remained significantly suppressed[16]. These differential effects observed may suggest that BGN-BMP2-ALK6 signaling may control the expression of specific osteogenic markers such as Akp2, BSP, and Osx.

In conclusion, in this study, we demonstrated that BGN binds to BMP-2 and its receptor, ALK6, and that BGN promotes BMP-2 induced osteoblast differentiation likely through its specific bindings. Further studies are obviously warranted to elucidate the mechanisms by which BGN potentiates the BMP-2 signaling pathway. Such understanding may lead to the development of efficient strategies for skeletal tissue engineering/regeneration.

7.5. ACKNOWLEDGMENTS

This study was supported by NIH grants AR052824, DE10489 and NASA grant NAG 2-1596.

7.6. REFERENCES

1. B. R. Olsen, A. M. Reginato, and W. Wang, Bone development, *Annu Rev Cell Dev Biol* **16**, 191-220 (2000).
2. G. Xiao, R. Gopalakrishnan, D. Jiang, E. Reith, M. D. Benson, and R. T. Franceschi, Bone morphogenetic proteins, extracellular matrix, and mitogen-activated protein kinase signaling pathways are required for osteoblast-specific gene expression and differentiation in MC3T3-E1 cells, *J Bone Miner Res* **17**(1), 101-110 (2002).
3. K. Miyazono, S. Maeda, and T. Imamura, BMP receptor signaling: transcriptional targets, regulation of signals, and signaling cross-talk, *Cytokine Growth Factor Rev* **16**(3), 251-263 (2005).
4. P. ten Dijke, O. Korchynskyi, G. Valdimarsdottir, and M. J. Goumans, Controlling cell fate by bone morphogenetic protein receptors, *Mol Cell Endocrinol* **211**(1-2), 105-113 (2003).
5. R. V. Iozzo, The biology of the small leucine-rich proteoglycans. Functional network of interactive proteins, *J Biol Chem* **274**(27), 18843-18846 (1999).
6. L. Ameye, and M. F. Young, Mice deficient in small leucine-rich proteoglycans: novel in vivo models for osteoporosis, osteoarthritis, Ehlers-Danlos syndrome, muscular dystrophy, and corneal diseases, *Glycobiology* **12**(9), 107R-116R (2002).
7. P. Bianco, L. W. Fisher, M. F. Young, J. D. Termine, and P. G. Robey, Expression and localization of the two small proteoglycans biglycan and decorin in developing human skeletal and non-skeletal tissues, *J Histochem Cytochem* **38**(11), 1549-1563 (1990).
8. T. Xu, P. Bianco, L. W. Fisher, G. Longenecker, E. Smith, S. Goldstein, J. Bonadio, A. Boskey, A. M. Heegaard, B. Sommer, K. Satomura, P. Dominguez, C. Zhao, A. B. Kulkarni, P. G. Robey, and M. F. Young, Targeted disruption of the biglycan gene leads to an osteoporosis-like phenotype in mice, *Nat Genet* **20**(1), 78-82 (1998).
9. X. D. Chen, S. Shi, T. Xu, P. G. Robey, and M. F. Young, Age-related osteoporosis in biglycan-deficient mice is related to defects in bone marrow stromal cells, *J Bone Miner Res* **17**(2), 331-340 (2002).
10. Y. Bi, C. H. Stuelten, T. Kilts, S. Wadhwa, R. V. Iozzo, P. G. Robey, X. D. Chen, and M. F. Young, Extracellular matrix proteoglycans control the fate of bone marrow stromal cells, *J Biol Chem* **280**(34), 30481-30489 (2005).
11. A. Hildebrand, M. Romaris, L. M. Rasmussen, D. Heinegard, D. R. Twardzik, W. A. Border, and E. Ruoslahti, Interaction of the small interstitial proteoglycans biglycan, decorin and fibromodulin with transforming growth factor beta, *Biochem J* **302** (Pt 2), 527-534 (1994).
12. Y. Hayashi, C. Y. Liu, J. J. Jester, M. Hayashi, I. J. Wang, J. L. Funderburgh, S. Saika, P. J. Roughley, C. W. Kao, and W. W. Kao, Excess biglycan causes eyelid malformation by perturbing muscle development and TGF-alpha signaling, *Dev Biol* **277**(1), 222-234 (2005).
13. E. Tufvesson, and G. Westergren-Thorsson, Tumour necrosis factor-alpha interacts with biglycan and decorin, *FEBS Lett* **530**(1-3), 124-128 (2002).
14. X. D. Chen, L. W. Fisher, P. G. Robey, and M. F. Young, The small leucine-rich proteoglycan biglycan modulates BMP-4-induced osteoblast differentiation, *Faseb J* **18**(9), 948-958 (2004).
15. M. Moreno, R. Munoz, F. Aroca, M. Labarca, E. Brandan, and J. Larrain, Biglycan is a new extracellular component of the Chordin-BMP4 signaling pathway, *Embo J* **24**(7), 1397-1405 (2005).
16. D. Parisuthiman, Y. Mochida, W. R. Duarte, and M. Yamauchi, Biglycan modulates osteoblast differentiation and matrix mineralization, *J Bone Miner Res* **20**(10), 1878-1886 (2005).

17. T. Imamura, M. Takase, A. Nishihara, E. Oeda, J. Hanai, M. Kawabata, and K. Miyazono, Smad6 inhibits signalling by the TGF-beta superfamily, *Nature* **389**(6651), 622-626 (1997).
18. T. Ebisawa, K. Tada, I. Kitajima, K. Tojo, T. K. Sampath, M. Kawabata, K. Miyazono, and T. Imamura, Characterization of bone morphogenetic protein-6 signaling pathways in osteoblast differentiation, *J Cell Sci* **112 (Pt 20),** 3519-3527 (1999).
19. A. Nishihara, T. Watabe, T. Imamura, and K. Miyazono, Functional heterogeneity of bone morphogenetic protein receptor-II mutants found in patients with primary pulmonary hypertension, *Mol Biol Cell* **13**(9), 3055-3063 (2002).
20. K. J. Livak, and T. D. Schmittgen, Analysis of relative gene expression data using real-time quantitative PCR and the 2(-Delta Delta C(T)) Method, *Methods* **25**(4), 402-408 (2001).
21. H. Itoh, M. Yamauchi, H. Kataoka, R. Hamasuna, N. Kitamura, and M. Koono, Genomic structure and chromosomal localization of the human hepatocyte growth factor activator inhibitor type 1 and 2 genes, *Eur J Biochem* **267**(11), 3351-3359 (2000).
22. T. Katagiri, A. Yamaguchi, M. Komaki, E. Abe, N. Takahashi, T. Ikeda, V. Rosen, J. M. Wozney, A. Fujisawa-Sehara, and T. Suda, Bone morphogenetic protein-2 converts the differentiation pathway of C2C12 myoblasts into the osteoblast lineage, *J Cell Biol* **127**(6 Pt 1), 1755-1766 (1994).
23. S. Maeda, M. Hayashi, S. Komiya, T. Imamura, and K. Miyazono, Endogenous TGF-beta signaling suppresses maturation of osteoblastic mesenchymal cells, *Embo J* **23**(3), 552-563 (2004).
24. S. Harada, and G. A. Rodan, Control of osteoblast function and regulation of bone mass, *Nature* **423**(6937), 349-355 (2003).
25. L. A. Sabourin, and M. A. Rudnicki, The molecular regulation of myogenesis, *Clin Genet* **57**(1), 16-25 (2000).
26. J. M. Wozney, V. Rosen, A. J. Celeste, L. M. Mitsock, M. J. Whitters, R. W. Kriz, R. M. Hewick, and E. A. Wang, Novel regulators of bone formation: molecular clones and activities, *Science* **242**(4885), 1528-1534 (1988).
27. T. Kirsch, W. Sebald, and M. K. Dreyer, Crystal structure of the BMP-2-BRIA ectodomain complex, *Nat Struct Biol* **7**(6), 492-496 (2000).
28. J. Garcia Abreu, C. Coffinier, J. Larrain, M. Oelgeschlager, and E. M. De Robertis, Chordin-like CR domains and the regulation of evolutionarily conserved extracellular signaling systems, *Gene* **287**(1-2), 39-47 (2002).
29. S. Hartwig, M. C. Hu, C. Cella, T. Piscione, J. Filmus, and N. D. Rosenblum, Glypican-3 modulates inhibitory Bmp2-Smad signaling to control renal development in vivo, *Mech Dev* **122**(7-8), 928-938 (2005).
30. T. A. Samad, A. Rebbapragada, E. Bell, Y. Zhang, Y. Sidis, S. J. Jeong, J. A. Campagna, S. Perusini, D. A. Fabrizio, A. L. Schneyer, H. Y. Lin, A. H. Brivanlou, L. Attisano, and C. J. Woolf, DRAGON, a bone morphogenetic protein co-receptor, *J Biol Chem* **280**(14), 14122-14129 (2005).
31. H. Nishitoh, H. Ichijo, M. Kimura, T. Matsumoto, F. Makishima, A. Yamaguchi, H. Yamashita, S. Enomoto, and K. Miyazono, Identification of type I and type II serine/threonine kinase receptors for growth/differentiation factor-5, *J Biol Chem* **271**(35), 21345-21352 (1996).
32. A. Nohe, S. Hassel, M. Ehrlich, F. Neubauer, W. Sebald, Y. I. Henis, and P. Knaus, The mode of bone morphogenetic protein (BMP) receptor oligomerization determines different BMP-2 signaling pathways, *J Biol Chem* **277**(7), 5330-5338 (2002).

8

USE OF NEOPTERIN AS A BONE MARROW HEMATOPOIETIC AND STROMAL CELL GROWTH FACTOR IN TISSUE-ENGINEERED DEVICES

E. Zvetkova[1*], Y. Gluhcheva[1], and D. Fuchs[2]

8.1. ABSTRACT

The *in vitro* response of early haematopoietic progenitors or stem cells (CD34+) — common for myeloid (granulocyte, eosinophil, megakaryocyte) and marrow stromal cell lineages, to neopterin, exogenously added to the liquid mouse bone marrow cultures, at doses 12.5–25 μg/ml culture medium, has been studied. The results obtained show a significant stimulation of common — myeloid and stromal/mesenchymal progenitor cell proliferation and differentiation, as early as 24h to the 96h after the *in vitro* treatment with neopterin. On day 4 of cultivation the granulocyte/macrophageal proliferation and differentiation has been attenuated giving place to the marrow stromal/mesenchymal cell growth and differentiation. A functional role of neopterin as hematopoietic growth factor — essential for the proliferation and differentiation of bone marrow common (hematopoietic and stromal) progenitors is not yet clear and remains to be elucidated. The *in vitro* and *ex vivo* applying of neopterin — alone or in specific combinations with other cytokines (e.g. FGF-2) for the induction of marrow stromal/mesenchymal cell proliferation and differentiation, merits further investigations with regards to its future use in regenerative medicine. The results provide a theoretical basis for the application of neopterin in tissue-engineered devices: incorporated into biodegradable polymer microparticles (with encapsulated early bone marrow progenitors and other special supplements), it could be experimentally applied for fast and easy induction of endothelial, osteoblastic/osteogenic, neuronal and other cell lineage differentiation as well as for improving tissue trophical processes and reparative microenvironment.

---

[1] Institute of Experimental Morphology and Anthropology with Museum, Bulgarian Academy of Sciences, Sofia, Bulgaria
[2] Division of Biological Chemistry, Biocentre, Innsbruck Medical University, Innsbruck, Austria
* To whom all correspondence should be directed – e-mail address: ezvetkova@hotmail.com

8.2. INTRODUCTION

Bone marrow cells from erythroid, granulocyte/macrophageal (G/M), megakaryocytic (Mg) and stromal/mesenchymal cell (S/MeC) lineages have a subset of common early marrow progenitors (CD34+) giving rise to blood- and stromal cell growth and differentiation. Several cytokines or cytokine cocktails contribute to marrow hematopoietic and/or stromal cell growth and differentiation — in normal and pathological conditions [2-7]. Recently, a functional role of neopterin for the proliferation and differentiation of bone marrow common hematopoietic and stromal/mesenchymal progenitors (early hematopoietic and stromal colony and cluster formation) was elucidated [1, 2, 12, 20-24].

Neopterin is a metabolite of guanosine triphosphate (GTP) in the synthetic pathway of biopterin and large amounts of it are produced by monocytes/macrophages — in response to stimulation with interferon-γ (IFN-γ) [15, 9, 17].

The aim of the study is to examine the in vitro response of mouse bone marrow stromal/mesenchymal progenitors to exogenously added neopterin as hematopoietic and stromal cell growth factor.

8.3. MATERIAL AND METHODS

8.3.1. Solutions and Media

IMDM and fetal calf serum (FCS) for cultivation *in vitro* were obtained from GIBCO.

8.3.2. Mouse Bone Marrow-Derived Cell (mBMCs) Suspension and In Vitro Cultivation

Mouse bone marrow cells (mBMCs) were isolated in IMDM from femurs of BALB/c mice. Cell suspension (10^6 nucleated cells/ml medium — IMDM) was cultivated in conditions of liquid marrow cultures, after modifications of previously reported methods [20,21,26].

The *in vitro* morphological/cytochemical characteristics of bone marrow hematopoietic and stromal cell progenitors — in response to neopterin (Schricks Laboratories, Jona, Switzerland), exogenously added to the liquid mouse bone marrow cultures at doses 12.5– 5 µg/ml (tested as optimal *in vitro* [20,21,23]), have been examined after 24-, 48-, 72- and 96 h of cultivation.

Control liquid mouse bone marrow cultures — without exogenously added neopterin, were also investigated.

8.3.3. Cytochemical Staining Methods

The non-adherent hematopoietic cells from control and neopterin-treated liquid mouse bone marrow cultures were collected and cytocentrifuged. Cytospin preparations obtained were stained in situ with methylene blue/fast green — for DNP, RNP and some basic (cytoplasmic and nuclear) proteins [25,26].

The same cytochemical staining methods [25,26] were additionally applied on the bottom of plastics (Nunc Petri dishes) — to visualize cell colonies and clusters of adherent stromal/mesenchymal marrow cells.

The hematopoietic cell groups – colonies and clusters, in the cytospin preparations (from the liquid parts of cultures), as well as the adherent stromal cells, stained *in situ* (on plastics), were examined by light microscopy (Opton).

8.4. RESULTS

The results of the control experiments (samples without stimulus — exogenously added neopterin), were negative: no proliferation, differentiation and blood cell colony-formation was observed.

The results obtained after addition of exogenous neopterin (at doses 12.5 to 25 μm) to the liquid marrow cultures show stimulated *in vitro* myeloid (granulocyte-, eosinophil-, monocyte/macrophage- and megakaryocyte-) cell proliferation, differentiation and colony formation as early as 24 hours (Figure 8.1).

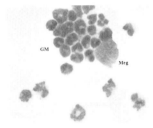

Figure 8.1. Cytospin preparation from the liquid mouse bone marrow culture exogenously treated (24h) with neopterin. GM-cluster (**GM**) with a single megakaryocyte (**Meg**) x 600.

At this time, the marrow stromal/mesenchymal cells were not yet proliferating and differentiating *in vitro*: they were not visible as groups adhering on the bottom of plastics and only individual stromal cells could be seen in cytospin preparations — around undifferentiated granulocyte- (G-) and granulocyte-macrophageal (GM-) colonies.

After 96h of *in vitro* cultivation (at the same doses of exogeneous neopterin treatment), the growth of G- and GM- colonies have been attenuated giving place to an intensive stromal/mesenchymal cell proliferation and differentiation: sporadic nodule-like stromal and endothelial cell groups appeared in liquid phase of cultures and/or adhered on the bottom of Petri dishes (Figure 8.2).

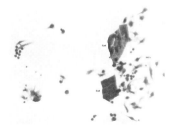

Figure 8.2. Proliferating stromal cells (**StCs**) and two groups of endothelial cells (**End**) on the bottom of plastic (Petri dishes) after 96h cultivation of mouse bone marrow in the presence of exogenously added neopterin x 450.

Since day 4 to day 7 of *in vitro* cultivation the bone marrow stromal/ mesenchymal cells — mainly with fibroblast-like morphology (spindle-shaped, with extending cytoplasmic processes), considerably enhanced their adhesiveness and attachment to the glass coverslips and/or to the bottom of plastics, forming abundant cytoplasmic protrusions and intercellular relationships and reaching confluency (Figures 8.3 and 8.4).

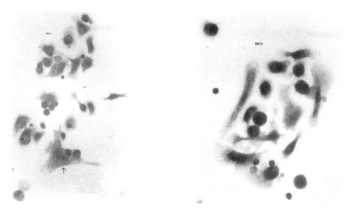

Figures 8.3. and 8.4. Stromal cells (**StCs**) from liquid mouse bone marrow cultures exogenously treated with neopterin: adherent on the bottom of plastics (Petri dishes) fibroblast-like cells with extending cytoplasmic processes and a stromal cell with dendrite-like cytoplasmic protrusions (**arrow**) x 1250

At the same time one could see also clusters of undifferentiated – lymphocyte-like cells (probably very early common progenitors), localized near and/or in direct contact with the stromal cells (Figure 8.5).

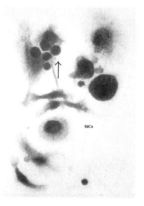

Figure 8.5. Bone marrow stromal cells (**StCs**) from neopterin treated cultures adhered on the bottom of plastics (Petri dishes) and are localized near the clusters of undifferentiated lymphocyte-like cells (**arrow**) x 1250

8.5. DISCUSSION

The induction of myeloid (granulocyte-macrophageal) and marrow stromal cell proliferation/differentiation and colony formation in liquid mouse bone marrow cultures and/or on the bottom of plastics — in the presence of exogenously added neopterin, characterized this biologically active substance as a hematopoietic (granulocyte-macrophageal) and marrow stromal / mesenchymal cell growth factor [1,2,20-24].

The significance of the selective clonal stimulation of myeloid and/or stromal bone marrow progenitors *in vitro* – under influence of exogenously added neopterin could be compared to the effects of other marrow hematopoietic and stromal cell growth factors and cytokine cocktails — M-CSF, GM-CSF, FGF-2 etc. [2-7]. The possible *ex vivo* or clinical application of neopterin — alone and/or in specific combinations with other cytokines and growth factors, in the induction of marrow stromal/mesenchymal cell proliferation and differentiation could be compared only with the *in vitro* use of FGF-2 [7] and merits further investigations.

In our study we focused on the *in vitro* stimulatory effects of neopterin on bone marrow stromal / mesenchymal and endothelial cell growth (proliferation and differentiation) from multipotent stem cells. It was shown the possibility for very early hematopoietic and stromal colony and cluster formation after exogenous addition of neopterin to mouse bone marrow cultures — probably of practical importance in the regenerative medicine and tissue engineering. The formation of stromal / mesenchymal cell cytoplasmic protrusions and cell-to-cell relationships under the *in vitro* influence of neopterin, correlate with the production of extracellular matrix and fibers with high adhesiveness (probably containing fibronectin and/or other cell adhesion molecules) and could be interpreted as a sign of complete (terminal) marrow stromal cell differentiation [19,22-24].

We suppose that the increased *in vitro* proliferation/differentiation of marrow stromal cells – in the presence of exogenous neopterin, could enhance (early in the culture period) the influence of other lineage specific stimuli (e.g. osteogenic, chondrogenic, neuronal, endothelial): it's well established that the marrow stromal/mesenchymal progenitors could give rise to fibroblasts, osteocytes, chondrocytes, myocytes, adipocytes, endothelial and neuronal cells [4,5,8,10,11]. This provides theoretical basis for the future use of neopterin in tissue-engineered devices. We suggest that neopterin, incorporated into biodegradable polymer microparticles – with encapsulated early bone marrow stromal progenitors and other specific supplements, could be applied for induction of endothelial, osteoblastic/osteogenic, chondrogenic and neuronal cell differentiation as well as for improving tissue trophical processes and reparative microenvironment [10,11,13].

In addition, it is well known [3,6,18] that marrow stromal/mesenchymal stem cells express the enzyme indoleamine 2,3 – dioxygenase (IDO): IDO degrades tryptophan and creates a tryptophan-depleted milieu, thus promoting immunosuppression. This suggests new approaches to determine the successful use of human marrow MSCs for the purposes of the regenerative medicine [3,13,14,16].

We supposed that exogenously increasing neopterin concentration in our culture system additionally may lead to lower tryptophan amount in the milieu which is essential for further tissue-engineering applications. In this sense, we hypothesize that better understanding of the molecular mechanisms of neopterin affecting the differentiation of marrow stromal cells will allow researchers to manipulate in a new manner adult marrow mesenchymal stem cells (*in vitro* and *ex vivo*). These results could be also quantified in other experimental designs (e.g. by flow cytometry in order to determine DNA, RNA and protein content of growing *in vitro* — in the presence of exogenous neopterin, hematopoietic and stromal cells).

8.6. CONCLUSION

The more important approaches currently utilizing mesenchymal stem cells are tissue engineering and gene therapy — both exploit the current knowledge in molecular/cellular biology and biomaterial science to direct MSCs to differentiate *in vivo* to desired lineages and tissues. In this regard, the functional role of neopterin as a marrow hematopoietic, stromal and endothelial cell growth factor – influencing *in vitro* the proliferation and differentiation of early common (hematopoietic and mesenchymal) marrow progenitors, is not yet clear and remains to be elucidated.

8.7. ACKNOWLEDGMENTS

This work is supported by Austrian Ministry of Education and Technology, under Contract with Austrian Science and Research Liaison, OSI, Office Sofia.

8.8. REFERENCES

1. S. Aizawa, M. Hiramoto, S. Araki, H. Hoshi, S. Kojima, K. Wakasugi, In vivo stimulatory effects of neopterin on hematopoiesis, Pteridines 9, 13-17 (1998).
2. S. Aizawa, M. Hiramoto, S. Araki, S. Negishi, Y. Kimura, H. Hoshi, S. Kojima, K. Wakasugi, Stimulatory effects of neopterin on hematopoiesis in vitro are mediated by activation of stromal cell function, Hematol Oncol 16(2), 57-67 (1998).
3. F. Barry, J. Murphy, K. English, B. Mahon, Immunogenicity of adult mesenchymal stem cells: lessons from the fetal allograft, Stem Cells Dev 14(3), 252 – 265 (2005).
4. J. Chen, S. Sotome, J. Wang, H. Orii, T. Uemura, K. Shinomiya, Correlation of in vivo bone formation capability and in vitro differentiation of human bone marrow stromal cells, J Med Dent Sci 52(1), 27 – 34 (2005).
5. H. Egusa, F. Schweizer, C. Wang, Y. Matsuka, I. Nishimura, Neuronal differentiation of bone marrow-derived stromal stem cells involves suppression of discordant phenotypes through gene silencing, J Biol Chem 280(25), 23691-23697 (2005).
6. B. Frick, K. Schroecksnadel, G. Neurauter, F. Leblhuber and D. Fuchs, Increasing production of homocysteine and neopterin and degradation of tryptophan with older age, Clin Biochem 37(8), 684 – 687(2004).
7. S. Hankemeier, M. Keus, J. Zeichen, M. Jagodzinski, T. Barkhausen, U. Bosch, C. Krettek, M. Van Griensven, Modulation of proliferation and differentiation of human bone marrow stromal cells by fibroblast growth factor 2: potential implications for tissue engineering of tendons and ligaments, Tissue Eng 11(1-2), 41 – 49 (2005).
8. N. Hibino, T. Shin'oka, G. Matsumura, Y. Ikada, H. Kurosawa, The tissue- engineered vascular graft using bone marrow without culture, J Thorac Cardiovasc Surg 129(5), 1064 – 1070 (2005).
9. C. Huber, J. Batchelor, D. Fuchs, A. Hausen, A. Lang, D. Niederwieser, G. Reibnegger, P. Swetly, J. Troppmair, H. Wachter, Immune response-associated production of neopterin. Release from macrophages primarily under control of interferon-gamma, J Exp Med 160(1), 310-316 (1984).
10. J. Hui, H. Ouyang, D. Hutmacher, J. Goh, E. Lee, Mesenchymal stem cells in the musculoskeletal tissue engineering: a review of recent advances in national University of Singapore, Ann Acad Med Singapore 34(2), 206-212 (2005).
11. I. Kan, E. Melamed, D. Offen, Integral therapeutic potential of bone marrow mesenchymal stem cells, Curr Drug Targets 6(1), 31-41 (2005).
12. Y. Kawakami, S. Aizawa, M. Hiramoto, I. Tsuboi, K. Wakasugi, Effects of neopterin on the proliferation and differentiation of hematopoietic progenitors derived from human umbilical cord blood, Pteridines 14(4), 129-132 (2003).
13. G. Pelled, G. Turgeman, H. Aslan, Z. Gazit, D. Gazit, Mesenchymal stem cells for bone gene therapy and tissue engineering, Curr Pharm Des 8(21), 1917-1928 (2002).
14. J. Plumas, L. Chaperot, M. Richard, J. Molens, J. Bensa, M. Favrot, Mesenchymal stem cells induce apoptosis of activated T cells, Leukemia 19(9), 1597-1604 (2005).
15. H. Rembold, W. Gyure, Biochemistry of the pteridines, Angew Chem Int Ed Engl 11(12), 1061-1072 (1972).
16. J. Ryan, F. Barry, J. Murphy, B. Mahon, Mesenchymal stem cells avoid allogeneic rejection, J Inflamm (Lond) 2(1), 8-18 (2005).

17. H. Wachter, D. Fuchs, A. Hausen, G. Reibnegger, G. Weiss, E. R. Werner, G. Werner-Felmayer, Neopterin: Biochemistry – Methods – Clinical application. De Gruyter, Berlin – New York, 1992
18. G. Werner-Felmayer, E. R. Werner, D. Fuchs, A. Hausen, G. Reibnegger, H. Wachter, Neopterin formation and tryptophan degradation by a human myelomonocytic cell line (THP-1) upon cytokine treatment, Cancer Res 50(10), 2863 – 2870 (1990).
19. W. Zhang, X. Walboomers, J. Wolke, Z. Bian, M. Fan, J. Jansen, Differentiation ability of rat postnatal dental pulp cells in vitro, Tissue Engineering 11(3-4), 357 – 368 (2005).
20. E. Zvetkova, E. Janeva, E. Nikolova, G. Milchev, A. Dikov, I. Tsenov, N. Bojilova, A. I. Hadjioloff, Hemopoietic colony-stimulating activity of ranopterins in murine bone marrow agar cultures, Compt Rend Acad Bulg Sci 44, 91-94 (1991).
21. E. Zvetkova, I. Tsenov, E. Katzarova, M. Bratanov, P. Angelova, I. Chowdhury, B. Nikolov, A. Dikov, In vitro proliferation of mouse bone marrow lymphocytes and stromal macrophages under the biological action of ranopterin (neopterin), Compt Rend Acad Bulg Sci 48, 81-84 (1995).
22. E. Zvetkova, Ranopterins — amphibia skin pteridines displaying hematopoietic, immunomodulatory and macrophageal proliferative biological activities, Pteridines 10, 178-189 (1999).
23. E. Zvetkova, D. Fuchs, E. Katzarova, M. Bakalska, M. Svetoslavova, B. Nikolov, Neopterin acting as a bone marrow stem cell factor on early common hematopoietic (myeloid) and stromal (dendritic, CD34+) cell progenitors in vitro, Pteridines 12, 135-139 (2001).
24. E. Zvetkova, D. Fuchs, E. Katzarova, M. Bakalska, M. Svetoslavova, B. Nikolov, I. Tsenov, I. Ilieva, Exogenously added in vitro neopterin is the bone marrow stem cell factor (BMSCF) acting on the early common hematopoietic (myeloid) and stromal (dendritic – CD34+) cell progenitors, Acta morphologica et anthropologica 6, 39-44 (2001).
25. E. Zvetkova, I. Zvetkov, A cytological method for the simultaneous staining of nucleoproteins and some cationic proteins, Acta Histochem 57, 1 – 13 (1976).
26. E. Zvetkova, J. Jelinek, Methylene blue-fast green staining of hematopoietic colonies in agar cultures, Gegenbaurs Morphol Jahrb 135, 779 – 793 (1989).

SECTION 3

SCAFFOLDS AND MATRIX DESIGN

9

INJECTABLE SYNTHETIC EXTRACELLULAR MATRICES FOR TISSUE ENGINEERING AND REPAIR

Glenn D. Prestwich[1,3,4], Xiao Zheng Shu[1,4], Yanchun Liu[1,4], Shenshen Cai[1,4], Jennifer F. Walsh[2,4], Casey W. Hughes[2,4], Shama Ahmad[2,4], Kelly R. Kirker[2], Bolan Yu[1,4], Richard R. Orlandi[3,4], Albert H. Park[3,4], Susan L. Thibeault[3,4], Suzy Duflo[3,4], and Marshall E. Smith[3,4]

9.1. INTRODUCTION

The development of novel biointeractive hydrogels for tissue engineering[1-3], tissue repair, and release of drugs[4] and growth factors[5] has attracted considerable attention over the past decade. Our attention has focused on hydrogels based on the extracellular matrix (ECM), a heterogeneous collection of covalent and noncovalent molecular interactions comprised primary of proteins and glycosaminoglycans (GAGs)[6]. In the ECM, covalent interactions connect chondroitin sulfate (CS), heparan sulfate (HS) and other sulfated GAGs to core proteins forming proteoglycans (PGs). Noncovalent interactions include binding of link modules of PGs to hyaluronan (HA), electrostatic associations with ions, hydration of the polysaccharide chains, and triple helix formation to generate collagen fibrils.

HA, a non-sulfated GAG present in all connective tissue as a major constituent of the ECM, has key roles in morphogenesis[7], and important factor for a potential scaffold for tissue engineering. HA, a versatile starting material for preparing biodegradable biomaterials,[8] has poor biomechanical properties, and its rapid degradation *in vivo* preclude many direct clinical applications. The literature on use of chemically-modified HA for drug delivery[9-11] and for biomaterials has been recently reviewed[12,13]. In order to develop hydrogel scaffolds that could perform the functions of an ECM *in vivo*, we

---

[1] Department of Medicinal Chemistry, The University of Utah, Salt Lake City, Utah, USA
[2] Department of Bioengineering, The University of Utah, Salt Lake City, Utah, USA
[3] Department of Surgery, The University of Utah, Salt Lake City, Utah, USA
[4] Center for Therapeutic Biomaterials, The University of Utah, Salt Lake City, Utah, USA

selected a chemical modification strategy that would allow a chemical simplification of the inherent complexity of the biological system.

Using this strategy, we recently developed a novel approach to prepare a covalently-crosslinked, synthetic ECM (sECM)[14]. The sECM material may be crosslinked *in situ* in the presence of cells in order to provide an injectable cell-seeded hydrogel for tissue repair. Alternatively, an injectable gel could be used with controlled-release, localized delivery of drugs or growth factors. Thiol-modified GAGs, proteins, and other carboxylate-containing polymers are the macromonomeric units that can be crosslinked with biocompatibile polyvalent electrophiles to form biocompatible, bioerodable hydrogels and porous sponges.

This overview focuses on the creation and use of sECMs based on crosslinked GAGs. We highlight selected applications of this technology, including *in vitro* and *in vivo* growth of healthy cellularized tissues using films, sponges, and hydrogels based upon the sECM technology. Specific examples of the *in situ* crosslinkable sECM include the *in vivo* repair of cartilage and bone defects, and the repair of tympanic membrane perforations. Other examples include the use of biointeractive, crosslinked heparin-containing GAG dressings for controlled release of basic fibroblast growth factor (bFGF) and concomitant re-epithelialization of full-thickness wounds in diabetic mice. Post-surgical adhesions can be prevented and sinus ostia can be maintained *in vivo* using crosslinked HA hydrogels, with or without covalently linked antiproliferatives.

9.2. A COVALENT, SYNTHETIC EXTRACELLULAR MATRIX (sECM)

9.2.1. The Vision

Figure 9.1 visualizes the strategy for creating covalently-crosslinked sECMs, as developed at the Center for Therapeutic Biomaterials. We envisaged three basic types of sECM, based on the clinical problem for which a solution was required. In the left panel of Figure 9.1, HA derivatives are crosslinked with different lengths and rigidities of crosslinkers to give HA-only sECMs with the stiffness, elasticity, and rate of degradation required for a specific clinical use. The crosslinked HA hydrogels were first developed as wound dressings for full-thickness[15] and partial-thickness wounds[16]. More recently, newer modification and crosslinking chemistries have provided materials for applications in which the clinical goal is scar-free healing. The crosslinked HA-only sECM provides hydration and a nonimmunogenic, non-inflammatory barrier to which normal cells cannot attach and through which they will not migrate. Such a biologically benign barrier has immediate uses for scar-free mucosal healing following endoscopic sinus surgery[17,18], for prevention of post-surgical abdominal adhesions[19], for vocal fold injections as a treatment for dysphonia[20], and as a potential coating for intubation tubes and airway stents to minimize subglottic stenosis[21]. A thiol-modified HA was employed as the building-block, with crosslinking by disulfide bond formation or crosslinking with difunctional electrophiles. The physical forms could be hydrogels, films, or injectable highly viscous solutions.

The center panel of Figure 9.1 illustrates an sECM biomaterial for 3-dimensional (3-D) cell growth *in vitro* or *in vivo*. The simplest version of this sECM was composed of thiol-modified HA and thiol-modified gelatin (Gtn), co-crosslinked by disulfide bonds or by conjugate addition. The hydrogels could be lyophilized to give implantable, cell-seeded porous sponge-like scaffolds, or the hydrogels could be used for *in vivo* cell delivery or as injectable devices for filling defects. Finally, the right panel shows a multi-component sECM in which thiol-modified HA, CS, Gtn, and heparin (HP) all co-crosslinked to give a better compositional mimic of the natural ECM that would also permit controlled release of a growth factor or small molecules.

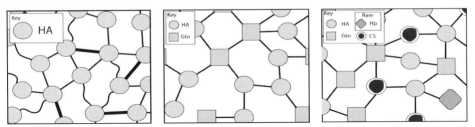

Figure 9.1 (see color insert, Fig. 9.1). Covalent, crosslinked, sECMs for different medical device applications (as drawn by Justin Chafe). **Left**, an HA-only material for scar-free healing and adhesion prevention; **Center**, a two-component sECM for 3-D cell growth *in vitro* and for tissue repair and engineering *in vivo*; **Right**, a multicomponent sECM for optimization of cell attachment as well as delivery of drugs and growth factors.

9.2.2. The Realization

To implement the vision of a modular, clinically versatile and readily-manufactured sECM, we developed a thiol-introduction chemistry based upon the modification of the carboxylate groups of GAGs, proteins, and other synthetic polymers by hydrazide formation. In the early1990s, we discovered that hydrazide derivatives, which maintain their nucleophilicity at low pH, can be efficiently condensed with GAG carboxyl groups at pH 4.5 using a water-soluble carbodiimid[22,23]. These mild aqueous conditions do not alter other chemical groups required for biological function of the GAG. Moreover, when the hydrazide reagent contains a disulfide bond[24], thiol-modified proteins and GAGs can be prepared and crosslinked into hydrogels under cytocompatible physio–logical conditions[25].

Thus, a three-step process is employed[25]. First, the disulfide hydrazide 3,3'-di(thiopropionyl) bishydrazide (DTPH) is used to modify the carboxyl groups of HA, CS, HP, or Gtn. Second, the disulfide bonds are reduced with dithiothreitol (DTT) to give, after dialysis, the thiol-modified macromonomers such as HA-DTPH, CS-DTPH, HP-DTPH, and Gtn-DTPH. Third, the monomers are crosslinked oxidatively to a hydrogel, which may be dried as a thin film or lyophilized to produce a porous sponge. Alternatively, crosslinking with difunctional electrophiles can be accomplished, in the presence or absence of cells, to give injectable and biocompatible hydrogels[14].

Figure 9.2 illustrates the basic chemistry of three types of injectable sECM that implement the vision diagrammed in Figure 9.1. The simplest form is a polyethylene glycol diacrylate (PEGDA)-crosslinked HA-DTPH (Figure 9.2A)[14]. Since cells cannot readily attach and spread on this material, it is best employed for adhesion prevention and scar-free healing of wounded tissues. To achieve an array of different physical properties and rates of biodegradation, we have examined and now control several parameters for the biocompatible HA-DTPH-PEGDA hydrogels[26]: (i) molecular weight of starting HA employed, from 20 kDa to 1,500 kDa; (ii) percentage DTPH modification (degree of substitution); (iii) concentration of HA-DTPH in the hydrogel; (iv) molecular weight of PEGDA; and (v) ratio of thiols to acrylates (an excess of thiol groups minimizes reactive electrophiles in the final product). We have also investigated polyfunctional acrylates, acrylamides, and additional thiol-reactive groups, e.g., PEG divinyl sulfone[27].

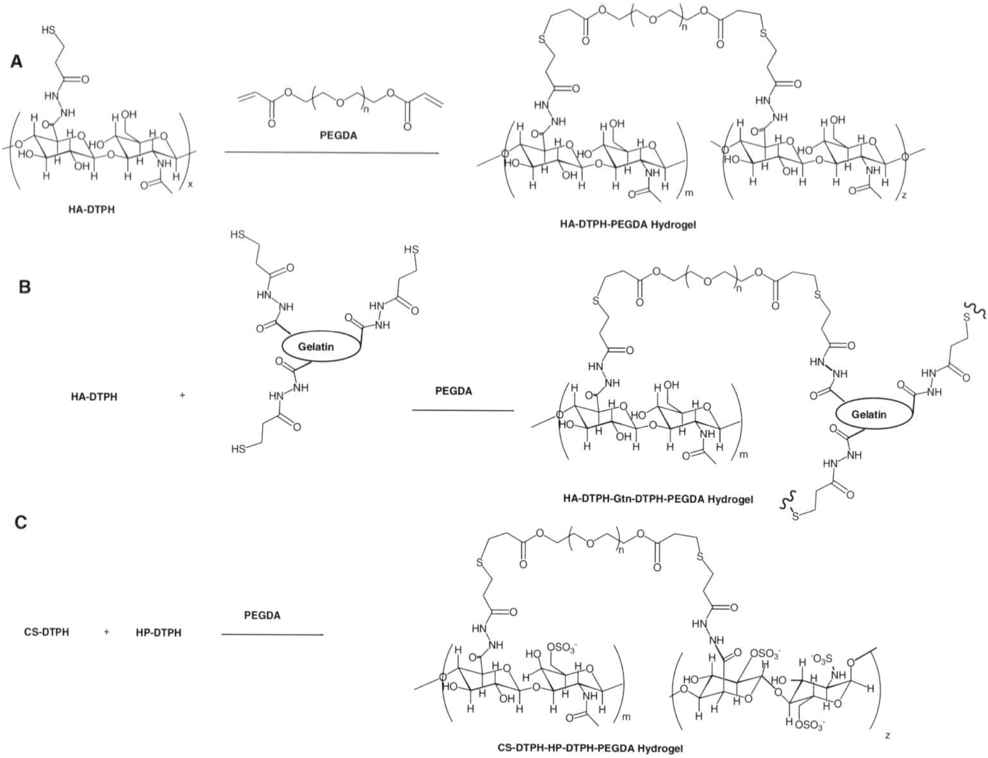

Figure 9.2. Chemical structures for the sECMs. **Panel A**, HA-DTPH-PEGDA for adhesion prevention and scar-free healing; **Panel B**, HA-DTPH-Gelatin-DTPH-PEGDA for 3-D cell growth; **Panel C**, CS-DTPH-HP-DTPH-PEGDA for controlled release of growth factors for angiogenesis and treatment of chronic wounds.

Figure 9.2B illustrates the minimal version of an sECM that is designed to support cell attachment, growth, and proliferation in 3D. By co-crosslinking the thiol-modified gelatin (Gtn-DTPH) with HA-DTPH, we obtained materials to which cells readily attached and spread[28]. This can be accomplished with lyophilized macroporous sponges based on disulfide co-crosslinking, or with injectable materials using PEGDA crosslinking. In this case, gelatin replaces the use of either an RGD peptide[29] or selected domains of fibronectin[30], both of which have been employed to convert HA-DTPH into an sECM capable of cell growth. For many applications, the 50:50 (w/w) HA-DTPH:Gtn-DTPH composition appears optimal[28]. The enzymatic processing of the co-crosslinked materials by hyaluronidase or collagenase is greatly reduced when the two biopolymers are covalently linked together in a hydrogel network.

A multifunctional sECM is required to both permit cell growth and simultaneously enhance the rate of neovascularization (Figure 9.2C). We have used sECMs composed of co-crosslinked HA-DTPH and HP-DTPH, CS-DTPH and HP-DTPH, and more recently formulations with thiol-modified HA, Gtn, and HP. These have been employed for controlled release of bFGF, vascular endothelial growth factor (VEGF)[31], and dual release of VEGF and keratinocyte growth factor (KGF)[32]. The addition of co-crosslinked HP-DTPH as low as 1% of the total GAG present gives a half-life for bFGF release of over one month *in vitro*[33].

Recently, the CTB has developed new biopolymer modification chemistries to improve the biological and physical properties of HA. Now licensed to Sentrx Surgical, Inc., the proprietary[34] Carbylan™-S is a biocompatible, thiol-modified semisynthetic glycosaminoglycan analogous to HA-DTPH[25]. When crosslinked with PEGDA, the resulting material, Carbylan™-SX, is analogous in function and physical properties to the HA-DTPH-PEGDA (Figure 9.2A). When mixed with gelatin-DTPH and crosslinked with PEGDA, the resulting co-crosslinked sECM hydrogel, Carbylan™-GSX, is obtained. Carbylan™-GSX is analogous in function to the HA-Gtn co-crosslinked material in Figure 9.2B. As discussed below, the Carbylan™-based materials perform in an equivalent or superior fashion *in vitro* and *in vivo* to the HA-derived materials.

9.3. BIOLOGICAL APPLICATIONS IN CELL CULTURE AND ANIMAL MODELS

9.3.1. *In Vitro* Applications

We have explored the growth of primary cells, untransformed cell lines, and cancer cell lines in the sECM hydrogels. As we adjust the chemistry of the modification, the chemistry of the crosslinkers, or the biomaterials properties, we use *in vitro* testing to confirm cytocompatibility and evaluate degradation rates. In general, each material is tested in three or four ways. First, we add the separate macromonomeric components in escalating doses to cells cultured on polystyrene plates in 2-D using normal serum-containing media. A viability assay, e.g., the MTS assay, provides a read-out for biocompability of the individual components prior to the crosslinking reaction for 8 to 24 h periods. Second, we form a 3-D hydrogel of a given sECM in the wells of a tissue culture plate, and seed cells on the surface of this hydrogel. This modified 2-D cell culture simply replaces the polystyrene surface with an sECM surface that has clearly defined biomaterial and chemical properties. In this test, we observe cell attachment, growth and proliferation each day for up to one week. Third, we add the cells and medium to the mixture of thiolated macromonomers and co-crosslink the components in the presence of cells. This is generally performed in tissue culture inserts that are seated into the wells of a plate and immersed in medium that is changed daily. An alternative to this cell encapsulation assay is the casting of the 3-D hydrogel in the insert followed by lyophilization. The resulting macroporous spongelike scaffolds are then seeded with cells and grown for several days. In both gels and sponges, viability is determined with MTS assays or cell growth and proliferation is determined by sectioning the materials and performing histological or immunocytochemical staining after a given growth period.

To date, we have cultured the following normal cells and cell lines *in vitro* in 3-D using either the co-crosslinked HA-Gtn or Carbylan™-GSX sECM hydrogels and sponges: T31 human tracheal scar fibroblasts, human dermal fibroblasts, human breast epithelial cells, human adipose-derived stem cells, L929 and NIH 3T3 murine fibroblasts, rat primary bone marrow stromal cells, rat primary hepatocytes, pig primary chondrocytes, and MCF10A human breast cells. In all cases, cells attachment and proliferation led to healthy tissue-like constructs. In addition, we have cultured a variety of human cancer cell lines in 3-D: breast (MCF-7, SK-Br-3, MDA-MB-231, MDA-MB-468), ovarian (OVCAR-3, SK-OV-3), colon (HCT-116, Caco-2), and pancreatic (MiaPaCa-2). In these examples, tumor-like masses result from *in vitro* cell culture if growth is allowed to proceed unchecked. These studies validated the 3-D injectable hydrogel for development of an *in vivo* xenograft model as discussed below.

Three studies will be highlighted that demonstrate the novel *in vitro* applications of the Carbylan™-GSX and HA-DTPH-Gtn-DTPH-PEGDA hydrogels and sponges. First, the unique features of this *in situ* crosslinkable and cytocompatible HA-DTPH-Gtn-DTPH-PEGDA system were recently demonstrated by using this material for centrifugal casting of a tubular construct containing quail endothelial cells expressing green fluorescent protein[34]. These experiments constituted a proof of concept for the ability to produce multilayer cellularized tubular constructs for engineering of vascular grafts and urethral replacements.

Second, we have been exploring the 3-D culture of primary rat hepatocytes to permit *in vitro* toxicological screening for drug discovery programs. Using Carbylan™-GSX, primary hepatocytes from perfused livers were grown *in vitro* and evaluated daily for the activity of the enzyme EROD, a cytochrome P-450 that demethylates ethoxyresorufin. Culture in 3-D was compared with primary hepatocytes grown in 2-D on Type I-coated polystyrene tissue culture plates. While the 2-D cultured cells lost enzyme activity gradually over a nine-day period, the 3-D cultured hepatocytes demonstrated a cyclical rise and fall of EROD activity that lasted beyond the 17-day test period.

Third, we have begun to use the 3-D system for both *in vitro* and *in vivo* evaluation of new anti-proliferative anti-cancer drugs[35]. The *in vitro* model uses the tissue culture insert method and permits medium-throughput evaluation of potential new drugs in 3-D as a pre-screen for efficacy prior to conducting animal studies. The *in vivo* application of this technique ultimately allows the orthotopic growth of either cancer cell lines or of unpassaged, human-derived biopsy materials in 3-D in a mouse xenograft model. The profound implications of the sECM for drug toxicity testing in 3-D and for personalized medicine have not escaped our notice.

9.3.2. *In Vivo* Applications

In addition to evaluating the sECMs shown in Figure 9.2 as reagents for *in vitro* cell culture or controlled release of growth factors[33] or antiproliferative agents[19,36], we have extensively evaluated the sECMs in specific animal models for human diseases. Several published and unpublished studies using these sECMs were cited in the introduction. Below we highlight several of the newest applications, and we note the increased use of the sECMs based upon the thiol-modified semisynthetic GAG known as Carbylan™-S or on sECMs using CS-DTPH and HP-DTPH.

For example, we used the heparin-containing gels that showed extended growth factor release (Figure 9.2C)[33] to examine the efficacy of this sECM in an animal model for chronic wound repair. Thus, we incorporated 2, 10, and 20 μg of bFGF into crosslinked CS or CS-HP sECMs and examined the effects of these bioresorbable, single application wound dressings on 1.6 cm full-thickness wounds in diabetic (*db/db*) mice. In a dose-dependent effect, the release of bFGF from a PEGDA-crosslinked 5% HP-DTPH: 95% CS-DTPH sECM resulting in dramatically accelerated healing. With 20 μg bFGF, the wound was 90% healed in two weeks, while untreated wounds reached less than 22% closure within the same time frame.

Moreover, we have shifted the majority of our studies to the replacement of HA-DTPH with Carbylan™-S. For the Figure 9.1A "HA-only" constructs, the PEGDA-crosslinked material Carbylan™-SX has been established as superior to HA-DTPH-PEGDA for prevention of post-surgical adhesions and promotion of scar-free healing in five animal models (unpublished results): rat uterine horn abrasion, rat caecal abrasion, rabbit sinus ostial maintenance,[17] and rabbit subglottic airway healing. In two published studies, Carbylan™-SX promoted healing in scoop-biopsied rabbit vocal folds[20].

Carbylan™-GSX serves as an excellent template for cell growth *in vivo*. For example, as yet unpublished work in progress has demonstrated *in vivo* efficacy (and in fact superiority to the HA-DTPH-Gtn-DTPH-PEGDA shown in Figure 9.2B) in several quite diverse animal models. First, we have found that Carbylan™-GSX hydrogels and sponges accelerate re-epithelialization and repair in a guinea pig model of tympanic membrane perforation (unpublished results). The new sECM reduced healing time from 4 days to less than 2 days, and significantly outperforms currently used products such as Epifilm™ and Gelfoam™. Indeed, these two materials show no difference from control myringotomies in this assay.

Second, injection of Carbylan™-GSX with varying amounts of gelatin showed that the viscoelasticity of biopsied rabbit vocal folds was substantially restored to normal with as little as 5% w/w gelatin present in the injectable hydrogel[37]. Third, we compared Carbylan™-GSX hydrogels and Carbylan™-GSX lyophilized sponges with and without human demineralized bone matrix (DBM) for repair of rat femoral defects. The dramatic results showed that although a 5-mm critical defect was less than 25% healed after 8 weeks in control animals, the Carbylan™-GSX-DBM sponge effectively gave complete bone defect repair in 6 weeks[38].

Fourth, we examined cell delivery models. Subcutaneous growth of primary human breast epithelial cells, human dermal fibroblasts, and human tracheal scar fibroblasts in nude mice showed excellent growth of normally vascularized tissues with diameters of up to 1 cm. In addition, installation of primary hepatocytes in a 3D sECM of Carbylan™-GSX restored liver structure and function in a 90% hepatectomy model in nude mice (unpublished results).

The ultimate goal of this research is the development of clinically-useful products that could achieve FDA approval as medical devices. Device-drug combinations that would permit localized release of growth factors, antibiotics, anti-inflammatory drugs, or anti-adhesive agents would be follow-on products for development. An example for adhesion prevention would be the inclusion of a small molecule anti-adhesive or anti-proliferative drug to improve the performance of adhesion-preventing barriers. A mitomycin-C (MMC) containing sECM has been prepared and tested *in vitro* for MMC release[36] and *in vivo* for prevention of adhesions in a rat uterine horn model[19]. Such drug-device combinations would likely require a 3 to 5 year timeline for an approvable product. Third, we imagined combination devices incorporating autologous or stem cells for tissue engineering and organ printing. We anticipated that these would have significantly longer timelines for product development and regulatory approval. Nonetheless, the clinical potential of the sECM technology will only be realized when cell-seeded hydrogels are used in applications such as the restoration of liver or pancreas function, or the implantation a new cardiovascular network or an engineered joint.

9.4. ACKNOWLEDGMENTS

Financial support was provided by Technology Commercialization Program of The University of Utah, by the NIH (1R01-DC 04336 to the late Steven D. Gray and G.D.P., and 2R01- DC 04336 to S.L.T. and G.D.P.), by NIH flow-through STTR funds from Sentrx Surgical, Inc., and by the Centers of Excellence Program of the State of Utah.

9.5. REFERENCES

1. Lee, K. & Mooney, D. Hydrogels for tissue engineering. *Chem. Rev.* **101**, 1869-1879 (2001).
2. Sakiyama-Elbert, S. & Hubbell, J.A. Functional biomaterials: design of novel biomaterials. *Annu. Rev. Mater. Res.* **31**, 183-201 (2001).
3. Anseth, K.S. et al. In situ forming degradable networks and their application in tissue engineering and drug delivery. *J. Control. Release* **78**, 199-209 (2002).
4. Langer, R. Biomaterial in drug delivery and tissue engineering: one laboratory's experience. *Acc. Chem. Res.* **33**, 94-101 (2000).
5. Lee, K.Y., Peters, M.C., Anderson, K.W. & Mooney, D.J. Controlled growth factor release from synthetic extracellular matrices. *Nature* **408**, 998-1000 (2000).
6. Knudson, C.B. & Knudson, W. Cartilage proteoglycans. *Semin. Cell Dev. Biol.* **12**, 69-78 (2001).
7. Toole, B.P. Hyaluronan in morphogenesis. *Semin. Cell Dev. Biol.* **12**, 79-87 (2001).
8. Prestwich, G.D. et al. Chemically modified hyaluronan: New biomaterials and probes for cell biology. in *New Frontiers in Medical Sciences: Redefining Hyaluronan* (ed. Weigel, P.H.) 181-194 (Elsevier Science, Padua, Italy, 2000).
9. Vercruysse, K.P. & Prestwich, G.D. Hyaluronate derivatives in drug delivery. *Crit. Rev. Ther. Drug Carr. Syst.* **15**, 513-555 (1998).
10. Luo, Y. & Prestwich, G.D. Novel biomaterials for drug delivery. *Exp. Opin. Ther. Patents* **11**, 1395-1410 (2001).
11. Luo, Y. & Prestwich, G.D. Cancer-targeted polymeric drugs. *Curr. Cancer Drug Targ.* **2**, 209-226 (2002).
12. Prestwich, G.D. Biomaterials from chemically-modified hyaluronan. *Glycoforum* http://glycoforum.gr.jp/science/hyaluronan/HA18/HA18E.html (2001).
13. Shu, X.Z. & Prestwich, G.D. Therapeutic biomaterials from chemically modified hyaluronan. in *Chemistry and Biology of Hyaluronan* (ed. Hales, C.A.) 475-504 (Elsevier Press, Amsterdam, 2004).
14. Shu, X.Z., Liu, Y., Palumbo, F., Luo, Y. & Prestwich, G.D. In situ crosslinkable glycosaminoglycan hydrogels for tissue engineering. *Biomaterials* **25**, 1139-1348 (2004).
15. Kirker, K.R., Luo, Y., Nielson, J.H., Shelby, J. & Prestwich, G.D. Glycosaminoglycan hydrogel films as biointeractive dressings for wound healing. *Biomaterials* **23**, 3661-3671 (2002).
16. Kirker, K.R., Luo, Y., Morris, S.E., Shelby, J. & Prestwich, G.D. Glycosaminoglycan hydrogel films as supplemental wound dressings for donor sites. *J. Burn Care Rehabil.* **25**, 276-286 (2004).
17. Proctor, M. et al. Composition of hyaluronan affects wound healing in the rabbit maxillary sinus. *Am. J. Rhinology*, in press (2005).
18. Gilbert, M.E. et al. Chondroitin sulfate hydrogel and wound healing in rabbit maxillary sinus mucosa. *Laryngoscope* **114**, 1406-1409 (2004).
19. Liu, Y., Li, H., Shu, X.Z., Gray, S.D. & Prestwich, G.D. Crosslinked hyaluronan hydrogels containing mitomycin C reduce post-operative abdominal adhesions. *Fertil. & Steril.* **83**, 1275-1283 (2005).
20. Hansen, J.K., Thibeault, S.L., Walsh, J.F., Shu, X.Z. & Prestwich, G.D. In vivo engineering of the vocal fold ECM with injectable HA hydrogels: Early effects on tissue repair and biomechanics in a rabbit model. *Ann. Otol. Rhinol. Laryngol.* **114**, 662-670 (2005).
21. Sondrup, C., Liu, Y., Shu, X.Z., Prestwich, G.D. & Smith, M.E. Bioactive stents in the prevention of airway stenosis. *Otolaryngol. Head & Neck Surg.*, in press (2005).

22. Pouyani, T. & Prestwich, G.D. Functionalized derivatives of hyaluronic acid oligosaccharides: Drug carriers and novel biomaterials. *Bioconjugate Chem.* **5**, 339-347 (1994).
23. Pouyani, T., Harbison, G.S. & Prestwich, G.D. Novel hydrogels of hyaluronic acid: Synthesis, surface morphology, and solid-state NMR. *J. Am. Chem. Soc.* **116**, 7515-7522 (1994).
24. Vercruysse, K.P., Marecak, D.M., Marecek, J.F. & Prestwich, G.D. Synthesis and *in vitro* degradation of new polyvalent hydrazide cross-linked hydrogels of hyaluronic acid. *Bioconjugate Chem.* **8**, 686-694 (1997).
25. Shu, X.Z., Liu, Y., Luo, Y., Roberts, M.C. & Prestwich, G.D. Disulfide crosslinked hyaluronan hydrogels. *Biomacromolecules* **3**, 1304-1311 (2002).
26. Liu, Y., Shu, X.Z. & Prestwich, G.D. Biocompatibility and stability of disulfide-crosslinked hyaluronan films. *Biomaterials* **26**, 4737-4746 (2005).
27. Ghosh, K. et al. Rheological characterization of in situ crosslinkable hyaluronan hydrogels. *Biomacromolecules* **6**, 2857-2865 (2005).
28. Shu, X.Z., Liu, Y., Palumbo, F. & Prestwich, G.D. Disulfide-crosslinked hyaluronan-gelatin hydrogel films: A covalent mimic of the extracellular matrix for *in vitro* cell growth. *Biomaterials* **24**, 3825-3834 (2003).
29. Shu, X.Z. et al. Attachment and spreading of fibroblasts on an RGD peptide-modified injectable hyaluronan hydrogel. *J. Biomed. Mat. Res.* **68A**, 365-375 (2004).
30. Ghosh, K., Ren, X.-D., Shu, X.Z., Prestwich, G.D. & Clark, R.A.F. Fibronectin functional domains coupled to hyaluronan stimulate primary human dermal fibroblast responses critical for wound healing. *Tissue Eng.*, in press (2005).
31. Peattie, R.A. et al. Stimulation of *in vivo* angiogenesis by cytokine-loaded hyaluronic acid hydrogel implants. *Biomaterials* **25**, 2789-2798 (2004).
32. Peattie, R.A. et al. Dual growth factor-induced angiogenesis in vivo using hyaluronan hydrogel implants. *Biomaterials*, **27**, 1868–1875 (2006).
33. Cai, S., Liu, Y., Shu, X.Z. & Prestwich, G.D. Injectable glycosaminoglycan hydrogels for controlled release of basic fibroblast growth factor. *Biomaterials* **26**, 6054-6067 (2005).
34. Mironov, V. et al. Fabrication of tubular tissue construct by centrifugal casting of cells suspended in an in situ crosslinkable hyaluronan hydrogel. *Biomaterials* **26**, 7628-7635 (2005).
35. Prestwich, G.D., Liu, Y., Shu, X.Z. & Xu, Y. 3-D culture of tumors in vitro and in vivo in a synthetic extracellular matris. in *American Association for Cancer Research* (Anaheim, CA, 2005).
36. Li, H., Liu, Y., Shu, X.Z., Gray, S.D. & Prestwich, G.D. Synthesis and biological evaluation of a cross-linked hyaluronan-mitomycin C hydrogel. *Biomacromolecules* **5**, 895-902 (2004).
37. Duflo, S., Thibeault, S.L., Li, W., Shu, X.Z. & Prestwich, G.D. Vocal fold tissue repair in vivo using a synthetic extracellular matrix. *Tissue Eng.*, in press (2005).
38. Liu, Y. et al. Accelerated repair of cortical bone defects using a synthetic extracellular matrix to deliver human demineralized bone matrix. *J. Orthoped. Res.*, in press (2005).

10

TEMPORAL CHANGES IN PEG HYDROGEL STRUCTURE INFLUENCE HUMAN MESENCHYMAL STEM CELL PROLIFERATION AND MATRIX MINERALIZATION

Charles R Nuttelman[1], April M Kloxin[1], and Kristi S Anseth[1,2]

10.1. INTRODUCTION

Preventing bone resorption or facilitating bone regeneration are major clinical challenges for several dental procedures, including ridge preservation after tooth extractions, integration of tooth implants, and the treatment of severe periodontal disease[1,2]. Many of the current treatments fail because of the inability of the materials and methods to heal osseous defects. Thus, recent directions in tissue engineering suggest strategies to design synthetic carriers for cell-based therapies that are targeted towards bone regeneration. For example, several groups[3-5] are interested in the development of injectable gel carriers that would allow simple and reproducible clinical delivery of human mesenchymal stem cells (hMSCs) to treat bone defects. From a bone tissue engineering perspective, hMSCs have many advantages. A large number of hMSCs can be easily obtained by aspiration of adult bone marrow[6], and these multipotent cells can then be coaxed to differentiate into osteoblasts by exposure to specific growth factors or hormones at the right time and with the right dose (e.g., dexamethasone, BMPs, others)[7-9]. During their differentiation to osteoblasts, hMSCs secrete significant amounts of extracellular matrix molecules, providing further advantages for tissue regeneration. Because of these properties, numerous groups are exploring the development of hydrogels for three-dimensional culture and expansion of hMSCs; controlled differentiation of hMSCs to osteoblasts[10], chondrocytes[11], and other cell types[12]; and the targeted delivery of hMSCs to bone defects[13].

Hydrogels are desirable cell carriers for numerous applications because of their high water content, which imparts unique properties with respect to biocompatibility, trans-

---

[1]Department of Chemical and Biological Engineering, University of Colorado, Boulder, Colorado, USA
[2]Howard Hughes Medical Institute, University of Colorado, Boulder, Colorado, USA

port, and elasticity. We are particularly interested in hydrogels formed from the photoinitiated chain polymerization of macromolecular poly(ethylene glycol) (PEG) monomers. These covalently crosslinked PEG hydrogels provide passive support for cell growth, and their synthetic nature allows control of the network's macroscopic properties and degradation mechanism. When combined with photopolymerization techniques, an aqueous cell-monomer suspension can be injected into a defect site and gelled *in situ* to form a cell-laden matrix. As an hMSC delivery vehicle for bone regeneration, the hydrogel must (i) maintain hMSC viability and permit proliferation, (ii) provide local cues that promote osteogenic differentiation, and (iii) degrade at a rate that supports the elaboration of a mineralized extracellular matrix by the delivered cells.

In general, the viability of anchorage-dependent hMSCs encapsulated in hydrogels decreases significantly with culture time due to the lack of important cell-matrix interactions. For example, in PEG-based gels, the viability of hMSCs drops to less than 15% after only one week of culture, but cell survival can be rescued by incorporation of epitopes that promote cell interactions, such as RGD[5, 14, 15], or functional groups that sequester cell secreted adhesion proteins, such as osteopontin[3, 5]. Beyond providing a microenvironment that permits cell viability and proliferation, hMSC differentiation to osteoblasts within gels can be achieved by incorporation of osteogenic signaling molecules within the network. For example, growth factor loaded microparticles are often embedded in gels to provide a localized and sustained release of proteins[16]. In an alternative approach, dexamethasone was incorporated into PEG hydrogels through hydrolytically cleavable pendant groups, and hMSCs encapsulated within these dexamethasone-releasing PEG hydrogels differentiated to osteoblasts *in vitro* in 2 weeks[17].

While important advances have been made in designing gels that promote hMSC viability and differentiation, less is known about the influence of gel degradation and temporal changes in the gel structure on tissue evolution. Here, we use a macromolecular monomer based on tri-block copolymers of poly(lactic acid)-b-PEG-b-poly(lactic acid) or polycaprolactone-b-PEG-b-polycaprolactone to synthesize gels with varying degradation profiles. To control the network degradation, the chemistry and number of degradable repeat units in the crosslinker was varied, with poly(lactic acid) repeats of 0, 2, 4, 6, 8, or 10 and poly(caprolactone) repeats of 2. To characterize the gel degradation behavior, the equilibrium water content was monitored and related to the hydrolysis of the gel crosslinks, and this information was used in a statistical-kinetic model to predict mass loss. To understand the effects of dynamic changes in the gel's macroscopic properties and mass loss on cell function, hMSCs were encapsulated in gels with varying degradation profiles, and hMSC proliferation and activity, expression of osteogenic genes, and mineralization of the gels were monitored.

10.2. MATERIALS AND METHODS

All chemicals were obtained from Sigma-Aldrich (St. Louis, MO) unless otherwise specified. All hydrogel samples were synthesized and characterized in triplicate, and error is represented as the standard deviation.

10.2.1. Macromer Synthesis

The tri-block copolymers, poly(lactic acid)-b-poly(ethylene glycol)-b-poly(lactic acid) (PEG4600-nLac) were synthesized as described elsewhere[18]. Briefly, poly(ethylene glycol) (M_n~4600 g/mol) was added to a 50-mL round bottom flask with a stir bar and combined with stoichiometric amounts of D,L-lactide (Polysciences) for the desired number of poly(lactic acid) repeating units. The components were melted at 140°C and purged with argon for 10 minutes, and 4.4 mg stannous octoate was added to the flask. The reaction was allowed to proceed for 4 hours at 140°C. The product was then dissolved in 20 mL CH_2Cl_2 (Fisher Scientific), precipitated three times in 200 mL ice-cold ethyl ether (Fisher Scientific), filtered, dried under vacuum, and stored at 4°C until use. PEG4600 and PEG4600-nLac macromolecular monomers were synthesized through the addition of methacrylate endgroups using a microwave-methacrylation procedure developed by Lin-Gibson et al. (2004)[19]. PEG4600-nLac or PEG4600 was placed in a microwave-resistant glass vial and purged with argon. The vial was sealed, and the contents were microwaved at 400W power for 5 minutes until molten. Methacrylic anhydride was then added to the glass vial; the vial was sealed, microwaved at 400W for 5 minutes, and cooled for 10 minutes at room temperature. The contents were microwaved again for 5 minutes. Finally, the vial was allowed to cool, and 5 mL CH_2Cl_2 was added. The product was precipitated three times in ice-cold ethyl ether, filtered, and dried under vacuum. Proton nuclear magnetic resonance (^{1}H-NMR) spectroscopy (500 MHz) was used to characterize the number of lactides added to the PEG4600 and to verify methacrylation. The ratio of lactide methyl group protons to ester PEG protons was used to determine the average amount of lactide groups per PEG molecule, and the ratio of methacrylate protons to ester PEG protons was used to verify methacrylation. PEG4600-2Cap-DMA was synthesized similarly to PEG4600-nLac-DMA, but ε-caprolactone was used in place of D,L-lactide. The chemical structures of PEG4600DMA, PEG4600-nLac-DMA, and PEG4600-2Cap-DMA are shown in Figure 10.1, and the NMR-verified number of degradable repeats (lactic acid or caprolactone) is reported in Table 10.1.

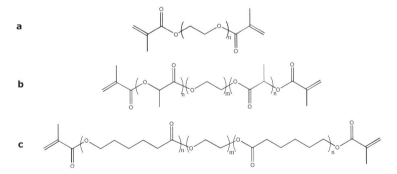

Figure 10.1. Chemical structures of the PEG-based non-degradable and degradable macromers: (a) PEG4600DMA, (b) PEG4600-nLac-DMA, and (c) PEG4600-nCap-DMA.

Table 10.1. Degradable PEG-based macromers containing varying numbers of lactic acid or caprolactone repeat units were synthesized. ^{1}H-NMR spectroscopy was used to determine the length of the degradable blocks (n) and to verify that methacrylation efficiency was >90%.

Product	Theoretical n	Actual n
PEG4600-2Lac-DMA	2	1.80
PEG4600-4Lac-DMA	4	3.57
PEG4600-6Lac-DMA	6	5.49
PEG4600-8Lac-DMA	8	7.77
PEG4600-10Lac-DMA	10	10.22
PEG4600-2Cap-DMA	2	1.84

10.2.2. Hydrogel Synthesis and Characterization

Hydrogel disks (5 mm in diameter, 2 mm in thickness) were fabricated using a solution based photopolymerization method. Briefly, 10 wt% of PEG4600-nLac-DMA or PEG4600-2Cap-DMA were dissolved in phosphate buffered saline (PBS), with 0.05 wt% of 2-hydroxy-1-[4-(hydroxyethoxy) phenyl]-2-methyl-1-propanone (I2959, Ceiba-Geigy) as a photoinitiator. The solutions were exposed to approximately 5 mW/cm^2 of 365 nm ultraviolet light (UVP, model XX-20) for 10 minutes[20]. For mass loss studies, the resulting hydrogels were degraded at 37°C in PBS, and at various time points, the gels were weighed, frozen, lyophilized, and weighed again. The mass swelling ratio was then calculated for each gel by dividing the equilibrium wet mass by the dry mass[21].

10.2.3. Human Mesenchymal Stem Cell Culture and Encapsulation

Human mesenchymal stem cells were obtained from Cambrex Biosciences (Walkersville, MD) and cultured in low glucose Dulbecco's modified eagle medium (Gibco) supplemented with 10% fetal bovine serum (Invitrogen), 1% penicillin/streptomycin (Gibco), 0.25% gentamicin (Gibco), and 0.25% fungizone (Gibco), hereafter referred to as CON media. Cells that had been passaged twice were used for encapsulations.

When confluent, hMSCs were trypsinized and centrifuged to collect the cells. Each cell pellet was then mixed with a 10-wt% PEG4600-nLac-DMA macromer solution and adjusted so that the final cell concentration in the hydrogels was 25 million cells/mL. The cell/macromer suspension was mixed carefully to minimize bubble formation, and then 40 µl of cell/macromer suspension was pipetted into 1-mL sterile syringes that had the tips cut off. The cell/macromer suspensions were then photopolymerized for 10 minutes (365 nm, 5 mW/cm^2). Upon polymerization, disks were pushed out of the syringe using the plunger, placed in hMSC media (CON), and cultured at 37°C with 5% CO_2. Disks were approximately 5 mm in diameter with a thickness of 2 mm. In addition, the effect of the weight percent of macromer in solution was investigated (i.e., 8 wt%, 12 wt%, 15 wt%, 20 wt%, etc.). Cells were also photoencapsulated in non-degrading PEG4600-DMA (n=0). In some instances, gels were cultured in osteogenic differentiation media (OST, CON media supplemented with 100 nM dexamethasone, 0.05 mM ascorbic acid phosphate, and 10 mM β-glycerophosphate).

10.2.4. Biochemical analysis of encapsulated hMSCs

At days 4 and 7, cell/hydrogel constructs were removed from culture; the constructs were rinsed three times with PBS; 1 ml of PBS was added; and the samples were manually homogenized and sonicated (Model W-380, Misonix, Inc., Farmingdale, NY) for 1 minute. Alkaline phosphatase (ALP) production was measured using an assay based on the change in absorbance of *o*-nitrophenol as it is enzymatically cleaved by ALP. When ALP is present, the substrate solution undergoes a change from colorless to yellow, which can be measured at 405 nm using a spectrophotometer. The assay was performed by combining 100 µl of sample with 100 µl of the ALP substrate. At 5-minute intervals, the absorbance at 405 nm was measured; absorbance versus time was a straight line, the slope of which is directly proportional to the concentration of ALP. By performing the assay using known concentrations of ALP in parallel with the samples, the concentrations of ALP for the samples were calculated. To normalize alkaline phosphatase production to a relative measure of cell number (DNA content), total DNA of the samples was determined using the PicoGreen assay (Molecular Probes), and the sonicated solutions described above. Alkaline phosphatase production is presented as alkaline phosphatase per nanogram of DNA.

10.2.5. Mineralization of Hydrogels by Encapsulated hMSCs

Gels containing photoencapsulated hMSCs were assessed for calcium content at 4 and 7 days. Cell/hydrogel constructs were removed from culture, rinsed three times with PBS, and placed in 1 mL 0.9 N H_2SO_4 (Fisher Scientific) overnight at 4°C. The next day, 2 µl of the supernatant was combined with 8 µl dH_2O, and this solution was added to 100µl of a solution containing 1 part calcium binding reagent (0.024% o-cresolphthalein complexone and 0.25% 8-hydroxyquinone in dH_2O) and 1 part calcium buffer (500 mmol/L 2-amino-2-methyl-1,3 propanediol in dH_2O). The absorbance of each solution was then measured at 560 nm using a plate reader, and based on a standard curve of known concentrations of calcium chloride, the total amount of calcium deposited in each hydrogel was determined.

10.2.6. Gene Expression of Encapsulated hMSCs

The gene expression of encapsulated hMSCs for the extracellular matrix proteins osteopontin and collagen type I, indicators of osteogenic differentiation, was assessed using real-time reverse transcription polymerase chain reaction (RT-PCR) in both non-degradable (PEG4600DMA) and degradable (PEG4600-nLac-DMA) gels. After 1 week in culture, cell/polymer hydrogel constructs were removed from culture and rinsed three times with PBS. Total RNA was isolated using a guanidinium thiocyanate/phenol reagent (TRI reagent) and standard manufacturer's protocols. After allowing the RNA pellet to dry, it was resuspended in nuclease-free water, and any residual genomic DNA in the samples was digested (DNase I, Invitrogen). RNA was then quantified using the RiboGreen assay (Molecular Probes) based on the manufacturer's instructions.

Reverse transcription was performed using the iScript cDNA Synthesis Kit (Bio-Rad). A 10-ng total RNA sample was used for the single strand cDNA synthesis. The reverse transcription reaction was incubated at 25 °C for 5 min, 42 °C for 30 min, and terminated at 85 °C for 5 min. PCR was conducted using the iCycler Real-Time PCR machine (Bio-Rad), and primers and probes were designed using the Beacon Designer primer design program (Table 10.2). Primers and probes (Integrated DNA Technologies) for osteopontin (OPN), collagen type I (COL I), and glyceraldehyde-3-phosphate dehydrogenase (GAPDH) were used in a multiplex format. The following PCR parameters were utilized: 95 °C for 90 sec followed by 45 cycles of 95 °C for 30 sec and 55 °C for 60 sec. Threshold cycle (C_T) analysis was used to quantify PCR products, normalized to GAPDH.

Table 10.2 a & b. (a) Forward (FWD) and reverse (REV) primers for genes assayed using real time RT-PCR. (b) Probe sequences, 5' end-labeled fluorophores, and 3' end-labeled quenchers used in real-time RT-PCR. The primers and probes could be multiplexed in the same reaction tube. Quenchers are Black Hole Quenchers (BHQ) produced by IDT Technologies.

a

Gene	FWD primer (5', 3')	REV primer (5', 3')
OPN	ATTCTGGGAGGGCTTGGTTG	TCTGGTCCCGACGATGCT
COL1	GGGCAAGACAGTGATTGAATACA	GGATGGAGGGAGTTTACAGGAA
GAPDH	GCAAGAGCACAAGAGGAAGAG	AAGGGGTCTACATGGCAACT

b

Gene	Probe sequence (5', 3)	Fluorophore	Quencher
OPN	CTCTGCCTCCTCCTGCTGCTGCTG	Texas Red X	BHQ-2
COL1	CCAAGTCCTCCCGCCTGCCCATC	Cy5	BHQ-2
GAPDH	ACCCTCACTGCTGGGGAGTCC	6-FAM	BHQ-1

10.3. RESULTS AND DISCUSSION

10.3.1. Hydrogel Characterization

The degradation behavior of gels synthesized from the PEG4600-nLac-DMA monomer was studied by following changes in the mass swelling ratio with time, and the results are shown in Figure 10.2. For all of the gel compositions studied, the initial water content was greater than 85%, which is typical for these PEG-based systems[22]. Because of the high water content, hydrolysis of the crosslinks is uniform throughout the gel and follows pseudo-first order reaction kinetics. Which means that the crosslinking density, ρ_{xl}, exponentially decreases with time as given below:

$$\rho_{xl} = \rho_{xlo} e^{-2nk't} \quad \text{(Equation 1)}$$

Here, ρ_{xlo} is the initial crosslinking density; k' is the pseudo first order hydrolysis kinetic constant for the lactide bond; n is the number of lactide bonds in the PLA block; t is the degradation time; and the factor of 2 arises from the fact that cleavage of the PLA block on either side of the PEG breaks the crosslink. While not reported here, a similar analysis for the PEG4600-2Cap-DMA gels has been undertaken.

For highly swollen gels, the equilibrium volume swelling ratio scales with the gel crosslinking density (ρ_{xl}) to the -3/5ths power[23], which means that the volume swelling ratio for bulk degrading gels should exponentially increase with time. The solid lines in Figure 10.2 are exponential fits to the experimentally measured mass swelling ratio with time. If one assumes constant density with degradation (e.g., approximately that of water), these gels appear to behave similarly to classic bulk degrading gels. Note that the deviations at later time points relate to changes in the gel chemistry at high extents of degradation, where the initially neutral gels become charged. In addition, the mass-swelling ratio increases at a faster rate for gels with longer PLA blocks in the crosslinks, as expected by the stoichiometry (i.e., n), and the degradation rate constant, k', was determined to be 4.13×10^{-6} min^{-1}. The value of understanding the degradation mechanism and determining degradation rate constant (k') is that numerous gel properties depend on the gel crosslinking density (e.g., diffusion, modulus, and others), and measuring one property can allow prediction of temporal changes in other properties[24].

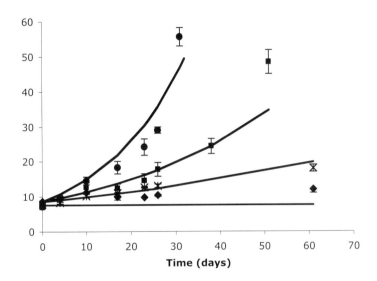

Figure 10.2. Degradation behavior of hydrogels made from PEG4600-nLac-DMA: n=8 (●), n=4 (■), n=2 (✕), and n=0 (♦). As ester bonds of PEG4600-nLac-DMA hydrolyze, the gel swells; as a result, the mass swelling ratio increases. At reverse gelation, the hydrogel becomes completely soluble, and the mass swelling ratio goes to infinity. The rate of degradation is greatest when n=8 and is the lowest when n=2. When there are no degradable lactide bonds present (PEG-nLac-4600 n=0), degradation is negligible under these *in vitro* experimental conditions. The degradation rate constant, k', for a poly(lactic acid) repeat unit was determined to be 4.13×10^{-6} min^{-1} and was used to predict the mass swelling ratio for each experimentally determined n, the solid lines on the above plot.

Of particular interest for many tissue engineering applications is understanding how mass loss occurs in biomaterial scaffolds and then manipulating the mass loss profile to support extracellular matrix deposition. Gel mass loss depends not only on the degradation kinetic constant, but also the overall connectivity of the macromolecules comprising the network. In the PEG-nLac-DMA gels studied here, the PEG molecules are connected to the network by two PLA blocks. In addition, polymerization through the methacrylate end groups leads to longer macromolecular kinetic chains that are linked to the network by numerous PEG crosslinks. One approach to understand, predict, and manipulate the gel mass loss profiles is to use statistical models to calculate the probability that the macromolecules are attached to the gel versus releasable. These models are described in detail elsewhere[25], but briefly, the basic equations depend upon three parameters: the hydrolysis kinetic constant (k'), the weight fraction of the network that resides in the crosslinks versus the kinetic chains, and the network connectivity of the macromolecules, which for PEG is 2 and for the kinetic chains is N in an ideal gel.

Figure 10.3 plots the predicted gel mass loss as a function of degradation time for a series of PEG-nLac-DMA gels, using the hydrolysis kinetic constant determined from the mass-swelling ratio. The kinetic chain connectivity, N, was determined by analysis of the time to complete dissolution of the gel, termed the reverse gel point. At the reverse gel point, fewer than two links exist per kinetic chain[25], and an estimate of the initial N can be determined. Here, N was fixed to 23 for all gel formulations, based on a fit of the reverse gel point. The general shape of the mass loss profile follows a slow, but steady loss of mass, which relates to the release of the PEG molecules as the PLA blocks are cleaved. Typically, >95% of the gel mass resides in the PEG molecules. The rate of this initial release depends strongly on the length of the PLA blocks. At later stages of degradation, a significant number of PLA blocks have degraded, and the kinetic chains, which are linked to the gels many times (N=23), begin to release. This region is shortly followed by the reverse gel point where the system transitions from an insoluble, crosslinked gel to a collection of soluble, highly-branched polymer chains. The trends in the mass loss profiles and time to complete degradation are supported by the experimental data presented in Table 10.3.

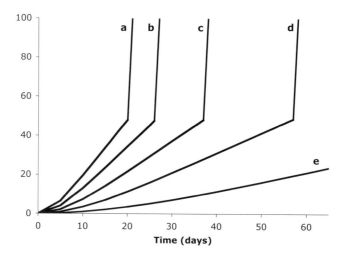

Figure 10.3. A statistical-kinetic model[25] was used to predict mass loss over time for the PEG4600-nLac-DMA gels with (a) n=10, (b) n=8, (c) n=6, (d) n=4, and (e) n=2 lactic acid repeat units. Since all gels were processed using similar polymerization conditions and the macromers have similar molecular weights, the kinetic chain length, N, should be the approximately same for each gel while the degradation rate increases proportionally with n. The model accurately predicts trends in this behavior and the complete degradation time for gels with n=2, 4, 6, 8, and 10 and N=23.

Table 10.3. Complete degradation times of PEG4600-nLac-DMA and PEG4600-2Cap-DMA hydrogels (i.e., when the gels have completely solubilized).

Gel compostion (10 wt% macromer)	Time for complete degradation	
	Observed	Predicted
PEG4600-2Lac-DMA	>62 days	>62 days
PEG4600-4Lac-DMA	51 days	58 days
PEG4600-6Lac-DMA	45 days	38 days
PEG4600-8Lac-DMA	31 days	27 days
PEG4600-10Lac-DMA	26 days	21 days
PEG4600-2Cap-DMA	>4 months	—

10.3.2. Human Mesenchymal Stem Cell Encapsulation and Proliferation

The temporal changes in the network structure described above directly influence hMSC proliferation and interaction with the hydrogel matrix. For example, Figure 10.4 shows the DNA content when hMSCs were photoencapsulated at the same initial cell seeding density (25×10^6 cells/mL) in non-degrading (PEG4600DMA) and degrading (PEG4600-4Lac-DMA and PEG4600-2Cap-DMA) hydrogels up to 14 days of culture in hMSC media (CON). The DNA content increases over three-fold after only 7 days in culture in the PEG4600-4Lac-DMA hydrogels. This is in stark contrast to the non-degrading and slowly degrading gels where proliferation is restricted by the gel microstructure.

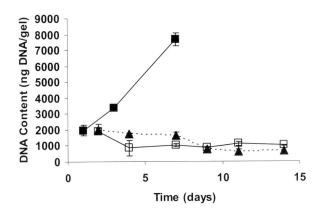

Figure 10.4. Human MSCs were photoencapsulated in non-degrading PEG4600DMA hydrogels (▲ and dotted line), PEG4600-2Cap-DMA hydrogels (□ and solid line), and PEG4600-4Lac-DMA hydrogels (■ and solid line) at a concentration of 25×10^6 cells/mL, and gels were cultured in hMSC media. DNA content (in triplicate) was measured after 7 days using the PicoGreen assay. As can be seen, DNA content increases in the PEG4600-4Lac-DMA gels, indicating that the cells are able to proliferate as gel degradation occurs.

During degradation, the gel is initially at its highest crosslinking density, and there is little room for cells to spread out and extend processes. Over time, ester bonds gradually hydrolyze. At some point, the gel is sufficiently degraded and the pore size is large enough that hMSCs are able to extend processes, spread out, and proliferate (as shown in Figure 10.4). Other groups have studied MSCs encapsulated in degradable [poly(ethylene glycol) fumarate] gels[3]. Unlike our results, where we saw high proliferation of hMSCs initially, Temenoff et al. (2004)[3] saw no evidence of rat MSC proliferation after encapsulation in oligo[poly(ethylene glycol) fumarate] hydrogels. This may be related to differences in the cell type.

10.3.3. Biochemical Activity of Encapsulated hMSCs

Figure 10.5 A shows the results of alkaline phosphatase activity assays conducted on PEG4600DMA and PEG4600-4Lac-DMA hydrogels containing photoencapsulated hMSCs and cultured in either CON or OST media. In all cases, ALP activity decreased from day 4 to day 7. Alkaline phosphatase is thought to aid in nucleation of mineral formation by removing nucleation inhibitors[26]. Increased expression of alkaline phosphatase by hMSCs usually indicates osteogenic differentiation. In developing osteoblasts, alkaline phosphatase activity disappears when the cells become embedded in the matrix as osteocytes[27]. Since there is already a matrix-like material (i.e., the PEG scaffold) present when hMSCs are encapsulated, we hypothesize that elevated alkaline phosphatase activity is not needed. Alkaline phosphatase is responsible for the initiation of matrix mineralization. It is possible that nucleation of mineral formation occurs quickly in these scaffolds, and since nucleation is already occurring in the gels, the cells decrease synthesis of alkaline phosphatase since it is simply not needed for nucleation or mineralization of the surrounding matrix. This would explain the decrease in ALP activity with time in all samples. However, alkaline phosphatase activity is likely modulated by two factors in PEG hydrogels: matrix-like interactions acting at the cell membrane that tend to down-regulate ALP expression and increases in ALP expression due to molecular changes brought about in response to the osteogenic differentiation media (i.e., dexamethasone stimulates the up-regulation of osteogenic genes, such as ALP).

10.3.4. Mineralization of Hydrogels by Encapsulated hMSCs

The ability of cells encapsulated in PEG4600-4Lac-DMA hydrogels to mineralize with time was assessed using an assay specific to calcium. Human MSCs were photoencapsulated in these hydrogels, and they were cultured in either CON or OST media. After 4 and 7 days, calcium content was measured, and the results are shown in Figure 10.5 B.

After 4 days, there is much greater mineralization in the degradable gels cultured in OST media than non-degradable gels cultured in either media or degradable gels cultured in CON media. After 7 days, the non-degradable gels are beginning to mineralize, which is consistent with our previously published results[5]. It has been shown that mineralization of polymers can be greatly enhanced by the presence of carboxylic acid groups[28, 29]. Hydrolysis of the lactide ester bonds yields a hydroxyl group and a carboxylic acid group. One reason for increased mineralization in the degradable hydrogels cultured in OST media may be due to increased presence of carboxylic acid groups upon hydrogel degradation. However, if this were the case (i.e., carboxylic acid groups lead to mineralization), one would also expect high mineralization in the gels cultured in CON media since carboxylic acid groups are also being generated upon degradation in these gels. The β-glycerophosphate present in OST media acts as a mineralization nucleator and probably contributes to the increased mineralization that is seen over constructs cultured in CON media.

An alternative explanation is that gel-encapsulated hMSCs are differentiating to the osteoblastic lineage in response to dexamethasone present in OST media. As a result, alkaline phosphatase activity increases and causes an increase in mineralization. However, the results of alkaline phosphatase activity assays disprove this hypothesis. Therefore, it is likely that the combined effects of β-glycerophosphate present in OST media and the carboxylic acid groups generated during gel degradation lead to increased mineralization in degradable hydrogels cultured in OST media.

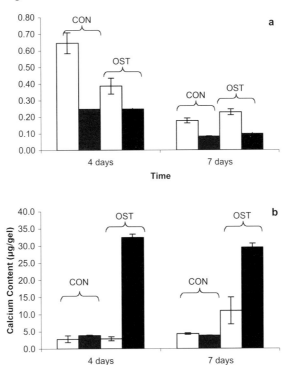

Figure 10.5 a & b.

(a) Human MSCs were photoencapsulated in PEG4600DMA hydrogels (non-degrading) and PEG4600-4Lac-DMA hydrogels (degrading), and gels were cultured in either control media (CON) or osteogenic differentiation media (OST). After 4 and 7 days in culture, alkaline phosphatase (ALP) activity was assessed and normalized to DNA: non-degradable gels cultured in CON media and OST media (white bars) and degradable gels cultured in CON media and OST media (black bars). ALP activity drops between day 4 and 7 in all samples, and ALP activity is higher in non-degradable gels than degradable gels cultured in the same media.

(b) Human MSCs were photoencapsulated as described in (a). After 4 and 7 days in culture, total calcium that had been deposited was measured using a calcium binding assay: non-degradable gels cultured in CON media and OST media (white bars) and degradable gels cultured in CON media and OST media (black bars). The rate of mineralization of degrading hydrogels was much faster (~10X) than non-degrading hydrogels. The high rate of mineralization was likely due to the formation of acidic groups within the hydrogel that form during ester hydrolysis.

10.3.5. Gene Expression of Encapsulated hMSCs

When hMSCs are encapsulated in the PEG hydrogel, the surrounding environment is foreign (i.e., no cellularly-recognized extracellular matrix *per se*). To respond to this foreign environment, the cells must produce their own matrix proteins; for bone matrix these are mainly collagen type I (COL1) and the adhesion protein osteopontin (OPN). OPN is implicated in general cell attachment to the extracellular matrix (ECM) by osteoprogenitor cells, such as MSCs[30]. To alter the hydrogel environment to a more native environment (i.e., containing recognizable ECM proteins), the cells must synthesize and secrete ECM components, such as OPN and COL1. Figure 10.6 A shows the gene expression of OPN as a function of scaffold composition (i.e., non-degradable vs. degradable) and media composition (control media or osteogenic differentiation media) as measured using real-time RT-PCR.

First, there is a large difference between gene expression of OPN in CON media and OST media in non-degradable gels. The dexamethasone in OST media generally leads to an increase in osteogenic genes, one of which is OPN. However, in Figure 10.6 A it is apparent that the gene expression of OPN is greater in both non-degradable and degradable gels when cultured in CON media than in OST media. When cultured in OST media, the β-glycerophosphate present leads to mineralization in the gel[5]. We hypothesize that this mineralization within the gel leads to sequestering of osteopontin within the hydrogel; therefore, cells encapsulated in the hydrogel and cultured in OST media would need to produce less OPN in order to adhere to the gel since any secreted OPN would more readily adsorb to the mineralized extracellular hydrogel environment. In contrast, cells in gels cultured in CON media need to produce extremely high levels of OPN to adhere to the extracellular hydrogel network since the secreted OPN does not adsorb well due to lack of mineral regions throughout the gel. This hypothesis is further supported by results published elsewhere[5].

However, in degradable gels the gene expression of OPN when the gels are cultured in CON media is much greater (5.3 in degradable gels as compared to 1.2 in non-degradable gels). This may be explained by the fact that these hydrogels are quickly degrading, and mass loss continues to increase with time. The cells need to produce increasing amounts of OPN in order to adhere to the non-mineralized gels. Interestingly, the gene expression of OPN in degradable gels cultured in OST media is much lower than the same gels cultured in CON media. This is likely due to mineralization occurring in these degradable gels cultured in OST media. In fact, the low OPN gene expression observed in both non-degradable and degradable hydrogels cultured in OST media may be directly related to the high mineralization seen in these same gels (see Figure 10.5 B).

Figure 10.6 B shows the gene expression of collagen type I in the same samples as Figure 10.6 A. We hypothesize that two factors govern the gene expression of COL1 in PEG hydrogels. First, COL1 expression can be up-regulated by osteogenic differentiation media. This is seen when comparing non-degradable gels cultured in CON media vs. OST media in Figure 10.6 B. The dexamethasone in OST media leads to up-regulation of osteogenic genes, and COL1 is a gene implicated in osteogenic differentiation of hMSCs. Second, we believe there is another component that regulates COL1 expression, which is implicated in the general hMSC surrounding extracellular matrix environment. According to our hypothesis, as the synthetic matrix is eroded, the hMSCs up-regulate the gene expression of COL1 in order to synthesize their own matrix for cell attachment, etc. Alternatively, since the synthetic matrix is quickly eroding away, this stimulates the production of more matrix material by the encapsulated hMSCs, leading to an even greater COL1 gene expression. In fact, COL1 gene expression is significantly higher in the degradable gels as compared to the non-degradable gels in both CON and OST media.

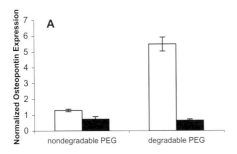
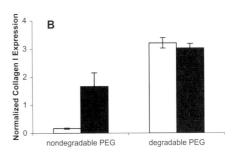

Figure 10.6 A & B.

(A) Gene expression of osteopontin was measured by real-time RT-PCR. Human MSCs were photoencapsulated in non-degradable hydrogels (PEG4600DMA) and degradable hydrogels (PEG4600-4Lac-DMA) and cultured in either CON media (white bars) or OST media (black bars) for 7 days. Gene expression was normalized to gene expression of glyceraldehyde-3-phosphate dehydrogenase.
(B) Gene expression of collagen type I was measured by real-time RT-PCR. Human MSCs were photoencapsulated in non-degradable hydrogels (PEG4600DMA) and degradable hydrogels (PEG4600-4Lac-DMA) and cultured in either CON media (white bars) or OST media (black bars). Gene expression was normalized to gene expression of glyceraldehyde-3-phosphate dehydrogenase.

10.6. CONCLUSIONS

Hydrogel degradation can be controlled by incorporation of hydrolytically labile bonds within a PEG crosslinker: poly(lactic acid) blocks for fast degradation or polycaprolactone blocks for slow degradation. Degradation of the network can be accurately predicted by a statistical-kinetic model and utilized to control gel properties for tailored cell-matrix interactions. Degradable hydrogels of PEG4600-4Lac-DMA allowed proliferation of encapsulated hMSCs, while hMSCs encapsulated in nondegradable or slowly-degradable hydrogels of PEG4600-DMA exhibited negligible proliferation over the same time period. The biochemical activity and gene expression of the encapsulated hMSCs were characterized as a function of the gel chemistry. Cellular response to the temporally changing network structure in different culture conditions, CON or OST media, was complex. Due to the presence of β-glycerophosphate and increased carboxylic acid groups within the network, increased mineralization of degradable gels in OST media was observed, which in turn decreased ALP activity and OPN gene expression as the hMSCs were able to interact with the mineralized matrix. Increased COL1 gene expression was observed in nondegradable gels in OST media, which indicates osteogenic differentiation, as well as in degradable gels in both CON or OST media.

10.5. ACKNOWLEDGMENTS

The authors would like to acknowledge the Howard Hughes Medical Institute and National Institutes of Health (DE16523) for research funding, the National Science Foundation and Department of Education's Graduate Assistantships in Areas of National Need (GAANN) for graduate research fellowships to CRN, and the National Aeronautics and Space Administration's Graduate Student Research Program (NASA GSRP) and GAANN for graduate research fellowships to AMK.

10.6. REFERENCES

1. K. Al-Hamdan, R. Eber, D. Sarment, C. Kowalski, H. L. Wang, Guided tissue regeneration-based root coverage: Meta-analysis, *J. Periodont.* **74**(10), 1520-1533 (2003).
2. L. Laurell, J. Gottlow, M. Zybutz, R. Persson, Treatment of intrabony defects by different surgical procedures. A literature review, *J. Periodont.* **69**(3), 303-313 (1998).
3. J. S. Temenoff, H. Park, E. Jabbari, T. L. Sheffield, R. G. LeBaron, C. G. Ambrose, A. G. Mikos, In vitro osteogenic differentiation of marrow stromal cells encapsulated in biodegradable hydrogels, *J. Biomed. Mater. Res. Part A* **70A**(2), 235-244 (2004).
4. B. Sharma, J. H. Elisseeff, Engineering structurally organized cartilage and bone tissues, *Ann. Biomed. Eng.* **32**(1), 148-159 (2004).
5. C. R. Nuttelman, M. C. Tripodi, K. S. Anseth, Synthetic hydrogel niches that promote hMSC viability, *Matrix Biol.* **24**(3), 208-218 (2005).
6. C. B. Ballas, S. P. Zielske, S. L. Gerson, Adult bone marrow stem cells for cell and gene therapies: Implications for greater use, *J. Cell. Biochem.* **38**(Supplement), 20-28 (2002).
7. A. I. Caplan, Mesenchymal Stem-Cells, *J. Orthop. Res.* **9**(5), 641-650 (1991).
8. S. E. Haynesworth, M. A. Baber, A. I. Caplan, Cell-Surface Antigens On Human Marrow-Derived Mesenchymal Cells Are Detected By Monoclonal-Antibodies, *Bone* **13**(1), 69-80 (1992).
9. M. F. Pittenger, A. M. Mackay, S. C. Beck, R. K. Jaiswal, R. Douglas, J. D. Mosca, M. A. Moorman, D. W. Simonetti, S. Craig, D. R. Marshak, Multilineage potential of adult human mesenchymal stem cells, *Science* **284**(5411), 143-147 (1999).
10. L. Wang, R. M. Shelton, P. R. Cooper, M. Lawson, J. T. Triffitt, J. E. Barralet, Evaluation of sodium alginate for bone marrow cell tissue engineering, *Biomaterials* **24**(20), 3475-3481 (2003).
11. W. J. Li, R. Tuli, C. Okafor, A. Derfoul, K. G. Danielson, D. J. Hall, R. S. Tuan, A three-dimensional nanofibrous scaffold for cartilage tissue engineering using human mesenchymal stem cells, *Biomaterials* **26**(6), 599-609 (2005).
12. W. J. Li, R. Tuli, X. X. Huang, P. Laquerriere, R. S. Tuan, Multilineage differentiation of human mesenchymal stem cells in a three-dimensional nanofibrous scaffold, *Biomaterials* **26**(25), 5158-5166 (2005).
13. H. Shin, P. Q. Ruhe, A. G. Mikos, J. A. Jansen, In vivo bone and soft tissue response to injectable, biodegradable oligo(poly(ethylene glycol) fumarate) hydrogels, *Biomaterials* **24**(19), 3201-3211 (2003).
14. H. Shin, K. Zygourakis, M. C. Farach-Carson, M. J. Yaszemski, A. G. Mikos, Modulation of differentiation and mineralization of marrow stromal cells cultured on biomimetic hydrogels modified with Arg-Gly-Asp containing peptides, *J. Biomed. Mater. Res. Part A* **69A**(3), 535-543 (2004).
15. F. Yang, C. G. Williams, D. A. Wang, H. Lee, P. N. Manson, J. Elisseeff, The effect of incorporating RGD adhesive peptide in polyethylene glycol diacrylate hydrogel on osteogenesis of bone marrow stromal cells, *Biomaterials* **26**(30), 5991-5998 (2005).
16. J. Elisseeff, W. McIntosh, K. Fu, T. Blunk, R. Langer, Controlled-release of IGF-I and TGF-beta 1 in a photopolymerizing hydrogel for cartilage tissue engineering, *J. Orthop. Res.* **19**(6), 1098-1104 (2001).
17. C. R. Nuttelman, M. C. Tripodi, K. S. Anseth, Dexamethasone-functionalized gels induce osteogenic differentiation of encapsulated hMSCs, *J. Biomed. Mater. Res.* **76A**,183–195 (2005).
18. A. S. Sawhney, C. P. Pathak, J. A. Hubbell, Bioerodible hydrogels based on photopolymerized poly(ethylene glycol)-co-poly(alpha-hydroxy acid) diacrylate macromers, *Macromolecules* **26**(4), 581-587 (1993).
19. S. Lin-Gibson, S. Bencherif, J. A. Cooper, S. J. Wetzel, J. M. Antonucci, B. M. Vogel, F. Horkay, N. R. Washburn, Synthesis and characterization of PEG dimethacrylates and their hydrogels, *Biomacromolecules* **5**(4), 1280-7 (2004).

20. S. J. Bryant, C. R. Nuttelman, K. S. Anseth, Cytocompatibility of UV and visible light photoinitiating systems on cultured NIH/3T3 fibroblasts in vitro, *J. Biomater. Sci.-Polym. Ed.* **11**(5), 439-457 (2000).
21. S. J. Bryant, K. S. Anseth, Photopolymerization of hydrogel scaffolds. In *Scaffolding in Tissue Engineering*, J. Elisseeff; P. X. Ma, Eds. Marcel Dekker, Inc.: Vol. In Press.
22. A. T. Metters, K. S. Anseth, C. N. Bowman, Fundamental studies of a novel, biodegradable PEG-b-PLA hydrogel, *Polymer* **41**(11), 3993-4004 (2000).
23. A. T. Metters, C. N. Bowman, K. S. Anseth, Verification of scaling laws for degrading PLA-b-PEG-b-PLA hydrogels, *Aiche J.* **47**(6), 1432-1437 (2001).
24. P. Martens, A. T. Metters, K. S. Anseth, C. N. Bowman, A generalized bulk-degradation model for hydrogel networks formed from multivinyl cross-linking molecules, *J. Phys. Chem. B* **105**(22), 5131-5138 (2001).
25. A. T. Metters, C. N. Bowman, K. S. Anseth, A statistical kinetic model for the bulk degradation of PLA-b-PEG-b-PLA hydrogel networks, *J. Phys. Chem. B* **104**(30), 7043-7049 (2000).
26. V. I. Sikavitsas, J. S. Temenoff, A. G. Mikos, Biomaterials and bone mechanotransduction, *Biomaterials* **22**, 2581-2593 (2001).
27. M. Holtrop, The ultrastructure of bone, *Annals of Clinical and Laboratory Science* **5** 264-271 (1975).
28. W. L. Murphy, D. J. Mooney, Bioinspired growth of crystalline carbonate apatite on biodegradable polymer substrata, *J Am Chem Soc* **124**(9), 1910-7 (2002).
29. J. Song, E. Saiz, C. R. Bertozzi, A new approach to mineralization of biocompatible hydrogel scaffolds: an efficient process toward 3-dimensional bonelike composites, *J Am Chem Soc* **125**(5), 1236-43 (2003).
30. H. Ohgushi, A. I. Caplan, Stem cell technology and bioceramics: from cell to gene engineering, *J Biomed Mater Res* **48**(6), 913-27 (1999).

11

NOVEL BIOPHYSICAL TECHNIQUES FOR INVESTIGATING LONG-TERM CELL ADHESION DYNAMICS ON BIOMATERIAL SURFACES

Z Feng[1], N Cai[2], V Chan[2], PS Mhaisalka[3], KS Chian[1*], BD Ratner[4], and K Liao[2]

11.1. ABSTRACT

Cell adhesion on biomaterial surface is crucial for the regeneration and function of clinically viable cell and tissues. In turn, the cellular phenotypes, following the mechano-chemical transduction of adherent cells on biomaterials, are directly correlated to the biophysical responses of cells. However, the lack of an integrated bio-analytical system for probing the cell-substrate interface poses significant obstacles to understanding the behavior of cells on biomaterial surface. We have developed a novel method, based on the principle of confocal reflectance interference contrast microscopy (C-RICM) that has enabled us to study the biomechanical deformation of cells on biomaterial surfaces. In this article, we would like to describe our recent development of the C-RICM system that integrates a confocal fluorescence microscope, phase contrast microscope and GFP expression system. We shall demonstrate the system by determining the adhesion contact kinetics, initial deformation rate, cytoskeleton structures of adherent cells on extracellular matrices (e.g., collagen and fibronectin) and biodegradable polymer (e.g., poly(lactic acid)) during long-term culture. We shall demonstrate that this unique approach could provide valuable biophysical information necessary for designing optimized biomaterial surfaces for cell/tissue regeneration applications.

---

[1] School of Mechanical and Aerospace Engineering, Nanyang Technological University, 50 Nanyang Avenue, Singapore 639798
[2] School of Chemical and Biomedical Engineering, Nanyang Technological University, 50 Nanyang Avenue, Singapore 639798
[3] BioMedical Engineering Research Centre, Research Technoplaza, Nanyang Technological University, Nanyang Avenue, Singapore 639798
[4] Department of Bioengineering, University of Washington, 484 Bagley, Box 351720, Seattle WA 98195-1720, USA

11.2. INTRODUCTION

Cell adhesion to extracellular matrix (ECM) plays a vital role in regulating key physiological processes including organogenesis, inflammation and endothelialization[1]. It is known that the biophysical responses of anchorage-dependent cells in contact with natural or synthetic materials directly trigger signal transduction cascades such as the focal adhesion kinase (FAK) phosphorylation, cytoskeleton remodeling, and gene expression. Thus, the control of cell adhesion on biomaterial is crucial to the design of cell therapy and engineered tissue equivalents. In the last decade, major attention was given to the design/synthesis of novel biomaterials with tailored physiochemical properties for promoting specific cellular responses. Increasingly, the interaction between cell and biomaterial surface has emerged as one of the most prominent processes leading to cell proliferation, differentiation and regeneration.

Several pertinent factors relating to biomaterials, including surface hydrophilicity, chemical functionality, biocompatibility, biological ligand, nanoscale topology, electro–statics and material properties, determined the physiological fate of the seeded cells[2]. The control of biological responses of adherent cells through surface modification has led to the emergence of biomaterial surface engineering. It is now known that the interaction of cell with ECM or biomaterial surface triggers a series of biological signaling cascades that eventually caters a forward feedback control loop of cellular functions. In particular, the molecular recognition of adhesion receptors (e.g., integrin) on cell membrane and ligand on biomaterial surfaces leads to the modulation of cytoskeleton structure and nucleus responses[3]. The above process is known as mechano-chemical transduction, which ultimately leads to the change of gene expressions and cellular phenotypes of adherent cells on biomaterials[4].

Our contribution to biomaterials surface engineering is in the development of a unique analytical system that is based on biophysical principles to elucidate the effect of substrates has on cell adhesion kinetics. For example, cell adhesion mechanism on biomaterial surfaces are influenced by polymer grafting, ligand immobilization, biopolymer modification or alteration to the cytoskeleton[5]. However, the measurement of fundamental forces that mediate cell adhesion on solid substrates poses significant challenges to the existing analytical techniques. In order to characterize the biophysical responses of cell upon adhesion, there is a need to monitor the formation of cell adhesion contact made with the biomaterial surface. Moreover, the contour of membrane-surface separation in the cohesive zone of adhering cells is correlated to the adhesion strength and membrane bending modulus. However, several optical techniques such as the side-view phase-contrast microcopy are incapable of probing the adhesion contact area (membrane-substrate distance < 50 nm) and separation in the range of 0.01 to 5µm between adhering cells or vesicles and solid substrate[6].

Recently, a novel technique, known as the reflectance interference contrast microscopy (RICM), for probing cell or vesicle adhesion and visualizing the complex contact patterns of bilayer vesicles or cells on supported planar membranes was reported[7]. Based on the interference of light reflected from the cell or biomembrane surface and that from the opposing solid surface, the RICM technique achieves a dynamics range of 0.05 to 1μm in measuring membrane-substrate separation. Despite this unique capability, the RICM fails to probe the membrane-substrate distance beyond 1μm and offers only limited spatial resolution in adhesion contact and membrane-substrate profile. These limitations are due to the non-coherence and non-ideal light profiles of the excitation sources such as mercury lamp and the CCD camera used for capturing the entire field of view in a defined time interval. In principle, these limitations of RICM can be overcome by improving the design of its optical and detection systems. By implementing the optical train found in the RICM with a confocal microscope, we have developed the Confocal-Reflection Interference Contrast Microscopy (C-RICM) to overcome the limitations of the current analytical techniques.

In this article, we aim to illustrate the usefulness of the C-RICM in investigating the responses of cells seeded on biomaterial surfaces quantitatively. Firstly, the determination of adhesion contact dynamics and cytoskeleton rearrangement of HepG2 cells on model ECM during long-term cell culture will be illustrated. Secondly, the biophysical responses of primary porcine esophageal fibroblasts seeded on poly(lactic acid) film, an important scaffold material for the tissue engineering of esophagus, are also described.

11.3. EXPERIMENTAL METHODS

11.3.1. Materials

CLONfectin reagent and p-enhanced green fluorescent protein (pEGFP)-actin plasmid were obtained from Clontech Inc. (Palo Alto, CA). Phosphate buffer saline, Dulbecco Modified Eagle Medium (DMEM), L-glutamine, collagen, streptomycin, penicillin, essential amino acids, fetal bovine serum (FBS), methanol, polylactic acid (PLA) were obtained from Sigma-Aldrich Chemical Inc. (USA). HepG2 cell was a gift from Johns Hopkins (Singapore). Fibronectin was obtained from Chemicon International Inc.

11.3.2. Substrate Preparations

Glass coverslips (30mm-diameter) are cleaned with the solution mixture of 30% 1N NaOH and 70% methanol in an ultra-sonic bath for 20 minutes at room temperature. The glass coverslips are then soaked in pure methanol solution for 15 minutes, sterilized by autoclaved followed by ultraviolet (UV) irradiation for 30 minutes.

To prepare a poly(lactic acid)-coated glass coverslip, approximately 0.4 ml of poly(lactic acid) solution (2 g/L in chloroform) was dispensed slowly and allowed to spread and dry onto a clean glass coverslip placed on a spin-coater. The spin coater was set at 3000 rpm and at room temperature.

To prepare collagen-coated substrates, 400 μL stock solution of collagen (1mg/ml in 0.012N HCl, 400 μL) was neutralized before use, by adding 50 μL of 0.1N NaOH and 50 μL of 10X PBS (final concentration of 0.8 mg/ml). A drop of neutralized collagen solution and allowed to spread evenly on the coated glass coverslip. The collagen was then allowed to adsorb onto the glass for 24 hours at 4°C. The collagen coated coverslip was then rinsed three times with PBS.

Same procedure, as described above for collagen-coated substrate, was used to prepare fibronectin-coated ones. However, a 0.8mg/ml fibronectin solution made by mixing fibronectin stock solution (1mg/ml, 50μL) and 12.5μL of PBS was used instead.

11.3.3. Cell Culture and Transfection

HepG2 cells were maintained in growth medium consisting of DMEM supplemented with 10% fetal bovine serum (FBS), 2 mM L-glutamine, 100μg/ml streptomycin, and 100U/ml penicillin (cell complete medium), at 37°C under 5% CO_2 and 100% humidity.

Transiently transfected HepG2 cells were established with pEGFP-actin by using CLONfectin delivery system (Clontech Inc., USA). CLONfectin reagent is a liposome-based system and promoted delivery of plasmid DNA into mammalian cells. pEGFP-actin plasmid encoded a fusion protein containing both green fluorescent protein and actin. Generally, 2μg of pEGFP-actin plasmid and 8μg of CLONfectin (1μg/μl in HBS) solution were incubated for 20min in 200μl serum free DMEM medium and then diluted with 1.8ml serum free medium. This solution was added to cells at 70% confluence in a 35 mm tissue culture plate. After 4 hours of incubation at 37°C, the entire medium was removed from the cell culture flask. The transfected cells were washed with PBS following by 2ml of fresh complete DMEM medium. Stable EGFP-actin expressing clones were obtained by using G418 (800μg/ml; Geneticin, Clontech) supplemented media. Clone expressing EGFP-actin was expanded and then detached by trypsin-EDTA solution, re-suspended in complete DMEM medium (Sigma-Aldrich Chemical Inc., USA) and were placed on collagen or fibronectin-coated coverslips for our biophysical measurements.

11.3.4. Primary Porcine Esophageal Fibroblasts

Primary porcine esophageal fibroblasts cells were freshly harvested from 5-6 month old pigs obtained from a local abattoir. About 5cm of the midsection portion of the esophagus was collected in sterile phosphate buffered saline. The sample was cut open longitudinally and rinsed several times in sterile saline. The tissue was further cut into smaller pieces and incubated at 4°C overnight in 0.25% trypsin-EDTA (Sigma). On the following day, the tissue was finely minced and further incubated for 15 minutes in trypsin-EDTA solution at 37°C. After incubation the tissue was aspirated several times and then passed through a 100μm pore size sterile nylon cell strainer (BD Falcon). Trypsin was then deactivated with high glucose DMEM media (HyClone, USA) containing 10% serum (JRH biosciences, USA). The cell suspension was then centrifuged at 1000rpm for 5 minutes. The supernatant was discarded and the cell pellet was re-suspended in culture media, which consisted of high glucose DMEM (HyClone) supplemented with 10% serum (JRH biosciences), penicillin 100U/ml, streptomycin 100μg/ml, amphotericin B 10U/ml and kanamycin 100μg/ml. Cells were seeded at density of 10^6 cells /5ml media. The plates were then incubated at 37°C in a 5% CO_2 atmosphere for 3 days. Plates were visually checked any microbial contamination. The culture medium was changed and replenished every 3 days.

11.3.5. Phase Contrast Microscopy

Pascal 5 confocal microscope system (Carl Zeiss, Germany) fitted with a 63X oil immersion objective, cross-polarizer and a transmitted light analyzer (Carl Zeiss, Germany) was used for imaging the adherent cells. Immediately following the seeding of cells, a series of cross-polarized light images were taken for up to 24hours to monitor the two-dimensional spreading kinetics of adherent cells. These images were analyzed using the Carl Zeiss image analysis software ZSM5 to determine the mid-plane diameter of the adhering cells.

11.3.6. Confocal Reflectance Interference Contrast Microscopy (C-RICM)

As shown in Figure 11.1, the C-RICM system is based on a laser scanning confocal microscope (Pascal 5, Carl Zeiss, Germany) equipped with one 80/20-filter set. The illumination source is a He-Ne laser with a maximum power of 1mM and excitation wavelength of 543nm. Either a 40X (Neofluar, N.A.: 1.35) or 63X (Neofluar, N.A.: 1.25) oil immersion objective is used in this study. The optical system carry the excitation light to the cell-substrate interface through the microscope objective and collected the direct reflected light simultaneously from the cell and glass surfaces. The pinhole for the scanning module is set at 69μm. The reflected light is eventually passed through the filter set and directed to a photo-multiplier tube. The constructive or destructive interference of reflected light from the two opposing surfaces resulted in the formation of fringes propagating from the interfacial region of strong contact zone to the peripheral region of the cell.

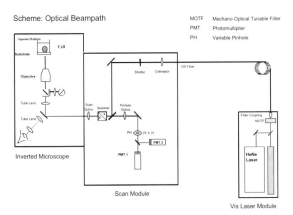

Figure 11.1. The optical path of the confocal reflectance interference contrast microscopy (C-RICM).

Mammalian cells cultured on various bio-mimetic surfaces are mounted on a temperature-controlled chamber at 37°C. All images are analysed using the ZSM5 image analysis software (Carl Zeiss, Germany). The raw data are then fitted with a previous and new model of adhesion. (11)

By combining the C-RICM and phase contrast microscope, the relative area of adhesion contact compared to the cell morphology is determined. Detail of the contact mechanics model of adherent cell is reported previously[8]. Briefly, the equilibrium geometry of a water-filled cell adhering on non-deformable substrate is modeled as a truncated sphere with a mid-plane radius R (see Figure 11.2) and $\sin\theta = (a/R) = \alpha$ where a is the contact zone radius and θ is the contact angle. Both "R" and "a" are measured by C-RICM and phase contrast microscopy, respectively.

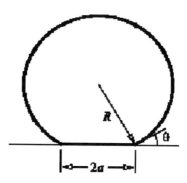

Figure 11.2. The contact mechanics model of an adherent cell. The values of R, a and θ correspond to the mid-plane radius, contact zone radius and contact angle respectively.

The assumption is that the cell wall is subjected to an uniform equi-biaxial stress, $\sigma = C\varepsilon$ where C is equivalent to $Eh/(1-v)$ in a linear system under small strain where E, h and v are the elastic modulus, membrane thickness and Poisson's ratio, respectively. The current model also assumes that the material is rigid with negligible bending deformation. In a related work, we have considered the effect of bending rigidity and showed that the truncated sphere model worked just as well as other theories based on the bending rigidity. The average biaxial strain ε directly calculated from experimental data including R and α, is shown as follows:

$$\varepsilon = \frac{1}{2}\left[\frac{2+2(1-\alpha^2)^{1/2}}{4/R^2 - \alpha^2} - 1\right] \quad (1)$$

In the absence of an external force, the cell spontaneously adjusts its distance of approach toward the substrate until equilibrium is achieved. As shown earlier that the adhesion energy, W, is given as shown below:

$$W = (1-\cos\theta)\,C\varepsilon + C\varepsilon^2 \quad (2)$$

Based on the experimental measurements of the mid-plane diameter R (phase contrast microscope), and the radius of contact zone, a (C-RICM), W is calculated using Equations (1) and (2) respectively. Elastic modulus E of the cell is obtained from biomechanical measurements such as micropipette aspiration and atomic force microscopy (AFM) indentation[9]. The ability to quantify and elucidate the adhesion mechanism of cell on various substrates provided important direction in the selection or modification of scaffold materials for tissue engineered scaffolds or biomedical applications.

11.3.7. GFP-Actin Imaging

HepG2 cells transfected with the pEGFP-actin plasmid are cultured on fibronectin- or collagen-coated coverglass and placed in a temperature-controlled chamber at 37°C. GFP is excited by an Argon-ion laser with a wavelength of 488nm and the fluorescence is detected between 506 and 538 nm. The temporal remodeling of the actin network in HepG2 cells is monitored by time-lapse, confocal microscopy with a 63X oil-immersion objective (Carl Zeiss).

11.4. RESULTS AND DISCUSSION

We have shown that our unique biophysical approach, based on C-RICM, is applicable to imaging live-cell on a model substrate during long-term cell culture. The first step involves measuring the average radii of adherent cells using phase contrast microscope, which is widely used in determining cell morphology. Figure 11.3 showed a series of phase-contrast images of GPP-actin expressing HepG2 cells adhering on collagen-coated coverglass at different seeding time at 37°C. In this case, HepG2 cell is chosen as a model for the validation of our new biophysical approaches for probing cell adhesion dynamics. The results showed that the shape of the cells remained rounded in the first 30 minutes after seeded on collagen-coated substrate. No significant change in the rounded morphology was observed even after seven hours. In a parallel experiment using the phase-contrast microscopy (C-RICM) to determine the adhesion contact area, i.e. which appeared as dark region in the image, the result indicated that strong cell adhesion contact evolved at around 30 minutes after seeding. From 30 minutes to seven hours after seeding, the adhesion contact area of the cells remained constant. Interestingly, the adhesion contact of all the cells concurrently evolved with time. The result implied that the adhesion of cells on collagen-mediated substrate is homogeneous. Figure 11.4 showed a series of C-RICM images for a typical group of GFP-actin HepG2 cells initially seeded on collagen-coated substrate.

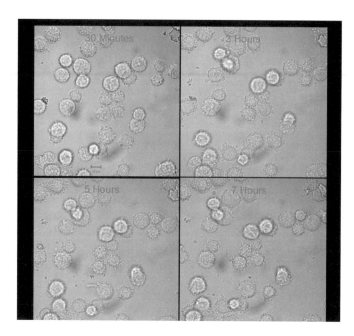

Figure 11.3. A series of phase contrast images GFP-actin HepG2 cells seeded on collagen-coated substrate.

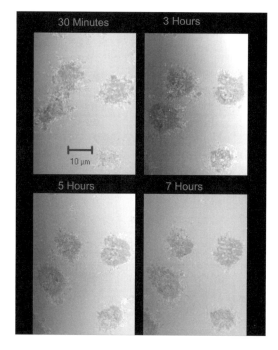

Figure 11.4. A series of C-RICM images for GFP-actin expressing HepG2 cells seeded on collagen-coated substrate.

It is known that different forms of integrin receptor on cell surface recognize distinct ligands on ECM or biomaterial surface. Figure 11.5 showed a series of phase contrast images for GFP-actin expressing HepG2 cells during a long-term cell culture on fibronectin-coated substrate at 37°C. During the first 30 minutes of seeding, the adherent cells remained rounded in shape. However, at 7.5 hours after seeding, the cell showed an extensively spreadout or flattened morphology. The extent of cell spreading on fibronectin was significantly higher compared to those on collagen-coated substrate. Figure 11.6 showed a series of C-RICM images for a typical group of GFP-actin expressing HepG2 cells on fibronectin-coated substrate during initial cell seeding. The result indicated that significant adhesion contact was formed at 30 minutes after cell seeding. From 30 minutes to 3.5 hours, the adhesion contact area was significantly increased until it reached a steady-state. After 3.5 hours, the adhesion contact area of the seeded cell did not change time.

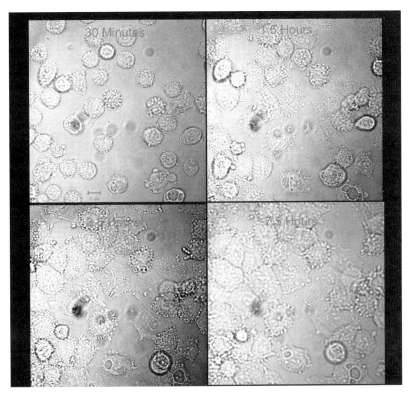

Figure 11.5. A series of phase contrast images for GFP-actin expressing HepG2 cells seeding on fibronectin-coated substrate.

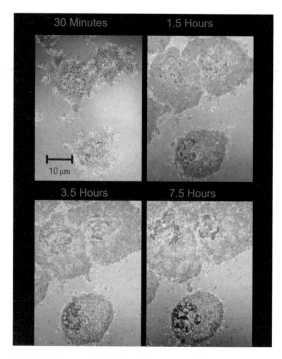

Figure 11.6. A series of C-RICM images for GFP-actin expressing HepG2 cell seeding on fibronectin-coated substrate.

By combining the data from phase-contrast microscopy and C-RICM, the degree of deformation a/R, which measures the exact geometry of adherent cells, can be determined. Figure 11.7 showed a/R of GFP-actin expressing HepG2 cells adhering on collagen or fibronectin-coated substrates against cell seeding time. Each error bars represented the standard deviation of the data from at least 60 cells on four identical samples. At the initial stage of cell seeding, the rate of a/R increased with time were 1.8 and 1.1 hr^{-1} on fibronectin- and collagen-coated surfaces, respectively. Beyond two hours, a/R reached steady-state values of 0.94 and 0.78 for fibronectin and collagen-coated surfaces, respectively. The results showed that the initial rate and the extent of cell deformation on fibronectin-coated surface were significantly higher than those on collagen-coated ones. Figure 11.8 showed the average adhesion energy of GFP-actin-expressing HepG2 cells with seeding time on fibronectin- and collagen-coated surfaces. Each error bars represented the standard deviation of the data from at least 60 cells on four identical samples. The results showed that the adhesion energy spans two orders of magnitude during long-term cell culture on both ligand-coated surfaces. The initial rate of increase in cell adhesion energy was significantly higher in the fibronectin-coated surface compared to collagen-coated one. Interestingly, the enhanced cell deformation and adhesion energy of HepG2 cells were accompanied with the higher degree cell spreading. The observed trend was probably related to the intricate signal transduction cascades of cell adhesion induced between integrin variants and different ligands on the model substrate.

BIOPHYSICAL TECHNIQUES FOR CELL ADHESION INVESTIGATIONS

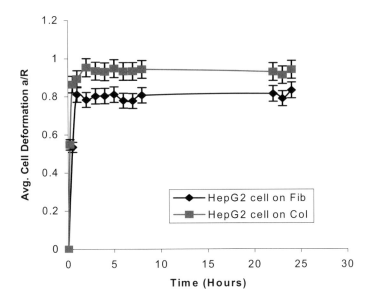

Figure 11.7. Average Degree of cell deformation, a/R, of GFP-actin expressing HepG2 cell on fibronectin and collagen coated surfaces. Each error bars represented the standard deviation of the data from at least 60 cells on four identical samples.

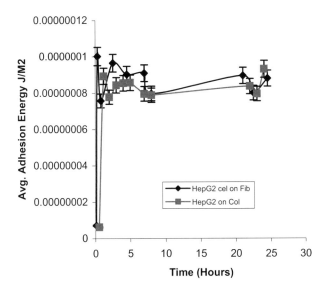

Figure 11.8. The average adhesion energy for a population of GFP-actin expressing HepG2 cells on collagen substrates against seeding time. Each error bars represented the standard deviation of the data from at least 60 cells on four identical samples.

Confocal fluorescence microscopy revealed the spatial organization of cytoskeleton of GPF-actin-expressing HepG2 cells during ECM protein-induced adhesion. Figure 11.9A showed a series of fluorescence images of stable GFP-actin- expressing HepG2 cells adhering to fibronectin-coated coverslips from 12 minutes to 22 hours after cell seeding. The phase contrast images of the same cells were also included for comparison. In the early stages of cell adhesion (12 minutes), the fluorescence image indicated that actin concentrated at the peripheral regions of the cell membrane. As cell spreading and adhesion continued, the spatial organization of actin transformed from a rounded morphology to a more extended one. The geometric transformation of actin network coincided with the morphological development of the adherent cell as shown by the phase contrast images. Specifically, cell-spreading on fibronectin was characterized by the localization of the actin filaments at the lamellapodia which is membrane blebbing during cell spreading. Figure 11.9B showed a series of fluorescence images of stable GFP-actin- expressing HepG2 cells seeded on collagen-coated coverslip at different time intervals. At 12 minutes after cell seeding, actin formed a donut-like structure around the edge of the adherent cell. As seeding time increased from 12 minutes to 22 hours, the thickness of the donut-like structure progressively reduced. In fact after 22 minutes, the actin molecules mostly concentrated at the periphery of the cell. It was noted that HepG2 cells that adhered to collagen substrates spread to a lesser extent compared to those on fibronectin-coated substrates. However, on both fibronectin and collagen-coated substrates, the actin filaments were localized in the cytoplasmic cortex. Our results concur with the data reported by Kusano et al. in P29 cells adhering on ECM proteins.

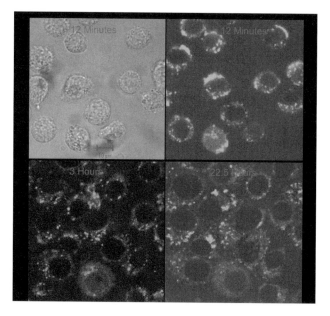

Figure 11.9.A. A series of GFP-actin images of HepG2 cell seeded on fibronectin substrate.

BIOPHYSICAL TECHNIQUES FOR CELL ADHESION INVESTIGATIONS

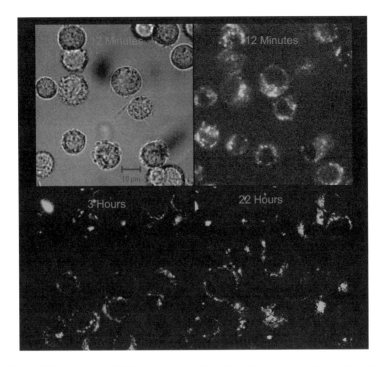

Figure 11.9.B. A series of GFP-actin images of HepG2 cell seeded on collagen substrate.

Based on both C-RICM and contact mechanics model, the change in the adhesion contact dynamics of anchorage-dependent cells on biomimetic surface for engineering tissue equivalents was shown. Figure 11.10 showed a sample series of C-RICM images taken at different times of several porcine esophageal fibroblasts within a cell population adhering on poly(lactic acid)-coated surface during transient cell attachment. In this case, porcine esophageal fibroblasts were chosen for the purposes of engineering esophageal tissue regeneration. At 50 minutes of seeding time, three surface-bound cells started to develop significant adhesion contacts with the PLA surface, as shown by the dark contact circles in the C-RICM images. Generally, two types of cell population were identified on the PLA surface. The first population of porcine esophageal fibroblasts (indicated by green arrows on Figure 11.10) showed significant cell adhesion contact within 50 minutes following seeding. From 50 minutes to 3.5 hours, the contact zones of the porcine esophageal fibroblasts progressively reduced in size. By 3.5 hours and beyond, no cell adhesion was observed.

In contrast, the second population of porcine esophageal fibroblast cells (red arrows in Figure 11.10) showed gradual increase in the cell adhesion contact area throughout the entire 3.5 hours of seeding period. From the above observations, it was evident that the development of a strong adhesion contact between the porcine esophageal fibroblast cell and the substrate was not necessarily accompanied by an increase in the degree of 2-dimensional cell spreading. This was shown by the similar 2-D morphology of adherent cells at the start and end of the transient cell attachment (Phase contrast images in Figure 11.10).

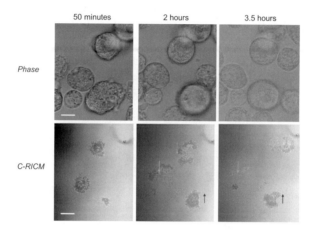

Figure 11.10. Biophysical measurements of esophageal fibroblast adhering on plain PLA surface (scale bar: 20 µm).

Figure 11.11 showed the temporal degree of deformation (a/R) for the strongly adhering porcine esophageal fibroblasts during the initial stage of cell seeding. The result indicated that the average a/R for the strongly adhering porcine esophageal fibroblasts (from at least 60 cells on three different samples) was significantly increased from 0 to 0.75 with seeding time from 0 to 140 minutes respectively. The increase of a/R is brought about by the emergence of strong adhesion contact during cell seeding under constant projected area of cell (from phase contrast image). Based on this new analytical and biophysical approach, we were able to obtain preliminary data to explore the intricate balance between 2-dimensional cell spreading and adhesion contact mechanics of the primary porcine esophageal cells which were relatively unknown.

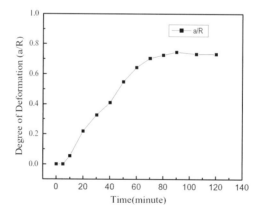

Figure 11.11. The average degree of deformation of porcine esophageal fibroblasts (rapidly adhering population) on plain PLA surface.

11.5. CONCLUSION

In this study, we aim to validate the use of our highly integrated biophysical analytical system (i.e. C-RICM) to determine quantitatively the cellular responses towards adhesion on model ligand- modified substrates. Our results showed that cell adhesion on substrate was a highly intricate process involving cell-spreading, adhesion contact evolution and cytoskeleton remodeling. At the same time, we had demonstrated the use of this C-RICM approach to study the adhesion characteristics of primary cells on our tissue engineering scaffold material of interest. Highly informative data on the adhesion dynamics of primary porcine esophageal fibroblasts involving heterogeneous biophysical responses, among a cell population, was demonstrated on an important biodegradable PLA surface.

11.6. ACKNOWLEDGMENTS

We would like to acknowledge the grant support received from (a) the Singapore Agency for Science & Technology Research (A*STAR) through the Singapore-University of Washington Alliance (SUWA) and (b) the Nanyang Technological University Tissue Engineering Research Initiative, Singapore.

11.7. REFERENCES

1. Iqbal J, Zaidi M, Molecular regulation of mechanotransduction, Biochem Biophys Res Commun., 2005; 328(3):751-5.
2. Wan Y, Qu X, Lu J, Zhu C, Wan L, Yang J, Bei J, Wang S., Characterization of surface property of poly(lactide-co-glycolide) after oxygen plasma treatment, Biomaterials, 2004; 25(19):4777-83.
3. Prasad NK, Decker SJ., SH2-containing 5'-inositol phosphatase, SHIP2, regulates cytoskeleton organization and ligand-dependent down-regulation of the epidermal growth factor receptor, J Biol Chem. 2005; 280(13):13129-36.
4. Inanlou MR, Kablar B., Abnormal development of the intercostal muscles and the rib cage in Myf5-/- embryos leads to pulmonary hypoplasia, Dev Dyn. 2005; 232(1):43-54.
5. Li F, Griffith M, Li Z, Tanodekaew S, Sheardown H, Hakim M, Carlsson DJ., Recruitment of multiple cell lines by collagen-synthetic copolymer matrices in corneal regeneration, Biomaterials. 2005; 26(16):3093-104.
6. Dong C, Lei XX , Biomechanics of cell rolling: shear flow, cell-surface adhesion, and cell deformability, J. Biomech., 33 (1): 35-43, 2000.
7. Feder TJ, Weissmuller G, Zeks B, Sackmann E, Fluctuation analysis of tension-controlled undulation forces between giant vesicles and solid substrates, Phys. Rev. E, 51 (4): 3427-3433 Part B, 1995.
8. Wan KT, Liu KK, Contact mechanics of a thin-walled capsule adhered onto a rigid planar substrate, Med. Biol. Eng. Comput., 2001; 39 (5): 605-608.
9. Mathur, A. B., Collinsworth, A. M., Reichert, W. M., Kraus, W. E., Truskey, G. A., Endothelial, cardiac muscle and skeletal muscle exhibit different viscous and elastic properties as determined by atomic force microscopy, J. Biomech., 2001; 34(12):1545-53.
10. Kusano Y, Oguri K, Nagayasu Y, Munesue S, Ishihara M, Saiki I, Yonekura H, Yamamoto H, Okayama M, "Participation of syndecan 2 in the induction of stress fiber formation in cooperation with integrin $\alpha 5\beta 1$: structural characteristics of heparin sulfate chains with avidity to COOH- terminal heparin-binding domain of fibronectin, Experimental Cell Research 256 (2000) 434-444.
11. Yin C, Liao K, Mao HQ, Leong KW, Zhuo RX, Chan V, Adhesion contact dynamics of HepG2 cells on galactose-immobilized substrates, Biomaterials 2003; 24:837-850.

12

EVALUATION OF VARIOUS TYPES OF SCAFFOLD FOR TISSUE ENGINEERED INTERVERTEBRAL DISC

Soon Hee Kim[1], Sun Jung Yoon[1], Bangsil Choi[1], Hyun Jung Ha[1], John M. Rhee[1], Moon Suk Kim[2], Yoon Sun Yang[3], Hai Bang Lee[2], and Gilson Khang[1*]

12.1. INTRODUCTION

Intervertebral discs (IVD) are specialized structures to anchor adjacent vertebral bodies conferring flexibility and providing mechanical stability during axial compression[1]. Degeneration of IVD results in discogenic low back pain and limited mobility. Very recently, to overcome limited success of current surgical treatment focused on fusion, few studies have been started by tissue engineering technique[2,3]. It has been recognized that tissue engineering offers an alternative techniques to whole organ and tissue transplantation for diseased, failed or malfunctioned organs[4,5]. In tissue engineering of IVD, presence of disc cells harvested from IVD tissue of donor and proper scaffold is needed[6-8].

For the scaffold materials, the family of poly(α-hydroxy acid)s such as polyglycolide (PGA), polylactide (PLA) and its copolymer like poly(lactide-*co*-glycolide) (PLGA) which are among the few synthetic polymers approved for human clinical use by FDA are extensively used or tested in the area of tissue engineered organs as a bioerodible material due to good biocompatibility, controllable biodegradabilitiy, and relatively good processability[1,2,9]. Also, inorganic biodegradable calcium polyphosphate was tested for the IVD scaffold material[2,3,5].

However, it is more desirable to endow with new functionality for the PLA, PGA and PLGA scaffold for the tissue engineered IVD[10-13]. For example, hydrophobic surfaces

---

[1] Department of Polymer/Nano Science and Technology, Chonbuk National University, 664-14, Dukjin, Jeonju 561-756, Korea
[2] Nanobiomaterials Laboratory, Korea Research Institutes of Chemical Technology, P.O.Box 107, Yuseong, Daejeon 305-600, Korea
[3] MEDIPOST Biomedical Research Institute., 7th Fl., Unit of Asan Institute for Life Science, 388-1, Pungnap 2 dong, Sonpagu, Seoul 138-736, Korea

of PLA, PGA, and PLGA possess high interfacial free energy in aqueous solutions, which tend to unfavorably influence their cell-, tissue- and blood-compatibility in initial stage of contact[12], so, it might be more favorable to hydrophilic surface resulting in more uniform cell seeding and distribution. Another example, the bioactive materials impregnated scaffolds might be better for the cell proliferation, differentiation, and migration due to the stimulation of cell growing from the sustained release of cytokine molecules such as nerve growth factor[14,15] and transforming growth factor[16].

One of the significant natural bioactive materials is demineralized bone particle (DBP) whose has a powerful inducer of new bone growth. Urist[17] described firstly the sequence of bone induction using demineralized cortical bone matrix and reported that bone morphogenetic protein acts as local mitogen to stimulate proliferation of mesenchymal stem cells[18]. Another natural one is small intestine submucosa (SIS) powder[7]. Badylak et al. described systematically that an acellular resorbable scaffold material derived from the SIS has been shown to be rapidly resorbed, support early and abundant new blood vessel growth, and serve as a template for the constructive remodeling of several body tissue including musculoskeletal structures, skin, bony wall, dura mater, urinary bladder and blood vessels. The SIS material consists of naturally occurring extracellular matrix (ECM) that has been shown to be rich in components which support angiogenesis such as fibronectin, glycosaminoglycans including heparin, several collagens including Types I, III, IV, V and VI, and angiogenic growth factors such as basic fibroblast growth factor and VEGF[19].

In this study, the novel natural/synthetic composite scaffold like DBP impregnated PLGA (DBP/PLGA), SIS impregnated PLGA (SIS/PLGA), SIS and DBP impregnated PLGA (SIS/DBP/PLGA) scaffolds and crosslinked SIS sponge have been developed and then compared with PLGA scaffold and PGA mesh for the possibility of the application of the tissue engineered IVD. PLGA, DBP/PLGA SIS/PLGA, and SIS/DBP/PLGA scaffolds were prepared by solvent casting/salt leaching method. Crosslinked SIS sponge was fabricated by freeze-drying method. Scaffolds were characterized by scanning electron microscopy (SEM) and mercury intrusion porosimeter. Disc cells which were harvested from rabbit IVD tissue, have been seeded in different scaffolds. To evaluate properties of examined scaffolds, *in vitro* and *in vivo* studies have been done. Proliferation ability assay and DNA quantification have been performed. At defined day scaffolds were implanted into the back of BALB/c nude mice. Influence of natural biomaterials from various types of scaffolds on disc tissue formation was investigated by H&E, Safranin-O, Masson's trichrome and immunochemical staining analysis on tissue section.

12.2. MATERIALS AND METHODS

12.2.1. Materials

PLGA (molecular weight: 90,000 g/mole, 75:25 by mole ratio of lactide to glycolide, Resomer® RG756) were purchased from Boehringer Ingelheim (Ingelheim, Germany). Human DBP was obtained from Osteotech, Inc. (Shrewsbury, USA). DBP with 10 ~ 30 μm size from 300 μm was milled to pulverize using freezer mill (SPEX 6700, USA). Sodium chloride (Oriental Chem. Co., Korea) and methylene chloride (MC, Tedia Co.

Inc., USA) were used as received. All other chemicals were a reagent grade. PGA nonwoven mesh (density: 53.3 mg/cc, porosity: above 95%, and thickness:3.1 mm) was purchased from Albany International Research Co. (NY, USA) and cut 5 x 5 mm^2.

12.2.2. Preparation of SIS Powder

Sections of porcine jejunum were harvested from market pigs within 10 minutes of sacrifice and prepared according to the method of Badylak *et al.*[19] Briefly, the harvested sections of intestine were rinsed free of contents and split in the longitudinal direction to form an elongated sheet[20,23]. The superficial layers of the tunica mucosa were then removed by mechanical delamination using back of knife. The tissue was then turned to the opposite side and the tunica muscularis externa and tunica serosa layers were mechanically removed again. The remaining tissue represented the SIS and consisted of the tunica submucosa and basilar layers of the tunica mucosa. The material consisted almost entirely of ECM. Following lysis of the few cellular remnants by exposure to 0.1% peracetic acid, the SIS materials were rinsed extensively in phosphate buffered saline (PBS, Sigma Chem. Co., St Louis, USA; pH = 7.4) and deionized water. The remaining SIS material was approximately 80 ~ 150 μm thickness. This acellular material consisted of the natural components of the ECM left in the normal three-dimensional architecture and then dried to evaporate water at -70°C for 24 hrs using freeze dryer (Model FDU-540, EYELA, Japan). Samples were stored in a vacuum dessicator at room temperature for at least 7 days. These dried SISs were pulverized using freezer mill at -198°C to get 10 ~ 20 μm size of SIS powder for the improvement of dispersivity into PLGA matrix.

12.2.3. Preparation of DBP/PLGA, SIS/PLGA, SIS/DBP/PLGA and PLGA Scaffolds by Solvent Casting/Salt Leaching Method

Hybrid scaffolds were prepared by solvent casting/salt leaching method[10,11,21] from mixtures composed of PLGA as biodegradable matrix, sodium chloride as porogen, and natural matrix containing bioactive molecule (Figure 12.1). First, 9 grams of sodium chloride particles sieved to a size range of 180 to 250 μm to 1 gram of PLGA were added to a solution of 0.2 w/v% concentration of PLGA in MC. Twenty percent of SIS, DBP and mixture of SIS/DBP was thoroughly dispersed into this PLGA solution, respectively, and then dispersions were cast in a silicon mold like circular disk (diameter: 5 mm and thickness: 5 mm). The samples were freeze-dried for 48 hrs and subsequently vacuum-dried for 24 hrs to remove any remaining solvent. The resulting natural biomaterials impregnated PLGA scaffolds were immersed in deionized water for 24 hrs with changed every 6 hrs to leach out sodium chloride, then finally vacuum-dried. These totally dried scaffolds were stored in a dessicator under vacuum until use.

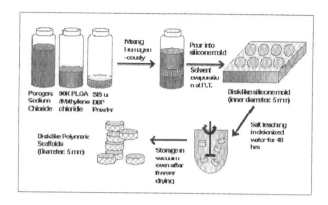

Figure 12.1. Schematic diagram of the fabrication method of DBP/PLGA, SIS/PLGA, DBP/SIS/PLGA, PLGA scaffold by solvent casting/salt leaching method.

12.2.4. Preparation of SIS Sponge [20]

The obtained SIS powders were added in 10 ml vial with aqueous solution consisting of 3% acetic acid and 0.1% pepsin, and then dissolved for 48 hrs. Two percent of SIS solution was carefully poured into homemade silicone mold to give SIS sponge shape, followed by freeze-drying (Figure 12.2). SIS sponges were crosslinked with 1-ethyl-(3,3-dimethylaminopropyl) carbodiimide hydrochloride (EDC, 50 mM) using a mixture of deionized water and ethanol (5/95 v/v) for 24 hrs. The crosslinked SIS sponges in the mold were dipped in water at 40°C for 1 hr to remove unreacted SIS, followed by freeze-drying to give finally SIS sponges. The scaffolds and sponges were sterilized by EO gas at low temperature.

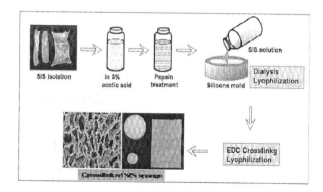

Figure 12.2. Schematic diagram of the fabrication method of SIS sponge crosslinked with EDC.

12.2.5. Characterizations of Scaffold

Surface and cross sectional morphology of various types of scaffolds were observed by SEM (Model S-2250N, Hitachi Co. Ltd., Japan) to investigate the pore structure. Samples sliced by sharp razor for SEM were mounted on metal stub with double-sided tape and coated with platinum for 30 second under argon atmosphere using plasma sputter (SC 500K, Emscope, UK). Scaffolds were analyzed by mercury intrusion porosimeter using an AutoPore II 9220 (Micromeritics Co. Ltd., USA) to determine pore size distributions, specific pore area, median pore diameter and porosity.

12.2.6. Isolation and Culture of Disc Cells

Disc was composed of 2 distinct anatomic regions as the annulus fibrosus (AF) and the nucleus pulposus (NP) in each containing an ECM surrounding cells with different morphologies. In this study, we did not separate AF and NP, that is, we co-isolated disc cells from NP and AF[2,3]. New Zealand white rabbit spine (female, 3 weeks of age) were harvested, and other tissue surrounding the disc were removed aseptically. Disc cells were digested successive enzyme by 0.5% protease (Sigma Chem. Co.) for 1 hr at 37°C, followed by 0.1% collagenase (Sigma Chem. Co.) overnight at 37°C. The cell suspension was then filtered through a sterile nylon mesh and then cultured in 45% Ham's F12 (Gibco BRL) and 45% Dulbecco's Modified Eagles Medium (DMEM, Gibco BRL) supplemented with 10% fetal bovine serum (FBS, Gibco BRL) and antibiotics (100 unit/ml penicilin and 100 μg/ml streptomycin, Gibco BRL).

12.2.7. Measurement of Cell Proliferation Rate and DNA Quantification

After subculture of 4 passages, cells were harvested from T75 flask by using trypsin-EDTA (Gibco BRL). Then cells were seeded into various types of scaffolds with 5×10^5 cells/scaffold and cultured for 7, 14, and 21 days. Cell viability was assessed by a modified 3-(4,5-dimethylthiazole-2-yl)-2,5-diphenyltetrazolium-bromide (MTT, Sigma Chem Co.) method which was converted to blue water insoluble product formazan accumulated in the cytoplasm of viable cells[22]. At defined day, scaffolds with seeded cells were transferred into new plate and inserted medium 1000 μl. One hundred μl of MTT solution (5 mg/ml stock in PBS) was added to each well for 4 hrs at 37°C. Scaffolds were moved into new plate, and crystal form was dissolved by using dimethylsulfoxide (DMSO, Sigma Chem. Co.) 1 ml per scaffold for 1 day. One hundred μl of solubilization solution was plated in 96-well microtiter plates and then the absorption intensity was analyzed ELISA plate reader at 590 nm (E-max, Molecular Device, USA).

For biochemical analysis[23], tissues were digested with papain (Sigma Chem. Co., 40 g/ml in buffer composed of 20 mmol/l dithiothreitol) for 48 hrs at 65°C. The DNA content of tissues was determined from aliquots of the papain digest using Heost 33258 dye binding assay (Polyscience, Warrington, PA, USA) and fluorometry (emission wavelength 365 nm and excitation wavelength 458 nm). The standard curve was generated using calf thymus DNA (Sigma Chem. Co.).

12.2.8. Histological Evaluation

Six groups as PLGA, DBP/PLGA, SIS/PLGA, DBP/SIS/PLGA, crosslinked SIS and PGA nonwoven scaffolds seeded disc cells with 5×10^5 cells/scaffold were implanted into the back of BALB/c-nu nude mouse (female, Orient Animal Co., Korea). The implants were removed after 1, 4 and 6 weeks and fixed in 10% buffered formalin. Thin sections were cut from paraffin embedded tissue and histological sections were stained hematoxylin and eosin (H & E), safranin-O, Masson's trichrome and type II collagen immunohistochemical staining. Photomicrographs were taken using a Nikon inverted microscope with 100 and 200 magnifications.

12.3. RESULTS AND DISSCUSSION

12.3.1. Characterization of Scaffolds

Gross pictures and SEM microphotographs of PLGA, SIS/PLGA, DBP/PLGA, and SIS/DBP/PLGA scaffolds by means of solvent casting/salt leaching method as well as SIS sponge by means of freeze-drying method and PGA nonwoven are shown in Figure 12.3. In natural/synthetic hybrid scaffolds, the amount of natural one fixed 20%. Also, for the solvent casting/salt leaching method, the amount of porogen fixed 90%. Surface, cross section, and side of six types of scaffolds were highly porous with good interconnections between pores in which can support the surface of cell growth, proliferation and differentiation. Particularly, a uniform distribution of well interconnected pores from the surface to core region has been investigated. Table 12.1 lists the porosity and mean pore diameter of scaffolds. It can be observed that the pore size was almost same for solvent casting/salt leaching method, however, SIS sponge was smaller and PGA nonwoven was larger than solvent casting/salt leaching method, in the order of above 200 µm (PGA nonwoven) > 76 µm (DBP/PLGA) ≒ 80 µm (SIS/PLGA) ≒ 83 µm (SIS/DBP/ PLGA) ≒ 74 µm (PLGA) > 50 µm (SIS sponge). Porosities also were almost similar trends in the range of 93.3 ~ 98.1 %.

Table 12.1. Mean pore diameter and porosity for various types of scaffolds.

Scaffolds	Mean pore diameter (µm)	Porosity (%)
PLGA	74.1	93.3
SIS/PLGA	80.3	93.6
DBP/PLGA	76.3	94.0
SIS/DBP/PLGA	83.7	95.2
SIS sponge	50.8	98.1
PGA nonwoven	> 200[a]	> 95.0[b]

a: by naked eye and b: manufacturer's guide

12.3.2. Measurement of Cell Proliferation Rate and DNA Quantification

Figure 12.4 shows the morphology of monolayer culture of disc cells co-isolated from NP and AF on 4 passages. After 4 passages, around 10 folds of disc cell could be harvested compare with 0 passage. We can observe the typical disc cells mixed with spindle-like AF cell and polygonal NP cell.

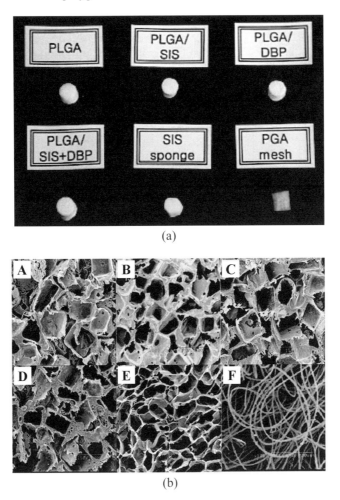

(a)

(b)

Figure 12.3. Gross pictures (a) and SEM microphotographs (b) of various types of scaffolds. (A) PLGA only, (B) SIS/PLGA, (C) DBP/PLGA, (D) SIS/DBP/PLGA, (E) SIS sponge and (F) PGA nonwoven.

Figure 12.5 shows the biological activity of proliferation rate into various scaffolds seeded with 5×10^5 disc cells. It has been observed that the hybrid scaffolds with natural biomaterials was higher than control and SIS sponge and PGA nonwoven in the order of DBP/PLGA ≥ SIS/DBP/PLGA ≅ SIS/PLGA > PLGA > SIS sponge ≅ PGA nonwoven.

Also, it was observed that the proliferation rate increased PLGA and PLGA/hybrid scaffolds whereas SIS sponge and PGA nonwoven decreased from 1 to 3 weeks. For the higher cell proliferation activity for the natural/synthetic hybrid scaffolds, it might be explained that cytokines containing DBP and SIS stimulate to proliferate disc cell activity[7,10,17,19]. For the lower activity for SIS sponge, it might be related with very short biodegradation time within 2 month resulting in lose of mechanical property[24]. SIS sponge scaffold was biodegraded prior to the enough cell proliferation and production of ECM from disc cells. For the PGA nonwoven fabric, the entrapment of disc cells into the scaffolds fabric was not enough at the cell seeding due to the larger porosity. In our previous studies[6,10,11,21,23], we confirmed that hydrophilization of PLGA scaffold causing from the blend with DBP and SIS affected to homogeneous cell seeding and adhesion on the surface of scaffold.

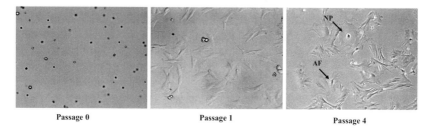

Figure 12.4. Typical disc cells mixed with spindle-like AF cell and polygonal NP cell from passage 0 to passage 4.

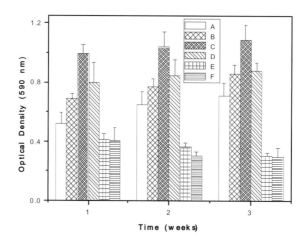

Figure 12.5. Activity of proliferation rate of disc cells analyzed by MTT assay after 1, 2 and 3 weeks in *in vitro*. (A) PLGA only, (B) SIS/PLGA, (C) DBP/PLGA, (D) SIS/DBP/PLGA, (E) SIS sponge and (F) PGA nonwoven.

Figure 12.6 shows DNA quantification of various types of scaffolds in *in vivo* and *in vitro* after 1 week. The DNA quantity of *in vivo* was higher than that of *in vitro* since the nutrition supply was enough in *in vivo* environment. For the *in vivo* and *in vitro* environment, SIS sponge shows the best DNA production among scaffold. It can be explained that SIS sponge scaffold consisted of 100 % of natural biomaterials, whereas other hybrid scaffolds contains only 20 % of natural biomaterials, resulting in the stimulation of DNA production by bioactive molecules in SIS. From the results of MTT and DNA analysis, we can conclude that DBP/PLGA scaffold is the best for the cell proliferation and SIS sponge is the best for the DNA production, respectively. It is very important information for the optimal design of the scaffold materials for the tissue engineered disc scaffolds.

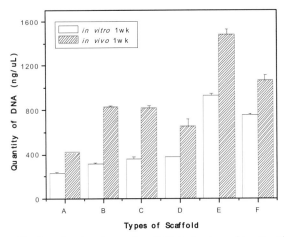

Figure 12.6. DNA quantification of various types of scaffolds in *in vivo* and *in vitro* after 1 week. (A) PLGA only, (B) SIS/PLGA, (C) DBP/PLGA, (D) SIS/DBP/PLGA, (E) SIS sponge and (F) PGA nonwoven.

12.3.3. Histological Evaluations

Figure 12.7 shows the gross pictures of tissue engineered disc implanted in nude mice after 1, 4 and 6 weeks. PLGA, SIS/PLGA, DBP/PLGA and SIS/DBP/PLGA scaffolds maintained theirs own original morphologies as cylinderical morphology due to relatively slow degradation rate of PLGA. However, SIS sponge and PGA nonwoven lose original morphology due to fast biodegradation. This relatively fast biodegradation results in the incomplete tissue formation. It might be suggested that the duration of biodegradation for SIS must prolong the application for the tissue engineered disc despite of its good biochemical and biological property.

Figure 12.8 shows the H&E staining of tissue engineered disc using scaffolds for 1, 4 and 6 weeks. Almost all of scaffolds, we could observe the density of disc cells increased from 1 week to 6 weeks. At 6 weeks, disc cells produced dense ECM which is wave pattern with pink color themselves resulting in firm anchorage between disc cell and scaffolds. We can observe the undegraded PLGA (p) interconnected area, SIS particle and interconnected area (s), DBP particle (d), undegraded PGA nonwoven (g), newly formed vascular capillary (v), disc cells (x) and many inflammatory cells (small and strong purple dot). For PLGA only scaffold, the number of disc cells was little bit increased with few amount production of ECM. We can see undegraded PLGA portion for 6 weeks. Figure 12.8(B) ~ (D) as SIS/PLGA, DBP/PLGA and SIS/DBP/PLGA scaffolds show relatively high density of disc cells surround with SIS and DBP powder with pink dot since SIS and DBP contain several cytokines for improving the cell proliferation compared with PLGA control.

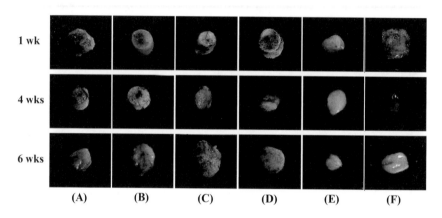

Figure 12.7. The gross pictures of disc cell seeded various types of scaffolds implanted on the back of nude mice after 1, 4 and 6 weeks. (A) PLGA only, (B) SIS/PLGA, (C) DBP/PLGA, (D) SIS/DBP/PLGA, (E) SIS sponge and (F) PGA nonwoven.

We could observe large portion of undegraded PLGA templates and SIS and DBP powders. For SIS sponge scaffolds, newly formed disc tissue was produced with relatively even and high density. The morphology of scaffolds between SIS manufactured by freeze-drying method and natural/synthetic hybrid scaffolds by solvent casting/salt leaching method appeared some differences as membrane thickness, pore shape and so on. For solvent casting/salt leaching method, pore was formed by dissolving salt resulting in thicker and irregular membrane wall thickness as well as heterogeneous pore shape. For freeze-drying method, almost all of pores were open structure and interconnected pore thickness was also very thin resulting in the easier cell intrusion and distribution into the scaffolds. Also, SIS sponge is more hydrophilic than natural/synthetic scaffolds. This hydrophilic property has positively influence on the cell adhesion and proliferation of disc cells. Despite several advantages of SIS, however, the fast biodegradation of SIS within 6 weeks was the cause of incomplete tissue formation as discussed earlier. Among six scaffolds, the disc tissue formation might be in the order of DBP/PLGA ≥ SIS/DBP/PLGA ≒ SIS/PLGA ≥ SIS sponge ≒ PGA nonwoven > PLGA. One of the significant indications for all scaffolds is the observation of inflammatory cell for 2 month due to acidic decomposition materials[25] such as lactic acid and glycolic acid from PLGA and PGA and some secretion of inflammatory agent from SIS. This inflammatory phenomenon must be solved in the near future for the application of scaffold materials.

Figure 12.9 shows Safranin-O staining, Masson's trichrome staining and type II collagen immunochemicalstaining for the detection of glycosaminoglycan/proteoglycan, collagen fiber and type II collagen, respectively, after 6 weeks. For Safranin-O staining, we can observe typical disc cell, one of the chondrocyte as stained glycolaminoglycan for all scaffolds. DBP and SIS containing scaffolds show more secretion of proteoglycan[2]. For Masson's trichrome staining, it was observed that the collagen synthesis of SIS sponge and PGA nonwoven was higher than that of natural/PLGA hybrid scaffolds due to

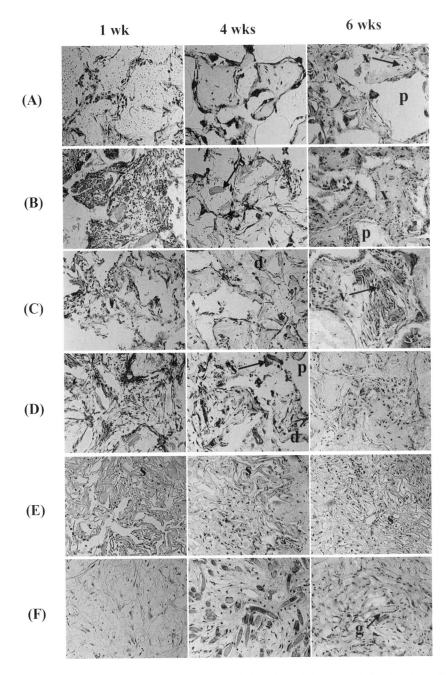

Figure 12.8. Photomicrographs from H & E histological sections of disc cell seeded various types of scaffolds implanted on the back of nude mice after 1, 4 and 6 weeks. (A) PLGA only, (B) SIS/PLGA, (C) DBP/PLGA, (D) SIS/DBP/PLGA, (E) SIS sponge and (F) PGA nonwoven. (200x). p:undegraded PLGA interconnected area, s:SIS particle and interconnected area, d:DBP particle, g:undegraded PGA nonwoven, v:newly formed vascular capillary, and x:disc cells.

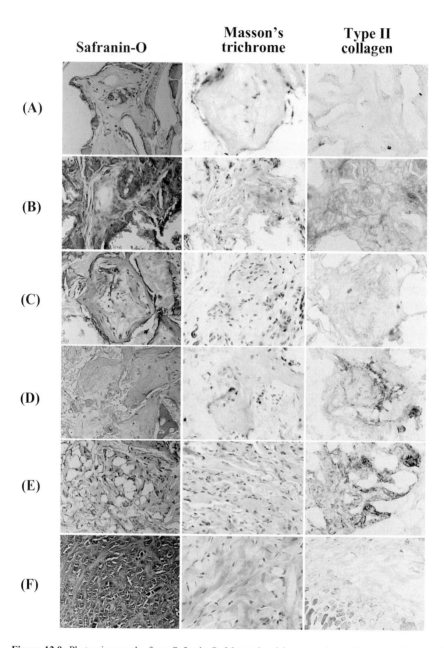

Figure 12.9. Photomicrographs from Safranin-O, Masson's trichrome and type II collagen immunochemical staining sections of disc cell seeded various types of scaffolds implanted on the back of nude mice after 1, 4 and 6 weeks. (A) PLGA only, (B) SIS/PLGA, (C) DBP/PLGA, (D) SIS/DBP/PLGA, (E) SIS sponge and (F) PGA nonwoven. (200x).

the bioactivity of cytokines from SIS and diffusion of nutrient media and waste through high porosity of nonwoven. For type II collagen mainly found disc cells (especially NP cells), the intensity of type II collagen of SIS sponge and natural/PLGA hybrid scaffolds was much higher than that of only synthetic materials as PLGA and PGA nonwoven due to bioactivity of natural biomaterials.

12.4. CONCLUSIONS

In order to the possibility for the application of tissue engineered disc, six types of scaffolds were tested. PLGA, SIS/PLGA (20:80), DBP/PLGA(20:80), and SIS/DBP/PLGA(10:10:80) were fabricated by solvent casting/particulate leaching method and SIS sponge was fabricated by freeze-drying method. From the results, we concluded as follows;

(1) It can be observed that the pore size was in the order of above 200 μm (PGA nonwoven) > 76 μm (DBP/PLGA) ≒ 80 μm (SIS/PLGA) ≒ 83 μm (SIS/DBP/PLGA) ≒ 74 μm (PLGA) > 50 μm (SIS sponge).
(2) The biological activity of proliferation rate by MTT into various scaffolds seeded with 5×10^5 disc cells in the order of DBP/PLGA ≥ SIS/DBP/PLGA ≒ SIS/PLGA > PLGA > SIS sponge ≒ PGA nonwoven.
(3) SIS sponge shows the best DNA production compared with other scaffolds due to the bioactive molecules from SIS.
(4) From the gross pictures of tissue engineered disc implanted in nude mice, PLGA, SIS/PLGA, DBP/PLGA and SIS/DBP/PLGA scaffolds maintained their own original morphologies as cylinderical morphology due to relatively slow degradation rate of PLGA, whereas SIS sponge and PGA nonwoven lose original morphology due to fast biodegradation.
(5) From the H & E staining of tissue engineered disc, the disc tissue formation might be in the order of DBP/PLGA ≥ SIS/DBP/PLGA ≒ SIS/PLGA ≥ SIS sponge ≒ PGA nonwoven > PLGA.
(6) One of the significant indications for all scaffolds is appearance of inflammatory cells during 6 weeks due to acidic decomposition materials such as lactic acid and glycolic acid from PLGA and PGA and some secretion of inflammatory agent from SIS. This inflammatory phenomenon needs to be solved in the near future, before any clinical application of scaffolds.
(7) SIS sponge and natural/PLGA hybrid scaffolds effectively synthesized proteoglycan, collagen, and type II collagen.

The physical and chemical requirements of ideal scaffolds for cell/tissue ingrowth are[1,5,26] (i) biocompatibility, (ii) promotion of cell adhesion, (iii) enhancement of cell growth, (iv) retention of differentiated cell function, (v) large surface area per volume, (vi) duration of adequate biodegradability, (vii) highly porosity to provide adequate space for cell seeding, growth and ECM production, and (viii) a uniformly distributed and interconnected pore structure. In terms of these requirements of scaffolds for the application of tissue engineered disc, natural/synthetic hybrid scaffolds have positive effects for the formation of disc tissue and biochemical activity due to the bioactivity of natural biomaterials.

Studies such as the isolation and culture of AF and NP, the optimization of content of natural biomaterials in hybrid scaffolds, the separated design and culture of AF and NP with different scaffolds, the characterization of mechanical properties and so on are in progress.

12.5. ACKNOWLEDGMENT

This work was supported by KMOHW (0405-BO01-0204-0006) and SCRC (SC3100).

12.6. REFERENCES

1. G. Khang, E. J. Kim, S. H. Kim, K. S. Park, C. W. Han, Y. S. Yang, and H. B. Lee, Recent development trend of artificial disc, *Tissue Eng. Regen. Med.*, **2**(1), 20-28 (2005).
2. H. Mizuno, A. K. Roy, C. A. Vacanti, K. Kojima, M. Ueda, and L. J. Bonassar, Tissue-engineered composites of annulus fibrosus and nucleus pulposus for intervertebral disc replacement, *Spine*, **29**(12), 1290-1298 (2004).
3. C. A. Seguin, M. D. Grynpas, R. M. Pillar, S. D. Walden and R. A. Kandal, Tissue engineered nucleus pulposus tissue formed on a porous calcium polyphosphate substrate, *Spine*, **29**(12), 1299-1307 (2004).
4. G. Khang, and H. B. Lee, Chap. 67, Cell-synthetic surface interaction: Physicochemical surface modification. In *Methods of Tissue Engineering*, Edited by A. Atala and R. Lanza, (Academic Press, New York, 2001), pp 771-780.
5. G. Khang, S. J. Lee, M. S. Kim, and H. B. Lee, Scaffolds; Tissue Engineering, In *Webster's Biomedical Engineering Handbook*, Edited by S. Webster, (John & Wiley Press, NY, 2005), in press.
6. G. Khang, S. J. Lee, C. W. Han, J. M. Rhee, and H. B. Lee, Chap. 17, Preparation and characterization of natural/synthetic hybrid scaffolds, In *Advances in Experimental Medicine and Biology*, vol. **657**, Edited by M. Elcin, (Kluwer-Plenum Press, London, 2003), pp 235-245.
7. G. Khang, M. S. Kim, S. H. Cho, I. Lee, J. M. Rhee, and H. B. Lee, Natural scaffolds biomaterials for tissue regeneration, *Tissue Eng. Regen. Med.*, **1**(1), 9-20 (2004).
8. G. Khang, S. K. Kim, K. D. Hong, W. Y. Jang, C. W. Han, I. Lee, and H. B. Lee, Recent advances for regeneration of the injured spinal cord, *Tissue Eng. Regen. Med.*, **1**(2), 136-142 (2004).
9. D. E. Perrin, and P. E. English, Chap.1, Polyglycolide and polylactide. In *Handbook of Biodegradable Polymers*, Edited by A. J. Domb, J. Kost and D. M. Wiseman, (Harwood Academic Publishers, Netherlands, 1997), pp 3-28.
10. G. Khang, C. S. Park, J. M. Rhee, S. J. Lee, Y. M. Lee, M. K. Choi, and H. B. Lee, Preparation and characterization of dimineralized bone particle impregnated PLA scaffold, *Macromol. Res.*, **9**, 267-276 (2001).
11. G. Khang, P. Shin, I. Kim, B. Lee, S. J. Lee, Y. M. Lee, H. B. Lee, and I. Lee, Preparation and characterization of small intestine submucosa particle impregnated PLA scaffold: The application of tissue engineered bone and cartilage, *Macromol. Res.*, **10**, 158-167 (2002).
12. S. J. Lee, G. Khang, Y. M. Lee, and H. B. Lee, Interaction of human chondrocyte and fibroblast cell onto chloric acid treated poly(α-hydroxy acid) surface, *J. Biomater. Sci., Polym. Ed.*, **13**, 197-212 (2002).
13. G. Khang, C. W. Choee, J. M. Rhee, and H. B. Lee, Interaction of different types of cells on physicochemically treated PLGA surface, *J. Appl. Polymer Sci.*, **85**, 1253-1262 (2002).
14. G. Khang, J. M. Rhee, J. K. Jeong, J. S. Lee, M. S. Kim, S. H. Cho and H. B. Lee, Development of local drug delivery system using biodegradable polymers, *Macromol. Res.*, **11**(4), 207-223 (2003).
15. E. K. Jeon, G. Khang, I. Lee, J. M. Rhee, and H. B. Lee, Preparation and release profile of NGF-loaded polylactide scaffolds for tissue engineered nerve regeneration, *Polymer(Korea)*, **25**, 893-901 (2001).

16. K. S. Park, E. J. Kim, C. W. Han, I. Lee, H. B. Lee, and G. Khang, Preparation and release profile of tranforming growth factor-β1 into alginate beads for tissue engineering, *Macromol. Res.,* **13**, 285-292 (2005).
17. M. R. Urist, Bone: formation by autoinduction, *Science*, **150**, 893-899 (1965).
18. S. Mizuno, and J. Glowacki, Three-dimensional composite of demineralised bone powder and collagen for in vitro analysis of chondroinduction of human dermal fibroblast, *Biomaterials*, **17**, 1819-1825 (1996).
19. S. L. Voytik-Harvin, A. O. Brightman, M. R. Kraine, B. Waisner, and S. F. Badylak, Identification of extractable growth factors from small intestine submucosa, *J. Cell. Biochem.,* **67**, 478-491 (1997).
20. M. S. Kim, K. D. Hong, H. W. Shin, S. H. Kim, S. H. Kim, M. S. Lee, W. Y. Jang, G. Khang, and H. B. Lee, Preparation of porcine small intestine submucosa sponge and their application as a wound dressing in full-thickness skin defect of rat, *Int J. Biological Macromolecules*, **36**, 54-60 (2005).
21. J. W. Jang, K. S. Park, S. H. Kim, C. S. Park, M. S. Kim, C. W. Han, J. M. Rhee, G. Khang and H. B. Lee, Tissue engineered bone regeneration using DBP-loaded PLGA scaffold in rabbit model, *Tissue Eng. Regen. Med.,* **2**(1), 34-40 (2005).
22. S. J. Lee, J. S. Choi, K. S. Park, G. Khang, Y. M. Lee and H. B. Lee, Surface roughness on MG63 osteoblast-like cells to the polycarbonate membrane surfaces with different micropore sizes, *Biomaterials*, **25**, 4699-4707 (2004).
23. S. J. Lee, I. Lee, Y. M. Lee, H. B. Lee and G. Khang, Macroporous biodegradable natural/synthetic hybrid scaffolds as small intestine submucosa impregnated poly(lactide-*co*-glycolide) for tissue engineered bone, *J. Biomater. Sci., Polym. Ed.*, **15**(8), 1003-1017 (2004).
24. M. Rosen, J. Ponsky, R. Petras, A. Fanning, F. Brody, and F. Duperier, Small intestinal submucosa as a bioscaffold for biliary tract regeneration, *Surgery*, **132**(3), 480-486 (2002).
25. C. A. Sundback, J. Y. Shyu, Y. Wang, W. C. Faquin, R. S. Langer, J. P. Vacanti, and T. A. Hadlock, Biocompatibility analysis of poly(glycerol sebacate) as a nerve guide material, *Biomaterials*, **26**, 5454-5464 (2005).
26. S. L. Ishaug, M. J. Yasemski, R. Bizios, and A. G. Mikos, Osteoblast function on synthetic biodegradable polymers, *J. Biomed. Mater. Res.*, **28**, 1445-1453 (1994).

13

PHYSICOCHEMICAL CHARACTERIZATION OF PHOTOPOLYMERIZABLE PLGA BLENDS

Biancamaria Baroli[1]

13.1. INTRODUCTION

Photopolymerizable systems have been proposed as good candidates for drug delivery [1-6] and tissue engineering [7-18] for their ability to be produced *in vivo* via minimally invasive surgery upon light or UV exposure. However, these systems might show poor light penetration or light scattering through the sample when macro-monomers are formulated with other molecules such as excipients and/or drugs, which might be responsible of hindering the passage of light [19]. In such circumstances, macro-monomers can polymerize better and faster close to the source of polymerizing light generating a gradient or an incomplete polymerization through the sample [19].

While testing if PLGA microspheres could be introduced into a photopolymerizable model macro-monomer, it was found that microspheres dissolved completely in the macro-monomer. It was very interesting to note that a hydrophobic polymer (PLGA) could dissolve into a hydrophilic macro-monomer (PEGDM) without the need of organic solvents and then producing transparent fluids. Therefore, the possibility of using PLGA as a biodegradable hydrophobic excipient for formulating photopolymerizable systems was investigated.

Consequently, a major formulative study where several different macro-monomers and PLGAs are used to produce and characterize photopolymerized networks has being undertaken. This contribution aims to describe the physico-chemical properties of one of these systems, which is composed of poly(D,L-lactide-*co*-glycolide) (PLGA) and the liquid macro-monomer poly(ethylene glycol) dimethacrylate (PEGDM). In particular, this manuscript reports the characterization of non-polymerized formulations in terms of (1) interactions occurring between PLGA and PEGDM, (2) viscosity and injectability, (3) transparency to the polymerizing light. Properties of non-polymerized PEGDM-PLGA blends will be discussed in view of possible drug delivery and tissue engineering applica-

---

[1] Dipartimento Farmaco Chimico Tecnologico, University of Cagliari, Cagliari, Sardinia, Italy.

tions, and product marketability. The characterization of photopolymerized PEGDM-PLGA networks in terms of (1) mechanical and superficial properties, (2) sterilizability, (3) cell attachment, and (4) delivery of hydrophilic model molecules will be instead presented elsewhere due to data space availability.

Nevertheless, the results of this study showed that PLGA dissolved in PEGDM up to a 44 % (w/w) without the need of organic solvents, giving transparent solutions that did not significantly absorb in the wavelength range of the commercial photopolymerizing blue-light lamps (400-520 nm). IR and NMR analyses revealed that PLGA interacts with PEGDM by hydrophobic/hydrophilic interactions and hydrogen bondings, and that new molecules are not formed during the dissolution process. Rheological measurements showed that shear viscosity of non-polymerized PEGDM-PLGA blends increased proportionally, up to 20,000 folds, with increasing the amount of PLGA in formulation composition. However, all tested PEGDM-PLGA blends deformed irreversibly by applying them an increasing shear stress (< 2,000), thus exhibiting a Newtonian behavior. Some other rheological measurements indicated that PEGDM-PLGA blends are viscous fluids. Finally, formulation injectability has been evaluated by using the Poiseuille law. Blends were easily photopolymerized with blue-light and a camphorquinone-amine photoinitiator system. The amount of PLGA in the blend composition did not affect polymerization.

These characterizations showed that PEGDM-PLGA formulations are stable, viscous but easily injectable fluids that can be rapidly photopolymerized under mild conditions, which are all appealing properties that allows these systems to be further developed for drug delivery and/or tissue engineering applications.

13.2. METHODS

13.2.1. Materials

Ethyl 4-dimethylaminobenzoate (4-EDMAB), camphorquinone (CQ), poly(ethylene glycol) dimethacrylate (PEGDM) were ordered from Aldrich (St. Louis, MO, USA). Two batches of poly(D,L-lactide-*co*-glycolide) 50:50 (PLGA; RESOMER® RG 503H) were purchased from Boehringer Ingelheim Chemicals, Inc. (Petersburg, VA, USA), while *N, N*-dimethylformamide-d_7 (DMF) from Cambridge Isotope Laboratories, Inc. (Andover, MA, USA). Chemicals were stored as specified by suppliers and used without further purification.

PLGA and PEGDM molecular weights (MWs) were assessed using a gel permeation chromatographer (GPC) equipped with an HPLC pump (model # 515), a refractive index detector (model # 2410), an auto-sampler (model # 717 plus), and a Styragel® HR4 THF column (all purchased from Waters Corporate, Milford, MA, USA), and calibrated with polystyrene standards (MWs 300,000 – 1,000).

13.2.2. Preparation of Photopolymerizable Formulations

PEGDM-PLGA blends were prepared as follows. For each formulation (Table 13.1), PEGDM was weighed in a screw-cap glass vial where the corresponding amount of PLGA was then added. Mixtures were left untouched and protected from light, at room temperature, until obtaining clear fluids, which occurred between one hour and three days depending on the percentage of PLGA. Formulations were supplemented with photoinitiators (1% each, w/w) only if they had to be used for the preparation of photopolymerized PEGDM-PLGA networks.

13.2.3. Characterization of Photopolymerizable Formulations

13.2.3.1. Ultraviolet-Visible Spectroscopy

Ultraviolet-visible (UV-vis) spectra of non-polymerized formulations (not all shown in Figure 13.1) were recorded, at room temperature, over a 190-1100 nm wavelength range (Varian, Palo Alto, CA, USA; model: Cary 50 Bio) using quartz cuvettes (path 1.000; Fisher Scientific, Pittsburgh PA, USA). Formulations were prepared using the first batch of PLGA, and then analyzed without further dilution.

13.2.3.2. Infrared Spectroscopy

Infrared (IR) spectra of non-polymerized formulations and their components were recorded –neat– using KBr crystal windows (Aldrich) and a FT-IR spectrometer (Thermo Electron Corporation, Waltham, MA, USA; model: Nicolet Series II Magna-IR 550). To obtain a neat sample of PLGA (first batch) that could be useful for IR analysis, few drops of a PLGA diluted solution (chloroform) were deposited onto one KBr window, and let evaporate in a dry cabinet. This procedure allowed a thin non-colored transparent film to be formed on the window.

13.2.3.3. Nuclear Magnetic Resonance Spectroscopy

Nuclear magnetic resonance (NMR) spectra of PLGA (first batch), PEGDM, and their blends were obtained in DMF, at 300° K, using a 400 MHz spectrometer (Bruker BioSpin Corporation, Billerica, MA, USA; model: Avance DPX-400) after a 15-minute acquisition.

13.2.3.4. Rheological Measurements

Flow properties and microstructure of non-polymerized formulations (Tables 13.2-13.4) were investigated, at room temperature, with the use of a rheometer (Bohlin Instrument Inc., East Brunswick, NJ, USA; model: CVOR), assembled with cone and plate geometry (plate: 60 mm diameter; cone: 40 mm diameter; cone angle: 4°; distance gap: 150 μm). Flow properties and microstructure were respectively studied with 'shear stress – shear rate' and 'oscillation frequency – strain' experiments. PEGDM-PLGA blends used for these measurements were formulated with the second batch of PLGA.

13.2.4. Photopolymerized PEGDM-PLGA Network Preparation

Photopolymerized PLGA-PEGDM networks were produced in different formulations (Table 13.1) and shapes. Non-polymerized blends were supplemented with 4-EDMAB and CQ (1% each, w/w), mixed until dissolution of the photoinitiators, poured in the appropriate Teflon mold, and exposed to a source of blue-light (3M Curinglight XL 1500, 420-500 nm, output 400 mW/cm^2, 3M Health Care, USA) at a distance of 3 mm for 5 minutes.

13.2.5. Statistical Analysis

Data reported as mean ± standard deviation (SD) were statistically analyzed by Student's *t*-test, where a p of < 0.05 was considered significant.

13.3. RESULTS

13.3.1. Non-Polymerized Formulations

Formulations were prepared using a macro-monomer (PEGDM) and a polymer (PLGA) that were, respectively, in the physical state of a liquid and a solid. GPC analysis showed that PEGDM MW was 1,069 Da whereas PLGA MWs were 44,792 Da (first batch), and 48,443 Da (second batch).

PLGA dissolved completely in PEGDM up to 44 % (w/w), and the resulting non-polymerized blends (Table 13.1) were very pale yellow and transparent fluids, which showed neither the Tyndall Effect nor deviation of a polarized light, which indicated that formulations were neither colloidal dispersions nor liquid crystals, respectively.

Table 13.1. Formulation composition

Formulation	Composition [a]	
	PEGDM	PLGA
PEGDM	100	0
PEGDM-PLGA 10	90.9	9.1
PEGDM-PLGA 20	83.3	16.7
PEGDM-PLGA 30	76.9	23.1
PEGDM-PLGA 40	71.4	28.6
PEGDM-PLGA 60	62.5	37.5
PEGDM-PLGA 80	55.6	44.4

[a] Composition is given in weight percentage (w/w). To obtain photopolymerized PEGDM-PLGA networks, each formulation was supplemented with CQ and 4-EDMAB (1% w/w each).

Macroscopically, blends differed from each other only in viscosity, which increased by increasing the amount of PLGA in their composition (Table 13.1), and decreased by increasing sample temperature.

13.3.2. Ultraviolet-Visible Spectroscopy

UV-vis spectra were recorded to verify whether formulations were transparent to the radiations emitted from commercial blue-light curing lamps. Thus, PEGDM-PLGA 40 spectrum was recorded and compared with that of PEGDM-PLGA 40 supplemented with 1% photoinitiators (PEGDM-PLGA 40+) to also establish whether PEGDM-PLGA blends might interfere with light absorption of photoinitiators (Figure 13.1).

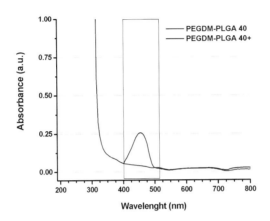

Figure 13.1. UV-vis spectra of PEGDM-PLGA 40 and PEGDM-PLGA 40+

Figure 13.1 showed that undiluted PEGDM-PLGA 40 did not significantly absorb within the normal range (400-520 nm) of blue-light curing lamps (square in Fig. 13.1), where no interference with photoinitiators' absorbing band was visible.

13.3.3. Infrared Spectroscopy

IR spectra of PEGDM, PLGA, and two PEGDM-PLGA blends (10 and 80), were recorded (not shown) to verify the presence of hydrogen bondings or other interactions occurring between PEGDM and PLGA, and to try to identify, by means of signal shifting, which groups of both molecules might be involved in such interactions [20].

In general, a hydrogen bond occurs between proton donor (carboxylic and hydroxylic groups, amine and amide) and proton acceptor (oxygen, nitrogen, and halogen atoms, which have a lone pair electrons, and/or unsaturated residues) groups. Hydrogen bonding is known to move stretching (more affected) and bending vibrations of both donor and acceptor groups to lower frequencies (differences of 10 to 300 cm^{-1}) [20].

By observing PEGDM and PLGA chemical structures (Figure 13.2), one can note that hydrogen bonding can theoretically occur between the terminal –OH residues of PLGA and either the two terminal conjugated carboxy-methacrylic groups or the several oxygen atoms of PEGDM.

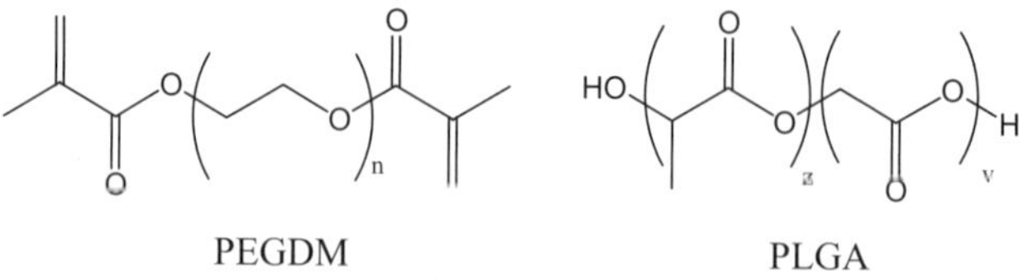

Figure 13.2. Chemical structure of PEGDM and PLGA, where n, z, and v are the repetitive unit numbers.

Nevertheless, analysis of vibration frequencies of terminal groups was unfruitful. In fact, PLGA terminal –OH groups were not clearly visible in the higher frequencies region of PLGA IR spectrum (normal value: 3650-3584 cm^{-1}) [20]. Thus, their certain identification was difficult because their second band, due to the stretching of C-OH signal (normal value: 1260-1000 cm^{-1}) [20], falls in the same region of another band that is due to the stretching of (CO)-OC groups (normal value: 1300-1000 cm^{-1}) [20], which are abundantly present in PLGA. Furthermore, it was also considered that the intensity of stretching vibrations of the two –OH end groups could be affected by the MW of the polymer (44,792 Da) and by the relative intensities of other bands (e.g., -C-COO-C-), which could in turn make the –OH groups not visible [21].

Consequently, it was concluded that PLGA dissolved in PEGDM mainly by hydrophobic-hydrophilic interactions, also known as intermolecular or secondary forces [22]. In addition, if hydrogen bondings occur, these are not identifiable by IR analysis.

Post-study experiments have shown that a 50:50 PLGA that has only one free hydroxylic group dissolved in PEGDM up to c.a. 20%. This additional result allows to redefine the aforementioned conclusion and to say that PLGA dissolves in PEGDM by both secondary forces and hydrogen bondings, but that hydrogen bondings are not identifiable by IR, using these particular formulations.

13.3.4. Nuclear Magnetic Resonance Spectroscopy

^{1}H-NMR spectra of PLGA, PEGDM, and of a PEGDM-PLGA blend were recorded to verify if PLGA, or a small amount of it, interacted with the monomer during the dissolution process forming new species. By analyzing NMR spectra, it was clear that PEGDM and PLGA did not form new molecules since peaks of both PLGA (1.50 ppm, -CH$_3$; 4.76 ppm, -COO-CH$_2$-COO-; 5.16 ppm, -COO-CH(CH$_3$)-COO-) and PEGDM (1.87 ppm, -CH$_3$; 3.57 ppm, -(OCH$_2$CH$_2$)$_n$-; 3.67 ppm, -COOCH$_2$-CH$_2$-; 4.22 ppm, -COOCH$_2$-CH$_2$-; 5.50 ppm, HCH=; 6.05 ppm, HCH=) spectra overlapped perfectly with those of PEGDM-PLGA blend spectrum (not shown).

NMR and IR results combined with sample dissolution and optical properties allowed to state that PLGA does dissolve in PEGDM, and that obtained fluids are most likely in the physical state of molecular solutions.

13.3.5. Rheological Properties of Non-Polymerized Mixtures

Rheological measurements, intended to illustrate flow properties of non-polymerized formulations, showed that shear viscosity was always independent of changes in shear rates (not shown), which indicated that, under the conditions of these experiments, formulations deformed irreversibly (Newtonian behavior) [21] under an applied stress (Table 13.2). Shear viscosities ranged from 0.04 ± 0.00 Pas (PEGDM) to 826.4 ± 19.1 Pas (PEGDM-PLGA 80) increasing up to 20,000 folds by increasing the amount of PLGA in formulation composition (Table 13.1).

Table 13.2. Rheological properties of non-polymerized formulations

Formulation	Stress-Strain experiments		
	Shear Rate (1/s)	Shear Stress (Pa)	Shear Viscosity (Pas)
PEGDM	3.0 – 1750	0.1 – 71.3	0.04 ± 0.0
PEGDM-PLGA 10	0.1 – 71.7	0.1 – 30	0.4 ± 0.0
PEGDM-PLGA 20	0.3 – 65.2	0.6 – 150	2.3 ± 0.0
PEGDM-PLGA 30	0.1 – 88.0	1 – 700	8.1 ± 0.1
PEGDM-PLGA 40	0.02 – 55.2	0.5 – 1500	28.2 ± 0.5
PEGDM-PLGA 60	0.003 – 5.3	0.5 – 1000	196.5 ± 3.5
PEGDM-PLGA 80	0.001 – 2.5	0.5 – 2000	826.4 ± 19.1

However, shear viscosity did not increase linearly, as demonstrated by plotting, in a log-log scale, shear viscosity values versus PLGA formulation amount (Figure 13.3).

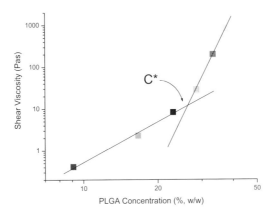

Figure 13.3. Shear viscosity (mean ± SD) dependence on PLGA concentration in PEGDM-PLGA formulations. C* indicates the percentage of PLGA (26.4 w/w) at which a slope change occurred.

The change in viscosity slope, occurring at a PLGA concentration of 26.4 % (w/w), reminds the typical behavior of polymeric particle solutions, where the concentration at which linearity is disrupted indicates the critical concentration from which particles start to strongly interact [23]. This same behavior is also common in polymer melts and solutions. In this case, the change in slope represents the concentration after which molecules do not diffuse separately any longer (molecules are entangled) [24]. Consequently, since other characterizations of this study indicated that non-polymerized formulations could be considered solutions of PLGA in PEGDM, the slope above C* could reveal the resultant of either molecule overlapping and entanglement, or strong molecule interactions/bondings. However, distinguishing between these two cases is pretty simple, since strong molecule interactions are associated with elastic or viscoelastic systems [23].

Consequently, to study the microstructure of non-polymerized formulations, some sinusoidal measurements were performed, where samples were subjected to a constant stress (0.5 or 1 Pa) and were oscillated with decreasing frequencies (10-0.005 Hz). Results of these measurements are shown in Table 13.3, and Figure 13.4 A-D where obtained complex modulus, elastic modulus, viscous modulus and complex viscosity have been plotted as a function of frequency (Figure 13.4; not all the results of Table 13.3 formulations are shown).

Table 13.3. Rheological properties of non-polymerized formulations

Formulation	Oscillatory experiments		
	Complex Viscosity (Pas)	Stress (Pa)	Phase angle (°)
PEGDM	---	---	---
PEGDM-PLGA 10	0.4 ± 0.0	0.5	87.2 ± 3.9
PEGDM-PLGA 20	---	---	---
PEGDM-PLGA 30	8.2 ± 0.1	1	89.6 ± 0.6
PEGDM-PLGA 40	28.1 ± 0.4	1	89.3 ± 0.6
PEGDM-PLGA 60	187.4 ± 9.3	1	86.0 ± 4.9
PEGDM-PLGA 80	750.3 ± 99.7	1	83.2 ± 8.8

Results showed that in all cases, (1) viscous moduli were dominant and overlapped respective complex moduli almost perfectly (Figure 13.4 A-D), (2) in the range of tested frequencies, complex viscosity remained quite stable and comparable ($p > 0.05$) with its corresponding shear viscosity (please confront shear viscosity and complex viscosity data in Tables 13.2 and 13.3), (3) all moduli decreased by decreasing oscillation frequency (Figure 13.4 A-D), (4) the phase angle was always greater than 80° (Table 13.3), (5) PEGDM-PLGA 30 and 40 showed a different relative arrangement of their elastic and viscous moduli, which were almost parallel among each other (Figure 13.4 B and 13.4 C). It is worth noting that parallel elastic and viscous moduli are found in polymeric systems showing some weak interactions among molecules [23]. In addition, it was observed that complex viscosity values of PEGDM-PLGA 60 and 80, although being very similar to their respective shear viscosity values, showed a greater SD that reflects a slight thinning behavior at higher frequencies (Tables 13.2 and 13.3). All these results indicate that non-polymerized PEGDM-PLGA formulations are viscous fluids.

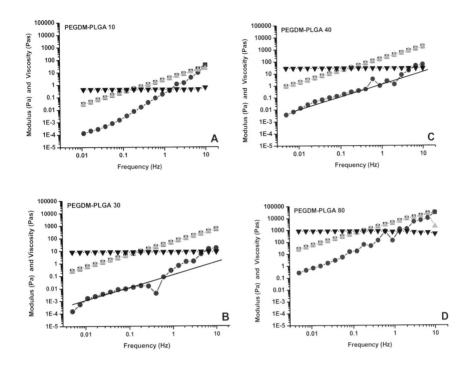

Figure 13.4. Modification of complex modulus (-■-), elastic modulus (-●-), viscous modulus (-▲-), and complex viscosity (-▼-) as a function of oscillation frequency, and composition PEGDM-PLGA 10 (Figure 13.4 A), PEGDM-PLGA 30 (Figure 13.4 B), PEGDM-PLGA 40 (Figure 13.4 C), and PEGDM-PLGA 80 (Figure 13.4 D). All values were recorded at 1 Pa stress.

Injectability was estimated using Poiseuille law [25], $(dV/dt) = [(\pi r^4)/(8\eta l)]\Delta p$, where dV/dt (m^3/s) is the rate at which a fluid of viscosity η (Pas) is flowed through a needle (or cannula) of radius r (m) and length l (m), when a difference in pressure Δp (Pa) is applied at the two extremities of the needle (or cannula).

Table 13.4. Rheological properties of non-polymerized formulations

Formulation	Injectability Δp^a (N/cm^2)
PEGDM	5.6 E-5
PEGDM-PLGA 10	5.6 E-4
PEGDM-PLGA 20	3.1 E-3
PEGDM-PLGA 30	1.1 E-2
PEGDM-PLGA 40	3.8 E-2
PEGDM-PLGA 60	2.7 E-1
PEGDM-PLGA 80	1.1 E+0

Table 13.4 reports the estimated Δp necessary to flow non-polymerized formulations (Table 13.1) at a rate of 1 mL/min through a cannula of 1 cm diameter and 20 cm length.

Values have to be considered estimated because, based on their Newtonian properties, it was hypothesized that PEGDM-PLGA blends moved through the cannula with a laminar flow.

In summary, rheological measurements described deformable, easy injectable, viscous systems whose PLGA molecules are non-associated or weakly associated with PEGDM ones.

13.3.6. Photopolymerized Polymer Network Preparation

Polymerization was unaffected by formulation composition (Table 13.1), showing a hardening time of a few seconds. Shrinking during polymerization was neglected by the presence of PLGA. Photopolymerized PEGDM-PLGA networks were translucent, and ranged from uncolored to a very pale white. It was observed that samples lost their translucent appearance and became whiter after being soaked in PBS or Milli-Q water for at least one day. The degree of color change followed the increasing concentration of PLGA in formulation composition (Table 13.1). Though, photopolymerized networks did not swell.

13.4. DISCUSSION

The results of this study clarified different properties of the photopolymerizable PEGDM-PLGA system. They will be now summarized and discussed in view of possible tissue engineering and drug delivery applications. It should not be forgotten that drug delivery and especially tissue engineering are multidisciplinary fields. Without underestimating the importance of all the other fields, a special emphasis is given in this manuscript to those formulative aspects that might compromise the marketability of a product.

UV-vis, IR and NMR analyses showed that PLGA dissolved in PEGDM mainly due to hydrogen bondings and other weak interactions caused by overlapping their respective hydrophobic and hydrophilic regions. However, the sum of many weak and few strong interactions might provide a reasonable amount of energy to maintain PLGA in solution. Such situation could explain why a hydrophobic molecule (PLGA) might dissolve in a hydrophilic one (PEGDM) but not in water. In addition, the possibility that PLGA molecules could arrange in supramolecular structures was questioned and rejected for the following considerations. First, non-polymerized formulations were perfectly transparent and did not scatter the light, indicating that formulations were not colloidal dispersions and further suggesting that they might be in a physical state of solution or liquid crystal [26,27]. Then, liquid crystals were excluded because PEGDM-PLGA blends were unable to deviate the path of a polarized light [26]. In addition, the observation that new molecules were not formed during the process of PLGA dissolution (NMR results) added further evidences that blends might be indeed solutions. Secondly, hypothesizing that there might be some supramolecular structures that do not cause the Tyndall Effect, if PLGA had arranged in clusters of different shape, it would have created solid domains since PLGA is a white powder at room conditions, which would have probably modified PEGDM-PLGA fluid's clarity, especially at higher PLGA concentrations. Further investigations have in fact shown that above the saturation concentration PLGA starts to precipitate as a fine powder within the blend, which turns opaque. In addition, presence of PLGA clusters would have also generated a system that could have been considered similar to a polymeric particle dispersions, and which are known to behave as elastic or viscoelastic fluids (see above in section 13.4.5). Thirdly, it was observed that photopolymerized matrices took on a whitish color upon incubation in PBS or Milli-Q water. It is reasonable to think that, in hydrated photopolymerized PEGDM-PLGA samples, water would be mostly associated with hydrophilic polyethyleneoxy units of PEGDM chain. In this circumstance, PEGDM and PLGA molecules will be spaced out decreasing the interactions between PEGDM and PLGA. All these observations led to conclude that PEGDM-PLGA blends are in fact solutions of PLGA in PEGDM.

From a formulative perspective, a formulation in a physical state of 'solution' would provide no, or at least lesser, stability concerns during storage and transportation [27]. In addition, the possibility to dissolve PLGA in PEGDM without adding organic solvent allows formulating photopolymerized drug delivery systems for proteic bioactive molecules. In fact, it is well known that even a short exposure to organic solvents is able to alter proteins and related molecules [28]. In addition, absence of organic solvents allows producing formulations (drug delivery systems and/or scaffolds for tissue engineering) that can be polymerized and implanted *in situ*, without risking toxicological responses of the surrounding tissues.

Rheological investigations showed that non-polymerized PEGDM-PLGA blends were fully deformable viscous fluids where macro-monomer and polymer molecules can get entangled and interpenetrated with each other as the concentration of PLGA increases. Viscosity, flow properties and microstructure have a great importance for some formulative and applicative issues. For instance, the viscosity of a system will determine how easy/difficult it would be to homogeneously suspend bioactive molecules or drug delivery systems in that particular formulation, and to avoid sedimentation or caking processes [27]. Avoiding these processes is usually important in the formulation of extemporaneous* and ready-to-use preparations, respectively. Another formulative-applicative challenge is related with injectability. Systems being concurrently physically stable, moderate viscous, irreversibly deforming and non-elastic, as PEGDM-PLGA blends, would have a whole supply of properties necessary for being also easily injectable, which is one of the most important properties for all the *in-vivo* applications (e.g.; *in-situ* formation of scaffold for tissue regeneration or drug delivery implants), when photopolymerization is carried out *in situ* through minimal invasive surgery. In fact, in this case, formulations, that may contain drugs and/or cells, are placed in the desired body location through a needle or a small cannula. Photopolymerization is successively initiated by an appropriated radiation. Finally and especially for tissue engineering purposes, rheological properties will also determine whether a non-polymerized formulation would perfectly fill all the possible asperities and/or canaliculi of a chosen cavity [29], and would be retained in place before its polymerization. It might be questioned whether rheological measurements should have been performed at body temperature. However, it has been thought that room temperature is the one that can have an effect on formulation injectability and stability. In addition, even hypothesizing any potential modifications of formulation physico-chemical properties at body temperature, these modifications would have no impact, since in a real situation non-polymerized formulations will be injected in the minimum amount of time and polymerized immediately after.

---

* Extemporaneous preparations are those where ingredients are mixed just before their administration.

Under this perspective, rheological data of non-polymerized PEGDM-PLGA blends allows for easily tuning the formulation viscosity for a desired application. Furthermore, it is anticipated in here that hydrophobicity and biodegradability of PLGA allowed to control the release of molecules from photopolymerized PEGDM-PLGA networks. Finally, the author would like to highlight that, to her knowledge, this is the first report about using PLGA as a hydrophobic and biodegradable viscosity modifier.

Studied PEGDM-PLGA formulations did not absorb in the common wavelength range, 400-520 nm, of commercial blue-light lamps (Figure 13.1). This is another important result of this study, because it signifies that these formulations are transparent to the wavelength of polymerization, or, in other words, that PLGA could be used to modify viscosity and hydrophobicity of a non-polymerized PEGDM-PLGA blend without affecting the penetration depth of the polymerizing blue-light. Consequently, during polymerization, the intensity of light will decrease through the thickness of the sample only as a function of photoinitiator concentration. The importance of these findings are also corroborated by the fact that there are no reports about how to modify rheological properties of a photopolymerizable formulation while maintaining its transparency to polymerizing radiations in literature so far.

The ability to maintain formulation transparency to the polymerizing light might be important with thick matrices, and especially in *in-vivo* implantations where there would be just one opening from which formulation would be injected and then polymerized. If a non-polymerized formulation (without photoinitiators) were not light conductive, the concern as to whether polymerization (in the presence of photoinitiators) would occur only near to the light source [19], would be legitimate. In this eventuality, potential toxicological risks due to the presence of non-polymerized macro-monomers should be considered as well.

Photopolymerization was carried out easily and in few minutes. Mechanism of polymerization has been described exhaustively elsewhere [30]. In brief, the process is initiated by CQ, which after absorbing the polymerizing light dissociates producing radical species. The process is accelerated by 4-EDMAB, and involves the polymerization of PEGDM methacrylic groups. Thus, PEGDM will form a cross-linked network within which PLGA will be entrapped. For this reason, resulting matrices can be considered semi-interpenetrating networks (semi-IPNs) [31]. It is well known that IPNs and semi-INPs are used in polymer chemistry to blend the properties of different polymers [31]. It can be anticipated that in the second part of this study it was found that properties of PLGA and PEGDM were indeed blended; these included all mechanical properties, surface properties, cell attachment and drug delivery.

From a formulative point of view, the possibility to simply combine materials to blend their properties might be advantageous and cheaper than to synthesize and characterize new materials.

13.5. CONCLUSIONS

The results of this study showed that PLGA could be blended with PEGDM without the use of organic solvents to produce viscous, easy injectable fluids that might be easily photopolymerized using a blue-light and a camphorquinone/amine photoinitiator system. The results presented and those anticipated in here showed that these formulations have some appealing features that might be useful in the formulative development of photopolymerized matrices to be used in tissue engineering and drug delivery.

13.6. ACKNOWLEDGMENTS

The author is indebted to Prof. D.A. Weitz for kindly allowing access to the rheometer facility at the division of Engineering and Applied Sciences (DEAS) of the Harvard University (Cambridge, MA, USA), and with Prof. M. Kilfoil for her enthusiastic assistance in the use of the equipment and valuable discussions. The author would like to express her immense gratitude to Prof. R. Langer for granting her several appointments at the Department of Chemical Engineering of the Massachusetts Institute of Technology (Cambridge, MA, USA), where this study was partially done. This research was also funded by MIUR (protocol number 2003033945_002) and by Fondazione Banco di Sardegna (protocol number 1255/5260).

13.7. REFERENCES

1. Y. An, J.A. Hubbell, Intraarterial protein delivery via intimally-adherent bilayer hydrogels, *J Control Rel* **64**(1-3), 205–215 (2000).
2. M.B. Mellott, C. Searchy, M.V. Pishko, Release of protein from highly cross-linked hydrogels of poly(ethylene glycol)diacrylate fabricated by UV polymerization, *Biomaterials* **22**(9), 929–941 (2001).
3. J. Elisseeff, W. McIntosh, K. Fu, T. Blunk, R. Langer, Controlled-release of IGF-I and TGF-b1 in a photopolymerizing hydrogel for cartilage tissue engineering, *J Orthop Res* **19**(6), 1098–1104 (2001).
4. K.S. Anseth, A.T. Metters, S.J. Bryant, P.J. Martens, J.H. Elisseeff, C.N. Bowman, In situ forming degradable networks and their application in tissue engineering and drug delivery, *J Control Rel* **78**, 199–209 (2002).
5. K.A. Davis, K.S. Anseth, Controlled Release from crosslinked degradable networks, *Critical Reviews in Therapeutic Drug Carrier Systems* **19**(4-5), 385-423 (2002).
6. D.J Quick, K.S. Anseth, DNA delivery from photocrosslinked PEG hydrogels: encapsulation efficiency, release profiles, and DNA quality, *J Control Rel* **96**(2), 341-351 (2004).
7. J. Elisseeff, K. Anseth, D. Sims, W. McIntosh, M. Randolph, R. Langer, Transdermal photopolymerization for minimally invasive implantation, *Proc Natl Acad Sci USA* **96**(6), 3104–3107 (1999).
8. A.K. Burkoth, K.S. Anseth, A review of photocrosslinked polyanhydrides: in situ forming degradable networks, *Biomaterials* **21**, 2395-2404 (2000).
9. R.H. Schmedlen, K.S. Masters, J.L. West, Photocrosslinkable polyvinyl alcohol hydrogels that can be modified with cell adhesion peptides for use in tissue engineering, *Biomaterials* **23**, 4325–4332 (2002).
10. K. Truong Nguyen, J.L. West, Photopolymerizable hydrogels for tissue engineering applications, *Biomaterials* **23**, 4307–4314 (2002).
11. J.A. Burdick, K.S. Anseth, Photoencapsulation of osteoblasts in injectable RGD-modified PEG hydrogels for bone tissue engineering, *Biomaterials* **23**, 4315–4323 (2002).
12. Y. Doo Park, N. Tirelli, J.A. Hubbell, Photopolymerized hyaluronic acid-based hydrogels and interpenetrating networks, *Biomaterials* **24**, 893–900 (2003).
13. D. Wang, C.G. Williams, Q. Li, B. Sharma, J.H. Elisseeff, Synthesis and characterization of a novel degradable phosphate-containing hydrogel, *Biomaterials* **24**, 3969–3980 (2003).
14. K.S. Masters, D.N. Shah, G. Walker, L.A. Leinwand, K.S. Anseth, Designing scaffolds for valvular interstitial cells: cell adhesion and function on naturally derived materials, *Journal of Biomedical Material Research* **71A**(1), 172-180 (2004).
15. F. Yang, C.G. Williams, D.A. Wang, H. Lee, P.N. Manson, J. Elisseeff, The effect of incorporating RGD adhesive peptide in polyethylene glycol diacrylate hydrogel on osteogenesis of bone marrow stromal cells, *Biomaterials* **26**(30), 5991-5998 (2005).
16. Q. Li, C.G. Williams, D.D.N. Sun, J. Wang, K. Leong, J.H. Elisseeff, Photocrosslinkable polysaccharides based on chondroitin sulfate, *Journal of Biomedical Material Research* **68A**(1), 28-33 (2004).

17. K.S. Masters, D.N. Shah, L.A. Leinwand, K.S. Anseth, Crosslinked hyaluronan scaffolds as a biologically active carrier for valvular interstitial cells, *Biomaterials* **26**(15), 2517-2525 (2005).
18. C.R. Nuttelman, M.C. Tripodi, K.S. Anseth, Synthetic hydrogel niches that promote hMSC viability, *Matrix Biology* **24**(3), 208-218 (2005).
19. M.D. Goodner, C.N. Bowman, Development of a comprehensive free radical photopolymerization model incorporating heat and mass transfer effects in thick films, *Chemical Engineering Science* **57**, 887–900 (2002).
20. R.M. Silverstein, G.C. Bassler, T.C. Morril, *Spectrometric Identification of Organic Compounds*, 5th edition, (John Wiley & Sons, Inc., New York, 1991).
21. F. Rodriguez, Analysis and identification of polymers, in: *Principles of Polymer Systems*, edited by J.V. Brown, V.M. Ziobro, and E. Dugger (Hemisphere publishing Corporation, Washington, 1982, 2nd edition), p. 482.
22. F. Rodriguez, Basic structure of polymers, in: *Principles of Polymer Systems*, edited by J.V. Brown, V.M. Ziobro, and E. Dugger (Hemisphere publishing Corporation, Washington, 1982, 2nd edition), pp. 17-32.
23. H.N. Naé, Introduction to rheology, in: *Rheological Properties of Cosmetics and Toiletries*, edited by D. Laba (Marcel Dekker. Inc., New York, 1993), pp.9-33.
24. F. Rodriguez, Viscous flow, in: *Principles of Polymer Systems*, edited by J.V. Brown, V.M. Ziobro, and E. Dugger (Hemisphere publishing Corporation, Washington, 1982, 2nd edition), pp. 155-198.
25. Department of Physics and Astronomy of Georgia State University, (Georgia, USA, August 2004); http://hyperphysics.phy-astr.gsu.edu/hbase/ppois.html
26. *Handbook of Microemulsion Science and Technology*, edited by P. Kumar and K.L. Mittal (Marcel Dekker, Inc., New York, 1999).
27. Remington. *The Science and Practice of Pharmacy*, 20th edition, (Philadelphia college of pharmacy and science. Philadelphia, 2000).
28. W. Wang, Instability, stabilization, and formulation of liquid protein pharmaceuticals, *Int J Pharm* **185**, 129–188 (1999).
29. M. Bohner, B. Gasser, G. Baroud, P. Heini, Theoretical and experimental model to describe the injection of a polymethylmethacrylate cement into a porous structure, *Biomaterials* **24**, 2721-2730 (2003).
30. W.D. Cook, Photopolymerization kinetics of dimethacrylates using the camphorquinone/amine initiator system, *Polymer* **33**(2), 600-609 (1992).
31. G.G. Odian. *Principles of Polymerization*, 3rd edition (John Wiley & Sons, Inc., New York, 1991).

14

POROUS TANTALUM TRABECULAR METAL SCAFFOLDS IN COMBINATION WITH A NOVEL MARROW PROCESSING TECHNIQUE TO REPLACE AUTOGRAFT

Xuenong Zou[1,2,*], Haisheng Li[1], Lijin Zou[1], Tina Mygind[1], Martin Lind[1], and Cody Bünger[1]

14.1. ABSTRACT

Introduction. Interbody fusion requires a structural member to carry load while the autograft or osteoinductive agent stimulates bone formation. In the present study, we evaluated the potential use of extracted nucleated cells from bone marrow mixed in hyaluronic acid gel as an osteoinductive agent, in comparison to Collagraft loaded with nucleated cells or rhBMP-2 in the porous tantalum ring, in an anterior lumbar interbody fusion (ALIF) in pigs.

Methods. Four 3-month-old female Danish landrace pigs were employed in the current study. Bone marrow was collected by means of aspiration, from the medullary cavity of the proximal tibia. The nucleated cells were isolated with a Ficoll step gradient centrifugation. The cell adhered rate after 24 hours of cultivation and ALP activity in the osteogenic medium following 4 days of cultivation were measured. Cell numbers in the porous tantalum discs were assessed by CyQuant measurement, and fluorescent live/dead cell staining in the porous tantalum discs was performed after periods of 24 hours and 7 days of cultivation. The nucleated cells mixed in hyaluronic acid gel were cultivated on slides for 24 hours, 7 days and 21 days. The live/dead cell staining, ALP staining or osteocalcin staining, were performed. A porous tantalum ring was loaded with nucleated cells in hyaluronic acid gel or packed with Collagraft strips also with nucleated cells or rhBMP-2. Immediately after preparation, one of three implants was inserted into L2-3,

---

[1] Orthopaedic Research Laboratory, Aarhus University Hospital, 8000 Aarhus C, Denmark
[2] Department of Orthopaedics, the 5th Affiliated Hospital of Sun Yat-sen University, Zhuhai, Guangdong, China
* Correspondence and reprint requests: zxnong@hotmail.com (X. Zou)

L4-5 or L6-7 respectively. The pigs were killed 3 months postoperatively. The lumbar spine specimens were prepared for histological evaluation.

Results. The adhered rate, of the nucleated cells, was 2.26 ± 0.56‰. ALP activity was no different in the osteogenic culture compared to DMEM/10%FBS alone. Cell numbers and live/dead cells showed no difference in the porous tantalum discs. Histological appearance showed that nucleated cells mixed with hyaluronic acid gel, had more mature bone in the central hole of the porous tantalum ring, compared to Collagraft strips with nucleated cells or rhBMP-2. Bone volume fraction did not differ within the three porous tantalum rings; however, more marrow space in the central hole of the porous tantalum ring was present when nucleated cells mixed with hyaluronic acid gel (57.4%) compared to Collagraft strips with rhBMP-2 (29.7%).

Conclusion. In the current study, we demonstrate that nucleated cells, which were isolated from bone marrow intraoperatively, could be used to replace autograft if nucleated cells mixed with hyaluronic acid gel or with Collagraft strips packed into the porous tantalum ring in the pig ALIF model.

14.2. INTRODUCTION

Porous tantalum Trabecular Metal (Trabecular Metal™; Zimmer Inc., Warsaw, IN.) is highly porous (70-80%) and has a structural stiffness in the relatively low range of about 2.5 to 4.0 GPa. The high porosity of the material makes it similar to cancellous bone. The quality of the materials can be advantageous as a structural member. As the material is non-degradable, this type of matrix and the high porosity of the material provide a highly controlled physical environment to support load, as an interbody fusion device for spinal fusion, and to serve as tissue engineering scaffolds for loading cells. Porous tantalum Trabecular Metal has been used successfully as an anterior cervical interbody fusion device (Wigfield et al., 2003) as well as implants in a variety of spinal animal studies (Sidhu et al., 2001; Zou et al., 2003; Zou et al., 2004b; Zou et al., 2005). Previous work in our laboratory has shown 91% fusion rates with the porous tantalum Trabecular Metal devices, when used in combination with pedicle screw fixation (Zou et al., 2005), as opposed to a fusion rate of 56% when used with anterior staple fixation (Zou et al., 2004b).

Interbody fusion requires a structural member to carry load while the autograft or osteoinductive agent stimulates bone formation. Although autogenous bone graft is the golden standard for spinal fusion, there are limits to its mass as well as complications associated with bone harvest (Banwart et al., 1995; Younger and Chapman, 1989). A variety of agents have been evaluated and shown to be equivalent to autograft, such as Collagraft (Cornell et al., 1991) and InFuse (Burkus et al., 2002). Nowadays, many researchers are particularly interested in progenitor cell sources such as bone marrow stromal cells (BMSCs), which is a very attractive cell source in tissue engineering due to their capacity to differentiate into lineages of the mesenchymal tissues, including bone, cartilage, fat and muscle (Ringe et al., 2002). Unfortunately, BMSCs sources are scarce and the number of BMSCs available in the bone marrow decreases with aging (Muschler and Midura, 2002). So far, conventional use of an autologous BMSCs construct in the clinical setting is time consuming, requiring aspiration of bone marrow from the patient, several weeks for cell expansion, including gene delivery and quality-control testing, and finally re-implantation. However, bone-forming efficiency of BMSCs *in vivo* is markedly reduced following extensive subcultivation *in vitro*. This progressive loss of proliferation and osteogenic differentiation *in vitro* drastically limits the potential use of BMSCs' clinical practice. Hence, further refinement is needed in order to improve the efficiency of BMSCs' clinical application.

In our previous *in vitro* study, it has been demonstrated that a low molecular weight of hyaluronic acid accelerated an *in vitro* cellular proliferation of porcine BMSCs with the increase of the concentration of hyaluronic acid. Hyalaronic acid also up-regulated endogenous cellular ALP activity and osteocalcin mRNA expression, and interacted with dexamethasone and rhBMP-2 (Zou et al., 2004a). A combination of bone marrow stromal cells, hyaluronic acid and dexamethasone applied to porous tantalum Trabecular Metal scaffolds resulted in ectopic bone formation in a subcutaneous pig model. However, the practical application of BMSCs in porous tantalum Trabecular Metal scaffolds is hampered due to an uneven cell distribution in *in vitro* cultivation after conventional static seeding (Zou et al., 2003). In the present study, we proposed that promotion of the *in vivo* expansion and osteogenic differentiation for primary BMSCs, which enriched nucleated cells intraoperatively, could be a better solution for cell-based tissue engineering. The aim of the present study was to evaluate the potential use of extracted nucleated cells from bone marrow mixed with hyaluronic acid gel as an osteoinductive agent in comparison to Collagraft strips loaded with the nucleated cells or rhBMP-2 in a porous tantalum interbody device in a pig spinal fusion model.

14.3. MATERIALS AND METHODS

14.3.1. Bone Marrow Aspiration and Isolation

Four 3-month-old female Danish landrace pigs weighing around 50 kg were employed in the current study. Bone marrow was obtained by means of aspiration from the medullary cavity of the proximal tibia before the operation. A low-density cell fraction of bone marrow (6 ml) was placed over a Ficoll (4 ml) step gradient solution (density 1.077 g/ml; Ficoll-Paque Plus, Amersham). After that, cell suspensions were centrifuged at $400 \times g$ at room temperature for 30 min. The nucleated cells were collected from the defined layer at the interface, diluted with two volumes of PBS, centrifuged twice at $100 \times g$ for 10 min and finally nucleated cells in number were counted by a haemocytometer.

14.3.2. Preparation of Porous Tantalum Rings and Discs

After cell counting, a suspension of 400×10^6 nucleated cells in 10 ml Dulbecco's modified Eagle's medium with Glutamix-1, sodium pyruvate, 4500 mg/l glucose and pyridoxine (DMEM; Gibco, BRL) were poured on one porous tantalum ring (23 mm x 15 mm x 11 mm) and 13 porous tantalum discs (10.2 mm in diameter, 5 mm in height). This was done in a 50 ml culture tube with 200 mg hyaluronic acid (Mw=800 kDa; Lifecore

Biomedical, Inc., Chaska, MN.), in which the scaffolds were mixed with hyaluronic acid gel and nucleated cells. A suspension of 100 x 10^6 nucleated cells were loaded into Collagraft strips (11 mm x 10 mm; Zimmer Inc., Warsaw, IN.) containing 65% hydroxyapatite/35% tricalcium phosphate powder-type I bovine fibrillar collagen matrices. Before cell loading, Collagraft strips were packed into the central hole of the porous tantalum ring. A solution containing 6 mg of rhBMP-2 (InFUSE™; Medtronic Sofamor Danek, Memphis, Tenn.) was loaded into the Collagraft strips, which were also packed into the porous tantalum ring (Figure 14.2.). Immediately after preparation, the porous tantalum ring was implanted into L2-3, L4-5, or L6-7 respectively. The surgical procedures are described below.

14.3.3. Measurements of Cell Adhered Rate and ALP Activity

For each pig, a suspension of 5 x 10^6 nucleated cells per well was cultivated in 2 wells of the 6-well plate (9.6 cm^2). After 24 hours of cultivation, the adhered cells were trypsinated and total adhered cells were counted by a haemocytometer. The adhered rate of nucleated cells was calculated. For alkaline phosphonatase (ALP) activity, 6000 cells/cm^2 were cultivated in 75-cm^2 flasks in DMEM and 10% fetal bovine serum (FBS Australian Origin; Bio Whittaker Europe, Belgium; Lot 8SB0001). After 20 hours, the medium was changed. The cells were cultivated in the osteogenic medium (dexamethasone 1×10^{-8} mol/l, ascorbate 82 mg/ml, ß-glycerophosphate 10 mmol/l) or in DMEM/10%FBS alone, for 4 days. ALP activity was measured in the cell layer after 30 min of incubation with p-nitrophenyl phosphate (Sigma) as a substrate at 37°C. Absorbance of p-nitrophenol was determined by microspectrophotometer at 405 nm. Intra-assay CV: 4.6%. Phenotype expression was estimated by the ratio of ALP in wells supplemented with 10% FBS. For adjustment of ALP value with cell number, parallel cell culture in the flasks was designed. Cell numbers were counted by CyQuant measurement.

14.3.4. The *In Vitro* Assays of Nucleated Cells in Hyaluronic Acid Gel

Each porous tantalum disc loaded with nucleated cells in hyaluronic acid gel was transferred to a well of 48-well culture plate and added 500 µl DMEM/10%FBS for a 24 hour period and a 7 day period of cultivation. Cell numbers on the porous tantalum discs were assessed by CyQuant measurement while live/dead cell staining on the porous tantalum discs were assessed by using the fluorescence LIVE/DEAD® Viability/Cytotoxicity Kit (L-3224; Molecular Probes, Inc., Eugene, OR) following the kit protocol. Samples were incubated for 45 min at room temperature in 5 ml of PBS containing 10 µl EthD-1 stock solutions, which stained green for live cells, and 2.5 µl calcein AM stock solution, which stained red for dead cells. Vortex, the resulting solution ensures thorough mixing. EthD-1 and calcein could be viewed simultaneously with a conventional fluorescein longpass filter under a light microscope (Olympus Denmark A/S, Albertslund, Denmark). The culture wells and surfaces of samples were evaluated immediately after staining. Following this procedure, the porous tantalum discs were fixed with formalin and embedded in methylmethacrylate. 20 μm serial sections were cut and viewed under the fluorescence microscope.

The nucleated cells in hyaluronic acid gel were cultivated on slides for period of 24 hours, 7 days and 21 days. The cells were also assessed by live/dead cell staining at 24 hours and at 7 days of cultivation. After 21 days of cultivation, the cells were treated by ALP staining and osteocalcin staining.

14.3.5. Surgical Procedures

Each pig performed a discontinuous three-level lumbar arthrodesis at L2-3, L4-5 and L6-7, with the employment of the porous tantalum ring, under general anesthesia. A detailed description of surgical procedures can be found in our preceding studies elsewhere (Zou et al., 2003; Zou et al., 2004b; Zou et al., 2005); only the brief description is reported here. A paramedian abdominal incision was chosen. Through a retroperitoneal approach, the anterior lumbar spine was exposed. After preparation of the intervertebral disc place, each level was implanted with one of the porous tantalum rings, which were prepared by the aforementioned description: (1) Collagraft strips loaded with nucleated cells (100 x 10^6 cells) in the central hole of the porous tantalum ring, (2) Hyaluronic acid gel with nucleated cells (40 x 10^6 cells) in the porous tantalum ring, or (3) Collagraft strips loaded with rhBMP-2 (6 mg) in the central hole of the porous tantalum ring. Each implant was temporarily secured with two titanium staples (22 mm in length x 16 mm in depth; Howmedica GmbH, Schönkirchen, Germany) in front of the implant. The abdominal muscle and the rectus abdominis sheath were carefully sutured, and the skin was closed by discontinuous sutures. Prophylactic ampicillin (1.0g, I.V., Anhypen; Gist-Brocades, Delft, the Netherlands) and analgesic buprenorphine (Temgesic, 0.02mg/kg, IM, TID; Hull, UK) were given before and immediately after surgery, and twice a day during the following 3 days. The pigs were housed individually with water *ad libitum*. Food was controlled with necessary nutrients to avoid rapid growth. After 3 months, the pigs were killed by intravenous injection by an overdose pentobarbital (0.4 mg/kg) given under general anesthesia. The spine segments were taken from L1 to sacrum, stripped of soft tissue, and frozen at -20°C until histological examination. All animal surgeries and experiments complied with the Danish Law on Animal Experimentation and were approved by the Danish Ministry of Justice Ethical Committee, J.nr.1998-561-67.

14.3.6. Histology and Histomorphometry

The implant specimen was dehydrated in graded ethanol (70-99%) containing 0.4% basic fuchsin and embedded in methylmethacrylate. 40 μm thick sections were cut sagittally, with 500 μm intervals between each section, to obtain the maximum range of sampling using a Microtome KGD 95 sawing (Meprotech, Heerhugowaard, the Netherlands). All surfaces were counterstained with 2% light green for 2 min. Four slides were produced from each specimen for qualitative and quantitative histological studies.

In the qualitative histological analysis, all sections were evaluated in a blind manner. Tissue types of bone, bone marrow, fibrous tissue, and residual HA/TCP were identified under the light microscope. Histological sections were used to define the state of interface histology in contact with the device at the cranial and caudal implant interfaces between the host bone and implant. Histological sections were also used to define the state of implant histology in the central hole of the porous tantalum ring.

For histomorphometry, a stereological software program (CAST-Grid®, Olympus Denmark A/S, Albertslund, Denmark) was used. The program is based on a user-specified grid applied to microscopic fields captured on the monitor (attached to a light microscope; objective x4, ocular x10). Four sections from each specimen were evaluated in a blind manner using the linear intercept technique and point counting. Bone volume, bone marrow space, fibrous tissue, or residual HA/TCP was calculated (as a percentage) in each region of interest (ROI). The ROIs on the section are defined as zone *A*: the central hole of the porous tantalum ring, zone *B*: the pores of the porous tantalum ring, zone *C*: the vertebrae implant interface, zone *D*: the vertebrae graft interface, zone *E*: the adjacent vertebral bone. Bone, bone marrow or fibrous tissue was counted using the point-counting technique counting approximately 600-1200 points per implant (4 sections) in each region of interest (Zou et al., 2004b; Zou et al., 2005).

14.4. RESULTS

The nucleated cells were isolated from 4 pigs. The adhered rate of the nucleated cells was calculated as 2.26 ± 0.56‰ during 24 hours of cultivation.

Cell numbers on the porous tantalum discs were assessed by CyQuant measurement. The average cell number was 98955.3 ± 14456.3 in a 24 hour period of cultivation and 92462.8 ± 17456.0 in a 7 day period of cultivation. No difference was evident between 24 hours and 7 days of cultivation, when the nucleated cells in hyaluronic acid gel were loaded into the porous tantalum discs.

The nucleated cells with hyaluronic gel in the porous tantalum discs, cultivated for 24 hours or 7 days, were assessed by using the fluorescence LIVE/DEAD staining. This demonstrated that live cells were not only on the surface of discs for 24 hours of cultivation, but also inside the discs after 7 days of cultivation. The nucleated cells in hyaluronic acid gel were cultivated on slides for periods of 24 hours, 7 days and 21 days. The live cells which adhered to the slide could be seen for 24 hours of cultivation and many cells became growth on the slide after 7 days of cultivation. After 21 days of cultivation on the slide, the cells were positive to ALP staining and osteocalcin staining (See Figure 14.1.).

All histological sections from the 4 pigs are depicted in Figure 14.2. Histological observation showed that nucleated cells mixed with hyaluronic acid gel had more mature bone in the central hole of the porous tantalum ring, compared to Collagraft strips with nucleated cells or rhBMP-2, due to residual HA/TCP in the latter. In each group, 50% had at least new bone ingrowth through the central hole of the porous tantalum ring. The histological appearance in the porous tantalum rings did not show any difference in the vertebrae implant/graft interface.

Histomorphometric results at the different locations are summarized in Table 14.1. Bone volume fraction was 19.8%, 18.5%, and 20.2% in the pore of the porous tantalum rings with the treatments of nucleated cells with hyaluronic acid gel, Collagraft strips with nucleated cells, and Collagraft strips with rhBMP-2, respectively. Bone volume fraction was 36.3%, 32.9%, and 38.2% in the central hole of the porous tantalum rings with above three treatments; however, there was more marrow space in the central hole

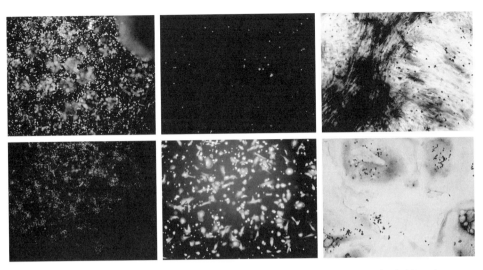

Figure 14.1 (see color insert, Figure 14.1). The nucleated cells in hyaluronic acid gel loaded into the porous tantalum discs after 24 hours (Left panel, top) and 7 days (Left panel, bottom) of cultivation. The nucleated cells in hyaluronic acid gel were cultivated on slides for duration of 24 hours (Middle panel, top) and 7 days (Middle panel, bottom). Live/dead cell staining showed that live cells were green, and dead cells were red. After 21 days of cultivation, the nucleated cells in hyaluronic acid gel show positive ALP staining (Right panel, top) and osteocalcin staining (Right panel, bottom).

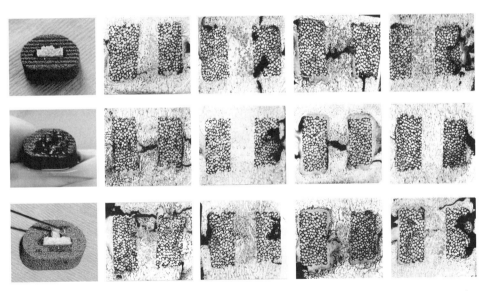

Figure 14.2 (see color insert, Figure 14.2). Porous tantalum rings with different graft materials, for an anterior lumbar interbody fusion in pigs, were implanted into L2/3 (top), L4/5 (middle) and L6/7 (bottom). First panel shows Collagraft strips with nucleated cells (100 millions) in the central hole of the porous tantalum ring (top), hyaluronic acid gel with nucleated cells (40 million /ml) in the porous tantalum ring (middle), and Collagraft strips containing 6 mg of rhBMP-2 in the central hole of the porous tantalum ring (bottom). The second to fifth panels shows histological sections from the porous tantalum rings, which correspond to implants in pig 1 to pig 4 three months after the initial operation. The histology in the porous tantalum rings depicts very similar appearances in the vertebrae implant/graft interfaces and in the central hole of the porous tantalum rings.

of the porous tantalum ring when nucleated cells were mixed with hyaluronic acid gel (57.4%), compared to Collagraft strips with rhBMP-2 (29.7%). Collagraft strips with the nucleated cells and Collagraft strips with rhBMP-2 still had 25.0% and 20.8% residual HA/TCP in the central hole of the porous tantalum ring, respectively. The tissue volume fractions were not different at the vertebrae implant interface, the vertebrae graft interface and the adjacent vertebrae bone.

Table 14.1. Histomorphometric results at the different locations (mean ± SEM)

Locations	Collagraft + cells	Hyaluronan + cells	Collagraft + rhBMP-2
A zone†			
Bone	32.9 ± 4.0	36.3 ± 8.3	38.2 ± 5.8
Bone Marrow	38.2 ± 4.2	57.4 ± 12.0	29.7 ± 4.6
Fibrous Tissue	3.1 ± 3.1	1.7 ± 1.7	10.3 ± 6.1
Residual HA/TCP	25.0 ± 3.2		20.8 ± 3.5
B zone‡			
Bone	18.5 ± 3.6	19.8 ± 5.2	20.2 ± 4.1
Bone Marrow	41.5 ± 10.2	38.5 ± 11.8	28.1 ± 8.9
Fibrous Tissue	40.0 ± 13.7	41.5 ± 17.1	51.7 ± 12.9
C zone§			
Bone	39.5 ± 1.4	35.9 ± 2.3	41.1 ± 1.0
Bone Marrow	56.6 ± 3.0	58.5 ± 6.0	54.4 ± 3.1
Fibrous Tissue	7.2 ± 2.9	5.6 ± 4.0	4.5 ± 2.4
D zone⟩⟩			
Bone	37.8 ± 3.6	34.9 ± 3.3	42.6 ± 3.1
Bone Marrow	61.1 ± 4.0	65.1 ± 3.3	55.7 ± 4.0
Fibrous Tissue	1.1 ± 1.1		1.7 ± 1.2
E zone¶			
Bone	34.9 ± 3.0	32.7 ± 1.3	41.1 ± 1.0
Bone Marrow	65.1 ± 3.0	67.2 ± 1.3	54.4 ± 3.1

† The central holes of the porous tantalum ring.
‡ The pores of the porous tantalum ring.
§ The vertebrae implant interface.
⟩⟩ The [[ertebrae graft interface.
¶ The adjacent vertebral bone.

14.5. DISCUSSION

In the current study, we demonstrated that bone volume fraction in the pore of the porous tantalum rings was 19.8%, 18.5%, and 20.2% when three different graft materials were used in the central hole of the porous tantalum ring. The various graft materials were hyaluronic acid gel with nucleated cells, Collagraft strips with nucleated cells and Collagraft strips with rhBMP-2. Bone volume fraction in the central hole of the porous tantalum rings were 36.3%, 32.9%, and 38.2% in the three treatments; however, hyaluronic acid gel with nucleated cells had more marrow space (57.4%) than Collagraft strips with rhBMP-2 (29.7%). In the 3-months follow-up study of pigs, bone volume fraction was 39.3% in the central hole of the porous tantalum ring and only 11.0% in the pores of the porous tantalum ring, when autograft was packed in the central hole of the porous tantalum ring (Zou et al., 2004b). Bone volume fraction was 38.0% in the central hole of the porous tantalum ring and 16.1% in the pores of the porous tantalum ring, when autograft was used in the central hole of the porous tantalum ring at the 6-months follow-up (Zou et al., 2005). In the present study, a novel marrow processing technique in the 3-months follow-up study of a pig spinal fusion model, produced results similar to the 6-months follow-up study in pigs with autograft used in the central hole of the porous tantalum ring (Zou et al., 2005). The results showed that a novel marrow processing technique for preparing graft materials could be used to replace autografts in the porous tantalum interbody device.

In our spinal fusion model with ALIF cages, the empty carbon fiber cage could not produce spinal fusion in 10 pigs with a 3-months follow-up (Xue et al., 2004). Empty porous tantalum rings could likewise not produce spinal fusion in pigs after 6-months follow-up with pedicle screw fixation (data not showing). β-TCP particles in the carbon fiber cages achieved poor results (only partly spinal fusion) when compared with autogenous bone graft, even if application of platelet-rich plasma of the certain concentration into the β-TCP particles did not demonstrate any effect on bone formation or β-TCP resorption (Li et al., 2004). In the present study, each treatment (4 porous tantalum rings) had at least 50% spinal fusion, which was defined as new bone ingrowth through the central hole of the porous tantalum ring. The findings showed that equivalent results within the three graft materials were produced due to enriched nucleated cells or rhBMP-2.

The porous tantalum ring is made of porous tantalum trabecular metal, which is fabricated via a chemical vapor infiltration (CVI) process in which pure tantalum metal is precipitated onto a reticulated vitreous carbon (RVC) skeleton resulting in encasement of the RVC within the tantalum. The quality of the materials could be advantageous in providing a highly controlled physical environment to support load for spinal fusion serving as an interbody fusion device. Furthermore, it could serve as tissue engineering scaffolds for loading cells, due to the high porosity of the material, which is fully interconnected with an average size of 400 to 500 μm. Clinically, porous tantalum trabecular metal offers a viable solution to several challenges in orthopaedic reconstructive surgery, including mono-block acetabular cups, avascular necrosis intervention devices, and total hip reconstruction in situations of massive femoral bone loss, as described by Christie (2002). Porous tantalum Trabecular Metal has been used successfully as an anterior cervical interbody fusion device (Wigfield et al., 2003). The literature would indicate that porous tantalum exhibits bone-ingrowth-promoting characteristics, and that the geometrical structure of the material and its biomechanical properties are suited for interbody fusion cages as for larger reconstruction procedures in the spine.

Several studies suggest that three-dimensional porous tantalum scaffolds may be useful in advancing the in vitro culture and transduction of hematopoietic stem and progenitor cells (Bagley et al., 1999; Ehring et al., 2003; Rosenzweig et al., 1997) and cell-based bone tissue engineering (Toh et al., 2005; Zou et al., 2003). However, the distribution of cells in the scaffold was uneven after the conventional cell seeding and the in vitro static culture, which corresponded to the in vivo bone formation in 3D scaffolds. The practical application of BMSCs in 3D scaffolds was hampered, due to a very low initial cell number and an uneven cell distribution in the in vitro culture, after conventional static seeding (Zou et al., 2003). There is a need to improve the seeding efficiency of BMSCs and to expand the limited cell numbers in 3D scaffolds.

Hyaluronic acid as biological hydrogels was used to improve the *in vitro* efficiency of static seeding, although its limitations were the same as fibrin glue (Bensaid et al., 2003; Ringe et al., 2003) and collagen (Ushida et al., 2002). For example, there is inherent variability in such biological materials and there is no precise control over the physiochemical parameters that triggers the gelation of these types of biological hydrogels. Hyaluronic acid gel may also have implications for the homogeneity of cell distribution and the diffusion limits of nutrients and wastes inside the scaffolds. Nevertheless, it has been found that hyaluronic acid could stimulate cellular proliferation following the increase of the concentration. Hyaluronic acid could also up-regulate endogenous cellular ALP activity and osteogenic maker gene expression, to generate direct and specific cellular effects (Huang et al., 2003; Zou et al., 2004a). Thus, we hypothesized that hyaluronic acid gel could entrap osteoprogenitor cells inside 3D scaffolds and promote the *in vivo* cell expansion, proliferation and differentiation in 3D scaffolds, which would then serve as bone substitute material to replace autograft.

In the present study, we collected bone marrow by means of aspiration from the medullary cavity of the proximal tibia in pigs, and isolated the nucleated cells with a Ficoll step gradient centrifugation. The nucleated cells could been grown in the porous tantalum trabecular metal scaffolds with hyaluronic acid gel for up to 7 days of cultivation. The nucleated cells in hyaluronic acid gel were cultivated on slides for periods of 24 hours, 7 days and 21 days. The results showed that nucleated cells remained alive in hyaluronic acid gel and continued to promote cell proliferation and osteogenic differentiation. After isolation of nucleated cells, a low density of nucleated cells in hyaluronic acid gel loaded into the porous tantalum ring, resulted in new bone formation similar to the high density of nucleated cells or rhBMP-2 loaded into Collagraft strips in the central hole of the porous tantalum ring in the pig ALIF model. The osteoinduction results in this model suggested that hyaluronic acid gel is vital, in part, due to its ability to maintain nucleated cells and to promote the *in vivo* cell expansion, proliferation and osteogenic differentiation in the porous tantalum trabecular metal scaffolds. In addition, with key interest for tissue regeneration application, fragments of hyaluronic acid have also been shown to promote angiogenesis (West et al., 1985). The incorporation of hyaluronic acid and the degradation of hyaluronic acid from a biomaterial can lead to more rapid vascularization and a greater chance for transplanted cells or regenerating tissues to remain viable (Collier et al., 2000). Therefore, the incorporation of hyaluronic acid and bone marrow stromal cells into 3D scaffolds would have a greater potential to the bone regeneration by tissue engineering strategies. From a clinical point of view, this could be a better solution for cell-based tissue engineering by enriching the nucleated cells from bone marrow intraoperatively and combining it with hyaluronic acid gel and 3D scaffolds, to replace autograft in the clinical setting.

To summarize in conclusion, this study demonstrates that nucleated cells, which were isolated from bone marrow intraoperatively, could be used to replace autograft when combined with hyaluronic acid gel or Collagraft strips and loaded into the porous tantalum trabecular metal scaffolds in a pig ALIF model.

14.6. ACKNOWLEDGMENTS

The authors thank Mrs. Anette Milton for histological technical assistance and Mrs. Anette Baatrup for cell culture technical assistance.

The authors are grateful for financial support from the Institute for Clinical Medicine and Aarhus Spine Research Foundation, The University of Aarhus, Aarhus, Denmark, and Zimmer Inc., Warsaw, IN. Porous tantalum Trabecular Metal discs, porous tantalum interbody devices, and Collagraft strips were manufactured and kindly provided by Zimmer Inc., Warsaw, IN., USA. rhBMP-2 was kindly provided by Medtronic Sofamor Danek, Memphis, Tenn., USA.

14.7. REFERENCES

Bagley, J., Rosenzweig, M., Marks, D.F., and Pykett, M.J., 1999, Extended culture of multipotent hematopoietic progenitors without cytokine augmentation in a novel three-dimensional device, *Exp. Hematol.* **27**(3):496-504.

Banwart, J.C., Asher, M.A., and Hassanein, R.S., 1995, Iliac crest bone graft harvest donor site morbidity. A statistical evaluation, *Spine* **20**(9):1055–1060.

Bensaid, W., Triffitt, J.T., Blanchat, C., Oudina, K., Sedel, L., and Petite, H., 2003, A biodegradable fibrin scaffold for mesenchymal stem cell transplantation, *Biomaterials* **24**(14):2497-2502.

Burkus, J.K., Transfeldt, E.E., Kitchel, S.H., Watkins, R.G., and Balderston, R.A., 2002, Clinical and radiographic outcomes of anterior lumbar interbody fusion using recombinant human bone morphogenetic protein-2, *Spine* **27**(21):2396-2408.

Christie, M.J., 2002, Clinical applications of Trabecular Metal, *Am. J. Orthop.* **31**(4):219-220.

Collier J.H., Camp J.P., Hudson T.W., and Schmidt C.E., 2000, Synthesis and characterization of polypyrrole-hyaluronic acid composite biomaterials for tissue engineering applications, *J. Biomed. Mater. Res.* **50**(4):574-584.

Cornell, C.N., Lane, J.M., Chapman, M., Merkow, R., Seligson, D., Henry, S., Gustilo, R., and Vincent, K., 1991, Multicenter trial of Collagraft as bone graft substitute, *J. Orthop. Trauma.* **5**(1):1-8.

Ehring, B., Biber, K., Upton, T.M., Plosky, D., Pykett, M., and Rosenzweig, M., 2003, Expansion of HPCs from cord blood in a novel 3D matrix, *Cytotherapy* **5**(6):490-499.

Huang, L., Cheng, Y.Y., Koo, P.L., Lee, K.M., Qin, L., Cheng, J.C., and Kumta, S.M., 2003, The effect of hyaluronan on osteoblast proliferation and differentiation in rat calvarial-derived cell cultures, *J. Biomed. Mater. Res. A* **66**(4):880-884.

Li, H., Zou, X., Xue, Q., Egund, N., Lind, M., and Bunger, C., 2004, Anterior lumbar interbody fusion with carbon fiber cage loaded with bioceramics and platelet-rich plasma. An experimental study on pigs, *Eur. Spine J.* **13**(4):354-358.

Muschler, G.F., and Midura, R.J., 2002, Connective tissue progenitors: practical concepts for clinical applications, *Clinical Orthop.* **395**:66-80.

Ringe, J., Kaps, C., Burmester, G.R., and Sittinger, M., 2002, Stem cells for regenerative medicine: Advances in the engineering of tissues and organs, *Naturwissenschaften.* **89**(8):338–351.

Ringe, J., Leinhase, I., Endres, M., Stich, S., Loch, A., and Sittinger, M., 2003, Human periosteal cells and mesenchymal stem cells for tissue engineering: A comparative study, *Tissue Eng.* **9**(4):783-784.

Rosenzweig, M., Pykett, M., Marks, D.F., Johnson, R.P., 1997, Enhanced maintenance and retroviral transduction of primitive hematopoietic progenitor cells using a novel three-dimensional culture system, *Gene Ther.* **4**(9):928-936.

Sidhu, K.S., Prochnow, T.D., Schmitt, P., Fischgrund, J., Weisbrode, S., and Herkowitz, H.N., 2001, Anterior cervical interbody fusion with rhBMP-2 and tantalum in a goat model, *Spine J.* **1**(5):331-340.

Toh, Y.C., Ho, S.T., Zhou, Y., Hutmacher, D.W., and Yu, H., 2005, Application of a polyelectrolyte complex coacervation method to improve seeding efficiency of bone marrow stromal cells in a 3D culture system, *Biomaterials* **26**(19):4149-4160.

Ushida, T., Furukawa, K., Toita, K., and Tateishi, T., 2002, Three-dimensional seeding of chondrocytes encapsulated in collagen gel into PLLA scaffolds, *Cell Transplant.* **11**(5):489-494.

West D.C., Hampson I.N., Arnold F., and Kumar S., 1985, Angiogenesis induced by degradation products of hyaluronic acid, *Science* **228**(4705):1324-1326.

Wigfield, C., Robertson, J., Gill, S., and Nelson, R., 2003, Clinical experience with porous tantalum cervical interbody implants in a prospective randomized controlled trial, *Br. J. Neurosurg.* **17**(5):418-425.

Xue, Q., Li, H., Zou, X., Christensen, F.B., Lind, M., and Bünger, C., 2005, Healing properties of allograft from alendronate-treated animal in lumbar spine interbody cage fusion, *Eur. Spine J.* **14**(3):222-226.

Younger, E.M. and Chapman, M.W., 1989, Morbidity at bone graft donor sites, *Orthop Trauma.* **3**:192-195.

Zou, X., Li, H., Baatrup, A., Lind, M., and Bunger, C., 2003, Engineering of bone tissue with porcine bone marrow stem cells in three-dimensional trabecular metal: in vitro and in vivo studies, *APMIS Suppl.* **111**(109):127-132.

Zou, X., Li, H., Baatrup, A., Bünger, C., and Lind, M., 2004a, Stimulation of porcine bone marrow stromal cells by hyaluronan, dexamethasone and rhBMP-2, *Biomaterials* **25**(23):5375-5385.

Zou, X., Li, H., Bünger, M., Egund, N., Lind, M., and Bünger, C., 2004b, Bone ingrowth characteristics of porous tantalum and carbon fiber interbody devices: an experimental study in pigs, *Spine J.* **4**(1):99-105.

Zou, X., Li, H., Teng, X., Xue, Q., Egund, N., Lind, M., and Bünger, C., 2005, Pedicle screw fixation enhances Aanterior lumbar interbody fusion with porous tantalum cages: an experimental study in gigs, *Spine* **30**(14):E392-E399.

Zou, X., Xue, Q., Li, H., Bünger, M., Lind, M., and Bünger, C., 2003, Effect of alendronate on bone ingrowth into porous tantalum and carbon fiber interbody devices: An experimental study on spinal fusion in pigs, *Acta Orthop Scand.* **74** (5):596-603.

15

PREPARATION OF SPONGE USING PORCINE SMALL INTESINAL SUBMUCOSA AND THEIR APPLICATIONS AS A SCAFFOLD AND A WOUND DRESSING

Moon Suk Kim[1], Min Suk Lee[1,2], In Bum Song[1,2], Sang Jin Lee[1], Hai Bang Lee[1]*, Gilson Khang[2]*, and Il Woo Lee[3]

15.1. INTRODUCTION

Small intestine submucosa (SIS) derived from the submucosal layer of porcine intestine cause minimum immune response as acellular collagen based matrix[1,2] and moreover is a biodegradable.[3] SIS consists of types I and III collagens above 90% and small amounts of types IV, V, and VI collagens.[4] In addition, SIS contains a wide variety of cytokine such as basic fibroblast growth factor (bFGF), transforming growth factor-β (TGF-β), epidermal growth factor (EGF), vascular endothelial growth factor (VEGF), and insulin-like growth factor-1 (IGF-1) as well as glycosaminoglycans, fibronectins, chondroitin sulfates, heparins, heparin sulfates, and hyaluronic acids.[5,6] These constituents are well known to play an important role for tissue remodeling and wound healing. SIS has been used as commercial goods in practical biomedical fields such as the repair of numerous body tissues including musculotendinous structures, lower urinary tract reconstruction, dura mater replacement, vascular reconstruction, and the repair of full and partial thickness skin wounds.[7-9]

In recent years, the development of novel biomaterials has been demanded in the implantable porous scaffolds.[10-13] To fulfill such demands, several studies have been investigated to fabricate the sponge with microstructure as scaffolds, which temporarily

---

[1] Nano-biomaterials Laboratory, Korea Research Institutes of Chemical Technology, P.O.Box 107, Yuseong, Daejeon 305-606, Korea
[2] Department of Polymer/Nano Science and Technology, Chonbuk National University, 664-14, Dukjin, Jeonju 561-756, Korea
[3] Department of Neurosurgery, Catholic University of Korea, 520-2, Daeheung 2 Dong, Jung Gu, Daejeon 301-723, Korea

acted as the supporting materials for ingrowths of the cells and degraded along with extracellular matrix (ECM) production. Naturally derived polymers such as collagen and chitosan have been widely utilized to construct porous scaffolds because of their good biocompatibility and biodegradability.[14-16] Based on particular properties ascribed above, SIS is an ideal biomaterial because it can promote cellular differentiation and support rapid host tissue ingrowths, and also provide comparably good mechanical properties to support structure shape as a scaffold.[5,17-19] SIS may also exhibits biodegradability less than 90 days.[20] Therefore, SIS have various potentials in biomedical application.

The aim of our research was to expand a utility of SIS in biomedical applications such as biomaterials and tissue engineering. In this paper, we approach to design three-dimensional SIS sponges by using chemical crosslinking that could be utilized to endow the desirable physical and mechanical properties into naturally derived SIS. The designed SIS sponges have been also examined by the physical properties such as pore size distribution, the effective crosslinking upon structure, and the water absorption ability for various buffers. Further study performed to investigate potential application as scaffolds for the attachment and proliferation of cells and wound dressing.

15.2. MATERIALS AND METHODS

15.2.1. Materials

Porcine jejunum was purchased from Woomi Food Company (Korea). 1-Ethyl-(3,3-dimethylaminopropyl) carbodiimide hydrochloride (EDC), pepsin, and 3-(4,5-dimethylthiazol-2-yl)-2,5-diphenyltetrazolium bromide (MTT) were purchased from Sigma Chemical Co. (St. Louis, MO, USA) and used as received. PGA nonwoven mesh was purchased from Albany International (NY, USA).

15.2.2. Preparation of SIS Powder

Sections of porcine jejunum were harvested from market pigs (Finish pig, F_1; Land race + Yorkshire, around 100 kg at 6 months) within 10 minutes of sacrifice and prepared according to the method of Badylak et al.[5] Briefly, to separate SIS in porcine jejunum, fat firstly removed from porcine jejunum, followed by carefully washing with water. The porcine jejunum cut in lengths of approximate 10 cm and then washed with a saline solution. SIS was obtained by mechanical removal of the tunica serosa and tunica muscularis. Finally, the obtained SIS washed again with a saline solution and freeze-dried at −55 °C for 48 hrs using freeze dryer (Model FDU-540, EYELA, Japan). The dried SIS was pulverized using freezer mill (6700, SPEX Inc., USA) at −198 °C to give 10 ~ 20 μm size of SIS powder

15.2.3. Preparation of SIS Sponge

The obtained SIS powders (1 or 2% concentration) were added in 10ml vial with aqueous solution consisting of 3% acetic acid and 0.1% pepsin, and then stirred for 48 h to cleave only non-triplehelical domains of collagen.[21,22] Accordingly, the collagen molecules which have native triplehelical structure were solubilized from tissue. The SIS solution was carefully poured into homemade silicone molder (30 mm x 5 mm) to give

SIS sponge shape, followed by freeze-drying. SIS sponges were crosslinked with EDC in various concentrations (1-100 mM) using solution of a mixture of deionized water and ethanol (5/95, v/v) for 24 h. The crosslinked SIS sponges (ex. 1S-50E, 2S-100E; 1S and 2S represent 1 and 2 wt.% SIS concentration, 50E and 100E represent EDC concentration used to prepare sponge) in the molder were dipped in water at 40 °C for 1 h, followed by freeze-drying to give finally SIS sponges.

15.2.4. Crosslinking Investigations of SIS Sponge

SIS sponge (0.05 g) crosslinked with EDC in various concentrations was fed into a molder. A small portion of the mixture was immediately introduced into a sample pan cell. The crosslinking process was monitored by differential scanning calorimeter (DSC, No2910, TA Instrument, USA) from room temperature to 250 °C at a heating rate of 10 °C/min under a nitrogen atmosphere. After crosslinking, the characteristic peaks of the crosslinked SIS sponges were also measured by FT-IR (Bio-Rad Digilab, FTS-165, Canada) using KBr.

15.2.5. Weight Change of SIS Sponge before and after Crosslinking

The weight changes of SIS sponges were determined by the comparison of initial weight and the lyophilized SIS sponge weight after crosslinking with different EDC concentrations (0-100 mM). After crosslinking, the crosslinked SIS sponges were washed with water at 40 °C, followed by freeze-drying. The weight changes of each sample were individually measured for five SIS sponges and then calculated as average value.

15.2.6. Measurement of Porosity and Pore Size

Porosimeter (Instruments Co. Model Auto Pore IV 9520 V 1.03, USA) was used to examine the porosity and mean pore diameter of the SIS sponge crosslinked with EDC of different concentrations. The porosimeter was capable of acquisition for continuous data up to 60,000 psi pressure for mercury intrusion into SIS sponges. Higher pressures used to intrude mercury into smaller pore sizes of 6-0.003 µm and low pressures did for pore diameter ranging of 360-3.6 µm. Penetrometer equipped with five consecutive capillary stems (1.5 cm diameter and 1.0 cm long) in intrusion volume of 0.38, 1.1, 1.7, 3.1, and 3.9 cm^2. Intrusion resolution was better than 0.1 µl. Incremental change in the applied pressure allowed for measurement of incremental volume of mercury intruded (pore volume) into the SIS sponges. Thus pore size distribution in the SIS sponges was determined by relating pore size to pore volume. The porosimeter was equipped with a computer-based acquisition system that generated data files on cumulative and incremental volumes of intruded mercury as function of pore sizes.

15.2.7. Measurement by Scanning Electron Microscope

Scanning electron microscope (SEM, S-2250N, Hitachi, Japan) was used to examine the pore structure of the SIS sponges crosslinked with EDC of different concentrations (1-100 mM) and to compare the NIH-3T3 cell morphology. SIS sponges were cut in vertical and horizontal section. The sample were mounted on metal stubs and coated with a thin layer of platinum using plasma-sputtering apparatus (Model SC 500K, Emscope,

UK) for 2 min under argon atmosphere. The obtained image was analyzed with image analysis program P-SEM (Mirero, Korea).

15.2.8. Water Absorption Ability of SIS Sponges

The water uptake amount of SIS sponge (0.05 g) was determined by weight change before and after dipping in beaker with deionized water (different pH or various buffers) of 20 ml for 2 min (or different times). Water absorption ability was calculated by equation 1:

$$W = \frac{F - 0.05}{0.05} \times 100 \qquad (1)$$

Where W is water absorption ability of SIS sponge and F is weight of SIS sponge after dipping for 2 min. The water uptake amount of five SIS sponges was individually measured and then calculated as average value.

15.2.9. Cell Culture

NIH-3T3 cell line was obtained by KCLB (Korea Cell Line Bank) and cultured in RPMI medium 1640 (Gibco BRL, USA) supplemented with 10% fetal bovine serum (Gibco BRL, USA) and 1% antibiotic-antimycotic (Gibco BRL), and maintained at 37 °C in 5% CO_2 humidified atmosphere. The cells were seeded into 75-cm^2 flasks, and cultured and changed medium every 2 days.

15.2.10. Cell Attachment

SIS sponge or PGA mesh was sterilized by EO gas at Catholic university of Korea, St. MARY'S Hospital. NIH-3T3 cell suspension (approximate 2 x 10^4 cells/sponge or mesh) was seed into SIS sponge or PGA mesh (5 mm x 5 mm) in a 24-well plate. The cells were incubated overnight to allow for cell attachment. Cell viability was determined by using water-soluble enzyme substrate MTT which was converted to blue water-insoluble product formazan accumulated in the cytoplasm of viable cells. Cell viability of five SIS sponges or five PGA mesh performed individually and then calculated as average value. In brief, 100 μl of PBS solution of the MTT tetrazolium substrate (50 mg/ml) was added after 1, 2, 4, 8, and 14 days. After incubation for 4 h at 37 °C, the resulting violet formazan precipitate was solubilized by the addition of 1 ml of DMSO and shaken for 4 h. The solutions were then read using a plate reader of an ELISA (E-max, Molecular Device, USA). The optical density of each well determined at 520 nm.

15.2.11. Wound Healing Using Sponges after Skin Defect

The Sprague-Dawley (SD) rats (150–160 g, 5 weeks), which were cared in accordance with the Catholic University of Korea Council on Animal Care Guidelines, were used in this animal test. Prior to the test, rats were anaesthetized by using ketamine and rompun (1:1 ratio, 3 ml/kg), followed by shaving. Full-thickness rectangular skin wound of 3.5 cm x 3.5 cm was prepared on the back of rats. Four rats for each dressing were used to examine wound healing behavior. Wound healing was observed for 4 weeks after skin defect. The wound was covered with SIS sponge. Then, a Tegaderm™ band

SMALL INTESTINAL SUBMUCOSA SPONGE

was employed above the sponges. As a control, Tegaderm™ band alone was applied on a skin wound to compare wound healing property with SIS sponge. Macroscopic photograph was taken for wound at a set day to biopsy wound surface.

15.2.12. Histological Analysis of Wound

The rats were sacrificed for histological analysis on post-surgery. A skin wound tissue of rat was excised. The section was immediately fixed in 10% buffered formalin, embedded in paraffin wax, sectioned in 4 µm size. The section was stained by hematoxylin-eosin (H&E) and Masson's Trichrome (MTS) staining to investigate the resulting healing effects. Photomicrographs were taken using an Olympus light microscope.

15.2.13. Statistical Analysis

The mean and standard derivations are reported for each experimental group. Statistic analysis was performed by Student's t-test (independent-difference). Results were considered significant at P<0.05.

15.3. RESULTS AND DISSCUSSION

15.3.1. Preparation of SIS Sponge

Schematic diagram of SIS sponge was represented in Figure 15.1. First, SIS fine powder was prepared by removal of inside and outside layer of porcine jejunum. The size of SIS powder exhibited the ranging of approximate 20 µm by SEM observation.

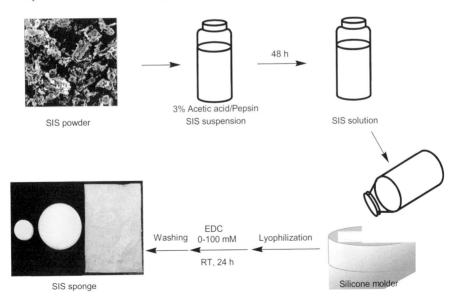

Figure 15.1. Schematic diagram for the preparation processing of SIS sponge.

SIS powder was only swelling not soluble in water as well as biological solution. To construct an intact SIS to a certain structure-remolded shape, SIS should be processed to make the dissolution of SIS powder. It was added in an aqueous mixture solution of 3% acetic acid and 0.1% pepsin, and stirred for 48 h. The suspension of SIS powder was changed to swelled form after 24 h and finally made a SIS solution after 48 h. This process gave 1 or 2% SIS solution.

Various SIS sponge shapes were formed in various molders after freeze-drying, but the sponge did not maintained the shape in water due to dissolving. Therefore, to keep the shape of the SIS sponge, we chose EDC as crosslinking agent between SIS chains, since EDC can be easily removed from the SIS sponge crosslinked after crosslinking.[23-26] The crosslinking was carried out with EDC of various concentrations (1-100 mM) at room temperature for 24 h.[27] The carboxylic acid group on SIS chain was activated by EDC and successively reacted with the amine group on intra and inter SIS chain. We examined a crosslinking process of the SIS with EDC by DSC. The thermograms in the presence of EDC showed broad exothermic peak corresponding to the crosslinking of SIS in the range of 150 - 170 °C, while it in absence of EDC showed no exothermic peak, indicating the progress of crosslinking of SIS on heating. The exothermic value increased from 9 to 18 J/g as EDC concentration increased (Table 15.1).[28]

Table 15.1. Thermogram values observed in the process of crosslinking and weight loss in the process of washing in water after crosslinking with different EDC concentrations

No	EDC concentration (mM)	ΔH (J/g)[2]	Weight loss (%)
1S-0E	Control[1]	2.1	~ 100
1S-1E	1	9.7	44
1S-5E	5	10.6	41
1S-10E	10	9.7	36
1S-50E	50	15.1	23
1S-100E	100	18.2	23

[1]Control : non-crosslinked SIS sponge, [2] Determined by DSC.

The IR spectra of the SIS sponges before and after crosslinking were examined with different EDC concentrations (1-100 mM). The intensity of characteristic peak assignable to stretching of carboxylic acid group in the SIS at 1406 cm^{-1} decreased according to increasing EDC concentrations. Meanwhile, the peaks assignable to the amide I, amide II, and amide III were also observed at 1653, 1543, and 1453 cm^{-1}, respectively,[29] and the peak intensity increased as EDC concentration increased. This result demonstrated that SIS sponges were prepared by the intra- and inter-crosslinking reaction of carboxylic acid group with the amine group on SIS chain via activation reaction of carboxylic acid by EDC. In addition, the crosslinked SIS sponges keep the shape in water even at 40 °C. To investigate crosslinking degree of the crosslinked SIS sponges, the weight change of the crosslinked SIS sponges was observed after washing with water at 40 °C. Uncrosslinked SIS sponge assigned as control could not determined the weight change because it did not keep the shape of sponge. The crosslinked SIS sponge showed the weight loss under keeping the sponge shape. It decreased from 44% to 23% as EDC concentration increased (Table 15.1), implying that uncrosslinked SIS chain dissolved in water. These results indicate that EDC served as a crosslinking agent of the SIS. In addition, the crosslinked SIS sponges were easy to handle due to good physical properties.

15.3.2. Structures of SIS Sponges

In the view of the microstructures of the porous scaffolds, high porosity (>90%) and interconnected pore network are desirable. The porosity and mean pore diameter of the SIS sponge crosslinked by EDC of different concentrations were examined. The pore size of SIS sponges showed values ranging up to 400 μm. All SIS sponges including the uncrosslinked SIS sponge have an almost similar porosity above 90%. The mean pore diameter of SIS sponges showed a rough increase tendency in the order of increasing EDC concentration. However, the SIS sponge prepared with 1 mM EDC concentration exhibited the mean pore diameter of 50 μm. As described above, uncrosslinked SIS chain was eliminated from SIS sponge in the process of washing with water after crosslinking. Therefore, the elimination of uncrosslinked SIS may induce a decrease in mean pore diameter of the SIS sponge crosslinked by 1 mM, probably due to the collapsing of pore in SIS sponge. The SIS sponges prepared with 1 and 2% SIS concentrations showed an almost similar porosity and mean pore diameter.

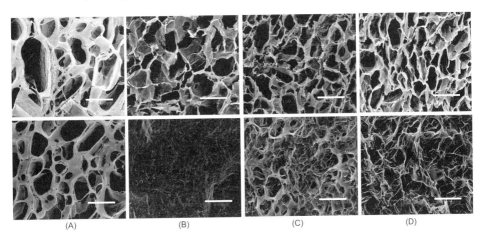

Figure 15.2. SEM pictures of 1% SIS sponges. (A) control (noncrosslinked SIS sponge) and SIS sponges crosslinked with EDC of (B) 1 mM, (C) 50 mM, and (D) 100 mM. (Upper: cross section, Bottom: surface, Magnification is 500, scale bar represents 100 μm)

The morphologic observation of the SIS sponges crosslinked with different EDC concentrations was measured by SEM. As shown in Figure 15.2, the cross section of SIS sponge exhibited highly porous structure with good interconnections between pores. The uncrosslinked SIS sponge exhibited irregular pore, while the crosslinked SIS sponges have maintained comparably regular pore even though their sizes slightly decreased as EDC concentration increased. In case of surface picture, the SIS sponge at 1 and 5 mM EDC exhibited almost closed pore structure. On the other hand, the pore of surface changed from closed to opened and interconnected structure as EDC concentration increased. The SIS sponge prepared with 2% SIS concentration showed slightly denser structure than that of 1%. This indicated that the SIS sponges with mean pore diameter around 100 μm and interconnective structure may support of cell growth, proliferation, and differentiation.

15.3.3. Water Uptake of SIS Sponges

A potential scaffold as substrate for cell should penetrate the nutrient in culture medium into scaffold in order to proliferate with cell. In addition, a potential wound dressing should adsorb the bleed and exudation at the wound site. Aforementioned, uncrosslinked SIS sponge dissolved in water, but the crosslinked SIS sponges absorbed only water without dissipation of the sponge shape by dissolving in water. Therefore, it was essential that wet and swelling property of SIS sponge examined to compare potential ability as scaffold and wound dressing.

First, surface wetting property of SIS sponge was examined by dropping of blue dye solution (10 µl). All crosslinked SIS sponges wetted rapidly within 2 min. The wetting rate was an order of SIS sponge crosslinked with 100 mM • 50 mM (10 sec) > 10 mM (30 sec) > 5 mM (1 min) > 1 mM (2 min). This result could be explained by the change of surface morphology from closed to open pore structure according to EDC concentration variation as shown in Figure 15.2.

Water absorption ability according to dipping time was also examined for 1S-100E sponge using deionized water for 2 min-24 h. The water absorption ability was calculated by equation 1 described in experimental part. Slight increasing in water uptake was observed from 8216% at 2 min to 8716% at 24 h (Figure 15.3A). SIS sponge was surprisingly reached at almost maximum water absorption state even at dipping for 2 min. This result indicates that SIS sponge absorbed the water at very fast speed and in addition at large amount, probably due to hydrophilic property and interconnective porous structures of SIS sponges. Therefore, the water uptake amount from next experiment was determined by dipping for 2 min to compare simply.

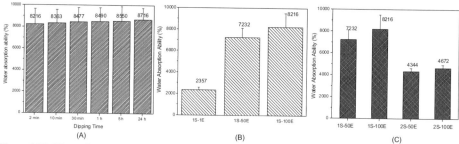

Figure 15.3. Water absorption ability (A) according to dipping times (2 min-24 h) for 1S-100E, (B) of 1% SIS sponge crosslinked with different EDC concentrations (1-100 mM) and (C) of SIS sponge prepared with different SIS sponge contents. Each number represents the average value of water absorption ability for five SIS sponges.

Next, a water uptake of SIS sponges prepared with different EDC concentrations and 1 or 2% SIS concentrations was examined by dipping SIS sponges in deionized water for 2 min. The water absorption ability of the crosslinked SIS sponges was an increase tendency as EDC concentration increased (Figure 15.3B). This is probably due to decrease pore size in order of increase EDC concentration. The SIS sponges crosslinked with 100 mM showed approximate 4 times higher water absorption ability than that of 1 mM. SIS sponges prepared with 2% SIS concentration exhibited slightly lower water absorption than that of 1% (Figure 15.3C), probably due to slightly denser structure. Finally, we examined the water uptake of 1% SIS sponge crosslinked with EDC 100 mM according to various pH and buffers. Although the pore structure in SEM picture was

SMALL INTESTINAL SUBMUCOSA SPONGE

changed slightly after dipping at high and low pH (data not shown), the SIS sponges at different pH showed almost similar water absorption ability above 8000% as shown in Figure 15.4A. In addition, there are no large differences for water uptake of the SIS sponges even in case of using various buffers (Figure 15.4B). These results may indicate that the crosslinked SIS sponges provided well-defined pore structures that could easily penetrate culture medium into the sponge.

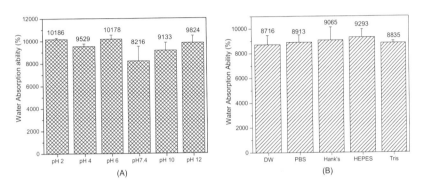

Figure 15.4. Water absorption ability of 1S-100E at (A) different pH and (B) different buffer solution. Each number represents the average value of water absorption ability.

15.3.4. Application as a Scaffold of SIS Sponges Using NIH-3T3

The SIS sponges showed the morphology of the porous structure with a high degree of interconnectivity, which allowed adequate environment in growth of the cells within the sponges. SIS sponges were examined as a scaffold in the view of the cell attachment and proliferation. The in vitro cell attachment and proliferation on SIS sponges were evaluated on the basis of cell morphology and cell viability using NIH-3T3 cells.[17] PGA mesh, which has been usually used in in vitro and in vivo because of its biodegradability and biocompatibility in spite of hydrophobic property, was also examined to compare with SIS sponges in views of the cell attachment and proliferation. Equal numbers of NIH-3T3 cells were seeded and cultured for 1-14 days. The cell morphology was measured by SEM (Figure 15.5). In case of SIS sponges, cells attached comparably uniformly on the surface or internal pores, indicating uniform spreading of cells. Cells in the SIS sponges exhibited a similar round cellular morphology, indicating cell attachment on pore of hydrophilic SIS sponges. On the other hand, cells in the PGA mesh showed irregularly aggregated cellular morphology on PGA mesh, due to another cell attachment upside cells initially attached onto hydrophobic PGA mesh.

As shown in Figure 15.6, cell attachment and proliferation were examined by MTT assay. Optical density assignable to cell viability for all SIS sponges was higher than that measured for PGA mesh. This result indicates that SIS sponges as a scaffold could significantly induce cell attachment and enhance the cell proliferation by providing probably enough spaces and natural environments. H&E staining was also performed at 14 day. The stained NIH-3T3 cells were obviously identified on SIS sponges (Data not shown).

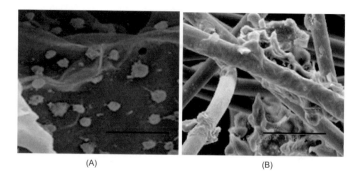

Figure 15.5. Cell morphology on (A) 1S-100E sponge and (B) PGA mesh. Magnification is 1000 and scale bar represents 50 μm.

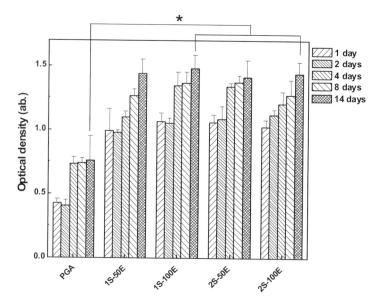

Figure 15.6. Cell viability for SIS sponges and PGA mesh. Control is PGA mesh (* $P<0.05$ compared with control).

15.3.5. Wound Healing

In wound healing test, full-thickness rectangular wounds were made on the back of each rat. SIS sponge (1S-100E) and Tegaderm™ as control to compare were used to study wound healing behavior.

SIS sponges absorbed the bleed and exudation at the wound site and attained uniform adherence to the wound surface. The SIS sponges exhibited higher extent of exudation absorption for wound than that covered with Tegaderm™. SIS sponges acted as hemostatic agent. Epithelialization of the wound was proceeding at postoperative day as shown in Figure 15.7. The wound at the 21st postoperative day was more contractive than that of the wound observed at the first postoperative day. However, no significant difference in wound contraction was observed between either of 1S-100E and control using Tegaderm™.

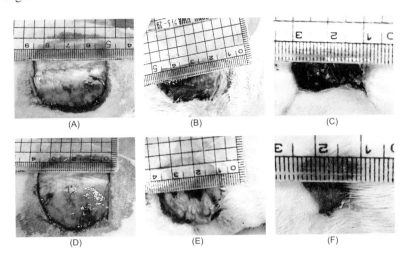

Figure 15.7. Wound healing process using (A-C) 1S-100E sponge and (D-F) Tegaderm™. (A,D) 1 day (B,E) 7 days, and (C,F) 21 days.

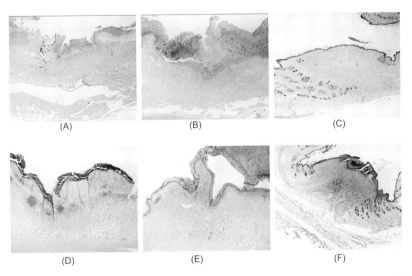

Figure 15.8. H&E stain of wound healing using (A-C) 1S-100E sponge and (D-F) Tegaderm™. (A, D) 7 day (B,E) 14 days, and (C,F) 21 days. Magnification is 100.

Histological evaluation performed for 1S-100E sponge-treated wounds and Tegaderm™ as control. Figure 15.8 shows H&E stain of wound. 1S-100E sponge-treated wounds exhibited little exudates and neutrophil at 7 days. Epithelialization process had started on the wound. At 21 days, the wound was almost completely covered with a thin layer of epidermis and in addition, new fibrous tissue was observed in the wounds treated with SIS sponges. On the other hand, a large exudate and neutrophil was found on the Tegaderm™-treated wounds, and the dermis was rich in macrophage inflammatory cells. Even by 21 days, Tegaderm™-treated wounds showed inflammation localized to the new dermis and little epidermal regeneration. In MTS stain (Figure 15.9), dermal collagen had regenerated at only SIS sponges treated wounds at 7 days. The deposition of new collagen in the wound was oriented along the same axis parallel to the skin surface, suggesting a repairing of the damaged tissue.

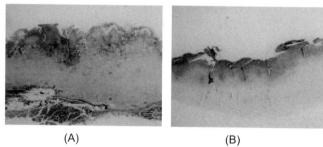

(A)   (B)

Figure 15.9. MTS stain of wound healing using (A) 1S-100E sponge and (B) Tegaderm™ at 7 days. Magnification is 100.

15.4. CONCLUSIONS

SIS sponge was prepared by crosslinking with EDC of various concentrations. The crosslinking was occurred by the intra- and inter-reaction of carboxylic acid group activated by EDC with the amine group on SIS chain. The broad exothermic peaks corresponding to the crosslinking of SIS observed in the range of 150-170 °C at DSC. The crosslinked SIS sponges maintained sponge structure with interconnective pore compared to that of uncrosslinked SIS after washing with water. SIS sponges possess relatively good physical properties and can easily handle. In addition, the crosslinked SIS sponges exhibited approximately several-order time's higher water absorptions. The higher absorbance of MTT assays at both initial and long culture was obtained when the SIS sponges were applied in comparison with PGA mesh. The crosslinked SIS sponges as a scaffold facilitated the attachment and proliferation of NIH-3T3 cells. In wound healing test, the SIS sponges exhibited higher extent of exudation absorption at wound. The SIS sponges appeared to be more organized, completely epithelialized, and devoid of inflammation compared to Tegaderm™. Although we did not determine the retention of cytokines in SIS sponges after proteolytic treatments and crosslinking, we believe that the SIS sponges could serve as a scaffold and a wound dressing.

15.5. ACKNOWLEDGMENT

This work was supported by KMOICE (N11-A08-1402-05-1-3).

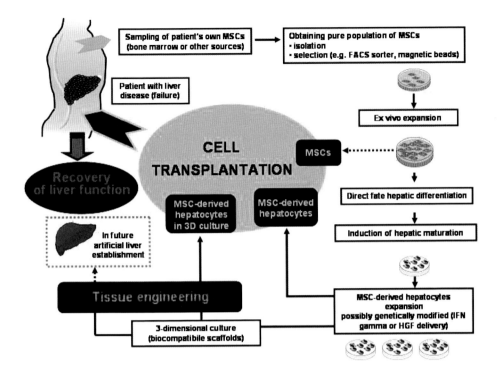

Figure 1.4. Schematic representation of mesenchymal stem cell (MSC)-based therapy and tissue engineering. MSCs can be obtained from patient's own tissue (bone marrow, adipose tissue), purified using MACS or FACS system and after expansion directly induced into hepatic lineage differentiation. Mature hepatocytes might be directly implanted or after genetic manipulations back into damaged liver of the patient or using tissue engineering technologies transplanted as small liver devices. Tissue engineering development holds promises for a future bioartificial liver establishment.

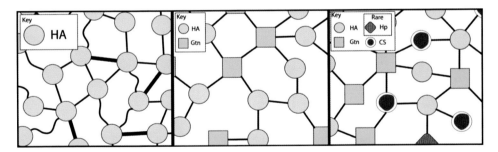

Figure 9.1. Covalent, crosslinked, sECMs for different medical device applications (as drawn by Justin Chafe). Left, an HA-only material for scar-free healing and adhesion prevention; center, a two-component sECM for 3-D cell growth in vitro and for tissue repair and engineering in vivo; right, a multicomponent sECM for optimization of cell attachment as well as delivery of drugs and growth factors.

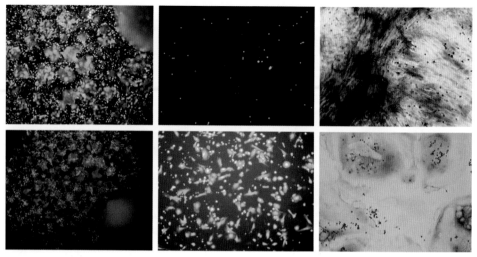

Figure 14.1. Nucleated cells in hyaluronic acid gel loaded into porous tantalum discs after 24 hours (Left panel, top) and 7 days (left panel, bottom) of cultivation. The nucleated cells in hyaluronic acid gel were cultivated on slides for 24 hours (middle panel, top) and 7 days (middle panel, bottom). Live/dead cell staining showed that live cells were green, and dead cells were red. After 21 days of cultivation, the nucleated cells in hyaluronic acid gel show positive ALP staining (right panel, top) and osteocalcin staining (right panel, bottom).

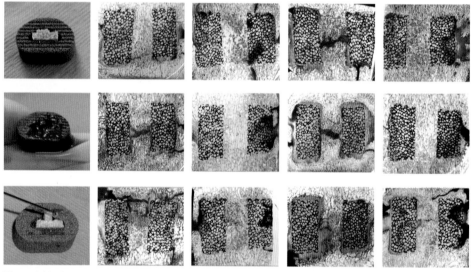

Figure 14.2 . Porous tantalum rings with different graft materials, for an anterior lumbar interbody fusion in pigs, were implanted into L2/3 (top), L4/5 (middle) and L6/7 (bottom). First panel shows Collagraft strips with nucleated cells (100 millions) in the central hole of the porous tantalum ring (top), hyaluronic acid gel with nucleated cells (40 million /ml) in the porous tantalum ring (middle), and Collagraft strips containing 6 mg of rhBMP-2 in the central hole of the porous tantalum ring (bottom). The second to fifth panels show histological sections from the porous tantalum rings, which correspond to implants in pigs 1-4 3 months after the initial operation. The histology in the porous tantalum rings depicts very similar appearances in the vertebrae implant/graft interfaces and in the central hole of the porous tantalum rings.

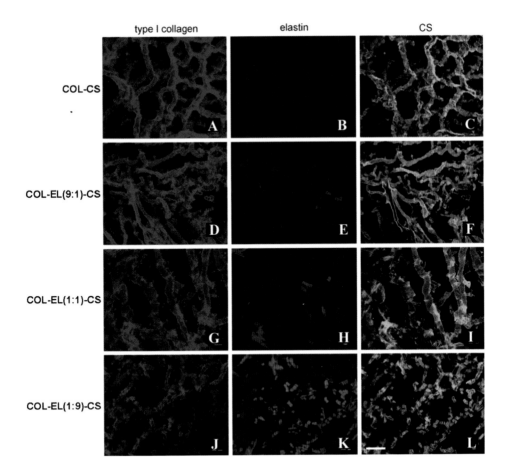

Figure 19.4. Immunostaining of scaffolds containing variable amounts of collagen and elastin with covalently attached chondroitin sulfate using immunostaining for type I collagen (red) and CS (green), whereas elastin was analysed by UV optics (blue). Bar is 50 μm. COL=collagen, EL=elastin, CS=chondroitin sulfate. Figure modified with permission from Daamen et al.

15.6. REFERENCES

1. E. M. Palmer, B. A. Beilfuss, T. Nagai, R. T. Semnani, S. F. Badylak, and G. A. Van Seventer, Human helper T cell activation and differentiation is suppressed by porcine small intestinal submucosa, *Tissue Eng.*, **8**, 893-900 (2002).
2. J. Allman, T. B. McPherson, S. F. Badylak, L. C. Merrill, B. Kallakury, C. Sheehan, R. H. Raeder, and D. W. Metzger, Xenogeneic extracellular matrix grafts elicit a TH2-restricted immune response, *Transplantation*, **71**, 1631-1640 (2001).
3. B. P. Kropp, Small-intestinal submucosa for bladder augmentation: a review of preclinical studies, *World J. Urol.*, **16**, 262-267 (1998).
4. M. F. Graham, R. F. Diegelmann, C. O. Elson, W. J. Lindblad, N. Gotschalk, S. Gay, and R. Gay, Collagen content and types in the intestinal strictures of Crohn's disease, *Gastroenterology*, **94**, 257-265 (1998).
5. S. L. Voytik-Harbin, A. O. Brightman, M. R. Krain, B. Waisner, and S. F. Badylak, Identification of extractable growth factors from small intestinal submucosa, *J. Cellular Biochem.*, **67**, 478-491 (1997).
6. J. Hodde, Naturally occurring scaffolds for soft tissue repair and regeneration, *Tissue Eng.*, **8**, 295-308 (2002).
7. Y. M. Bello, A. F. Falabella, and W. H. Eaglstein, Tissue-engineered skin. Current status in wound healing, *Am. J. Clin. Dermatol.*, **2**, 305-313 (2001).
8. Y. Zhang, B. P. Kropp, P. Moore, R. Cowan, P. D. 3rd Furness, M. E. Kolligian, P. Frey, and E. Y. Cheng, Coculture of bladder urothelial and smooth muscle cells on small intestinal submucosa: Potential applications for tissue engineering technology, *J. Urol.*, **164**, 928-935 (2000).
9. J. A. Gastel, W. R. Muirhead, J. T. Lifrak, P. D. Fadale, M. J. Hulstyn, and D. P. Labrador, Meniscal tissue regeneration using a collagenous biomaterial derived from porcine small intestine submucosa, *Arthroscopy*, **17**, 151-159 (2001).
10. D. W. Hutmacher, Scaffold design and fabrication technologies for engineering tissues state of the art and future perspectives, *J. Biomater. Sci. Polym. Ed.*, **12**, 107-124 (2001).
11. C. M. Agrawal and R. B. Ray, Biodegradable polymeric scaffolds for musculoskeletal tissue engineering, *J. Biomed. Mater. Res.*, **55**, 141-150 (2001).
12. W. L. Murphy and D. J. Mooney, Controlled delivery of inductive proteins, plasmid DNA and cells from tissue engineering matrices, *J. Periodontal Res.*, **34**, 413-419 (1999).
13. S. K. Kim, K. D. Hong, J. W. Jang, S. J. Lee, M. S. Kim, G. Khang, I. Lee, and H. B. Lee, Tissue engineered spinal cord using bone marrow stromal stem cells seeded PGA scaffolds; Preliminary study, *Tissue Eng. Regen. Med.*, **1(2)**, 149-156 (2004).
14. G. Khang, P. Shin, I. Kim, B. Lee, S. J. Lee, Y. M. Lee, H. B. Lee, and I. Lee, Preparation and characterization of small intestine submucosa particle impregnated PLA scaffold: The application of tissue engineered bone and cartilage, *Macromolecular Res.*, **10**, 158-167 (2002).
15. D. W. Hutmacher and M. Sittinger, Periosteal cells in bone tissue engineering, *Tissue Eng.*, **9**, S45–64 (2003).
16. G. Khang, M. S. Kim, S. H. Cho, I. Lee, J. M. Rhee, and H. B. Lee, Natural scaffolds biomaterials for tissue regeneration, *Tissue Eng. Regen. Med.*, **1(1)**, 9-20 (2004).
17. K. Lindberg and S. F. Badylak, Porcine small intestinal submucosa (SIS): a bioscaffold supporting in vitro primary human epidermal cell differentiation and synthesis of basement membrane proteins, *Burns*, **27**, 254-266, (2001).
18. S. F. Badylak, The extracellular matrix as a scaffold for tissue reconstruction, *Seminars in Cell & Developmental Biology*, **13**, 377-383 (2002).
19. S. F. Badylak, B. T. Kropp, B. McPherson, H. Liang, and P. W. Snyder, Small intestinal submucosa: a rapidly resorbed bioscaffold for augmentation cystoplasty in a dog model, *Tissue Eng.*, **4**, 379-387 (1998).
20. E. H. Ledet, A. L. Carl, D. J. DiRisio, M. P. Tymeson, L. B. Andersen, C. E. Sheehan, B. Kallakury, M. Slivka, and H. Serhan, A pilot study to evaluate the effectiveness of small intestinal submucosa used to repair spinal ligaments in the goat, *The Spine Journal*, **2**, 188-196 (2002).
21. K. Sato, T. Tanahashi-Shiina, F. Jun, A. Watanabe-Kawamura, M. Ichinomiya, Y. Minegishi, Y. Tsukamasa, Y. Nakmura, M. Kawabata, K. Ohtsuki, Simple and rapid chronaographic purification of type V collagen from a pepsin digest of porcine intedtinal connective tissue, an unmanageable starting material for conventional column chromatography, *Journal of Chromatography B*, **790**, 277-283 (2003).
22. M. T. Sheu, J. C. Huang, G. C. Yeh, and H. O. Ho, Characterization of collagen gel solutions and collagen matrices for cell culture, *Biomaterials*, **22**, 1713-1719 (2001).
23. Y. Chang, C. C. Tsai, H. C. Liang, and H. W. Sung, In vivo evaluation of cellular and acellular bovine pericardia fixed with a naturally occurring crosslinking agent (genipin), *Biomaterials*, **3**, 2447-2457 (2002).

24. V. Charulatha and A. Rajaram, Influence of different crosslinking treatments on the physical properties of collagen membranes, *Biomaterials*, **24**, 759-767 (2003).
25. J. S. Pieper, T. Hafmans, J. H. Veerkamp, and T. H. Van Kuppevelt, Development of tailor-made collagen-glycosaminoglycan matrices: EDC/NHS crosslinking, and ultrastructural aspects, *Biomaterials*, **21**, 581-593 (2000).
26. G. T. Hermanson, Bioconjugate Techniques; Academic Press: San Diego, 1996.
27. S. N. Park, J. C. Park, H. O. Kim, M. I. Song, and H. Suh, Characterization of porous collagen/hyaluronic acid scaffold modified by 1-ethyl-3-(3-dimethylaminopropyl)carbodiimide cross-linking, *Biomaterials*, **23**, 1205-1212 (2002).
28. H. W. Shin, S. H. Kim, J. W. Jang, M. S. Kim, S. H. Cho, H. B. Lee, and G. Khang, Preparation and characterization of sponge using porcine small intestinal submucosa, *Polymer(Korea)*, **28**, 194-200 (2004).
29. L. A. Forato, R. B. Filho, and L. A. Colnago, Protein structure in KBr pellets by infrared spectroscopy, *Anal. Biochem.*, **5**, 136-141 (1998).

SECTION 4

BIOREACTOR AND ASSESSMENT TECHNOLOGIES

16

MODULATION OF CELL DIFFERENTIATION IN BONE TISSUE ENGINEERING CONSTRUCTS CULTURED IN A BIOREACTOR

Heidi L. Holtorf[1], John A. Jansen[2], and Antonios G. Mikos[1]

16.1. INTRODUCTION

There is a significant need for therapies to enhance healing in large skeletal defects because there exist over 1 million cases each year of patients requiring bone graft procedures to correct such defects[1]. These defects can arise for a variety of reasons including trauma, congenital deformity, and tumor resection and thus exist in a wide range of shapes, sizes, and functional locations. The most successful of current treatments for large bone defects is autologous bone graft. This therapy is attractive because there is no risk of immune rejection to the transplanted tissue; however, there are two major drawbacks associated with this procedure. First, there is a limited supply of donor bone, which is harvested primarily from the trabecular bone of the iliac crest, or from a whole rib or fibula. Thus, there may not be enough donor tissue for proper shape reconstruction of the defect that can also support the necessary mechanical load during healing.[2] Second, autologous bone graft therapies are associated with a risk of morbidity at the donor site which was healthy to begin with. Due to these issues, there is a need for alternative strategies to bone healing that allow exact shape reconstruction, are mechanically strong, and are biocompatible in both the short and long term. To this end, bone tissue engineering has evolved as a practical method of regenerating large bony defects.

Tissue engineering strategies for bone regeneration must factor in the biological, mechanical and surgical issues involved with the specific application of each construct. Currently, these strategies utilize solid support scaffolds, bioactive molecules, and osteogenic cells either alone or in various combinations with one another. The solid support provides a space filling function to provide a surface for anchorage dependent bone cells on the perimeter of the defect to infiltrate the space and begin the healing process within the defect. Bioactive molecules can act as chemoattractants to recruit bone

---

[1] Department of Bioengineering, Rice University, Houston, TX, USA
[2] Department of Periodontology and Biomaterials, Radboud University Medical Center, Nijmegen, The Netherlands

forming cells to the site of the defect or to encourage the osteodifferentiation of bone precursor cells already at the defect site. Osteogenic cells are the prime ingredient for healing of large bone defects as they are the tool that will lay down the new bone tissue and eventually integrate the defect site with the surrounding healthy tissue. A strategy that incorporates all three of these components would likely have the best possibility of regenerating a defect in an appropriate amount of time.

In order to contrive the best possible tissue engineered scaffold for bone regeneration, it is important to understand the physiological process of natural bone formation such that the body's natural healing mechanisms can be exploited to their utmost potential. Consequently, this review first gives an overview of bone biology and the natural course of bone formation in vivo. Next, an in vitro model of bone formation is presented to put into context the following sections on bone tissue engineering scaffolds and bioreactors. Finally, we present our most recent work on development of integrated bone tissue engineering constructs. In this approach, osteoprogenitor cells are seeded on solid porous scaffolds and these scaffold/cell constructs are cultivated *in vitro* in a specially designed flow perfusion bioreactor to create an extracellular matrix rich in bioactive molecules. These scaffold/cell/extracellular matrix constructs can then be implanted to induce bone tissue formation *in vivo*.

16.2. BONE STRUCTURE

All mature bones in the human skeleton are composed of a central marrow cavity surrounded by bone tissue which is covered by periosteum. The bone marrow contains extensive blood vessels which supply the bone tissue with nutrients as well as a store of cells capable of initiating bone repair.

Bone tissue exists in two forms, cancellous and cortical bone. Cancellous bone is highly porous (50-90%) and is capable of deformation in order to absorb high mechanical loads and distribute them evenly over a wider area.[3] The major part of the cancellous bone that exists within the skeleton is located within short and flat bones as well as at the end of long bones near synovial joints. Because of the highly porous nature of cancellous bone, it possesses a high surface area and a majority of cells in cancellous bone rest on this surface in close proximity to the marrow and its blood vessels. In contrast, cortical bone is only about 10% porous resulting in a much stiffer and much stronger tissue than cancellous bone.[3] About 80% of the human skeleton is composed of cortical bone which is the main type of bone found within weight bearing regions of the skeleton, but also surrounds cancellous bone in all types of bones. Because of the low porosity of cortical bone, the majority of bone cells are completely embedded within the bone matrix resulting in limited access to the marrow and its blood vessels. Despite these limitations, cortical bone is still a highly active tissue, although cancellous bone tends to have a much higher metabolic rate than cortical bone and responds more rapidly to changes in mechanical loads.[3]

Cortical and cancellous bone may consist of two different arrangements, woven bone or lamellar bone.[3] Woven bone is sometimes referred to as primary bone in that it is the first type of bone laid down during embryonic development as well as after fracture. In time, this woven bone is remodeled into lamellar bone resulting in a very small amount of woven bone present in the adult skeleton. These two types of bone exhibit differences in regard to their formation, composition, organization and mechanical properties. Woven bone forms quite rapidly due to a high cell number per unit volume and has a random arrangement of collagen fibrils, resulting in isotropic behavior of the bone. Because of the random collagen arrangement, mineralization of woven bone is quite irregular as well, thereby resulting in a tissue that is relatively flexible and weak. In contrast, lamellar bone, also referred to as secondary bone, forms at a much lower rate and is much more ordered than woven bone. Instead of a random arrangement, the collagen fibrils of lamellar bone are of relatively uniform diameter and are aligned into parallel sheets, forming lamellae. Due to the regularity of collagen fiber orientation, mineralization proceeds in a much more uniform manner compared to woven bone. The highly order structure of cortical bone results in a tissue that is stiffer and stronger than woven bone and behaves anisotropically, allowing the bones to be stronger in the direction of higher mechanical loads.[3]

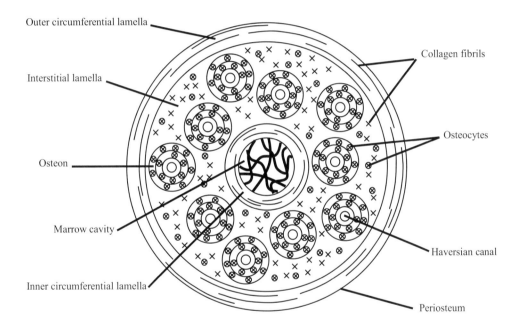

Figure 16.1. Organization of lamellar cortical bone

Because the majority of the adult skeleton is composed of lamellar bone, it is important to understand the structure and organization of lamellar bone. Lamellar bone is composed of four main types of lamellae; trabecular, circumferential, interstitial, and osteon. The highly porous bone composing both the central marrow cavity and cancellous bone is organized into trabecular lamellae. Alternatively, the highly dense bone composing cortical bone is organized into inner and outer circumferential lamellae, interstitial lamellae and lamellae of osteons (Figure 16.1). Each of these lamellae is composed of highly oriented collagen fibrils; however, they are oriented differently in each lamella. The inner circumferential lamella is adjacent to and surrounds the trabecular lamellae composing the central marrow cavity of the bone. In this lamella, the collagen fibrils are oriented perpendicular to the axis of the bone, forming a circle, or circumference, around the central marrow cavity. The outer circumferential lamella is organized in the same manner as the inner circumferential lamella but is located at the outer perimeter of the bone near the periosteum.[3]

Between these two circumferential lamellae lie the osteons, which form the majority of cortical bone. Each osteon is arranged into a cylindrical bundle with the collagen fibrils oriented longitudinally to the bone axis. At the center of each osteon is a canal, referred to as a haversian canal, which contains blood vessels, lymphatic vessels, and in some cases nerves. Each haversian canal is surrounded by several lamellae, and within each lamella lie osteocytes responsible for the metabolic activity of bone. Very small canals called canaliculi house the cell processes of osteocytes and radiate outward from the central haversian canal. The canaliculi connect osteocytes from different lamellae to each other and to the central canal. Because nutrient diffusion through mineralized bone matrix is minimal, the canaliculi allow for nutrient transport to cells in all lamellae of the osteon as well as a means for rapid cell-cell communication. The outer lamella of each osteon is covered with a thin layer of organic matrix or cement line. This cement line separates each osteon from the next as canaliculi and collagen fibrils do not cross cement lines. This separation prevents crack propagation across the bone, allowing the bone to repair cracks before fracture occurs.[3]

The interstitial lamella makes up the irregularly shaped spaces that exist between osteons of cortical bone. The collagen fibrils of the interstitial lamellae are oriented longitudinally allowing efficient space filling of bone tissue between the cylindrically shaped osteons. Throughout the length of cortical bone there are also intermittent vascular canals that run crosswise between the marrow space and osteons, osteon to osteon, and osteon to periosteum. These vascular canals, or Volkmann canals, allow nutrient transport to the osteons near the perimeter of the cortex as well as to the periosteum, thus connecting all of the lamellae into a single unified bone tissue.[3]

The outer surface of bone tissue is covered by periosteum. This thin membranous-like tissue comprises two layers, an outer fibrous layer and an inner vascular and cellular layer. While the function of the outer layer is mainly connectivity of one bone to the next, the inner layer has important functions in regard to regular bone metabolism as well as wound healing. This inner layer, or cambium layer, has a dense vascular bed that supplies nutrients to the surface of the bone and also contains a store of progenitor cells that are capable of differentiating into osteoblasts for normal bone growth and maintenance or on a larger scale for bone repair in response to injury.[3]

The highly vascular nature of the periosteum, the extensive vascular network within cortical bone lamellae, and the extremely vascularized bone marrow are indicative of the highly metabolic nature of bone tissue. The close proximity of cells to the marrow in cancellous bone and the extensive vascular canals lying within the lamellae of cortical bone allow that no bone cell is more than 300 µm from a blood vessel. This is especially important as the dense mineralized extracellular matrix of bone severely hinders diffusion of nutrients from and waste products to the blood vessels.[3]

16.3. BONE COMPONENTS

Bone is a highly organized tissue that consists of several different components that interact with one another to create the complex tissue. These three main components are bone cells, organic extracellular matrix and inorganic extracellular matrix.

The bone cells are responsible for the formation, resorption, remodeling and repair of bone tissue and are composed of three main cell types; osteoblasts, osteocytes, and osteoclasts. Osteoblasts are the cells responsible for the formation of new bone. These cells are derived from undifferentiated mesenchymal cells that reside within the vast network of bone canals, the bone marrow and the periosteum. When needed, these cells are recruited to the necessary site where they proliferate and then differentiate into the osteoblasts required to start forming new bone. The primary role of osteoblasts is the synthesis and secretion of organic extracellular matrix molecules, although they also function to balance electrolyte levels in the extracellular fluid with the osseous fluid and aid the mineralization of the bone matrix. During bone synthesis, there are large numbers of active osteoblasts present that may follow one of three different fates when they are no longer actively forming bone. First, they may remain on the surface of the bone in a resting state until needed to once again initiate bone formation. Second, they may become embedded within the extracellular matrix and become osteocytes, performing tissue maintenance. Finally, they may disappear from the site. Because many more cells are present during active bone formation than become osteocytes or resting surface osteoblasts, the majority of cells are removed by some unknown mechanism.

Those osteoblasts that become osteocytes account for more than 90% of the bone cells found in the mature skeleton.[3] These cells have many processes that extend outward through the canaliculi and connect with other cells within the bone, allowing for good cell-cell communication within the tissue. This is vitally important in that those cells that lie on the surface of the bone are very sensitive to stresses on the bone and require a speedy network to transfer these signals to osteocytes so they may adjust their activity. The interconnected cell network allows the cells to sense bone deformations and to coordinate bone resorption and formation as well as the flow of ions between the mineralized matrix and the extracellular fluid space in response to these stimuli. In this manner, bone tissue will increase when exposed to higher stresses and decrease when exposed to lower stresses over a long period of time.

The third type of cell found within bone tissue is the osteoclast, which is responsible for the resorption of old bone for repair and remodeling purposes. Unlike the osteoblasts and osteocytes, these cells do not originate from mesenchymal stem cells, but rather from hematopoietic stem cells as do other cells from the monocyte family. These precursor cells can be found in the marrow as well as in the circulating blood and when activated will proliferate and then fuse to form large multinucleated cells. These giant cells are very efficient at resorbing bone by attaching to the surface of bone and creating a sealed off space between the cell and the bone matrix. Endosomes containing large amounts of proton pumps move to the cell membrane bordering this space where the pumps work to lower the pH of the extracellular pocket from 7 to about 4. This acidic environment allows the mineral components of the bone matrix to dissolve and activates acid proteases released from the cell to digest the organic matrix. In this manner, osteoclasts form characteristic resorption cavities in the bone matrix to allow for deposition of new bone. Once completing its resorptive function, an osteoclast may divide into mononuclear cells and remain in a resting state until reactivated to form new osteoclasts.

The cellular component of bone comprises only a fraction of the total volume of bone tissue. The largest portion of bone tissue is the extracellular matrix, constituting more than 90% of the tissue volume. It is composed of both an organic and inorganic component and is responsible for the mechanical properties of bone. The inorganic component consists primarily of calcium, carbonate, and acid phosphate ions arranged in a crystalline-like structure to give bone its ability to resist compression and to also serve as an ion reservoir. The organic component consists primarily of collagen fibrils that give bone its form and ability to resist tension. Other components of the organic matrix include non-collagenous proteins such as osteocalcin, osteonectin, and bone sialoproteins that effect matrix organization and matrix mineralization. In addition, bone matrix also contains a variety of growth factors including transforming growth factor-β, insulin-like growth factors 1 and 2, bone morphogenic proteins, platelet-derived growth factors, interleukins 1 and 6, and colony stimulating factors that primarily affect cell behavior. Such cell behaviors as recruitment of stem cells, differentiation of stem cells, bone formation, and bone resorption can be effected by these growth factors.

Like all tissues, bone tissue is highly hydrated and thus consists of an extracellular fluid to fill in the void spaces between the cells and the extracellular matrix molecules. Recall from the earlier discussion of bone structure that there exist vast networks of small canaliculi which allow cell processes to penetrate through the dense mineralized matrix to communicate with other cells. These small canals are filled with fluid which flows in response to mechanical stimuli to the bone tissue, creating shear stresses and streaming potentials within the bone tissue that may affect cell behavior. In response to a mechanical load, these micropores will deform with some increasing in volume while others decrease, leading to a difference in pressure which results in fluid flow. This fluid flow leads to streaming ion potentials as well as cellular deformations. Thus, the osteocytes are able to sense mechanical stimuli and react in an appropriate manner.[4]

16.4. BONE FORMATION *IN VIVO*

The normal course of bone formation in vivo, whether it stems from embryonic development, normal growth, remodeling or fracture healing, follows a specific pathway. It begins with aggregation of undifferentiated mesenchymal cells or preosteoblasts followed by a period of proliferation to provide sufficient cell numbers for tissue formation. After this period of initial cell proliferation, the cells start to synthesize and secrete a loose organic matrix and they begin to differentiate toward osteoblasts. As these cells continue to differentiate, they lay down organic bone matrix that then mineralizes. This mineralization takes place in an organized fashion, with crystals first forming in specific hole zone regions of collagen. These crystals then grow along the collagen fibrils, eventually connecting the hole zone regions together. Once it begins, the mineralization process proceeds quite rapidly, with 60% of the final mineral content being formed within hours of initiation. However, after this initial blast of mineralization, the rate decreases and mineral continues to deposit slowly over an extended period of time. During mineralization, the water and non-collagenous protein concentrations in the bone matrix may change, but the collagen amounts and organization does not change appreciably. Osteoblasts cover the surface of this newly formed bone matrix and continue to rapidly lay down more bone matrix until many of these cells are engulfed within the matrix, becoming osteocytes, and the bone volume has reached a sufficient level. This primary, or woven, bone has a relatively random configuration and after initial deposition, osteoclasts come to the site of formation and start the remodeling process in order to produce secondary or mature lamellar bone.

During embryogenesis, the size and shape of newly formed bone is determined primarily by gene expression; however, movement and mechanical forces play an increasing role as growth continues. In fact, changes in mechanical loading in the adult skeleton can result in remodeling of bone to accommodate the new mechanical environment. In order to retain normal bone density, bone tissue requires repetitive mechanical loading and changes in this loading pattern over extended periods of time lead to alterations in bone mass. Decreased loading from such phenomena as extended bed rest or long-term exposure to the microgravity of outer space leads to decreased bone mass. Increased mechanical loading due to, for example, large weight gain leads to increased bone mass. Thus, the body is able to equilibrate bone mass with the necessary mechanical integrity to support daily functions through the coordinated efforts of bone formation and bone resorption.

This process of bone formation is mediated by cells which generally originate in the bone marrow. The marrow is composed of a variety of cell types including adherent stromal cells, endothelial cells, and non-adherent hematopoietic cells. Of these three cell types, the stromal cells are considered to be the osteogenic precursor cells while the haematopoietic cells may play a helper role in osteodifferentiation.[5] The process begins with proliferation of marrow stromal cells, characterized by the up-regulation of proliferative genes such as histones and protooncogenes. After a period of logarithmic growth, proliferation slows and there is an up-regulation of genes associated with the osteoblast phenotype including alkaline phosphatase, type I collagen, osteopontin, bone sialoprotein, and osteocalcin. Alkaline phosphatase levels initially increase, then peak, and finally decrease when mineralization is underway.[6] Osteopontin is up-regulated throughout the differentiation process with peaks during proliferation and again near the onset of matrix mineralization.[7] Bone sialoprotein is first detectable during matrix deposition, while osteocalcin appears during bone mineralization[6]. This differentiation process which occurs *in vivo* also follows the same process when marrow stromal cells are cultivated *in vitro*[5] and the protein markers mentioned above can be used to determine the extent of osteodifferentiation during *in vitro* cell culture experiments.

16.5. BONE-LIKE TISSUE FORMATION *IN VITRO*

The natural process of bone-like tissue formation can be recapitulated through *in vitro* experiments utilizing osteoprogenitor cells from a typical animal model such as the rat. These osteoprogenitor cells typically consist of either fetal calvaria cells or marrow stromal cells. Fetal calvarial cells are isolated via collagenase digestion of minced fetal calvarial bones whereas marrow stromal cells are isolated by flushing the marrow cavities of femora and tibiae of young adult rats.[5] The cells of several animals are pooled together and plated in tissue culture flasks for subsequent culture in 2-dimensions. To promote the osteodifferentiation of these precursor cells, several factors have been identified as crucial elements in the cell culture process. The batch of fetal bovine serum (FBS) used in the culture medium has a strong effect on the ability of the progenitor cells to differentiate into osteoblasts due to the wide variability in different serum lots to support mineralization. The culture medium must also be supplemented with 3 factors in order to promote osteodifferentiation. These factors include L-ascorbic acid, which induces collagen synthesis and deposition; β-glycerophosphate, which provides a source of inorganic phosphate for mineralization; and dexamethasone, a synthetic glucocorticoid that promotes bone nodule formation.[5, 7] While the first two components are relatively inactive additives that serve as reservoirs for molecules necessary for osteodifferentiation, dexamethasone is a potent chemical that exerts a powerful influence on mineralization, and the formation of nodules in rat marrow stromal cell cultures is entirely dependent on the presence of this glucocorticoid.[8]

It is necessary to grow marrow stromal cells in 2-dimensions for a brief period following initial harvest for several reasons. First, it allows isolation of the adherent cell population from the heterogeneous mixture of cells found within the bone marrow. Second, it allows removal of cell and bone particulates from the bone marrow aspirate. Third, the number of marrow stromal cells initially obtained can be expanded to a quantity sufficient for successful tissue formation. After this initial culture phase, the cells can be lifted from the 2-D culture surface and seeded onto a scaffold material for 3-D culture. The subsequent 3-D bone tissue formation will eventually serve as a tissue engineered bone replacement for large bone defects. During the initial cell isolation and expansion phase of culture, marrow stromal cells may or may not be exposed to the assortment of medium supplements previously described, as early exposure to dexamethasone can result in an up to 5-fold reduction in cell number.[8] In either case, marrow stromal cells that have undergone this initial primary culture have been utilized in a variety of ways in order to promote the growth of bone-like tissue *in vitro*.

16.6. SCAFFOLD MATERIALS FOR BONE TISSUE ENGINEERING

Three main classes of scaffold materials have been investigated for the creation of bone tissue engineering constructs. Each of these scaffold materials has inherent advantages and disadvantages toward the tissue engineering of new bone.

Polymers are attractive scaffold materials in that their chemical and mechanical properties can be varied through synthesis and processing procedures to match a specific defect need. In addition, many polymers offer the advantage of being biodegradable, thus eliminating the potential hazards of a permanent implant such as chronic inflammation, infection, or bone resorption due to stress shielding. A variety of polymer scaffolds have been investigated as solid support structures for marrow stromal cell growth and osteodifferentiation toward the development of tissue engineered bone grafts. Poly(propylene fumarate-co-ethylene glycol) hydrogels were shown to resist cell attachment, yet when modified with short adhesion peptides such as RGD allowed attachment and migration of marrow derived osteoblasts in a dose dependent manner.[9] Furthermore, when these hydrogels were formed into macroporous 3-dimensional structures, seeded marrow stromal cells differentiated into osteoblasts over 28 days in static culture with osteogenic medium.[10] Similarly, oligo[poly(ethylene glycol) fumarate] (OPF) hydrogels were able to support marrow stromal cell adhesion and migration in a dose dependent fashion when modified with an adhesion peptide.[11] In addition, marrow stromal cells encapsulated within unmodified OPF hydrogels differentiated into osteoblasts over 28 days of static culture in osteogenic medium.[12] Poly(propylene fumarate) (PPF) was shown to be a suitable surface for 2-dimensional culture and osteodifferentiation of marrow stromal cells. Moreover, when the marrow stromal cells were encapsulated within gelatin microspheres to protect them from the harsh chemical environment, they attached, proliferated and differentiated into osteoblasts on PPF surfaces that were not yet fully crosslinked.[13] Poly(D,L-lactic acid)-poly(ethylene glycol)-monomethyl ether (Me.PEG-PLA) films were shown to support marrow stromal cell adhesion and osteodifferentiation over 20 days in osteogenic medium.[14] Marrow stromal cells showed enhanced osteodifferentiation on Me.PEG-PLA surfaces over plain poly(lactic acid) or poly(lactic-co-glycolic acid) surfaces when cultivated under the same conditions.[14]

In addition to polymers, calcium phosphate ceramic materials that imitate the inorganic component of bone, particularly the mineralized matrix, have been used as scaffolding for tissue engineered bone constructs. Normal mineralized bone matrix is composed primarily of carbonated apatite and the majority of synthetic calcium phosphate ceramics used in bone regeneration applications consist of thermally processed hydroxyapatite or tricalcium phosphate.[15,16] Although these materials are meant to imitate the mineral component of bone, they are more crystalline and are therefore resorbed more slowly than native bone mineral or not at all. Calcium phosphate ceramic materials are also quite brittle with poor tensile strength, making them unsuitable for filling load-bearing defects. However, these materials are very attractive as bone defect fillers because they do not elicit a foreign body reaction and are tolerated well by host tissues.[17] A variety of calcium phosphate materials are currently used by surgeons as stand alone materials for filling bone voids and their potential as scaffold materials for tissue engineered bone constructs has recently been investigated.[17-19] These ceramic materials are osteoconductive, meaning they will allow bone ingrowth when placed adjacent to normal host bone. Some calcium phosphate ceramics are claimed to be osteoinductive, meaning they will actively induce bone formation. However, the amount of bone they induce is very limited.[20] Therefore, much work has been aimed at making calcium phosphate ceramics more osteoinductive by adding growth factors[21-23] and/or osteoprogenitor cells to the scaffolds[24-27].

A third class of scaffold materials for bone tissue engineering constructs includes metals. Metals differ from both polymers and ceramics in that they are nonresorbable and thus will remain at the defect site indefinitely. Despite this drawback, metals are attractive scaffold materials in that they are inert, do not provoke an immune response, and are mechanically strong, making them suitable for load bearing bone regeneration applications. Indeed, metals, particularly titanium, have been used for many years for total joint replacement in both the hip and knee due to their superior mechanical properties. Surface modifications to these implants have furthered their success by facilitating integration with host bone to stabilize the implants. Recently, porous titanium scaffolds in the form of a fiber mesh have been investigated as a suitable scaffold material for facilitating bone regeneration. Titanium fiber mesh has been shown to be osteoconductive but not osteoinductive as a stand alone material and much effort has been aimed at increasing osteoinductivity by addition of coatings, growth factors, and/or osteoprogenitor cells.[28,29] In vitro, titanium fiber mesh can support the osteodifferentiation of marrow-derived progenitor cells, induced by dexamethasone or bone morphogenetic protein-2 (BMP-2) in the culture medium.[30,31] In vivo, titanium fiber mesh can support bone in-growth from surrounding tissue in an orthotopic site, but can induce bone formation in an ectopic site when modified with a calcium phosphate coating,[28,32] BMP-2 loading,[30,33] transforming growth factor β-1 (TGF-β1),[29] or seeded with marrow stromal cells.[31, 34] Thus, a combination approach combining a scaffold, cells and signaling molecules should be more successful in bone regeneration.

16.7. CELL SEEDING ONTO TISSUE ENGINEERING SCAFFOLDS

Many of the scaffold materials mentioned above have been used in conjunction with osteoprogenitor cells to create more osteoinductive tissue engineering constructs. An effective method of cell seeding is critical for promoting uniform cell distribution throughout the scaffold. Good cell distribution promotes uniform extracellular matrix distribution and thus uniform tissue formation within the construct. A variety of cell seeding techniques have been investigated for their effectiveness in promoting uniform seeding, the simplest of which involves placing a droplet of cell suspension on the top of the scaffold and letting the liquid slowly drip through the porosity of the scaffold. However, if measures are not taken to force the liquid through the scaffold, the droplet may spread and run over the side of the scaffold resulting in very little cell attachment to the scaffold itself. Thus, better consistency in seeding may be achieved by placing the scaffolds in a concentrated cell suspension combined with gentle agitation.[35] This method, while allowing better consistency of seeding, is not ideal in that cells are not distributed evenly throughout the thickness of the scaffolds, but rather are concentrated near the surface of the scaffold.

In an attempt to improve the cell seeding distribution, several types of bioreactors have been investigated including spinner flasks, rotating wall vessels, and perfusion reactors. A spinner flask is a simple bioreactor consisting primarily of a flask with two side arms. Scaffolds are suspended within the medium by needle-like shafts anchored to the cap of the flask. Medium is mixed with either a magnetic stir bar or a shaft with an impeller rotating at low speed to provide the lowest possible shear. Cells are suspended in medium, mixing is begun and cells are allowed to attach to the scaffolds for a given period of time. Vunjak-Novakovic et al.[36] seeded chondrocytes onto porous poly(glycolic acid) scaffolds in a spinner flask and found that 90-100 % of cells in suspension were seeded on the scaffolds within 24 hours and that cells were uniformly distributed throughout the thickness of the scaffolds. Kim et al.[37] studied the cell attachment of smooth muscle cells to poly(glycolic acid) fiber mesh scaffolds by three different seeding methods including a spinner flask. They showed greater cell attachment to the scaffolds in a spinner flask compared to both droplet and gentle agitation methods, as well as better cell distribution throughout the scaffold. Mauney et al.[38] studied attachment of human bone marrow stromal cells on partially demineralized bone matrix and also saw more uniform cell distribution and greater cell seeding efficiency in a spinner flask compared to a static droplet/cell suspension method. Thus, the spinner flask resulted in better uniformity of cell seeding for a variety of cell types in several different scaffolds. However, despite the enhancement of cell attachment and uniformity of seeding in the spinner flask, Carrier et al.[39] showed that some damage to the cells occurred due to shear from mixing of the vessel and Wendt et al.[40] showed low cell seeding efficiency. This method of seeding is also very time-consuming, typically requiring a 24 hour period of cell attachment.

These drawbacks inspired these and other researchers to develop other dynamic cell seeding methods. Carrier et al.[39] found that cardiac myocytes had greater cell attachment and suffered less cell damage when seeded onto poly(glycolic acid) fiber meshes in a rotating wall vessel compared to a spinner flask. Wendt et al.[40] developed a novel oscillating perfusion system where the scaffolds were press-fitted into flow chambers and a cell suspension was forced through the porosity of the scaffold. Flow of medium was continually reversed such that the cell suspension traveled back and forth through the scaffolds to increase opportunity for cell attachment. They showed a small increase in overall cell seeding efficiency, but immense increases in cell viability and uniformity of seeding over both a spinner flask and static seeding. Godbey et al.[41] utilized the centrifugal force generated by a common laboratory centrifuge to seed bladder smooth muscle cells or human foreskin fibroblasts onto poly(glycolic acid) scaffolds from a dilute cell suspension. They showed better cell seeding efficiency and greater cell survival for a 10 min seeding time in the centrifuge compared to a 24 hour seeding time in a spinner flask.

16.8. BIOREACTORS FOR BONE TISSUE ENGINEERING

As discussed above, several types of bioreactors have been utilized for dynamic cell seeding of a variety of cell types onto a variety of scaffolds. These and other bioreactors have been more often used for the long term culture of cell-seeded scaffolds. The simplest method of 3-dimensional cell culture entails placing the scaffold/cell constructs into a well plate, covering with medium and simply placing in an incubator. However, the usefulness of this static culture method is severely limited in creating large tissue constructs *in vitro* as a result of poor mass transport of nutrients to and waste products from cells near the center of the scaffolds. Recall from the discussion of bone vascularity that no cell in bone tissue is more than 300 μm from a blood vessel and that the most active cells are located on the surface of the bone tissue where there is an abundance of vessels for nutrient transport. Thus, in creating bone tissue engineering constructs *in vitro*, the actively proliferating and differentiating cells initially located at the center of a thick scaffold will suffer from nutrient deprivation and waste product buildup if the medium filling the porosity of the scaffold does not move in and out at an acceptable rate. In static culture, there is no bulk fluid movement and as such, cells must rely on the process of diffusion to carry nutrients from the medium surrounding the scaffold, through the porous network to the cell surface. As the nutrients diffuse inward, cells along the perimeter of the scaffold will take what they need first, leaving less and less available for cells in the interior creating a concentration gradient that will ultimately limit cell survival to a small region near the scaffold surface. The need for alternate methods of cultivating these scaffold/cell constructs that reduce or eliminate the mass transport limitations inherent in static culture has spurred the development of a variety of bioreactors.

The spinner flask was the first type of bioreactor used for the long term cultivation of scaffold/cell tissue engineering constructs. In this simple design, a stirring mechanism is used to mix the medium exterior to the scaffold, creating a flow field to the surface of the scaffold for nutrient transport. Although nutrient transport within the scaffold is still governed by diffusion, the fluid flow around the scaffold exterior effectively moves the concentration gradient inward as the nutrient concentration at the scaffold surface is now the same as that in the bulk of the medium, allowing cell survival at a greater distance from the scaffold interior. This small increase in nutrient transport has resulted in great increases in cell survival and differentiation. Sikavitsas et al.[42] cultivated marrow stromal cells on poly(D,L-lactic-*co*-glycolic acid) (PLGA) scaffolds in both static and spinner flask culture in osteogenic medium for 21 days. They found increased cellularity over the first 2 weeks of culture in the spinner flask indicating a greater capacity to support cell growth as well as greater alkaline phosphatase activity and mineralization at 2 and 3 weeks of culture, indicative of osteoblastic differentiation. However, the mineralization front was still limited to the perimeter of the scaffold in spinner flask culture, although the layer of calcified matrix was thicker than in static culture. Others have found similar results when cultivating MSCs on porous scaffolds in spinner flasks.[43, 44]

A second type of bioreactor for long term culture of musculoskeletal tissues is the rotating wall vessel; a bioreactor developed by NASA to create a simulated microgravity environment while providing good mixing to the medium within the vessel. The rotating wall vessel is a horizontally mounted hollow cylinder housing an oxygenator membrane along the central axis of rotation. The space between the membrane and the outer vessel wall is filled with medium and the whole vessel is rotated. The medium rotates at a speed equivalent to the rotational speed of the vessel wall and this angular momentum offsets the pull of gravity on particles within the vessel. These particles can be microcarriers, scaffolds, or tissue aggregates and the speed of rotation can be adjusted to balance the gravitational force on particles of differing sizes. As for the spinner flask, the rotating wall vessel provides good mixing of medium to the scaffold surface while relying on diffusion to transport nutrients within the scaffold. Sikavitsas et al.[42] compared the osteogenic differentiation of marrow stromal cells cultivated on PLGA scaffolds in a rotating wall vessel to both spinner flask and static culture. They found decreased scaffold cellularity over the first week compared to static culture and similar cellularity at 2 and 3 weeks of culture indicating an initial suppression of proliferation in the rotary vessel. There was also much less alkaline phosphatase activity and calcification in the rotary vessel compared to static culture suggesting that there was a detrimental effect of this bioreactor on the osteoblastic differentiation of marrow stromal cells. Similar results were also observed by Goldstein et al.[43] These results are not entirely surprising as bone cells *in vivo* require mechanical stimulation to form and remodel bone. Astronauts who are in space for long periods of time lose substantial bone mass due to the absence of the gravitational force which normally provides the mechanical loading which signals bone growth and remodeling. Since the rotating wall vessel was designed to minimize the effects of gravity, creating a nearly weightless environment, these progenitor cells lack even the minimal mechanical signals provided by static culture. These results emphasize that while good mass transport is essential for developing tissue engineered constructs, the mechanical environment experienced by the cells plays an equally important role in osteoblast differentiation.

The third type of bone tissue engineering bioreactor is a perfusion bioreactor which, by forcing medium through the porosity of the scaffold, completely mitigates the mass transport limitations inherent in static, spinner flask, and rotary vessel culture and introduces a mechanical stimulation to the cells in the form of fluid shear. Marrow stromal cells seeded on porous PLGA foams and cultivated in a flow perfusion bioreactor resulted in increased alkaline phosphatase activity and more uniform cell distribution throughout the thickness of the scaffold compared to static culture.[43, 44] Using a novel flow perfusion bioreactor design developed in this laboratory[45], marrow stromal cells were cultivated on titanium fiber mesh scaffolds of 8 mm diameter and cultivated at a medium flow rate of 0.5 ml/min for up to 16 days. There was enhanced alkaline phosphatase activity at day 8, increased calcium deposition at day 16, and improved cell and extracellular matrix distribution under flow perfusion compared to static controls.[46]

Further studies with marrow stromal cell/titanium fiber mesh composites in this flow perfusion bioreactor revealed that increasing the flow rate of medium resulted in increasing calcified matrix deposition in a dose dependent fashion.[47] Increased fluid flow rate results in both better mass transport through the scaffold as well as increased mechanical forces in the form of fluid shear. In a subsequent study where fluid shear rate was increased without changing the fluid flow rate, increasing fluid shear resulted in increasing calcified matrix deposition and increased spatial distribution of cells and matrix within the titanium fiber mesh.[48] These studies highlight the importance of mechanical environment on the differentiation of marrow stromal cells. Additionally, in this bioreactor system, fluid flow rate and fluid shear can be easily modulated to accommodate specific mechanical requirements. Furthermore, when marrow stromal cells were seeded onto starch-based polymer fiber mesh scaffolds[49] or resorbable poly(L-lactic acid) fiber mesh scaffolds[50] there were similar increases in calcium deposition and cellular spatial distribution at a low flow rate of 0.3 ml/min, showing that the perfusion bioreactor system can accommodate a variety of scaffold materials.

16.9. FLOW PERFUSION CULTURE FOR BONE TISSUE ENGINEERING

Recent work in our laboratory has focused on further characterization of this flow perfusion bioreactor for development of bone tissue engineering constructs. Specifically, we investigated the effects of adhesion molecules, extracellular matrix molecules, culture supplements, and scaffold pore size on the osteoblastic differentiation of marrow stromal cells seeded onto titanium fiber mesh scaffolds.

To determine if cell differentiation could be enhanced by promoting integrin specific cell binding to the scaffold, a titanium fiber mesh was coated with the adhesion peptide sequence RGD. We discovered that cell adhesion was much stronger to the RGD coated fiber mesh and that this stronger adhesion tended to delay osteoblastic differentiation, rather than promote it in static in vitro culture.[51] We also investigated the osteoinductive potential of either plain titanium fiber mesh or RGD peptide surface modified titanium fiber mesh scaffolds seeded with marrow stromal cells for 1 day prior to subcutaneous implantation. We found that ectopic bone formation required the presence of marrow stromal cells that had already started down the osteoblast differentiation pathway.[51] These results indicate that cell differentiation state plays an important role in bone formation. Further studies are required to continue evaluating the angiogenic potential of these scaffold/cell constructs as well as the role of initial bone-like extracellular matrix on inducing de novo bone formation in vivo.

We then hypothesized that a combination of adhesion sequences and other extracellular matrix molecules would enhance the osteoblastic differentiation of marrow stromal cells. To test this hypothesis, marrow stromal cells were cultivated on titanium fiber mesh scaffolds under conditions known to result in the deposition of bone-like extracellular matrix. After 12 days of culture, this matrix was at the onset of mineralization. At this point, the cellular component of the scaffold/cell/ECM constructs was removed to yield titanium fiber mesh scaffolds with a bone-like extracellular matrix deposited on its surface. This pre-formed bone-like extracellular matrix was shown to enhance the osteoblastic differentiation of freshly seeded marrow stromal cells even in the absence of the osteogenic supplements normally required, specifically dexamethasone.[52]

Knowing MSC osteoblast differentiation is enhanced by fluid shear in a flow perfusion bioreactor and by bone-like extracellular matrix in the absence of dexamethasone, we hypothesized that fluid shear stress would be sufficient to induce the osteoblast phenotype in a flow perfusion bioreactor in the absence of dexamethasone. Marrow stromal cells were seeded on titanium fiber mesh scaffolds and cultivated in a flow perfusion bioreactor in the absence of dexamethasone. Our results supported the initial hypothesis and showed a synergistic effect between the two components, though dexamethasone was a greater enhancer of the osteoblast phenotype than fluid shear alone.[53]

Lastly, we evaluated the effect of scaffold pore size on the osteoblastic differentiation of marrow stromal cells seeded on titanium fiber mesh scaffolds and cultivated in a flow perfusion bioreactor. We hypothesized that the difference in scaffold pore size would result in alterations in fluid flow and subsequently fluid shear stress experienced by the seeded cells that would affect their osteoblastic differentiation. Our results showed that differentiation was indeed dependent on scaffold pore size, however the dependence was not linear with respect to time. Larger pore size was conducive to early osteoblast differentiation while smaller pore size was conducive to later differentiation and matrix deposition.[54] These studies indicate that physical properties of titanium fiber mesh scaffolds have a large influence on the behavior of cells seeded onto their surfaces and that these properties can be tailored to induce the osteoblastic differentiation pathway of progenitor cells harvested from bone marrow.

16.10. SUMMARY

In summary, many factors can influence the osteoblastic differentiation of marrow stromal cells when cultivated on three-dimensional tissue engineering scaffolds. In creating ideal bone tissue engineering constructs consisting of a combination of a scaffold, cells, and bioactive factors; a flow perfusion bioreactor is a much more suitable culture environment than static culture in well plates. The bioreactor eliminates mass transport limitations to the scaffold interior and provides mechanical stimulation to the seeded cells through fluid shear. Scaffold properties such as pore size impact cell differentiation, especially in flow perfusion culture. In addition, the bone-like extracellular matrix created by the in vitro culture of marrow stromal cells on porous scaffolds creates an osteoinductive environment for the differentiation of other marrow stromal cell populations. Therefore, bone tissue engineering constructs created by in vitro culture have excellent potential for bone regeneration applications in the clinic. However, more work is required to optimize this tissue engineering strategy. A biodegradable material with mechanical integrity similar to native bone and degradation properties similar to the rate of bone formation would be a more ideal scaffold material. It is also yet unclear what the optimum scaffold pore size and amount of in vitro generated extracellular matrix are to maximize bone formation. Finally, better characterization of the flow patterns within the flow perfusion bioreactor is needed to better understand the relationship between fluid shear and cell differentiation for creation of the ideal scaffold/culture combination.

16.11. ACKNOWLEDGMENTS

The work on bone tissue engineering has been supported by the National Institutes of Health (R01 AR42639).

16.12. REFERENCES

1. R. Langer and J. P. Vacanti, Tissue Engineering, *Science* **260**(5110), 920-926 (1993).
2. M. J. Yaszemski, J. B. Oldham, L. Lu and B. L. Currier, Clinical Needs for Bone Tissue-Engineering Technology, in: *Bone Engineering*, edited by J. E. Davies (em squared incorporated, Toronto, 2000), pp. 541-546.
3. J. A. Buckwalter, M. J. Glimcher, R. R. Cooper and R. Recker, Bone Biology, *J. Bone Joint Surg. Am.* **77-A**(8), 1256-1289 (1995).
4. V. I. Sikavitsas, J. S. Temenoff and A. G. Mikos, Biomaterials and Bone Mechanotransduction, *Biomaterials* **22**(19), 2581-2593 (2001).
5. J. E. Aubin and A. Herbertson, Osteoblast lineage in experimental animals, in: *Marrow Stromal Cell Culture*, edited by J. N. Beresford and M. Owen (Cambridge University Press, Cambridge, 1998), pp. 88-110.
6. J. E. Aubin, The Osteoblast Lineage, in: *Principles of Bone Biology*, edited by J. P. Bilezikian, L. G. Raisz and G. A. Rodan (Academic Press, San Diego, 1996), pp. 51-67.
7. J. E. Aubin, Osteogenic Cell Differentiation, in: *Bone Engineering*, edited by J. E. Davies (em squared incorporated, Toronto, 2000), pp. 19-29.
8. C. Maniatopolous, J. Sodek and A. H. Melcher, Bone formation in *in vitro* by stromal cells obtained from bone marrow of young adult rats, *Cell Tissue Research* **254**(2), 317-330 (1988).
9. E. Behravesh, K. Zygourakis and A. G. Mikos, Adhesion and migration of marrow-derived osteoblasts on injectable *in situ* crosslinkable poly(propylene fumarate-*co*-ethylene glycol)-based hydrogels with a covalently linked RGDS peptide, *J. Biomed. Mater. Res.* **65A**(2), 261-271 (2003).
10. E. Behravesh and A. G. Mikos, Three-dimensional culture of differentiating marrow stromal osteoblasts in biomimetic poly(propylene fumarate-*co*-ethylene glycol)-based macroporous hydrogels, *J. Biomed. Mater. Res.* **66A**(3), 698-706 (2003).
11. H. Shin, S. Jo and A. G. Mikos, Modulation of marrow stromal osteoblast adhesion on biomimetic oligo[poly(ethylene glycol) fumarate] hydrogels modified with Arg-Gly-Asp peptides and a poly(ethylene glycol) spacer, *J. Biomed. Mater. Res.* **61A**(2), 169-179 (2002).
12. J. S. Temenoff, H. Park, E. Jabbari, D. E. Conway, T. L. Sheffield, C. G. Ambrose and A. G. Mikos, Thermally Cross-Linked Oligo(poly(ethylene glycol) fumarate) Hydrogels Support Osteogenic Differentiation of Encapsulated Marrow Stromal Cells In Vitro, *Biomacromolecules* **5**(1), 5-10 (2004).
13. R. G. Payne, J. S. McGonigle, M. J. Yaszemski, A. W. Yasko and A. G. Mikos, Development of an injectable, in situ crosslinkable, degradable polymeric carrier for osteogenic cell populations. Part 3. Proliferation and differentiation of encapsulated marrow stromal osteoblasts cultured on crosslinking poly(propylene fumarate), *Biomaterials* **23**(22), 4381-4387 (2002).
14. E. Lieb, J. Tessmar, M. Hacker, C. Fischbach, D. Rose, T. Blunk, A. G. Mikos, A. Gopferich and M. B. Schulz, Poly(D,L-lactic acid)-Poly(ethylene glycol)-Monomethyl Ether Diblock Copolymers Control Adhesion and Osteoblastic Differentiation of Marrow Stromal Cells, *Tissue Eng.* **9**(1), 71-84 (2003).
15. M. J. Gilmcher, L. C. Bonar, M. D. Grynpas, W. J. Landis and A. H. Roufosse, Recent studies of bone mineral: Is the amorphous calcium phosphate theory valid?, *J. Cryst. Growth* **53**(1), 100-119 (1981).
16. B. R. Constantz, I. C. Ison, M. T. Fulmer, R. D. Poser, S. T. Smith, M. VanWagoner, J. Ross, S. A. Goldstein, J. B. Jupiter and D. I. Rosenthal, Skeletal Repair by in Situ Formation of the Mineral Phase of Bone, *Science* **267**(5205), 1796-1799 (1995).
17. C. G. Finkemeier, Bone grafting and bone graft substitutes, *J. Bone Joint Surg. Am.* **84A**(3), 454-464 (2002).
18. S. N. Parikh, Bone graft substitutes in modern orthopedics, *Orthopedics* **25**(11), 1301-1309 (2002).
19. J. A. McAuliffe, Bone Graft Substitutes, *J. Hand Ther.* **16**(2), 180-187 (2003).
20. H. Yuan, M. van den Doel, S. Li, C. A. van Blitterswijk, K. de Groot and J. D. de Bruijn, A comparison of the osteoinductive potential of two calcium phosphate ceramics implanted intramuscularly in goats, *J. Mater. Sci. Mater. Med.* **13**(12), 1271-1275 (2002).

21. P. Q. Ruhé, H. C. Kroese-Deutman, J. G. C. Wolke, P. H. M. Spauwen and J. A. Jansen, Bone inductive properties of rhBMP-2 loaded porous calcium phosphate cement implants in cranial defects in rabbits, *Biomaterials* **25**(11), 2123-2132 (2004).
22. E. J. Blom, J. Klein-Nulend, C. P. A. T. Klein, K. Kurashina, M. A. J. van Waas and E. H. Burger, Transforming growth factor-ß1 incorporated during setting in calcium phosphate cement stimulates bone cell differentiation *in vitro*, *J. Biomed. Mater. Res. A* **50**(1), 67-74 (2000).
23. P. Laffargue, P. Fialdes, P. Frayssinet, M. Rtaimate, H. F. Hildebrand and X. Marchandise, Adsorption and release of insulin-like growth factor-1 on porous tricalcium phosphate implant, *J. Biomed. Mater. Res.* **49A**(3), 415-421 (2000).
24. J. Toquet, R. Rohanizadeh, J. Guicheux, S. Couillaud, N. Passuti, G. Daculsi and D. Heymann, Osteogenic potential *in vitro* of human bone marrow cells cultured on macroporous biphasic calcium phosphate ceramic, *J. Biomed. Mater. Res.* **44A**(1), 98-108 (1999).
25. T. Kai, G. Shao-qing and D. Geng-ting, In vivo evaluation of bone marrow stromal-derived osteoblasts-porous calcium phosphate ceramic composites as bone graft substitute for lumbar intervertebral spine fusion, *Spine* **28**(15), 1653-1658 (2003).
26. J. Goshima, V. M. Goldberg and A. I. Caplan, Osteogenic potential of culture-expanded rat marrow cells as assayed *in vivo* with porous calcium phosphate ceramic, *Biomaterials* **12**(2), 253-258 (1991).
27. H. Ohgushi, M. Okumura, S. Tamai, E. C. Shors and A. I. Caplan, Marrow cell induced osteogenesis in porous hydroxyapatite and tricalcium phosphate: a comparative histomorphometric study of ectopic bone formation, *J. Biomed. Mater. Res.* **24A**(12), 1563-1570 (1990).
28. J. W. M. Vehof, P. H. M. Spauwen and J. A. Jansen, Bone formation in calcium-phosphate-coated titanium mesh, *Biomaterials* **21**(2003-2009 (2000).
29. J. W. M. Vehof, M. T. Haus, A. E. de Ruijter, P. H. M. Spauwen and J. A. Jansen, Bone formation in transforming growth factor beta-I-loaded titanium fiber mesh implants, *Clin. Oral Implants Res.* **13**(1), 94-102 (2002).
30. J. W. M. Vehof, A. E. de Ruijter, P. H. M. Spauwen and J. A. Jansen, Influence of rhBMP-2 on rat bone marrow stromal cells cultured on titanium fiber mesh, *Tissue Eng.* **7**(4), 373-383 (2001).
31. J. van den Dolder, J. W. M. Vehof, P. H. M. Spauwen and J. A. Jansen, Bone formation by rat bone marrow cells cultured on titanium fiber mesh: effect of in vitro culture time, *J. Biomed. Mater. Res.* **62A**(3), 350-358 (2002).
32. J. W. M. Vehof, J. van den Dolder, J. E. de Ruijter, P. H. M. Spauwen and J. A. Jansen, Bone formation in CaP-coated and noncoated titanium fiber mesh, *J. Biomed. Mater. Res.* **64A**(417-426 (2003).
33. J. W. M. Vehof, J. Mahmood, H. Takita, M. A. van't Hof, Y. Kuboki, P. H. M. Spauwen and J. A. Jansen, Ectopic bone formation in titanium mesh loaded with bone morphogenetic protein and coated with calcium phosphate, *Plast. Reconstr. Surg.* **108**(2), 434-443 (2001).
34. J. van den Dolder, E. Farber, P. H. M. Spauwen and J. A. Jansen, Bone tissue reconstruction using titanium fiber mesh combined with rat bone marrow stromal cells, *Biomaterials* **24**(1745-1750 (2003).
35. J. van den Dolder, P. H. M. Spauwen and J. A. Jansen, Evaluation of Various Seeding Techniques for Culturing Osteogenic Cells on Titanium Fiber Mesh, *Tissue Eng.* **9**(2), 315-325 (2003).
36. G. Vunjak-Novakovic, B. Obradovic, I. Martin, P. M. Bursac, R. Langer and L. E. Freed, Dynamic cell seeding of polymer scaffolds for cartilage tissue engineering, *Biotechnol. Prog.* **14**(2), 193-202 (1998).
37. B.-S. Kim, A. J. Putnam, T. J. Kulik and D. J. Mooney, Optimizing seeding and culture methods to engineer smooth muscle tissue on biodegradable polymer matrices, *Biotechnol. Bioeng.* **57**(1), 46-54 (1998).
38. J. R. Mauney, J. Blumberg, M. Pirun, V. Volloch, G. Vunjak-Novakovic and D. L. Kaplan, Osteogenic differentiation of human bone marrow stromal cells on partially demineralized bone scaffolds *in vitro*, *Tissue Eng.* **10**(1-2), 81-92 (2004).
39. R. L. Carrier, M. Papadaki, M. Rupnick, F. J. Schoen, N. Bursac, R. Langer, L. E. Freed and G. Vunjak-Novakovic, Cardiac tissue engineering: cell seeding cultivation parameters, and tissue construct characterization, *Biotechnol. Bioeng.* **64**(5), 580-589 (1999).
40. D. Wendt, A. Marsano, M. Jakob, M. Heberer and I. Martin, Oscillating perfusion of cell suspensions through three-dimensional scaffoldsd enhances cell seeding efficiency and uniformity, *Biotechnol. Bioeng.* **84**(2), 205-214 (2003).
41. W. T. Godbey, B. S. S. Hindy, M. E. Sherman and A. Atala, A novel use of centrifugal force for cell seeding into porous scaffolds, *Biomaterials* **25**(14), 2799-2805 (2004).
42. V. I. Sikavitsas, G. N. Bancroft and A. G. Mikos, Formation of three-dimensional cell/polymer constructs for bone tissue engineering in a spinner flask and a rotating wall vessel bioreactor, *J. Biomed. Mater. Res.* **62A**(1), 136-148 (2002).

43. A. S. Goldstein, T. M. Juarez, C. D. Helmke, M. C. Gustin and A. G. Mikos, Effect of convection on osteoblastic cell growth and function in biodegradable polymer foam scaffolds, *Biomaterials* **22**(11), 1279-1288 (2001).
44. L. Meinel, V. Karageorgiou, R. Fajardo, B. Snyder, V. Shinde-Patil, L. Zichner, D. L. Kaplan, R. Langer and G. Vunjak-Novakovic, Bone tissue engineering using human mesenchymal stem cells: effects of scaffold material and medium flow, *Ann. Biomed. Eng.* **32**(1), 112-122 (2004).
45. G. N. Bancroft, V. I. Sikavitsas and A. G. Mikos, Design of a Flow Perfusion Bioreactor System for Bone Tissue-Engineering Applications, *Tissue Eng.* **9**(3), 549-554 (2003).
46. J. van den Dolder, G. N. Bancroft, V. I. Sikavitsas, P. H. Spauwen, J. A. Jansen and A. G. Mikos, Flow perfusion culture of marrow stromal osteoblasts in titanium fiber mesh, *J. Biomed. Mater. Res.* **64A**(2), 235-241 (2003).
47. G. N. Bancroft, V. I. Sikavitsas, J. van den Dolder, T. L. Sheffield, C. G. Ambrose, J. A. Jansen and A. G. Mikos, Fluid flow increases mineralized matrix deposition in 3D perfusion culture of marrow stromal osteoblasts in a dose-dependent manner, *Proc. Natl. Acad. Sci. U. S. A.* **99**(20), 12600-12605 (2002).
48. V. I. Sikavitsas, G. N. Bancroft, H. L. Holtorf, J. A. Jansen and A. G. Mikos, Mineralized matrix deposition by marrow stromal osteoblasts in 3D perfusion culture increases with increasing fluid shear forces, *Proc. Natl. Acad. Sci. U. S. A.* **100**(25), 14683-14688 (2003).
49. M. E. Gomes, V. I. Sikavitsas, E. Behravesh, R. L. Reis and A. G. Mikos, Effect of Flow Perfusion on the Osteogenic Differentiation of Bone Marrow Stromal Cells Cultured on Starch-Based Three-Dimensional Scaffolds, *J. Biomed. Mater. Res.* **67A**(87-95 (2003).
50. V. I. Sikavitsas, G. N. Bancroft, J. J. Lemoine, M. A. K. Liebschner, M. Dauner and A. G. Mikos, Flow perfusion enhances the calcified matrix deposition of marrow stromal cells in biodegradable non-woven fiber mesh scaffolds, *Ann. Biomed. Eng.* **33**(1), 63-70 (2005).
51. H. L. Holtorf, J. A. Jansen and A. G. Mikos, Ectopic bone formation in rat marrow stromal cell/titanium fiber mesh scaffold constructs: Effect of initial cell phenotype, *Biomaterials* **26**(31), 6208-6216 (2005).
52. N. Datta, H. L. Holtorf, V. I. Sikavitsas, J. A. Jansen and A. G. Mikos, Effect of bone extracellular matrix synthesized in vitro on the osteoblastic differentiation of marrow stromal cells, *Biomaterials* **26**(9), 971-977 (2005).
53. H. L. Holtorf, J. A. Jansen and A. G. Mikos, Flow perfusion culture induces the osteoblastic differentiation of marrow stromal cell-scaffold constructs in the absence of dexamethasone, *J. Biomed. Mater. Res.* **72A**(3), 326-334 (2005).
54. H. L. Holtorf, N. Datta, J. A. Jansen and A. G. Mikos, Scaffold Mesh Size Affects the Osteoblastic Differentiation of Seeded Marrow Stromal Cells Cultured in a Flow Perfusion Bioreactor, *J. Biomed. Mater. Res.* **74A**(2), 171-180 (2005).

17

BIOREACTORS FOR TISSUES OF THE MUSCULOSKELETAL SYSTEM

Rita I Abousleiman[1] and Vassilios I Sikavitsas[1,2]

17.1. SUMMARY

Muskuloskeletal tissue includes bone, cartilage, ligament, skeletal muscle and tendons. These tissues malfunction either due to a natural injury, trauma, or a disorder. In all cases natural regeneration needs to be enhanced by medication and, in many instances, by surgery. Surgical techniques are limited to suturing, autografts or allografts. Tissue engineering stems from the challenge presented by the limited resources for natural implants and the ineffectiveness of previous curing techniques. The challenge in tissue engineering resides in the design of a functional bioreactor that would: (1) house the engineered construct under sterile conditions; and (2) provide the appropriate stimuli that would result in a neotissue with biochemical and biomechanical properties comparable to *in situ* tissue. The various types and designs of bioreactors for the regeneration of musculoskeletal tissue, including spinner flask, rotating wall vessel, flow perfusion, and mechanical loading devices are presented in this paper.

17.2. INTRODUCTION

In the year 2000, the major reason for physicians' office visits was musculoskeletally related[1]. Sixty two percent of all physicians' visits for injury were musculoskeletal, accounting for 56 million patients, out of which 7 million were hospitalized[2]. Comparably, the National Center for Health Statistics reported that 7.3 million orthopaedic surgeries were conducted in 1996[2]. One in every seven Americans have a musculoskeletal detriment that limits or decreases their ability to function normally at home, work, sports, or at play[3]. Each year, orthopaedic injuries in the U.S. cause children to miss 21 million days of school and workers more than 147 million days of labor[3].

---

[1] Oklahoma University Bioengineering Center, The University of Oklahoma, Norman, OK 73019

[2] Chemical, Biological, and Materials Engineering, The University of Oklahoma, Norman, OK 73019

From the above figures it is clear that musculoskeletal disorders should be a major concern for the scientific community. The Academy of Orthopaedic Surgeons reported that musculoskeletal conditions cost the economy more than $215 billion a year; however, only $92 million is dedicated to orthopaedic research out of which $15 million is for clinical research[2].

Musculoskeletal tissues malfunction either due to a natural injury, trauma, or a disorder. In all cases natural regeneration needs to be enhanced by medication and, in many instances, by surgery. Surgical techniques are limited to suturing, autografts or allografts[4]. Tissue engineering stems from the challenge presented by the limited resources for natural implants and the ineffectiveness of previous curing techniques. In order to engineer neotissue successfully there is a need to mimic the *in vivo* environment and engulf the *de novo* grown tissue or "construct" in a sterile chamber equipped with a specific stimulatory mechanism depending on the tissue of interest. Thus bioreactors were introduced. The various types and designs of bioreactors for the regeneration of musculoskeletal tissue are herein described and presented.

17.3. PROPERTIES AND PATHOLOGIES OF THE MUSCULOSKELETAL SYSTEM

Muskuloskeletal tissue includes bone, cartilage, ligament, skeletal muscle and tendons. All these types of tissue are strong and durable. Bone and cartilage are hard and have high compressive strength, while ligaments and tendons are considered soft tissue and poses high tensile strength[5]. Proliferation of tissue could be of two kinematically different types: appositional and interstitial[5]. In appositional growth the new matrix is deposited on the surface causing the tissue to grow from the outside. On the other hand, in interstitial growth cells multiply and deposit new matrix from within the tissue. Soft tissue develops solely by interstitial growth, while in hard tissue bone grows mainly appositionally and cartilage proliferates by both phenomena. In this section a summary of the properties and pathologies of each tissue is presented.

17.3.1. Bone

Bone is a very durable and strong tissue. It is vascularised and has the capability for healing. Bone tissue growth follows two general mechanisms; (1) intramembranous ossification where cells of the inner layer of the periostium differentiate into oteoblasts and start laying down bone matrix and (2) endochondral bone formation where chodrocytes of the epiphyseal plate undergo hypertrophy resulting in the resorption of the cartilage matrix which is replaced by spongy bone. Eventually the calcified spicules udergo osteoclastic remodeling and new bone matrix is formed by osteoblastic activity[6]. Osteocytes, mature bone cells, do not have the ability to multiply. As a result, osteoblasts, osteoclasts and multipotent cells are responsible for bone regeneration. However, like any other tissue in our body, bone might undergo trauma or a disorder under which condition the tissue would need help in healing.

Overstress of bone due to an injury or trauma results in stress fractures, bone shattering and inflammation conditions such as apophysitis and periostitis[7]. Osteonecrosis is a bone disorder in which osteocytes lyse and die causing the degradation of a bone segment[8]. Osteonecrotic bone eventually looses its mechanical properties, fractures and sometimes even shatters. If osteonecrosis involves the sub–

chondral bone, the eventual fracture and collapse of the bone leads to irregularities in the articular surface and subsequently to degenerative arthiritis[8]. The most common methods to support healing of bone are cast and brace immobilization. However, many fractures require additional internal or external support, and if a large segment of bone is shattered eminently immobilization would not solve the problem[8]. In this case a bone graft would be essential to provide the injured area with structural support and allow the bone to restore itself adequately. The main types of grafts currently used are autografts and allografts, however they both have their shortcomings. Limited supply and donor site morbidity are major concerns in autografts; allografts may induce an immune response or inflammatory reaction[4]. In order to enhance fracture healing osteogenic methods using tissue engineering were employed.

17.3.2. Cartilage

Cartilage, composed mainly of water, collagen type II, and proteoglycans, is a strong resistant tissue that is high is compressive strength[6]. It is described[9] to be a tangle of collagen fibrils intermingling with electrically charged proteoglycan molecules balanced by inorganic ions. Cartilage grows by two principal methods: (1) interstitial growth where the mature cartilage cells, chondrocytes, divide and proliferate; and (2) appositional growth where cells of the inner layer of the perichondrium differentiate into chondroblasts and start laying down cartilage matrix. To maintain its viability, being an avascular tissue, cartilage depends on the diffusion of nutrients from the surrounding connective tissue[6].

Cartilage is subjected to osmotic pressure accrued due to the large amounts of water bound to hyaluronic proteoglycan molecules[9]. The tension present in the intermingling collagen fibers resists this pressure build up[9]. During physical motion, stress is usually applied unevenly to joints inducing the development of osmotic pressure due to the movement of water along the ion concentration gradient[10]. As a result, dynamic flow and mechanical stimulation are necessary in culturing cartilage-like tissue *in vitro*.

Cartilage is in general of three types: elastic, fibrous, and hyaline. Elastic cartilage contains elastic fibers in its extra cellular matrix giving the tissue elastic properties. It is mainly found in the auricle of the external ear, auditory tube, epiglottis, and in part of the larynx[6]. Fibrocartilage is a combination of cartilage and dense connective tissue and therefore, it has collagen type I in its matrix. Intervertebral discs, knee and shoulder joints, and symphysis pubis all contain fibrocartilage. The presence of fibrocartilage gives the tissue resilience which helps to absorb physical shocks and stresses[6]. In addition to collagen type II, hyaline cartilage contains large amounts of glycosaminoglycans. It provides structural framework for the larynx, trachea and bronchi[6]. It also covers the articular ends of ribs and synovial joints, in which case it is called articular cartilage. Articular cartilage covers the surface of bone mainly in joints. It is a very durable tissue, however, it has poor healing capacity after injury[11,12] due to its avascular nature, low cellularity, and lack of undifferentuiated cells within the tissue[12,14]. Lack of vascularization deprives cartilage of the normal response to injury that starts by a fibrin clot formation and causes inflammatory cells to rush to the scene followed by undifferenciated cells that would lie new matrix and help rejuvenate the tissue[15]. This tissue may be damaged by trauma, inflammation or may undergo progressive degeneration eventually exposing the underlying bone and causing osteoarthiritis[15]. In many cases this leads to defective joint function resulting in prosthetic joint replacement. However, prosthetic replacements lack the durability of natural joints and are only appropriate for a limited number of patients that are in severe pain conditions[15]. Marrow-stimulation techniques, such as drilling, microfracture, or abrasion arthroplasty, to promote cartilaginous tissue regeneration have been attempted. Nevertheless, they failed to yield long-term solutions since they resulted in the production of fibrocartilage, which lacks the biomechanical properties of articular cartilage[16]. Due to the lack of a proper solution for the injuries and diseases of articular cartilage there is a need for tissue engineering and bioreactors to device new techniques for cartilage regeneration.

17.3.3. Tendons

Tendons are inelastic collagenous anatomical soft tissues[9] that connect muscles to bone. Tenocytes are spindle shaped cells, sparsely spaced, and sandwiched between parallel layers of collagen type I[17,18]. Tendons have different anatomical locations in the body and thus different cross sectional areas relative to the muscles they are connected to. Depending on the muscle they serve, tendons are subjected to different stress levels and therefore their tensile strength varies remarkably[9]. Tendons possess high tensile strength (σ: 50-105 MPa)[17-19] but have poor intrinsic healing capabilities[20]. Most tendon injuries result in the degeneration and morphological alteration of collagen fibers. The exact causes of collagen degeneration are still not very well understood.

Tendon injuries affect several individuals yearly and in many cases prevent participation in daily activities[2]. These injuries could be a result of an accident or overuse. Overuse of soft tissue, tendons in particular, causes progressive damage where the repetitive strain overcomes the ability of the tissue to repair itself[7,21]. This might lead to tendinosis (tendon tissue degeneration without inflammatory response), tendonitis (tendon tissue degeneration with inflammatory response), edema, partial tears, or complete ruptures[20,21]. Common examples include tennis elbow, swimmer's shoulder, little league elbow, runner's knee, jumper's knee, and Achilles tendinitis[7,20]. In most sports and activities, overuse injuries, termed as "tendinopathies", are the most common and challenging to diagnose and treat[20]. They produce a great diagnostic and therapeutic problem because the symptoms are often dispersed and non-specific[7]. Common treatments to tendinosis and tendonitis include, but are not limited to, rest, strengthening, non-steroidal anti-inflammatory drugs, corticosteroids, braces, cryotherapy, and surgery [20]. Suturing techniques provide adequate mechanical strength for the tendon and diminishes the gap between the tendon stumps. However, tendon replacement might be a necessity in case of peripheral nerve injury and for patients with rheumatoid arthiritis[21]. Tissue engineering provides several choices for tendon replacements and thus a functional solution for the common and recurring tendon pathologies.

17.3.4. Ligaments

Ligaments, classified as dense connective tissue, have similar morphology to tendons. They are composed mainly of fibroblasts sandwiched between layers of collagen type I. However, since ligaments connect bone to bone they experience traction forces from several angles giving their collagen fibers more varied directionality than in tendons[4]. In addition, ligaments are shorter and wider than tendons, and contain less collagen and more ground substance in their extracellular matrix. Ligament injuries can be classified as being partial or complete and sometimes can include underlying bone injury and lead to osteoarthiritis[18]. Ligament regeneration is not always successful and the problem could become chronic.

One of the major causes of ligament trauma is sports. Sport injuries result in a great number of knee injuries including the anterior and posterior cruciate ligaments (ACL and PCL)[4,18,22]. In the year 2002, 12,400 ACL tear cases were recorded in in-patient care in the United States[2]. According to the department of Human Health Services the number of patients undergoing total knee replacement surgery increased from 257,000 in 1998 to 365,000 in 2002[23], reflecting a 42% increase. ACL injuries are considered problematic because the tissue usually does not heal. If kept un-treated, an injured ACL could lead to meniscal damage and joint instability and eventually osteoarthiritis[18]. To reduce knee instability in affected individuals immobilization and suturing techniques have been attempted, however they lead to decreased mechanical properties in the long-term[24]. Autografts and allografts have resulted in extended viability but also decreased mechanical properties compared to innate tissue[18]. The patellar tendon has been frequently used to replace the ACL but the potency of this repair mechanism is completely dependent on the revascularization of the transplanted tissue that is progressively surrounded by the synovial membrane[4,25]. Due to limitations associated with current graft methods for ACL reconstruction and lack of capacity for self-repair, interest in tissue engineered solutions has increased[22].

17.4. FUNCTIONAL TISSUE ENGINEERING

Tissue engineering uses the principles of engineering, biology, and chemistry in designing a neotissue that would augment a malfunctioning *in vivo* tissue[26]. Since the traditional methods of treating orthopaedic injuries and disorders are not completely effective and have several limitations, tissue engineering has gained remarkable support as an approach to treat musculoskeletal disorders circumventing the limitations of existing therapies[4].

The main requirements for functional engineered tissue include reparative cellular components that proliferate on a biocompatible scaffold grown within a bioreactor which provides specific biochemical and physical signals to regulate cell differentiation and tissue assembly[25,27-29]. There are several approaches to tissue engineering. One possibility is to seed the scaffold with auotologous cells *in vitro* and then implant it into the defective site. Another approach is to engineer the whole tissue or organ *in vitro*, using a biodegradable scaffold for integrity and support, and only implant it in the patient when the morphological, biological and biomechanical properties of the engineered construct match those of the natural tissue. It is imperative, however that cells synthesize a functional matrix at a rate sufficient to balance the loss of mechanical integrity of the resorbed scaffold material[30,31]. A third application of tissue engineering is to implant a non- biodegradable conductive scaffold. The drawback of this method is that another surgical procedure may be needed to remove the scaffold when the tissue heals. Further explanation and elaboration on the different components of tissue engineering are included herein.

17.4.1. Cells

Cells are by far the most important component of an engineered tissue. They are the living component of the construct. Given the suitable biomechanical and biophysical environment cells would start secreting matrix that would eventually form the neotissue. The type and properties of secreted matrix depend on the different stimuli that cells are subjected to. For musculoskeletal tissue engineering several types of cells have been used. For example, osteoblastic cells have been widely employed in bone regeneration[32], chondrocytes for cartilage[33-35], and fibroblasts for tendon and ligament repair[36,37].

It is imperative that cells used in the tissue construct have the ability to proliferate and deposit matrix at a high rate in order to be able to implant the neotissue in the patient soon after the injury. Osteoblasts and chondrocytes are almost mature and do not proliferate at a high rate[38]. As a result, the best and most abundant source of cells is mesenchymal stem cells (MSC). MSC's are undifferentiated pluripotent cells that have the potential to differentiate into a number of mature cells of different lineages, depending on the biochemical and biophysical stimuli that they are subjected to[38-39]. These lineages include, but not limited to, osteoblasts (bone), chondocytes (cartilage), and fibroblasts (tendon and ligament). MSC's have been widely used as a musculoskeletal repair therapy[40-44]. The most popular source of MSC's is bone marrow, however MSC-like cells have also been extracted from other anatomical locations including subcutaneous adipose tissue[12]. It is necessary to mention that although the number of MSC's decline dramatically with age, their ability to differentiate and repair tissue is retained[41]. Being intermediate between embryonic and adult tissue MSC's may provide an *in situ* source of healing cells throughout an adult's lifetime[45].

17.4.2. Scaffolds

Cells are greatly affected by the surface to which they adhere. The type and properties of the scaffold used for seeding cells could alter the proliferation rate and extracellular matrix deposited by cells, and thus affect the final biomechanical and morphological properties of the engineered tissue[28]. The primary objective of using a scaffold is to provide mechanical stability and integrity to the construct and to supply a template for three-dimensional organization of the developing tissue[28]. The final goal is to obtain *de novo* tissue with biomechanical properties comparable to the damaged tissue. Scaffolds with high stiffness like ceramic hydroxyapatite are thus used for growing bone[28], while polymers that are more compliant are often chosen as scaffolds for cartilage, tendon, and ligament[28].

17.4.2.1. Scaffolds Used for Musculoskeletal Tissue Engineering

The scaffold used for tissue engineering must be non-toxic and biocompatible, i.e. evades the immune response. Biocompatible scaffolds could be either non-biodegradable or biodegradable. As mentioned earlier, a second surgery might be necessary to remove the implanted non-biodegradable scaffold after the tissue heals. If using a biodegradable polymer it is imperative that (1) the degradation products be biocompatible as well, and (2) the degradation rate of the scaffold be comparable to the tissue repair rate so that the implanted construct does not loose its mechanical integrity[4,25].

Non-biodegradable scaffolds include ceramics, metal (titanium), minerals (hydroxyapatite) and bioactive glasses[46]. Biodegradable scaffolds include synthetic poly (α-hydroxy ester) polymers[8,47] such as polylactic acid (PLA), polyglycolic acid (PGA)[33,48], poly (L-lactic acid) PLLA[49], poly(lactic-co-glycolic acid) PLGA[32,50,51], and polycaprolactone (PCL)[52]. Extensive research is being conducted on the regeneration of *in vivo* tissue using poly (α-hydroxyl esters)[47,53]. Since PLLA and its degradation products are non-toxic and biocompatible, and since its degradation rate is balanced by the rate of formation of human tissue[54], this material has gained the approval of the U.S. Food and Drug Administration for a variety of human clinical applications[55].

PGA scaffolds are widely used for cartilage tissue engineering[33,48,56,57]. Cartilage implants on PGA had a morphology, cellularity and matrix composition (collagen and glycosaminoglycan) comparable to normal cartilage[49]. Furthermore, the rate of proliferation of chondrocytes seeded on PGA scaffolds was twice as high compared to that of cells seeded on porous PLLA scaffolds[49]. PLLA scaffolds coated with fibronectic have been shown to be a better scaffold for ligament tissue reconstruction than PGA which has a very rapid degradation rate that could not be balanced by cell matrix production *in vivo*[22,36].

The use of natural acellular biomaterials as scaffolds for tissue engineering is very desirable since these materials, when processed properly, elude the immune response. Some of the natural biomaterials that are incorporated in designing scaffolds for bone and cartilaginous tissues are hyaluronic acid[58-60], agarose hydrogels[14,61] and alginate gels[62]. Collagen gel is used extensively as scaffolding material for tendon and ligament applications[31,37,63,64].

Composite scaffolds, designed by mixing synthetic polymers with natural biomaterials, created a favorable environment for cellular proliferation. For example cartilaginous constructs were engineered by using benzylated hyaluronan and PGA[65]. Additionally, collagen microsponges were formed in the pores of a PLGA sponge[66]. Chondrocytes seeded on the composite scaffold adhered to the collagen microsponges, proliferated, and filled up the pores between the collagen and PLGA.

17.4.2.2. Surface Modifications

To make biomaterial surfaces more conducive to cell attachment and spreading, some surface modifications were incorporated to polymeric scaffolds[47]. Two examples of such modifications include enriching surfaces with fibronectin, a protein widely present in the extracelluar matrix[22], or incorporating RGD, a small adhesion peptide, on the surface of the substrate[51].

17.4.2.3. Seeding Techniques

A large number of cells is required on the scaffold to achieve successful extracellular matrix deposition *in vitro*[49,67]. The final construct cellularity has been found to be relatively independent of cell seeding number; however, extracellular matrix components deposited were optimized with increased cell seeding density[57,68]. Uniform cell seeding is required[69] to obtain homogeneous tissue formation throughout the scaffold especially in the middle part.

Culturing techniques widely affect the cell distribution throughout the scaffold. One of the most common seeding techniques in the past is static culture; however, it has been reported repeatedly to yield low seeding efficiencies[70-73] and non-uniform cell distribution within scaffolds[46,56,70,72-75]. Dynamic systems on the other hand, yielded significantly higher seeding efficiency and homogeneity than static culture[46,57].

17.4.3. Stimulation Techniques

Cells within a construct respond and adapt to the chemical and mechanical stimuli to which they are exposed *in vivo*[28,76]. To achieve efficient cell proliferation, proper differentiation and sufficient matrix deposition it is necessary to replicate the actual tissue environment.

17.4.3.1. Chemical Stimulation

Growth factors are polypeptides that support various terminal phenotypes and stimulate cell proliferation[28,77]. Some of the most commonly used growth factors are transforming growth factors-β (TGF-β)[8,78-80] which regulate stem cell differentiation; bone morphogenetic proteins (BMP) induce *in vivo* osteogenesis[8,81-84]; and fibroblast growth factors (FGF) are known to support angiogenesis especially in tendon and ligament tissue[8,42,79,85].

17.4.3.2. Mechanical Stimulation

In vivo, cells and tissues are continuously subjected to mechanical stimuli that affect the tissue's developing morphology[5] and its biomechanical properties[86]. Recent research suggests that mechanostimulus may significantly increase the biosynthetic activity of cells cultured *in vitro*[29].

In vitro mechanical stimulation, by subjecting the scaffold to dynamic flow, has been shown to provide a uniform cell distribution throughout the three dimensional seeded construct resulting in a homogeneous matrix deposition[48,67]. Moreover, it has been reported that direct mechanical strain applied on seeded silicone scaffolds induces the differentiation of MSC's into a ligament-like cell lineage in preference to bone or cartilage cell lineages[27].

17.5. BIOREACTOR APPLICATIONS

A bioreactor is a device that provides a controlled sterile environment for the development of engineered tissue[69]. It confines the cultured cells within barriers that mimic the physiological conditions and provide mechanical stimulation to enhance mass transfer and nutrient transport within the seeded cells[25]. The dynamic environment within bioreactors has been shown to affect the phenotype of differentiated MSC's, the deposition of extracellular matrix components, and the growth and development of tissue[48]. Currently several designs of bioreactors are employed for different types of tissue culture. Some of the most favored bioreactor designs for growing orthopaedic tissue are those based on dynamic flow (for bone and cartilage) and on mechanical cyclic stretching (for tendon, ligament, and bone). The different existing bioreactors for culturing tissue of the musculoskeletal system are included henceforth.

17.5.1. Autologous Cell Transplantation

Autologous cell transplantation includes harvesting functional cells from the patient, proliferating them *in vitro*, and implanting the expanded cell culture in the defective or injured segment of tissue. The transplanted cells secrete healthy natural extracellular matrix that would augment the deficiency in the tissue. Human bone marrow MSC's were cultured and expanded *in vitro* and then loaded onto a ceramic carrier, and implanted into critical-sized segmental defects in the femurs of adult rats[39]. The MSC's demonstrated the capacity to rejuvenate defective bone and induce osteogenesis and therefore could provide an alternative to synthetic or autogenous bone grafts. Autologous chondrocytes were transplanted to defective knee sites, using microbeads coated with collagen type I[11]. The transplanted autologous chondrocytes were able to survive and yield hyaline-like cartilage. However, the mechanical properties of the resulting matrix were inferior to that of native cartilage.

17.5.2. *In Vivo* Bioreactors

In vivo bioreactors is a bioengineering approach that depends on the conductive properties of the implanted scaffold to recruit MSC's from neighboring tissue. This approach takes advantage of the physiological environment to supply the necessary growth factors and nutrients to the construct. The main challenge is to find the appropriate scaffolding material that would induce the differentiation of MSC's into an adequate lineage.

Several *in vivo* bioreactors were developed in an attempt to generate vascularized host bone tissue[62,81,87]. For example, in the design of one *in vivo* bioreactor the scaffold was composed of coralline cylinders and supplemented with BMP-2, a growth factor that was shown to influence osteogenesis and osteoblastic differentiation[88,89]. A vascular pedicle was incorporated into the scaffold to supply a channel for the MSC's recruited by BMP-2 from the blood circulation and into the bioreactor. To isolate the bioreactor from the surrounding environment the scaffold was coated with silicone. This would ensure the isolation of osteogenesis within the bioreactor, thus bone formation would depend solely on the internal scaffold and the invading cells with osteogenic potential. The designed *in vivo* bioreactors were implanted into 12 male rats and harvested after 6 weeks. The extracted implants demonstrated neovascular ingrowth and new bone formation of 11.3%.

Another *in vivo* bioreactor was incorporated into the tibia of New Zealand white rabbits. An artificial space was created between the tibia and the periosteum using alginate gel[62]. Preosteoblastic cells were recruited from the inner layer of the periosteum. The engineered bone tissue was found to be biomechanically identical to native bone. When harvested and implanted into tibial defects, the engineered bone completely integrated within the native bone tissue after 6 weeks with no apparent morbidity at the donor site. It was hypothesized that by inhibiting angiogenesis and promoting a more hypoxic environment within the bioreactor space, cartilage formation could be exclusively promoted.

17.5.3. Static Culture

Static cell culture has been widely used in the past. The cells are deposited on a scaffold, supplied with the appropriate growth media, and cultured in an incubator. However, numerous studies have shown that static culture results in a non-homogeneous cell distribution[35]. Moreover, transport of nutrients into large scaffolds have been proven to be problematic[67] and consequently cells may grow preferentially at the periphery of the scaffold[32,46]. In this case extracellular matrix components would be deposited only on the external surface giving the engineered construct non-uniform morphological and biomechanical properties. The presence or absence of dynamic mixing primarily affects the final exracellular matrix deposited in the engineered constructs[33].

Most of musculoskletal tissue *in vivo* is subjected to some kind of mechanical stimulation, and thus static cultures cannot mimic the physiological environment and will not be capable of replicating the *in vivo* tissue. For example, chondrocytes *in vivo* are heavily influenced by mechanical forces, and bone tissue is subjected to continuous mechanical stimuli caused by interstitial fluid flow. As such it is imperative to apply a mechanical force during the culturing process to produce a phenotypically correct tissue[33,35,90].

17.5.4. Spinner Flask

In the spinner flask bioreactor seeded scaffolds covered with medium are attached to needles and suspended from the top cover of the flask. Mixing of the medium is sustained with a magnetic stir bar placed at the bottom of the flask[91]. Turbulent mixing of nutrients in a spinner flask bioreactor significantly enhances the biochemical compositions and alters morphologies of engineered constructs[56].

Compared to static culture, constructs cultured in a spinner flask had higher cell seeding densities and a more uniform distribution of cells[57]. However, for cartilage tissue engineering the rotating wall vessel bioreactor has proven to optimize nutrient transport and promote tissue growth and differentiation. For bone tissue the flow perfusion method was found to enhance *in vitro* osteogenesis when compared to the spinner flask[32,92,93].

17.5.5. Rotating Wall Vessel

The rotating bioreactor was developed at NASA[94]. It is composed of two concentric cylinders, with the outside wall capable of rotating. Scaffolds are freely suspended in the annular space between the two cylinders and are subjected to dynamic laminar flow[35]. Scaffolds tend to float in the annular space by balancing gravitational forces with centrifugal forces, thus establishing microgravity-like culturing conditions[91].

The rotating wall vessel (RWV) bioreactor provides a favorable hydrodynamic environment conductive to cartilage phenotype differentiation and cartilage tissue growth[68,95]. RWV systems induce chondrogenesis[34] and provide a superior method for studying chondrogenic mutations[96]. Accordingly, this system is widely used for culturing cartilage tissue *in vitro*[65]. Differentiated chondrocytes were inoculated in a RWV, without the use of any scaffolding material. After 90 days of cultivation, cartilage-like neotissue was formed, encapsulated by fibrous tissue that closely resembled the perichondrium[34]. Bovine calf articular chondrocytes were seeded onto biodegradable polymer scaffolds and cultured in a RWV bioreactor[97]. After 40 days of cultivation constructs had cellularities comparable to natural cartilage. Additionally, in comparison with the native cartilage tissue the engineered construct had 68% as much glycosaminoglycan (GAG) content and 33% of the content of type II collagen.

Although turbulence in spinner flasks provides good uniform mixing, it seems to result in unfavorable tissue growth[98]. For cartilage tissue engineering the RWV bioreactor appears to optimize nutrient transport and promote cartilage growth and differentiation superior to other currently tested culturing techniques[98]. Conversely, the spinner flask bioreactor seems to support osteogenesis more than RWV. Rat MSCs were cultured on polymeric scaffolds for a period of 21 days using static, spinner flask and RWV systems[44]. Cells cultured in the spinner flask had the highest alkaline phosphatase (AP) activity, and osteocalcin (OC) secretion among the three culturing systems. Additionally spinner flask constructs had higher proliferation rate and calcium content than statically cultured constructs.

17.5.6. Flow Perfusion

Flow perfusion bioreactors utilize a pump to percolate medium continuously through the scaffold's interconnected pores[46,90] resulting in improved mass transfer[91], homogeneous cell distribution and high seeding efficiency[46] throughout the thickness of the scaffold. Even though dynamic culturing techniques such as the spinner flask and the RWV alleviate the external circulation limitations, only the flow perfusion system eliminates the internal transport limitations since it forces media to flow through the interior of the scaffold[91,99].

Mechanical stimulation provided by fluid shear forces in flow perfusion culture was shown to enhance the expression of the osteoblastic phenotype[43]. It has been widely reported that fluid shear enhances *in vitro* osteogenesis[32,92,93]. Bone Marrow MSC's were cultured statically and in a perfusion system[92]. Only a surface layer of cells was observed for statically cultured constructs as opposed to a homogeneous cell distribution throughout the scaffold for perfused constructs. The proliferation rate and AP activity patterns were similar for both types of culture techniques; while scaffolds that were cultured under perfused conditions showed a significant increase in calcium deposition. Osteoblastic cells were seeded on PLGA foams and cultured for two weeks in three different bioreactors (RWV, spinner flask and flow perfusion)[32]. Cell seeding efficiencies and OC content were similar for the three systems. However, the spinner flask produced the least uniform cell distribution throughout the foams and the RWV system resulted in the lowest levels of AP activity. Consequently, the flow perfusion system appears to be a very attractive culturing technique for bone constructs[32]. Interstitial flow plays a major role in bone homeostasis[93]. As a result, engineered bone grafts must be adequately perfused for successful cell stimulation, nutrient transportation, and bone regeneration[93].

17.5.7. Mechanical Loading

Mechanical loading can enhance mass transport of nutrients through scaffolds and directly stimulates cell differentiation, proliferation and molecular expression[25]. Some of the techniques used for mechanostimulation of cell cultures *in vitro* include compressive loading, longitudinal stretching, and substrate bending systems[100]

Since immobilization lowers the ultimate strength of ligaments and tendons eminently, tissue engineers incorporated cyclic and continuous stretching in their soft tissue replacement designs[18]. Several traction machines have been designed to study the effect of stretching on fibroblast seeded collagen gels[27,37,53,64,101,102]. Designing a bioreactor that would apply the mechanical stimulus to the construct and yet keep it under sterile conditions is not a trivial task.

Collagen gels have long been used as scaffolds for tissue engineered constructs, especially of dense connective tissue such as tendon and ligament. The magnitude and form of stress applied during culture significantly affects the biomechanical properties of collagen fascicles and other extracellular components[30,103,104]. Three hours after stretching fibroblast seeded collagen gels, cells started aligning parallel to the direction of the applied forces[105]. Fibroblasts continued to orient several hours after suspension of stretch[106] giving the construct a tendon-like appearance[64]. Due to their highly developed actin cytoskeleton fibroblasts could be more responsive to stretching than other types of cells[105]. Moreover, mechanical stretching increased the secretion pattern of important growth factors (TGF-β, basic FGF and platelet derived growth factor) in tendons[79]. This reveals that stretching may have a positive influence on tendon and ligament healing[79]. Human tendon fibroblasts from patellar tendon were cultured on silicone dishes[37]. Subsequently, cyclic biaxial mechanical strain was applied to the dishes for 15, 30, and 60 minutes using a specially developed cell stretching system. Stretching for 15 minutes and 30 minutes resulted in an increase in DNA synthesis after 6 and 24 hours. However, a cyclic biaxial strain of 30 minutes resulted in a decrease of cell proliferation. The authors[37] hypothesized that this duration of stress induced cell damage and apoptosis.

Cyclic strain could direct Human MSC's to differentiate into ligament-like cells in the absence of specific ligament growth and regulatory factors[27]. Mechanical stimulation of cultured ligament fibroblasts increased the expression of ligament markers, namely collagens type I and type III[27,107], fibronectin[27,107], and tenascin-C[107].

Since bone is subjected to mechanical stresses *in vivo* it would be postulated that mechanostimulus elicits differentiation, proliferation and regeneration of bone tissue[102,108]. Brighton et al.[109] observed a significant increase in the DNA content of cultured rat osteoblasts at a strain of 0.04% applied for 15 minutes and for 24 and 48 hours. However, mechanical stretching at this strain rate resulted in a decrease in collagen synthesis, proteoglycan levels, and AP activity. The proliferation rate of human osteoblasts increased significantly after being subjected to a strain rate of 1% for 15 minutes per day on three consecutive days[102]. The authors reported that AP activity was not notably influenced by the level of cyclic strain applied. Osteoblasts strained cyclically, at 15 minute intervals for one hour, experienced significant decrease in AP activity and increase in DNA and calcium deposition versus cells strained continuously for one hour[110]. Osteoblasts were seeded on silicone dishes and cultured for three days[102]. Uniform and cyclic biaxial strains were applied on the surface of the scaffolds for duration of 15 minutes per day. Applying 1% strain increased osteoblasts proliferation significantly. Strain rates above 1% caused a 20% reduction in cell proliferation. The authors also observed that cyclic strains did not affect AP activity noticeably. In another study, the authors[108] further studied the effects of applying 1% strain to their seeded scaffolds by stimulating the osteoblastic constructs 30 minutes per day for two days. Similarly to their previous results, a significant increase in osteoblast proliferation and collagen type I release was observed. However, AP activity and OC release were remarkably reduced. From these findings it can be concluded that cyclic strain at physiological levels leads to an increase in osteoblast activities related to matrix production but a decrease in activities related to matrix mineralization[108].

Contrarily to the previous findings, Palvin et. al. reported that AP activity is an early marker of mechanically-induced differentiation of osteoblasts[111]. Osteoblasts were exposed to cyclic pressure for one hour per day for up to 19 days[112]. Mechanostimulation increased the collagen and calcium deposition in the tissue matrix. Human bone MSC's were cultured on a silicone dish and subjected to 8% strain for a total of six hours per day for three days[82]. AP activity and OC levels were increased and collagen type I and II synthesis were upregulated. It seems that straining osteoblastic constructs for longer durations and at higher strain rates enhances the osteogenic differentiation of MSC's and bone tissue regeneration.

Rat bone MSC's were cultured in porous polylactic acid scaffolds and subjected to four point bending deformation of 2500 microstrain at 0.004 Hz for sixteen days[53].

Using a medium strain rate and long straining duration, it would have been expected to get an increase in AP activity and mineral deposition as mentioned above. However, the reported results were contrary to the earlier findings. A potential explanation for this discrepancy is that in the first experiment the cells where exposed to stretching on a silicone dish with 1Hz frequency. The latter involved the application of a four point loading, with low frequency (0.004 Hz), to a polymeric scaffold[53]. As a result, the experimental variability could be due to frequency differences, the type of loading, or the scaffolding material.

17.5.8. Electric and Magnetic Stimulation

Since ultrasound has a strong influence on biologic activity, it has been widely used in medicine as a therapeutic and surgical tool[8,113]. A single application of low energy laser therapy on the middle cruciate ligament of a rat model significantly increased the collagen fibril size[113], thus promoting the healing process. Bone cells modulate the activity of hormones, growth factors and cytokines when exposed to electromagnetic stimuli[114]. Moreover, it is documented that electric stimulation promotes osteogenesis[115,116]. An increase in osteoblast proliferation and AP activity was reported when rabbit bone marrow was electrically stimulated[116]. Osteoblasts cultured on nanocomposite scaffolds were electrically stimulated for six hours/day for up to 21 days[115]. To apply electric current to their construct the authors designed a bioreactor to house the culturing media during stimulation under sterile conditions. After two days of stimulation a 46% increase in osteoblasts' proliferation was recorded. After 21 days of stimulation calcium deposition increased by 307% and upregulation of mRNA expression for collagen type-I was noted.

17.6. CONCLUSIONS

Tissue engineering provides a functional solution for the limited resources of natural implants and the ineffectiveness of present curing techniques for musculoskeletal disorders. The challenge in tissue engineering resides in the design of a functional bioreactor that would: (1) house the engineered construct under sterile conditions; and (2) provide the appropriate stimuli that would result in a neotissue with biochemical and biomechanical properties comparable to *in situ* tissue.

Several bioreactor designs have been employed to engineer orthopaedic tissue including dynamic flow and mechanical loading models. Using sophisticated conceptions researchers were successful in engineering tissue with cellular density and morphology that closely resembled cartilage, bone, tendon and ligament. However, the mechanical properties of the *neotissue* were inferior to that of *in vivo* tissue. As a result, there is a need to further explore the effects of biochemical and biomechanical stimulations on the microenvironment of cells and innovate techniques to optimize the mechanical properties of engineered tissue.

Moreover, scaling up bioreactor designs is a major challenge. Present *in vitro* bioreactor designs exploit scaffolds that are in the scale of several millimeters for cartilage and bone or a few centimeters for ligament and tendon. It is not possible to predict the behavior of cells when cultured in a larger environment. Would dynamic flow and fluid shear be sufficient enough to transport nutrients along the scaffold? What about cell distribution and matrix homogeneity? These issues need to be thoroughly addressed and investigated in order to achieve bioreactor designs that would mimic the *in vivo* microenvironment and yield constructs with morphology and biomechanical properties comparable to the native tissue.

17.7. REFERENCES

1. D.K. Cherry and D.A. Woodwell, National ambulatory medical care survey: 2000 summary, *Adv Data*, (328), 1-32 (2002).
2. AAOS, Aaos bulletin, 34-36 (1999).
3. A. Praemer, et al., Musculoskeletal conditions in the united states, 2nd ed, Park Ridge, IL, American Academy of Orthopaedic Surgeons, 182 (1999).
4. C.T. Laurencin, et al., Tissue engineering: Orthopedic applications, *Annu Rev Biomed Eng*, **1**, 19-46 (1999).
5. S.C. Cowin, Tissue growth and remodeling, *Annu Rev Biomed Eng*, **6**, 77-107 (2004).
6. M.H. Ross, G.I. Kaye and W. Pawlina, Histology : A text and atlas, 4th ed, Philadelphia, Pa., Lippincott Williams & Wilkins, 875 (2002).
7. P. Renstrèom and R.J. Johnson, Overuse injuries in sports. A review, *Sports Med*, **2**(5), 316-33 (1985).
8. S.M. Day, et al., Bone injury, regeneration, and repair, in *Orthopaedic basic science : Biology and biomechanics of the musculoskeletal system*, J.A. Buckwalter, et al., Editors, American Academy of Orthopaedic Surgeons, Rosemont, IL, 372-399 (2000).
9. R.F. Ker, The design of soft collagenous load-bearing tissues, *J Exp Biol*, **202**(Pt), 3315-24 (1999).
10. W.D. Comper, Water: Dynamic aspects, in *Extracellular matrix*, W.D. Comper, Editor, Harwood Academic Publishers, Amsterdam, 1-21 (1996).
11. H. Chiang, et al., Repair of porcine articular cartilage defect with autologous chondrocyte transplantation, *J Orthop Res*, **23**(3), 584-93 (2005).
12. G.R. Erickson, et al., Chondrogenic potential of adipose tissue-derived stromal cells in vitro and in vivo, *Biochem Biophys Res Commun*, **290**(2), 763-9 (2002).
13. E.G. Lima, et al., Functional tissue engineering of chondral and osteochondral constructs, *Biorheology*, **41**(3-4), 577-90 (2004).
14. R.L. Mauck, et al., Functional tissue engineering of articular cartilage through dynamic loading of chondrocyte-seeded agarose gels, *J Biomech Eng*, **122**(3), 252-60 (2000).
15. H.J. Mankin, V.C. Mow and J.A. Buckwalter, Articular cartilage repair and osteoarthiritis, in *Orthopaedic basic science : Biology and biomechanics of the musculoskeletal system*, J.A. Buckwalter, et al., Editors, American Academy of Orthopaedic Surgeons, Rosemont, IL, 472-488 (2000).
16. T. Minas and S. Nehrer, Current concepts in the treatment of articular cartilage defects, *Orthopedics*, **20**(6), 525-38 (1997).
17. D.L. Butler, N. Juncosa and M.R. Dressler, Functional efficacy of tendon repair processes, *Annu Rev Biomed Eng*, **6**, 303-29 (2004).
18. S.L.-Y. Woo, et al., Anatomy, biology, and biomechanics of tendon and ligament, in *Orthopaedic basic science : Biology and biomechanics of the musculoskeletal system*, J.A. Buckwalter, et al., Editors, American Academy of Orthopaedic Surgeons, Rosemont, IL, 582-616 (2000).
19. M.R. Dressler, et al., A potential mechanism for age-related declines in patellar tendon biomechanics, *J Orthop Res*, **20**(6), 1315-22 (2002).
20. K.M. Khan, et al., Histopathology of common tendinopathies. Update and implications for clinical management, *Sports Med*, **27**(6), 393-408 (1999).
21. L.G. Jâozsa and P. Kannus, Human tendons : Anatomy, physiology, and pathology, Champaign, IL, Human Kinetics, 574 (1997).
22. H.H. Lu, et al., Anterior cruciate ligament regeneration using braided biodegradable scaffolds: In vitro optimization studies, *Biomaterials*, **26**(23), 4805-16 (2005).
23. N.H.D. Survey, Number of patients, number of procedures, average patient age, average length of stay, U.S.D.o.H.a.H.S.C.f.D.C.a.P.N.C.f.H. Statistics., Editor, (2002).
24. S. Rupp, et al., Ligament graft initial fixation strength using biodegradable interference screws, *J Biomed Mater Res*, **48**(1), 70-4 (1999).
25. G. Vunjak-Novakovic, et al., Tissue engineering of ligaments, *Annu Rev Biomed Eng*, **6**, 131-56 (2004).
26. R. Langer and J.P. Vacanti, Tissue engineering, *Science*, **260**(5110), 920-6 (1993).
27. G.H. Altman, et al., Cell differentiation by mechanical stress, *FASEB J*, **16**(2), 270-2 (2002).
28. L.J. Bonassar and C.A. Vacanti, Tissue engineering: The first decade and beyond, *J Cell Biochem Suppl*, **30-31**, 297-303 (1998).
29. D.L. Butler, S.A. Goldstein and F. Guilak, Functional tissue engineering: The role of biomechanics, *J Biomech Eng*, **122**(6), 570-5 (2000).
30. C. Cacou, et al., A system for monitoring the response of uniaxial strain on cell seeded collagen gels, *Med Eng Phys*, **22**(5), 327-33 (2000).

31. M.G. Dunn, et al., Development of fibroblast-seeded ligament analogs for acl reconstruction, *J Biomed Mater Res,* **29**(11), 1363-71 (1995).
32. A.S. Goldstein, et al., Effect of convection on osteoblastic cell growth and function in biodegradable polymer foam scaffolds, *Biomaterials,* **22**(11), 1279-88 (2001).
33. K.J. Gooch, et al., Effects of mixing intensity on tissue-engineered cartilage, *Biotechnol Bioeng,* **72**(4), 402-7 (2001).
34. S. Marlovits, et al., Chondrogenesis of aged human articular cartilage in a scaffold-free bioreactor, *Tissue Eng,* **9**(6), 1215-26 (2003).
35. G. Vunjak-Novakovic, et al., Bioreactor cultivation conditions modulate the composition and mechanical properties of tissue-engineered cartilage, *J Orthop Res,* **17**(1), 130-8 (1999).
36. J.A. Cooper, et al., Fiber-based tissue-engineered scaffold for ligament replacement: Design considerations and in vitro evaluation, *Biomaterials,* **26**(13), 1523-32 (2005).
37. J. Zeichen, M. van Griensven and U. Bosch, The proliferative response of isolated human tendon fibroblasts to cyclic biaxial mechanical strain, *Am J Sports Med,* **28**(6), 888-92 (2000).
38. J.D. Enderle, S.M. Blanchard and J.D. Bronzino, Introduction to biomedical engineering. *Academic press series in biomedical engineering.*, ed., San Diego, Academic Press, 1062 (2000).
39. S.P. Bruder, et al., Bone regeneration by implantation of purified, culture-expanded human mesenchymal stem cells, *J Orthop Res,* **16**(2), 155-62 (1998).
40. S.P. Bruder, et al., The effect of implants loaded with autologous mesenchymal stem cells on the healing of canine segmental bone defects, *J Bone Joint Surg Am,* **80**(7), 985-96 (1998).
41. M.R. Dressler, D.L. Butler and G.P. Boivin, Effects of age on the repair ability of mesenchymal stem cells in rabbit tendon, *J Orthop Res,* **23**(2), 287-93 (2005).
42. S. Hankemeier, et al., Modulation of proliferation and differentiation of human bone marrow stromal cells by fibroblast growth factor 2: Potential implications for tissue engineering of tendons and ligaments, *Tissue Eng,* **11**(1-2), 41-9 (2005).
43. V.I. Sikavitsas, et al., Mineralized matrix deposition by marrow stromal osteoblasts in 3d perfusion culture increases with increasing fluid shear forces, *Proc Natl Acad Sci U S A,* **100**(25), 14683-8 (2003).
44. V.I. Sikavitsas, G.N. Bancroft and A.G. Mikos, Formation of three-dimensional cell/polymer constructs for bone tissue engineering in a spinner flask and a rotating wall vessel bioreactor, *J Biomed Mater Res,* **62**(1), 136-48 (2002).
45. S.P. Bruder, N. Jaiswal and S.E. Haynesworth, Growth kinetics, self-renewal, and the osteogenic potential of purified human mesenchymal stem cells during extensive subcultivation and following cryopreservation, *J Cell Biochem,* **64**(2), 278-94 (1997).
46. D. Wendt, et al., Oscillating perfusion of cell suspensions through three-dimensional scaffolds enhances cell seeding efficiency and uniformity, *Biotechnol Bioeng,* **84**(2), 205-14 (2003).
47. Y.L. Cui, et al., Biomimetic surface modification of poly (l-lactic acid) with gelatin and its effects on articular chondrocytes in vitro, *J Biomed Mater Res,* **66A**(4), 770-8 (2003).
48. P. Sucosky, et al., Fluid mechanics of a spinner-flask bioreactor, *Biotechnol Bioeng,* **85**(1), 34-46 (2004).
49. L.E. Freed, et al., Neocartilage formation in vitro and in vivo using cells cultured on synthetic biodegradable polymers, *J Biomed Mater Res,* **27**(1), 11-23 (1993).
50. E.A. Botchwey, et al., Bone tissue engineering in a rotating bioreactor using a microcarrier matrix system, *J Biomed Mater Res,* **55**(2), 242-53 (2001).
51. K. Eid, et al., Effect of rgd coating on osteocompatibility of plga-polymer disks in a rat tibial wound, *J Biomed Mater Res,* **57**(2), 224-31 (2001).
52. J.M. Williams, et al., Bone tissue engineering using polycaprolactone scaffolds fabricated via selective laser sintering, *Biomaterials,* **26**(23), 4817-27 (2005).
53. D.A. Shimko, et al., A device for long term, in vitro loading of three-dimensional natural and engineered tissues, *Ann Biomed Eng,* **31**(11), 1347-56 (2003).
54. B. Saad and U.W. Suter, Biodegradable polymeric materials, in *Encyclopedia of materials science and technology*, K.H.J. Buschow, et al., Editors, Elsevier, Oxford, UK, 551-555 (2001).
55. M.J. Yaszemski, et al., Evolution of bone transplantation: Molecular, cellular and tissue strategies to engineer human bone, *Biomaterials,* **17**(2), 175 (1996).
56. G. Vunjak-Novakovic, et al., Effects of mixing on the composition and morphology of tissue-engineered cartilage, *AIChE Journal,* **42**(3), 850-860 (1996).
57. G. Vunjak-Novakovic, et al., Dynamic cell seeding of polymer scaffolds for cartilage tissue engineering, *Biotechnol Prog,* **14**(2), 193-202 (1998).
58. J.A. Burdick, et al., Controlled degradation and mechanical behavior of photopolymerized hyaluronic acid networks, *Biomacromolecules,* **6**(1), 386-91 (2005).
59. L.A. Solchaga, et al., Treatment of osteochondral defects with autologous bone marrow in a hyaluronan-based delivery vehicle, *Tissue Eng,* **8**(2), 333-47 (2002).
60. T. Taguchi, T. Ikoma and J. Tanaka, An improved method to prepare hyaluronic acid and type ii collagen composite matrices, *J Biomed Mater Res,* **61**(2), 330-6 (2002).

61. C.T. Hung, et al., A paradigm for functional tissue engineering of articular cartilage via applied physiologic deformational loading, *Ann Biomed Eng,* **32**(1), 35-49 (2004).
62. M.M. Stevens, et al., In vivo engineering of organs: The bone bioreactor, *Proc Natl Acad Sci U S A,* **102**(32), 11450-5 (2005).
63. Z. Feng, et al., Investigation on the mechanical properties of contracted collagen gels as a scaffold for tissue engineering, *Artif Organs,* **27**(1), 84-91 (2003).
64. J. Garvin, et al., Novel system for engineering bioartificial tendons and application of mechanical load, *Tissue Eng,* **9**(5), 967-79 (2003).
65. M. Pei, et al., Bioreactors mediate the effectiveness of tissue engineering scaffolds, *FASEB J,* **16**(12), 1691-4 (2002).
66. G. Chen, et al., Tissue engineering of cartilage using a hybrid scaffold of synthetic polymer and collagen, *Tissue Eng,* **10**(3-4), 323-30 (2004).
67. L.E. Freed, G. Vunjak-Novakovic and R. Langer, Cultivation of cell-polymer cartilage implants in bioreactors, *J Cell Biochem,* **51**(3), 257-64 (1993).
68. S. Saini and T.M. Wick, Concentric cylinder bioreactor for production of tissue engineered cartilage: Effect of seeding density and hydrodynamic loading on construct development, *Biotechnol Prog,* **19**(2), 510-21 (2003).
69. I. Martin, D. Wendt and M. Heberer, The role of bioreactors in tissue engineering, *Trends Biotechnol,* **22**(2), 80-6 (2004).
70. C.E. Holy, M.S. Shoichet and J.E. Davies, Engineering three-dimensional bone tissue in vitro using biodegradable scaffolds: Investigating initial cell-seeding density and culture period, *J Biomed Mater Res,* **51**(3), 376-82 (2000).
71. Y.L. Xiao, J. Riesle and C.A. Van Blitterswijk, Static and dynamic fibroblast seeding and cultivation in porous peo/pbt scaffolds, *J Mater Sci Mater Med,* **10**(12), 773-7 (1999).
72. Y. Li, et al., Effects of filtration seeding on cell density, spatial distribution, and proliferation in nonwoven fibrous matrices, *Biotechnol Prog,* **17**(5), 935-44 (2001).
73. B.S. Kim, et al., Optimizing seeding and culture methods to engineer smooth muscle tissue on biodegradable polymer matrices, *Biotechnol Bioeng,* **57**(1), 46-54 (1998).
74. K.J. Burg, et al., Comparative study of seeding methods for three-dimensional polymeric scaffolds, *J Biomed Mater Res,* **51**(4), 642-9 (2000).
75. K.J. Burg, et al., Application of magnetic resonance microscopy to tissue engineering: A polylactide model, *J Biomed Mater Res,* **61**(3), 380-90 (2002).
76. R.L. Mauck, et al., Synergistic action of growth factors and dynamic loading for articular cartilage tissue engineering, *Tissue Eng,* **9**(4), 597-611 (2003).
77. H.F. Lodish, Molecular cell biology, 5th ed, New York, W.H. Freeman and Company, (2004).
78. E.B. Hunziker and L.C. Rosenberg, Repair of partial-thickness defects in articular cartilage: Cell recruitment from the synovial membrane, *J Bone Joint Surg Am,* **78**(5), 721-33 (1996).
79. M. Skutek, et al., Cyclic mechanical stretching modulates secretion pattern of growth factors in human tendon fibroblasts, *Eur J Appl Physiol,* **86**(1), 48-52 (2001).
80. P.C. Yaeger, et al., Synergistic action of transforming growth factor-beta and insulin-like growth factor-i induces expression of type ii collagen and aggrecan genes in adult human articular chondrocytes, *Exp Cell Res,* **237**(2), 318-25 (1997).
81. G.E. Holt, et al., Evolution of an in vivo bioreactor, *J Orthop Res,* **23**(4), 916-23 (2005).
82. M. Jagodzinski, et al., Effects of cyclic longitudinal mechanical strain and dexamethasone on osteogenic differentiation of human bone marrow stromal cells, *Eur Cell Mater,* **7**, 35-41; discussion 41 (2004).
83. E.A. Wang, et al., Recombinant human bone morphogenetic protein induces bone formation, *Proc Natl Acad Sci U S A,* **87**(6), 2220-4 (1990).
84. H.D. Zegzula, et al., Bone formation with use of rhbmp-2 (recombinant human bone morphogenetic protein-2), *J Bone Joint Surg Am,* **79**(12), 1778-90 (1997).
85. F.W. Sellke, et al., Therapeutic angiogenesis with basic fibroblast growth factor: Technique and early results, *Ann Thorac Surg,* **65**(6), 1540-4 (1998).
86. A.J. Grodzinsky, et al., Cartilage tissue remodeling in response to mechanical forces, *Annu Rev Biomed Eng,* **2**, 691-713 (2000).
87. R.C. Thomson, et al., Guided tissue fabrication from periosteum using preformed biodegradable polymer scaffolds, *Biomaterials,* **20**(21), 2007-18 (1999).
88. S.D. Boden, Bioactive factors for bone tissue engineering, *Clin Orthop Relat Res,* (367), S84-94 (1999).
89. S.D. Boden, J.H. Schimandle and W.C. Hutton, 1995 volvo award in basic sciences. The use of an osteoinductive growth factor for lumbar spinal fusion. Part ii: Study of dose, carrier, and species, *Spine,* **20**(24), 2633-44 (1995).
90. E.M. Darling and K.A. Athanasiou, Articular cartilage bioreactors and bioprocesses, *Tissue Eng,* **9**(1), 9-26 (2003).
91. G.N. Bancroft, V.I. Sikavitsas and A.G. Mikos, Design of a flow perfusion bioreactor system for bone tissue-engineering applications, *Tissue Eng,* **9**(3), 549-54 (2003).

92. M.E. Gomes, et al., Effect of flow perfusion on the osteogenic differentiation of bone marrow stromal cells cultured on starch-based three-dimensional scaffolds, *J Biomed Mater Res,* **67A**(1), 87-95 (2003).
93. M.V. Hillsley and J.A. Frangos, Bone tissue engineering: The role of interstitial fluid flow, *Biotechnol Bioeng,* **43**(7), 573-81 (1994).
94. G. Vunjak-Novakovic, et al., Microgravity studies of cells and tissues, *Ann N Y Acad Sci,* **974**, 504-17 (2002).
95. G. Vunjak-Novakovic, et al., Bioreactor studies of native and tissue engineered cartilage, *Biorheology,* **39**(1-2), 259-68 (2002).
96. P.J. Duke, E.L. Daane and D. Montufar-Solis, Studies of chondrogenesis in rotating systems, *J Cell Biochem,* **51**(3), 274-82 (1993).
97. L.E. Freed, et al., Chondrogenesis in a cell-polymer-bioreactor system, *Exp Cell Res,* **240**(1), 58-65 (1998).
98. K.A. Williams, S. Saini and T.M. Wick, Computational fluid dynamics modeling of steady-state momentum and mass transport in a bioreactor for cartilage tissue engineering, *Biotechnol Prog,* **18**(5), 951-63 (2002).
99. L. Meinel, et al., Bone tissue engineering using human mesenchymal stem cells: Effects of scaffold material and medium flow, *Ann Biomed Eng,* **32**(1), 112-22 (2004).
100. T.D. Brown, Techniques for mechanical stimulation of cells in vitro: A review, *J Biomech,* **33**(1), 3-14 (2000).
101. E. Langelier, et al., Cyclic traction machine for long-term culture of fibroblast-populated collagen gels, *Ann Biomed Eng,* **27**(1), 67-72 (1999).
102. C. Neidlinger-Wilke, H.J. Wilke and L. Claes, Cyclic stretching of human osteoblasts affects proliferation and metabolism: A new experimental method and its application, *J Orthop Res,* **12**(1), 70-8 (1994).
103. E. Yamamoto, et al., Effects of static stress on the mechanical properties of cultured collagen fascicles from the rabbit patellar tendon, *J Biomech Eng,* **124**(1), 85-93 (2002).
104. E. Yamamoto, S. Tokura and K. Hayashi, Effects of cyclic stress on the mechanical properties of cultured collagen fascicles from the rabbit patellar tendon, *J Biomech Eng,* **125**(6), 893-901 (2003).
105. C. Neidlinger-Wilke, et al., Cell alignment is induced by cyclic changes in cell length: Studies of cells grown in cyclically stretched substrates, *J Orthop Res,* **19**(2), 286-93 (2001).
106. C. Neidlinger-Wilke, et al., Fibroblast orientation to stretch begins within three hours, *J Orthop Res,* **20**(5), 953-6 (2002).
107. R. Chiquet-Ehrismann, et al., Tenascin-c expression by fibroblasts is elevated in stressed collagen gels, *J Cell Biol,* **127**(6), 2093-101 (1994).
108. D. Kaspar, et al., Dynamic cell stretching increases human osteoblast proliferation and cicp synthesis but decreases osteocalcin synthesis and alkaline phosphatase activity, *J Biomech,* **33**(1), 45-51 (2000).
109. C.T. Brighton, et al., The inositol phosphate pathway as a mediator in the proliferative response of rat calvarial bone cells to cyclical biaxial mechanical strain, *J Orthop Res,* **10**(3), 385-93 (1992).
110. L.C. Winter, et al., Intermittent versus continuous stretching effects on osteoblast-like cells in vitro, *J Biomed Mater Res,* **67A**(4), 1269-75 (2003).
111. D. Pavlin, et al., Mechanical loading stimulates differentiation of periodontal osteoblasts in a mouse osteoinduction model: Effect on type i collagen and alkaline phosphatase genes, *Calcif Tissue Int,* **67**(2), 163-72 (2000).
112. J. Nagatomi, et al., Cyclic pressure affects osteoblast functions pertinent to osteogenesis, *Ann Biomed Eng,* **31**(8), 917-23 (2003).
113. D.T. Fung, et al., Effects of a therapeutic laser on the ultrastructural morphology of repairing medial collateral ligament in a rat model, *Lasers Surg Med,* **32**(4), 286-93 (2003).
114. J.A. Spadaro, Mechanical and electrical interactions in bone remodeling, *Bioelectromagnetics,* **18**(3), 193-202 (1997).
115. P.R. Supronowicz, et al., Novel current-conducting composite substrates for exposing osteoblasts to alternating current stimulation, *J Biomed Mater Res,* **59**(3), 499-506 (2002).
116. K. Yonemori, et al., Early effects of electrical stimulation on osteogenesis, *Bone,* **19**(2), 173-80 (1996).

18

NON-INVASIVE MONITORING OF TISSUE-ENGINEERED PANCREATIC CONSTRUCTS BY NMR TECHNIQUES

Ioannis Constantinidis, Nicholas E. Simpson, Samuel C. Grant, Stephen J. Blackband,* Robert C. Long, Jr.,† and Athanassios Sambanis‡

18.1. INTRODUCTION

Tissue engineering is an expanding field that combines the principles of engineering and the life sciences towards the fundamental understanding of structure/function relationships in normal and pathological mammalian tissues, and the development of biological substitutes to restore, maintain, or improve function (1). There are several critical issues that hamper the development of tissue engineered constructs. These include, but may not be limited to: (i) the source and function of cells employed within the constructs; (ii) the biomaterials used to build the constructs; (iii) the ability to scale up production to a medically relevant scale; (iv) the immune acceptance of a construct; (v) the preservation and subsequent off-the-shelf availability of the construct, and (vi) the ability to monitor the function and integrity of the construct *in vivo*. In this review we will focus on the issue of non-invasive monitoring.

The main criterion in assessing the therapeutic efficacy of a tissue engineered construct is the successful restoration of the host physiology. Although accomplishment of such end point is critical, direct and non-invasive monitoring of the construct's function is important in assessing and possibly predicting construct efficacy. There are several imaging modalities that have been applied to monitor tissue engineered constructs, such as optical[1-3], radionuclide[4], computed tomography (CT)[5,6], and nuclear magnetic resonance (NMR)[7-11].

---

* University of Florida, Gainesville, FL 32610, USA
† Emory University, Atlanta, GA 30322, USA
‡ Georgia Institute of Technology, Atlanta, GA 30320, USA

Optical techniques were revolutionized during the past 10 years by the ability to incorporate fluorescent (e.g., green fluorescent protein)[12,13] and luminescent (e.g., luciferase)[14] proteins in cells, the development of novel fluorescing agents[15], and the development of new detection techniques[16]. Optical imaging is very sensitive and can generate images with sub-cellular resolution. However, they are hindered by the limited transmission of light through the body, and consequently, it may not be suitable to image deep-seated constructs. Thus, they have been used primarily *in vitro*, while their *in vivo* applications are restricted to sites close to the surface. Currently, they have not been applied to pancreatic constructs, although they have been used to assess islet cell mass *in vivo* following transplantation to a peripheral site[17,18].

Radionuclide imaging techniques, Positron Emission Tomography (PET) and Single Photon Emission Tomography (SPECT), are used readily in nuclear medicine to diagnose a variety of pathologies. However, at the present time, there is a paucity of reports describing their use in tissue engineering[4]. Both techniques are highly sensitive and benefit from a diverse group of radio nuclei that can be used on a broad range of ligands. However, both techniques suffer from low spatial resolution. Even microPET systems designed to provide enhanced resolution in small rodents have a spatial resolution of 1 mm or slightly less[19]. Neither of these techniques has been used to monitor pancreatic constructs.

Computed tomography (CT) and in particular microCT has been used extensively to monitor musculoskeletal tissue engineered constructs. The most common application of microCT is the *ex-vivo* analysis of bone architecture. MicroCT instruments can generate 2D images of excised bone samples with an isotropic resolution up to 10 μm. The recent development of *in vivo* microCT instruments will facilitate the monitoring of musculoskeletal constructs *in vivo* albeit at lower resolution and at higher power deposition than *in vitro*. MicroCT techniques have not been utilized to monitor pancreatic constructs.

NMR is an analytical technique that has been used for chemical and physical analyses by scientists since its inception in 1946[20,21]. It is noninvasive and does not require the genetic modification of the cells (i.e., expression of GFP), the introduction of radioactive labels (i.e., PET agents), or the deposition of harmful x-rays. Furthermore, magnetic fields penetrate uniformly throughout the sample, thus NMR is ideally suited to monitor constructs implanted at deep-seated locations. Its disadvantage is its low sensitivity. Whereas optical and radionuclide imaging techniques can detect tracer quantities, NMR requires millimolar or sub-millimolar concentrations for detection. However, it provides both anatomical and metabolic information, it can generate images with an isotropic resolution of 10 μm or less, and it can perform longitudinal studies of the same sample over a long period of time.

NMR data are acquired in a form of a frequency modulated spectrum. Advances in magnet and gradient technologies have made possible the generation of images[22,23] as well as the acquisition of spectra. Currently, NMR imaging can be applied to a variety of living systems ranging from a single cell[24] to human beings[25]. There are several biologically relevant nuclei that are NMR sensitive and can be applied to examine a tissue engineered construct. These include, but are not limited to: ^{1}H, ^{13}C, and ^{31}P. NMR techniques have been applied extensively to the study of perfused cells[26]. Some of the culture methods at the microscale that have been explored include: cells on microcarriers[27], or gel threads[28], cell entrapped in alginate or agarose beads[29], or collagen sponge[30], and cells cultivated as multicellular spheroids[31]. Other bioreactor designs have also been used, such as hollow fibers[32], and packed beds[33]. In addition, NMR techniques have been used to investigate the physiology of both isolated perfused and intact organs[34] as well as neoplastic tissues[35]. Despite this wide use of NMR in cell physiology, it has rarely been utilized in tissue engineered constructs[7-9]. In the context of a bioartificial pancreas the literature is limited to a few NMR studies[11,33,36-42], mostly by our laboratory.

Our research over the past decade has focused on monitoring pancreatic constructs by NMR techniques both *in vitro* and *in vivo*. *In vitro* experiments are designed to assess: (i) construct integrity, (ii) cell organization within the construct, (iii) metabolic activity of encapsulated cells in response to exogenous stimuli, and (iv) cell viability. *In vivo* experiments are designed to assess: (i) cell viability, (ii) construct integrity, and (ii) implant function. In this review we will highlight some of the NMR techniques that we have applied to monitor tissue engineered pancreatic constructs *in vitro* and *in vivo*. These techniques are not unique to our pancreatic constructs, but they can be applied to other types of constructs as well.

18.2. *IN VITRO* EXPERIMENTS

18.2.1. Construct Integrity

The most common design of a pancreatic construct is that of microencapsulation[43]. Insulin secreting cells are encapsulated in alginate beads, then coated with a poly-L-lysine (PLL) layer to improve the mechanical stability of the bead and to create a permselective membrane for immunoprotection of the encapsulated cells, and then dipped in alginate once more to improve their biocompatibility. The preparation of such alginate/poly-L-lysine/alginate (APA) beads is easy to perform and has the advantage that the molecular weight cutoff of the matrix can be manipulated by varying the exposure time between alginate beads and poly-L-lysine. One issue of critical importance to the development of an optimum pancreatic construct is the long-term integrity of APA beads. At present, visualization of the PLL layer using optical or electron microscopy techniques requires the chemical modification or fixation of the alginate matrix. We have recently developed non-invasive protocols based on ^{1}H NMR imaging techniques to visualize the PLL layer. Figure 18.1 illustrates three NMR images of alginate beads. The image on the left illustrates an alginate bead without a PLL layer, the image in the middle illustrates an APA bead, while the right image is that of an alginate bead that is coated with multiple PLL (APAPAPA) layers. All three images were acquired with 800 μm beads composed of MVM alginate (62% mannuronic acid, 38% guluronic acid content). Images were acquired at 17.6 T and have an isotropic resolution of 12.5 μm. Our data show that NMR imaging techniques can successfully detect the PLL layer. The PLL layer is depicted as a dark circle due to the magnetic susceptibility between the PLL layer and the alginate matrix. The thickness of the PLL layer in our images ranged from 35-45 μm. This is in agreement with data presented by Strand et al. and is attributed to the infiltration of PLL into the alginate matrix[44]. The image on the right was acquired from a preparation where the alginate beads were coated with three PLL layers. However, only two are detected in this image. This is attributed to the difference in thickness between the first and subsequent two layers. The ability to detect a single or multiple PLL layers is quite important because it allows us to perform longitudinal studies to assess temporal changes in the integrity of the PLL layer(s) with prolonged culture.

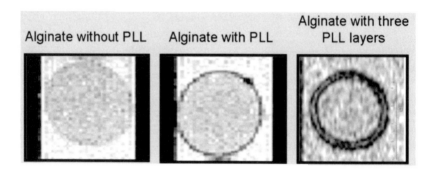

Figure 18.1. ^{1}H NMR images of an alginate bead without a PLL layer, with a PLL layer, and with multiple PLL layers.

18.2.2. Cell Organization

Another issue of critical importance in the development of the optimum pancreatic construct is the growth and rearrangement of encapsulated cells. This is particularly important for surrogate β-cells that have the propensity to grow without exhibiting contact inhibition. Over the past 5 years we have investigated the effects that alginate composition has on the growth potential and pattern of encapsulated cells[45-47]. Furthermore, we have demonstrated that although encapsulated cells may proliferate continuously, the number of viable cells that is sustained within APA beads is proportional to the available oxygen[38]. These results were reached by measuring changes in the metabolic activity of the cultures and examining histology cross sections of APA beads. The ability to non-invasively visualize this proliferation and growth pattern can facilitate the *in vitro* testing and development of new constructs. Figure 18.2 shows data acquired from βTC3 cells encapsulated in APA beads composed with the same alginate composition (LVM: low viscosity 62% mannuronic acid, 38% guluronic acid content) but varying diameter (0.75 and 0.46 mm). The data show that there are no differences in the metabolic activity of the cultures, as depicted by the glucose consumption rate (GCR). However, histology examinations and ^{1}H NMR images show that there is a difference in the pattern of growth between the two types of beads. Whereas βTC3 cells encapsulated in large beads grew in the periphery of the beads leaving a large necrotic center, cells encapsulated in smaller beads grew throughout the bead. The thickness of the viable cell layer in the larger beads is approximately 200 µm, which is equivalent to the diameter of the smaller beads (230 µm). Since both bead preparations were cultured under the same conditions and since environmental conditions such as oxygen tension and nutrient concentrations at the surface of the beads, dictate the thickness of viable cells at the periphery of the beads regardless of bead size, the observed difference may not represent a true change in growth pattern. However, analysis of these images reveal differences in T_2 as a function of time between the two types of beads that may reflect differences in cell density.

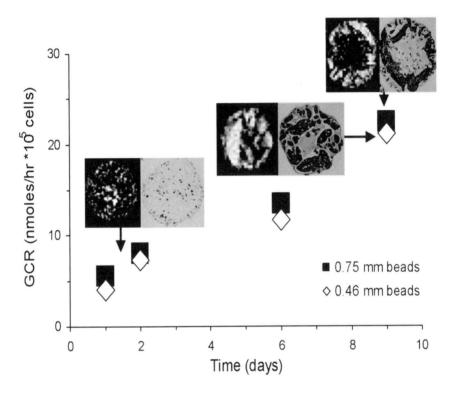

Figure 18.2. Temporal changes in glucose consumption by APA beads of two different diameters. ^{1}H NMR images and histology cross-section show the distribution of cells at the beginning and at the end of the experiment. The images were acquired at 17.6T at an in plane resolution of 20x20 µm and a slice thickness of 60 µm.

18.2.3. Metabolic Activity

One of the advantages of NMR is the diverse metabolic information that can be obtained by using different nuclei. As we stated earlier there are several biologically relevant nuclei (e.g. ^{1}H, ^{13}C, and ^{31}P) that are NMR sensitive and can be applied to examine a tissue engineered construct either *in vitro* or *in vivo*. ^{31}P is the nucleus most commonly used to examine biological samples and provides information about the bioenergetic status of cells, their phospholipid metabolism and intracellular pH. Figure 18.3 shows a ^{31}P NMR spectrum of βTC3 cells encapsulated in APA beads and perfused in a packed bed bioreactor. The perfusion system and its bioreactor are described in detail elsewhere[37]. The spectrum shows resonances assigned to the three phosphate groups of ATP, inorganic phosphate (P_i), phosphorylethanolamine (PE), phosphorylcholine (PC), glycerolphosphorylethanolamine (GPE), glycerolphosphorylcholine (GPC), NADP, and diphosphodiglycerides (DPDG). Since insulin secretion is an energy requiring process we have utilized ^{31}P NMR spectroscopy to monitor changes in the bioenergetic status of our constructs as they responded to changes in glucose concentration[36,37] and partial oxygen pressure[38,39]. Changes in ATP and P_i were then correlated with changes in insulin secretion. Our data have shown that, (i) for βTC3 cells, changes in insulin secretion were not always coupled with changes in ATP. Although this may contradict our previous statement that insulin secretion is an energy requiring process, it supports studies on mammalian islets that have demonstrated that insulin secretion is coupled to the ratio of ATP/ADP and not to ATP. (ii) The number of viable cells sustained within a bioreactor is proportional to the pO_2 of the perfusion medium, and (iii) transformed cells may be better suited as the source of insulin than mammalian islets in a diffusion limited pancreatic construct. This conclusion was reached based on the observations that insulin secretion by βTC3 cells was affected at a pO_2 level much lower than that of mammalian islets. Furthermore, reversing hypoxic conditions returned insulin and ATP to prehypoxic levels.

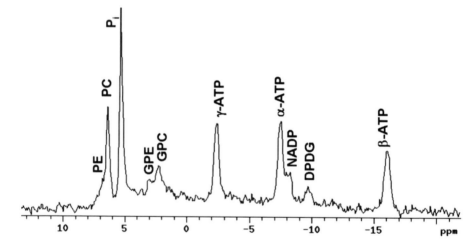

Figure 18.3. ^{31}P NMR spectrum of APA encapsulated βTC-tet cells. The spectrum was acquired within 20 min at 4.7T using a packed bed bioreactor.

^{13}C is another commonly used nucleus. However, the natural abundance of the ^{13}C isotope is low, and thus substrates enriched in ^{13}C are required. In biological samples, ^{13}C NMR spectroscopy is used to study the metabolic fate of labeled glucose or other nutrients and to determine fluxes through pathways like glycolysis and the TCA cycle[48,49]. In our laboratory we have used ^{13}C NMR spectroscopy to study the effect of alginate entrapment on the metabolic activity of encapsulated βTC3 cells[50] and to investigate the role of the TCA cycle and the electron transport chain on insulin secretion by encapsulated cells. Figure 18.4 is a ^{13}C NMR spectrum of APA encapsulated βTC-tet cells perfused with media containing glucose enriched with ^{13}C at the carbon-1 (C_1) position ($^{13}C_1$-glucose). Since glucose is metabolized through glycolysis to form pyruvate, glucose molecules labeled at the C_1 position become pyruvate molecules labeled at the C_3 position, which then are converted to $^{13}C_3$-lactate, $^{13}C_3$-alanine and $^{13}C_4$-glutamate. In addition, $^{13}C_2$-glutamate and $^{13}C_3$-glutamate are also detected due to anaplerotic entrance of pyruvate to the TCA cycle. Our spectra show the presence of a large $^{13}C_3$-lactate resonance, suggesting that βTC-tet cells metabolize pyruvate primarily via lactate dehydrogenase to form lactate. This is not unusual for transformed cell lines although native β-cells in islets produce very little lactate. Also the presence of $^{13}C_3$-alanine indicates that alanine aminotransferase is active, while $^{13}C_4$-glutamate indicates that pyruvate enters the TCA cycle predominantly through the acetyl-CoA. Small quantities of the $^{13}C_3$- and $^{13}C_2$-glutamate are indicative of the presence of anaplerosis. All of theses resonances are the result of metabolic activity by the encapsulated cells, however the two large resonances between 90-100 ppm are attributed to the C_1-glucose introduced in the media and are assigned to the α- and β- conformations of glucose.

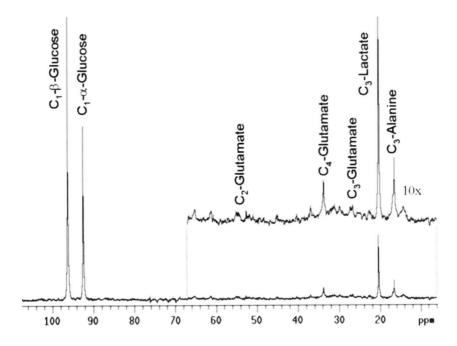

Figure 18.4. ^{13}C NMR spectrum of APA encapsulated βTC-tet cells. The spectrum was acquired within 1 hour at 4.7T using a packed bed bioreactor.

One of the advantages of NMR is the ability to acquire data from the same sample longitudinally to assess dynamic changes in response to exogenous stimuli or changing environmental conditions. Figure 18.5 shows temporal changes in ^{13}C and ^{31}P NMR detectable metabolites acquired from βTC-tet cells encapsulated in APA beads. βTC-tet cells were encapsulated at a cell density of 3.5x10[7] cells/ml alginate and APA beads were placed in a 10 ml packed bed bioreactor where they were perfused continuously for 4.5 days using a single pass perfusion system that is described elsewhere[37]. NMR data acquisition was initiated within a few hours from completion of the encapsulation protocol. The bioreactor was perfused with fully supplemented DMEM media containing 10 mM $^{13}C_1$-glucose for 2.5 days, followed by a medium containing 1 mM 2,4-dinitrophenol (2,4-DNP) and 10 mM $^{13}C_1$-glucose for 24 hours returning to the initial medium for the remainder of the experiment. ^{13}C NMR spectra were acquired on an hourly basis while ^{31}P NMR spectra were obtained at the beginning and at the end of each perfusion period. In addition to the metabolic information detected by NMR, oxygen partial pressure in the perfusion medium was measured at the output of the bioreactor continuously throughout the experiment while the amount of insulin secreted in the perfusion media was measured at the end of each perfusion period. Our data show that ^{13}C NMR detectable metabolites lactate and glutamate increased with time in culture during the first 2.5 days and reached a steady state concentration within 48 hours of perfusion. An increase in signal intensity was also observed for the ATP resonances detected in the ^{31}P NMR spectra. Conversely, the glucose resonances decreased until a steady state was reached because of the continuous consumption by the cells. In support of this data is an increase in the amount of insulin secreted during the first 48 hours and a progressive decrease in the pO_2 at the output of the bioreactor. All of this data suggest that encapsulated βTC-tet cells proliferated during the first 2.5 days of the experiment. Exposure to 2,4-DNP cause a dramatic change in the metabolic activity of the encapsulated cells. This was expected since 2,4-DNP is a strong uncoupler of oxidative phosphorylation inhibiting the production of ATP. Our data show that lactate production (increase in C_3-lactate resonance) and glucose consumption (decrease in C_1-glucose resonances) by the encapsulated cells increases dramatically with exposure to 2,4-DNP while oxygen consumption, glutamate and ATP synthesis, and insulin secretion decreased dramatically. This metabolic activity is attributed to the inhibitory effect of 2,4-DNP on ATP synthesis. Since oxidative phosphorylation is effectively shut down in an effort to sustain viability, encapsulated cells are forced to increase glucose consumption via anaerobic glucolysis producing large quantities of lactate. By removing the 2,4-DNP from the perfusion media, the metabolic activity of the cells recovered to their pre-2,4-DNP levels within 24 hours. The only exception was the low insulin secretion suggesting that the secretory pathway was not restored. This experiment highlights the utility of NMR spectroscopy to obtain dynamic information about the metabolic activity of tissue engineered constructs.

A potential pitfall with the use of packed bed bioreactors or other bioreactor designs is that the acquired NMR spectra represent the average metabolic activity over the entire bioreactor. If the tissue engineered construct under investigation contains cells that are proliferating during a prolonged period examination, then it is possible that cells located in the proximity of the bioreactor's inlet may proliferate faster than cells located at the bioreactor's outlet. This heterogeneous cell distribution across the bioreactor translates into a gradient in metabolic activity along the length of the bioreactor. We have demonstrated that such gradients develop within 5-10 days of continuous perfusion in a packed bed bioreactor for APA encapsulated βTC3 cells[37,40]. However, when encapsulated cells did not display significant growth, as was the case for AtT-20 spheroids, such gradients were not observed[33]. It is also important to note that gradients in metabolic activity may also develop in short term experiments for which cellular proliferation is not an issue, if the bioreactor is not operated differentially.

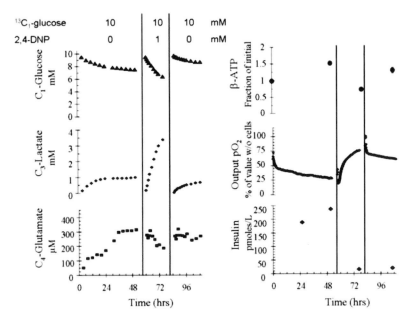

Figure 18.5. Temporal changes of various metabolites detected by ^{13}C and ^{31}P NMR spectra of APA encapsulated βTC-tet cells perfused for 4.5 days in a packed bed bioreactor. 10 mM ^{13}C$_1$-glucose was used throughout the experiment while media containing 1 mM 2,4-DNP was used for a 24 hour period between 56 and 80 hours.

18.2.4. Viable Cell Number

The ability to non-invasively measure cell viability is of great importance in assessing the functionality of a tissue engineered construct *in vivo* or *in vitro*. We have recently demonstrated the means of doing that with the use of ^{1}H NMR spectroscopy[41]. Figure 18.6 shows a ^{1}H NMR spectrum of βTC3 cells encapsulated in APA beads and perfused in a packed bed bioreactor. The spectrum was acquired within 5 min and displays two strong resonances: one attributed to methyl protons of lactate (assigned as Lactate) and the other to trimethylamine protons of the choline related metabolites choline, phosphorylcholine and glycerophosphorylcholine. This resonance is known as "Total Choline" and it is assigned on the spectrum as TCho. The remaining resonances are attributed to protons in the perfusion medium. Specifically, resonances indicated with an asterisk correspond to the methyl protons of the various amino acids in DMEM; the two resonances indicated as "Glx" correspond to various protons in glutamine and/or glutamate and finally the cluster of resonances indicated as "Glucose" correspond to various protons within the glucose molecule. It is important to note that methylene protons attached to C_6-glucose resonate close to the TCho resonance and appear as a shoulder of the TCho peak. Our data have shown that the area under the TCho resonance, once contamination from the glucose resonance has been accounted for, correlates to the number of viable cells within a construct[41]. This was validated with the independent colorimetric assay, MTT. Furthermore, the area under the TCho resonance was also correlated to the amount of insulin secreted. Since the ^{1}H is the most NMR sensitive nucleus and it is used routinely for *in vivo* imaging studies, we proceeded to test the *in vivo* efficacy of this assay.

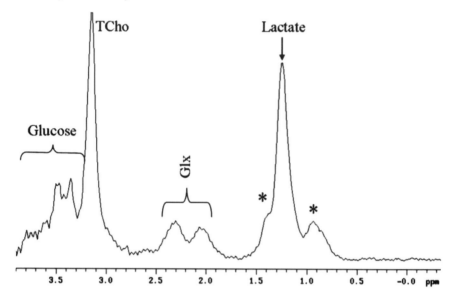

Figure 18.6. ^{1}H NMR spectrum of APA encapsulated βTC3 cells. The spectrum was acquired within 5 min at 4.7T using a packed bed bioreactor.

18.3. *IN VIVO* EXPERIMENTS

18.3.1. Viable Cell Number

Currently, the site most commonly used for the implantation of microencapsulation-based pancreatic constructs is the peritoneal cavity. Such implantations are performed with a simple injection of microcapsules and have been shown to successfully restore normoglycemia in diabetic animals for prolonged periods of time[51,52]. One of the problems with this type of implantation is that microcapsules distribute through out the abdominal area rendering their retrieval exceedingly difficult. Furthermore, it is currently impossible to monitor, via the techniques described above, every capsule in an effort to assess the metabolic activity and viability of the entire implanted volume. To alleviate these concerns, i.e. retrievability and detectability, we recently developed a macroencapsulation pancreatic construct[41,53]. This construct has a disk shape that measures approximately 16 mm in diameter and 3 mm in thickness. The construct can then be implanted surgically in the peritoneal cavity of the host animal and can be easily retrieved. It has the added benefit that by using localized spectroscopic techniques we can perform *in vivo* the same NMR examinations we highlighted above in our *in vitro* discussion. Our first objective was to determine whether we can acquire ^{1}H NMR spectra localized from within the construct and detect the TCho resonance, and to assess whether the correlation between TCho and cell viability is also valid under *in vivo* conditions. Figure 18.7 shows a sagittal and a coronal NMR image acquired at 4.7T of a C57BL/6J mouse with the construct clearly illustrated. Also shown on the figure is the ^{1}H NMR

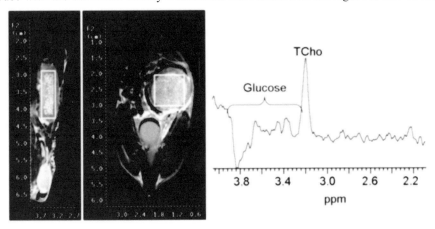

Figure 18.7. Sagittal and coronal ^{1}H NMR images of a C57BL/6J mouse implanted with APA encapsulated βTC3 cells encased within an agarose disk shaped macroconstruct. The rectangle overlaid over the construct corresponds to the volume used to acquire the ^{1}H NMR spectrum on the right.

spectrum acquired within 15 min from a predetermined volume within the construct. The boundaries of the volume of interest are highlighted with a white rectangle. The spectra clearly show the presence of the TCho and glucose resonances. To assess whether the correlation between TCho and viable cell number is valid under *in vivo* conditions, a series of implantations were performed on C57BL/6J mice. In this experiment constructs were seeded with either 14×10^6, 8×10^6, or 4×10^6 cells. Over a period of two weeks animals were examined by NMR spectroscopy followed by an *ex vivo* analysis of the construct by MTT to determine cell viability by an independent technique. Figure 18.8 shows the temporal changes in the average number of viable cells for a group of animals (n>3 per time point) examined at a specific time point after implantation. Day 0 represent measurements performed immediately after implantation. These data represent constructs seeded with 14×10^7 cells. Viability measurements are based on the area of the TCho resonance of the ^{1}H NMR spectrum after accounting for the overlapping glucose resonance (solid bars), and by an independent colorimetric assay (MTT). Both NMR and MTT measurements were performed on the same constructs. The data show a rapid decrease in viable cell numbers with time after implantation. With the exception of Days 1 and 2 there are no differences between the number of viable cells determined by the two techniques. It is not clear why the TCho measurements were lower during the first 2 days after implantation, but it may be related to the effects of hypoxia on the TCho resonance[40]. However, when constructs were explanted and measured by ^{1}H NMR ex vivo, the area of the TCho resonance correlated 1:1 with the area measured *in vivo*[11]. Regardless, this experiment demonstrates that detection of a ^{1}H NMR spectrum *in vivo* from within a tissue engineered construct is feasible and the TCho resonance can be used to non-invasively assess the number of viable cells within a construct. However, a limitation of our NMR setup (i.e. a 4.7T instrument and a surface coil to detect the signal) is the high number of cells needed, approximately 2×10^6 cells, to detect the TCho resonance. This is illustrated by the Day 14 data point where TCho based viable cell numbers were statistically higher than MTT based viable cell numbers. This limit was

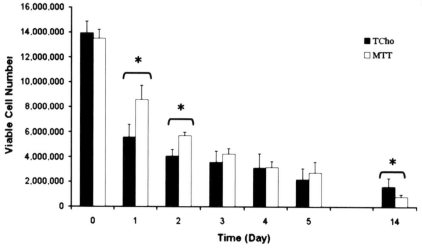

validated by implanting constructs at different seeding densities[11].

Figure 18.8. Temporal changes in the number of viable cells measured by TCho resonance (solid bars) and MTT assay (white bars). All time points from Days 1-14 were statistically different versus Day 0. Asterisks indicates statistical significance between TCho and MTT measurements at a given time.

18.3.2. Construct Integrity

One of the key issues in tissue engineering is the immune acceptance of an implanted construct. The mechanism by which the immune system attacks an implanted construct is complex. However, one of the trademark end points of implant rejection is the development of a fibrous layer. Being able to detect the development of this layer may be beneficial to the management of the implant. Figure 18.9 shows a sagittal image from two C57BL/6J mice implanted with an agarose macroconstruct. Images were obtained 12 and 13 days after implantation. Whereas mouse #1 appears to have only a thin layer of fibrous cells, mouse #2 has a thick layer of fibrous cells. This difference in the thickness of the fibrous layer is also depicted in the NMR images by a bright layer around the construct of mouse #2. It is not clear why one construct elicited such a response while the

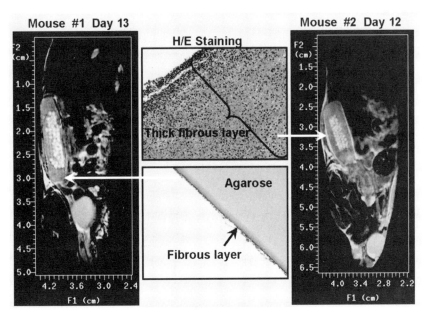

other did not. Neither do we know the limits of the NMR technique in detecting a fibrous layer.

Figure 18.9. Sagittal ^{1}H NMR images of two C57BL/6J mice implanted with an agarose macroconstruct. Note that the bright signal at the periphery of the construct in mouse #2 is lacking from the construct in mouse #1. Histology examination of the constructs revealed that the construct in mouse #2 was completely surrounded by a fibrous layer which was minimal on the construct of mouse #1.

18.3.3. Construct Function

Currently, the focal point of our research is to improve the sensitivity of our NMR setup in order to enhance our ability to monitor the function and possibly predict the rejection of an implanted pancreatic construct. Whereas *in vivo* experiments reported thus far from our laboratory were performed at 4.7T using a surface coil as a receiving antenna, we are currently in the process of enhancing the sensitivity of our experiment by performing *in vivo* experiments at 11.1T and developing custom made RF antennae for our pancreatic construct. Such modification yield an improvement in signal to noise in excess of 5:1 (unpublished data) allowing us to perform *in vivo* experiments with more physiologically relevant cell densities in our pancreatic constructs.

18.4. CONCLUSIONS

Over the past 10 years we have applied NMR techniques to monitor pancreatic constructs *in vitro* and *in vivo*. Our data have provided unique information regarding the metabolic activity and structural integrity of these constructs. It is our conclusion that

NMR is indeed a valuable tool in the non-invasive assessment of a pancreatic construct. Furthermore, we would like to point out that although experiments described in this review are focused on a pancreatic construct they are applicable to other tissue engineered constructs, provided that their architecture and composition are compatible with the NMR requirements, including complete absence of metals and air pockets from the constructs under examination.

18.5. ACKNOWLEDGMENTS

The authors would like to acknowledge the contributions of the students and assistants that worked in our labs during the past decade: Klearchos Papas, Cheryl Stabler, Vilje-Mia Peltonen, Suzanne Celper, Nelly Volland and others that their data are not discussed in this review. Work presented in this manuscript was supported by NIH grants: DK47858, DK56890, RR16105, RR13003, GM08433; and NSF grants: EEC-9731643 and the National High Magnetic Field Laboratory. This financial support is greatly appreciated.

18.6. REFERENCES

1. Mason, C., Markusen, J.F., Town, M.A., Dunnill, P. & Wang, R.K. The potential of optical coherence tomography in the engineering of living tissue. *Physics Medicine Biology* **49**, 1097-1115 (2004).
2. Kirkpatrick, S.J., Hinds, M.T. & Duncan, D.D. Acousto-optical characterization of the viscoelastic nature of a nuchal elastin tissue scaffold. *Tissue Engineering* **9**, 645-656 (2003).
3. Blum, J.S. et al. Development and characterization of enhanced green fluorescent protein and luciferase expressing cell line for non-destructive evaluation of tissue engineering constructs. *Biomaterials* **25**, 5809-5819 (2004).
4. Mertsching, H., Walles, T., Hofmann, M., Schanz, J. & Knapp, W.H. Engineering of a vascularized scaffold for artificial tissue and organ generation. *Biomaterials* **In Press, Corrected Proof**(2005).
5. Guldberg, R.E. et al. Analyzing bone, blood vessels, and biomaterials with microcomputed tomography. *IEEE Eng Med Biol Mag* **22**, 77-83 (2003).
6. Jones, A.C. et al. Analysis of 3D bone ingrowth into polymer scaffolds via micro-computed tomography imaging. *Biomaterials* **25**, 4947-4954 (2004).
7. Constantinidis, I. & Sambanis, A. Non-invasive monitoring of tissue engineered constructs by nuclear magnetic resonance methodologies. *Tissue Engineering* **4**, 9-17 (1998).
8. Hartman, E.H. et al. In Vivo Magnetic Resonance Imaging Explorative Study of Ectopic Bone Formation in the Rat. *Tissue Engineering* **8**, 1029-1036 (2002).
9. Burg, K.J. et al. Application of magnetic resonance microscopy to tissue engineering: a polylactide model. *J Biomed Mater Res* **61**, 380-390 (2002).
10. Neves, A.A., Medcalf, N. & Brindle, K. Functional assessment of tissue-engineered meniscal cartilage by magnetic resonance imaging and spectroscopy. *Tissue Engineering* **9**, 51-62 (2003).
11. Stabler, C.L., Long, R.C., Jr., Constantinidis, I. & Sambanis, A. In vivo noninvasive monitoring of viable cell number in tissue engineered constructs using 1H NMR spectroscopy. *Cell Transplantation* **14**, 139-149 (2005).
12. Chalfie, M., Tu, Y., Euskirchen, G., Ward, W.W. & Prasher, D.C. Green fluorescent protein as a marker for gene expression. *Science* **263**, 802-805 (1994).
13. Hadjantonakis, A.-K., Dickinson, M.E., Fraser, S.E. & Papaioannou, V.E. Technicolour transgenics: imaging tools for functional genomics in the mouse. *Nature Genetics* **4**, 613-625 (2003).
14. Greer III, L.F. & Szalay, A.A. Imaging of light emission from the expression of lucoferases in living cells and organisms: a review. *Luminescence* **17**, 43-74 (2002).

15. Gee, K.R., Zhou, Z.-L., Qian, W.-J. & Kennedy, R. Detection and imaging of zinc secretion from pancreatic β-cells using a new fluorescent zinc indicator. *Journal of the Americal Chemical Society Communications* **124**, 776-778 (2002).
16. Piston, D.W. Imaging living cells by two-photon excitation microscopy. *Trends in Cellular Biology* **9**, 66-69 (1999).
17. Lu, Y. et al. Bioluminescent monitoring of islet graft survival after transplantation. *Molecular Therapy* **9**, 428-435 (2004).
18. Fowler, M. et al. Assessment of Pancreatic Islet Mass after Islet Transplantation Using In Vivo Bioluminescence Imaging. *Transplantation* **79**, 768-776 (2005).
19. Tai, Y.C. et al. MicroPET II: design, development and initial performance of an improved microPET scanner for small-animal imaging. *Physics in Medicine and Biology* **48**, 1519-1537 (2003).
20. Purcell, E.M., Torrey, H.C. & Pound, R.V. Resonance absorption by nuclear magnetic moments in a solid. *Physical Review* **69**, 37-38 (1946).
21. Bloch, F., Hansen, W.W. & M., P. Nuclear induction. *Physical Review* **69**, 127 (1946).
22. Lauterbur, P.C. Image information by induced local interactions. Examples employing nuclear magnetic resonance. *Nature* **242**, 190-191 (1973).
23. Mansfied, P. & Grannell, P.K. NMR "difraction" in solids? *Journal of Physics C: solid state physics* **6**, L422-L426 (1973).
24. Aguayo, J.B., Blackband, S.J., Schoeniger, J., Mattingly, M.A. & Hintermann, M. Nuclear magnetic resonance imaging of a single cell. *Nature* **322**, 190-191 (1986).
25. Norris, D.G. High field human imaging. *Journal of Magnetic Resonancne Imaging* **18**, 519-529 (2003).
26. Szwergold, B.S. NMR spectroscopy of cells. *Annual Review Physiology* **54**, 775-798 (1992).
27. Neeman, M., Rushkin, E., Kadouri, A. & Degani, H. Adaptation of culture methods for NMR studies of anchorage-dependent cells. *Magn. Reson. Med.* **7**, 236-242 (1988).
28. Lyon, R.C., Faustino, P.J. & Cohen, J.S. A perfusion technique for ^{13}C NMR studies of the metabolism of ^{13}C-labeled substances by mammalian cells. *Magn. Reson. Med.* **3**, 663-672 (1986).
29. Narayan, K.S., Moress, E.A., Chatham, J.C. & Barker, P.B. 31P NMR of mammalian cells encapsulated in alginate gels utilizing a new phosphate-free perfusion medium. *NMR Biomed.* **3**, 23-26 (1990).
30. Gamcsik, M.P., Forder, J.R., Millis, K.K. & McGovern, K.A. A versatile oxygenator and perfusion system for magnetic resonance studies. *Biotechn. Bioeng.* **49**, 348-354 (1996).
31. Sillerud, L.O., Freyer, J.P., Neeman, M. & Mattingly, M.A. Proton NMR microscopy of multicellular tumor spheroid morphology. *Magn. Reson. Med.* **16**, 380-389 (1990).
32. Gillies, R.J. et al. Design and application of NMR-compatible bioreactor circuits for extended perfusion of high-density mammalian cell cultures. *NMR Biomed.* **6**, 95-104 (1993).
33. Constantinidis, I. & Sambanis, A. Towards the development of artificial endocrine tissues: 31P NMR spectroscopic studies of immunoisolated, insulin-secreting AtT-20 cells. *Biotechnology and Bioengineering* **47**, 431-443 (1995).
34. Koretsky, A.P. & Williams, D.S. Application of localized in vivo NMR to whole organ physiology in the animal. *Annu. Rev. Physiol.* **54**, 799-826 (1992).
35. Negendank, W. Studies of human tumors by MRS: a review. *NMR Biomed.* **5**, 303-324 (1992).
36. Papas, K.K., Long Jr, R.C., Constantinidis, I. & Sambanis, A. Role of ATP and P_i on the mechanism of insulin secretion in the mouse insulinoma βTC3 cell line. *Biochemical Journal* **326**, 807-814 (1997).
37. Papas, K.K., Long Jr, R.C., Constantinidis, I. & Sambanis, A. Development of a bioartificial pancreas: I. Long-term propagation and basal and induced secretion from entrapped βTC3 cell cultures. *Biotechnology and Bioengineering* **66**, 219-230 (1999).
38. Papas, K.K., Long Jr, R.C., Constantinidis, I. & Sambanis, A. Development of a bioartificial pancreas: II. Effects of oxygen on long-term entrapped βTC3 cell cultures. *Biotechnology and Bioengineering* **66**, 231-237 (1999).
39. Papas, K.K., Long Jr, R.C., Sambanis, A. & Constantinidis, I. Effects of short-term hypoxia on a bioartificial pancreatic construct. *Cell Transplantation* **9**, 415-422 (2000).
40. Long, R.C., Jr., Papas, K.K., Sambanis, A. & Constantinidis, I. In vitro monitoring of total choline levels in a bioartificial pancreas: ^{1}H NMR spectroscopic studies of the effects of oxygen level. *Journal of Magnetic Resonance* **146**, 49-57 (2000).
41. Stabler, C.L., Long, R.C., Jr., Constantinidis, I. & Sambanis, A. Noninvasive measurement of viable cell number in tissue engineered constructs in vitro using 1H NMR spectroscopy. *Tissue Engineering* **11**, 404-414 (2005).

42. Gimi, B. et al. NMR Spiral Surface Microcoils: Applications. *Concepts in Magnetic Resonance Part B (Magnetic Resonance Engineering)* **18**, 1-8 (2003).
43. Lim, F. & Sun, A.M. Microencapsulated islets as bioartificial endocrine pancreas. *Science* **210**, 908-910 (1980).
44. Strand, B.L., Yrr, A.M., Espevik, T. & Skjak-Braek, G. Visualization of alginate-poly-L-lysine-alginate microcapsules by confocal lazer scanning microscopy. *Biotechnology and Bioengineering* **82**, 386-394 (2003).
45. Constantinidis, I., Rask, I., Long Jr, R.C. & Sambanis, A. Effects of alginate composition on the metabolic, secretory, and growth characteristics of entrapped βTC3 mouse insulinoma cells. *Biomaterials* **20**, 2019-2027 (1999).
46. Stabler, C., Wilks, K., Sambanis, A. & Constantinidis, I. The effects of alginate composition on encapsulated βTC3 cells. *Biomaterials* **22**, 1301-1310 (2001).
47. Simpson, N.E., Stabler, C.L., Sambanis, A. & Constantinidis, I. The role of the $CaCl_2$-guluronic acid interaction on alginate encapsulated βTC3 cells. *Biomaterials* **25**, 2603-2610 (2004).
48. Malloy, C.R., Sherry, A.D. & Jeffrey, F.M.H. Evaluation of carbon flux and substrate selection through alternative pathways involving the citric acid cycle of the heart by ^{13}C-NMR spectroscopy. *Journal Biological Chemistry* **263**, 6964-6971 (1988).
49. Sherry, A.D., Jeffrey, F.M.H. & Malloy, C.R. Analytical solutions for 13C isotopomer analysis of complex metabolic conditions: substrate oxidation, multiple pyruvate cycles, and gluconeogenesis. *Metabolic Engineering* **6**, 12-24 (2004).
50. Constantinidis, I., Mukundan, N.E., Gamcsik, M. & Sambanis, A. Towards the development of a bioartificial pancreas: A ^{13}C NMR study on the effect of alginate/poly-L-lysine/alginate entrapment on glucose metabolism by βTC3 mouse insulinoma cells. *Cellular Molecular Biology* **43**, 721-729 (1997).
51. Hicks, B.A. et al. Transplantation of β cells from transgenic mice into nude athymic diabetic rats restores glucose regulation. *Diabetes Res. Clin. Pract.* **14**, 157-164 (1991).
52. Lanza, R.P. et al. Transplantation of islets using microencapsulation: studies in diabetic rodents and dogs. *J. Mol. Med.* **77**, 206-210 (1999).
53. Constantinidis, I., Stabler, C.L., Long, R.J. & Sambanis, A. Noninvasive monitoring of a retrievable bioartificial pancreas in vivo. *Annals New York Academy Sciences* **961**, 298-301 (2002).

SECTION 5

ANIMAL MODELS AND CLINICAL STRATEGIES

19

FROM MOLECULES TO MATRIX: CONSTRUCTION AND EVALUATION OF MOLECULARLY DEFINED BIOSCAFFOLDS

Paul J. Geutjes[1], Willeke F. Daamen[1], Pieter Buma[2], Wout F. Feitz[3], Kaeuis A. Faraj[1,4], Toin H. van Kuppevelt[1*]

19.1. SUMMARY

In this chapter, we describe the fundamental aspects of the preparation of molecularly-defined scaffolds for soft tissue engineering, including the tissue response to the scaffolds after implantation. In particular, scaffolds prepared from insoluble type I collagen fibres, soluble type II collagen fibres, insoluble elastin fibres, glycosamino–glycans (GAGs) and growth factors are discussed. The general strategy is to prepare tailor-made "smart" biomaterials which will create a specific microenvironment thus enabling cells to generate new tissues. As an initial step, all biomolecules used were purified to homogeneity. Next, porous scaffolds were prepared using freezing and lyophilisation, and these scaffolds were crosslinked using carbodiimides. Crosslinking resulted in mechanically stronger scaffolds and allowed the covalent incorporation of GAGs. Scaffold characteristics were controlled to prepare tailor-made scaffolds by varying e.g. collagen to elastin ratio, freezing rate, degree of crosslinking, and GAGs attachment. The tissue response to scaffolds was evaluated following subcutaneous implantations in rats. Crosslinked scaffolds maintained their integrity and supported the formation of new extracellular matrix. Collagen-GAG scaffolds loaded with basic fibroblast growth factor significantly enhanced neovascularisation and tissue

---

[1] Radboud University Nijmegen Medical Centre, Department of Biochemistry, P.O. Box 9101, 6500 HB Nijmegen, The Netherlands
[2] Radboud University Nijmegen Medical Centre, Department of Orthopaedics, P.O. Box 9101, 6500 HB Nijmegen, The Netherlands
[3] Radboud University Nijmegen Medical Centre, Department of Urology, P.O. Box 9101, 6500 HB Nijmegen, The Netherlands
[4] European Medical Contract Manufacturing, Middenkampweg 17, 6645 CH Nijmegen, The Netherlands
*Corresponding author TvK (a.vankuppevelt@ncmls.ru.nl).

remodelling. Animal studies of two potential applications of these scaffolds were discussed in more detail, i.e. for bladder and cartilage regeneration.

19.2. ABBREVIATIONS

bFGF	basic fibroblast growth factor
COL	collagen
CS	chondroitin sulfate
DEAE	diethylaminoethyl
DNA	deoxyribonucleic acid
DS	dermatan sulfate
ECM	extracellular matrix
EDC	1-ethyl-3-(3-dimethyl aminopropyl) carbodiimide
EGF	epidermal growth factor
EL	elastin
GAG	glycosaminoglycans
HA	hyaluronic acid
HE	haematoxylin eosin
HS	heparan sulfate
KS	keratan sulfate
LMW	low molecular weight
MES	2-morpholinoethane sulphonic acid
NHS	N-hydroxysuccinimide
PBS	phosphate buffered saline
rr	recombinant rat
SDS-PAGE	sodium dodecyl sulfate polyacrylamide gel electrophoresis
SEM	scanning electron microscopy
SIS	small intestinal submucosa
TEM	transmission electron microscopy
VEGF	vascular endothelial growth factor

19.3. INTRODUCTION

Tissue engineering is a rapidly growing area that aims to create, repair and/or replace tissues and organs by using combinations of biomaterials and cells. All tissues are composed of cells embedded in extracellular matrix. Tissue engineered constructs should have the capacity to become structurally integrated with the surrounding tissue, and to initiate restoration of essential functions of the lost or damaged tissue[1,2]. Most techniques of tissue engineering rely either on biocompatible scaffolds alone or a combination of scaffolds with cells to achieve new tissue formation. The scaffolds need to be compatible and designed to meet the nutritional and biological needs of the cell populations involved in the formation of new tissue[3]. Ideally, scaffolds should be able to guide cells, which may be achieved by signals that sustain cellular growth, migration and differentiation[4]. Engineered molecularly-defined smart scaffolds that resemble tissue-specific microenvironments may provide a means to accomplish this goal.

Major extracellular matrix (ECM) components in tissue and organs are collagens, elastin, proteoglycans, laminin, fibronectin and glycosaminoglycans (GAGs). Each tissue has its own unique set and content of scaffold biomolecules[5]. By selectively incorporating biologically active molecules into tissue-engineering constructs, cellular behaviour may be fine-tuned[6]. Since scaffolds are to be used inside the human body, special demands are put upon preparations used for this purpose. These include: purity (to avoid immunological response due to contaminants), porosity (for cellular ingrowth), biocompatibility and biodegradability. In this study, scaffolds were constructed on basis of collagen and/or elastin, and combined with GAGs and growth factors. We will first focus on the properties of the individual components, next on the purification/production of these components, then on the preparation, characterisation and evaluation of porous matrices. Finally, we will discuss some potential applications for clinical use.

19.3.1. Collagen

Collagen provides strength and structural integrity to almost all organs in the body, especially skin, ligaments, cartilage, bone, tendon and dental elements[7-9]. Fibrillar collagen is a 'triple helical' molecule (1.5 x 300 nm) with a molecular mass of about 300 kDa. It is composed of three left-handed polypeptides (α-chains) which are wrapped together to form a right-handed helical structure. The tight wrapping into a triple helix provides great tensile strength with virtually no capacity to stretch. Collagen molecules are grouped into fibrils in a head to tail alignment, and are covalently crosslinked to each other. At least 26 genetically distinct types of collagen are known. Type I collagen is the main fibrillar collagen of bone, tendon, and skin and provides tissues with tensile strength. Insoluble type I collagen has found ample usage in the biomedical field[2,4,10-12]. Type II collagen is the principal collagenous component of cartilage, intervertebral discs and the vitreous body. Its mechanical function is to provide tensile strength and resists shearing forces[13].

19.3.2. Elastin

Elastin provides elasticity to organs, especially skin, lung, arteries and ligaments[14]. Elastin can stretch to several times its normal length. Despite its remarkable mechanical properties, elastin has found little use as a biomaterial[5,15,16]. Elastin is a desirable protein for tissue engineering[15,17]. Due to its remarkable mechanical properties, elasticity and long term stability, elastin fibres maybe important in a wide variety of applications, including skin substitutes, vascular grafts, heart valves, and elastic cartilage. The high content of hydrophobic amino acids and intermolecular crosslinks (desmosine and isodesmosine) makes elastin one of the most chemically resistant proteins in the body. The precursor, tropoelastin, is composed of a 72 kDa single polypeptide chain. Individual molecules are secreted into the extracellular space, in association with microfibrillar components and crosslinked to each other to form elastic fibres[18].

19.3.3. Glycosaminoglycans (GAGs)

GAGs mediate many biological functions, e.g. hydration of tissue and the binding and modulation of effector molecules such as growth factors and cytokines[19,20]. These characteristics are essential for basic cellular phenomena like cell adhesion, growth differentiation and activation, and implicate a role for GAGs in wound healing, inflammation, tissue morphogenesis and homeostasis. GAGs are linear polysaccharides compromised of alternating hexuronic acid and hexosamine residues[21]. Due to the high degree of carboxylation and sulfation, GAGs are highly negatively charged molecules. Based on there backbone structure, GAGs can be grouped in four major classes; these are heparan sulfate (HS)/heparin, chondroitin sulfate (CS)/dermatan sulfate (DS), keratan sulfate (KS), and hyaluronic acid (HA). With the exception of HA, GAG chains are covalently attached to a core protein, forming proteoglycans. GAGs absorb water, causing osmotic swelling which provides the tissue with stiffness, strength and shock absorption[13]. Characteristics like growth factor binding and biocompatibility can be exploited in biomaterials.

19.3.4. Growth Factors

Growth factors are polypeptides that modulate cellular activities. Growth factors can either stimulate or inhibit cellular adhesion, migration, proliferation, and differenti–ation[22,23]. Growth factors initiate their action by binding to specific receptors on target cells. Hundreds of growth factors have been identified, characterised and, based on structural homologies, grouped into at least twenty families and superfamilies[24]. The ECM serves as a reservoir for growth factors, and promotes their long term bioavailability. Growth factors are stabilised and protected from proteolytic degradation by their interactions with e.g. GAGs. A sustained release of growth factors may be established by GAGs of ECM. HS for example, is a natural polysaccharide which stores and protects bFGF[25].

Specific control of tissue regeneration is achieved by controlled growth factor release from devices. Vascularisation of bioscaffolds is commonly a prerequisite for achieving appropriate tissue regeneration and function. Angiogenic factors like basic fibroblastic growth factors (bFGF) and vascular endothelial growth factor (VEGF) have a great potential for biomedical applications[26]. bFGF stimulates the growth of smooth muscle cells and fibroblasts as well as endothelial cells, whereas VEGF primarily stimulates endothelial cells. Interestingly, combining VEGF and bFGF produces a greater and more rapid improvement in angiogenesis than administration of either VEGF or bFGF alone[27]. bFGF is an 18 kDa protein with a length of 155 amino acids which does not contain disulfide bonds and is not glycosylated[28]. VEGF is a 34- to 42-kDa heparin-binding dimeric ligand which appears in different isoforms[29]. Since both growth factors have heparin binding sites, they can be specifically attached to GAG-containing scaffolds to improve neovascularisation and tissue generation.

The biocharacteristics of collagen, elastin, GAGs and growth factors make them valuable molecules to be incorporated into biomaterials. In the following, we will discuss the construction of tailor-made and biocompatible collagen-GAG and collagen-elastin-GAG scaffolds combined with growth factors, with defined physical, chemical, and biological characteristics, for use as a biomaterial for tissue engineering. Porous collagen or collagen-elastin scaffolds were fabricated by freezing and subsequently lyophilisation of a suspension of highly purified collagen and elastin. GAGs were covalently attached by using carbodiimide crosslinking, thus offering the opportunities to exploit GAG-mediated phenomena such as binding, modulation, and release of growth factors, and allowing the construction of bioactive smart scaffolds (Fig. 19.1).

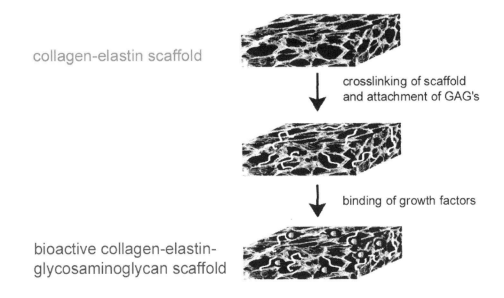

Figure 19.1. Overview of the preparation of a bioactive scaffold.

19.4. PREPARATION OF BIOACTIVE SCAFFOLDS

19.4.1. Isolation/Production of Components and Purity Assessment

Insoluble type I collagen was purified from bovine achilles tendon. Briefly, tendons were cleared from surrounding tissue, pulverised under liquid nitrogen conditions and extensively rinsed using diluted acetic acid, NaCl, urea, acetone and demineralised water as described[30]. The purity and fibril structure of the type I collagen preparation was analysed by sodium dodecyl sulfate polyacrylamide gel electrophoresis (SDS-PAGE), amino acid analysis, transmission electron microscope (TEM) and scanning electron microscope (SEM). SDS-PAGE indicated that the isolated collagen was essentially free of other proteins, and CNBr digestion of collagen revealed a specific type I collagen profile. TEM and SEM showed intact thin collagen fibrils with its characteristic striated pattern (Fig. 19.2A).

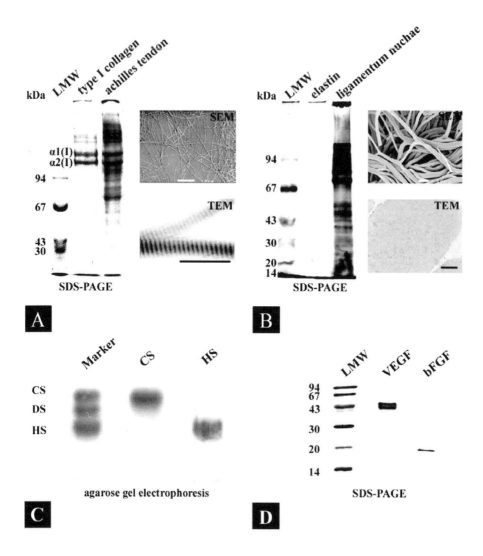

Figure 19.2. Purity of scaffold components. Shown are: A) Type I collagen. SDS-PAGE of low molecular weight marker (LMW), purified type I collagen α_1, α_2 and β chains, and bovine achilles tendon. Scanning and transmission electron microscopy showed intact collagen fibrils. B) Elastin. SDS-PAGE of low molecular weight marker (LMW), purified insoluble elastin, and equine ligamentum nuchae. After purification, no contaminants could be detected using SDS-PAGE, scanning and transmission electron microscopy. C) Chondroitin sulfate (CS) and heparan sulfate (HS). Agarose gel electrophoresis of GAG marker (CS, dermatan sulfate (DS) and HS) and isolated CS and HS. No other GAGs could be found. D) Vascular endothelial growth factor 164 (VEGF-164) and basic fibroblast growth factor (bFGF). No contaminants could be detected in VEGF-164 and bFGF with SDS-PAGE under non-reducing conditions. Bar is 10 μm in SEM micrographs and 0.5 μm in TEM micrographs.

Soluble type II collagen was isolated from bovine tracheal cartilage. Trachea were defatted, stripped from surrounding conjunctiva, cut into small pieces (0.5 cm^3) and washed/treated with Tris-HCl, guanidinium chloride, acetic acid, pepsin, and specific salt precipitation followed by dialysis against phosphate buffer[31]. The purity of the type II collagen preparation was analysed by SDS-PAGE, amino acid analysis, and immunohistochemistry. No contaminating proteins could be detected by SDS-PAGE, and after CNBr digestion a profile typical for type II collagen was obtained. Amino acid composition revealed an increase in glycine, hydroxyproline and hydroxylysine residues, relative to tracheal cartilage. No chondroitin sulfate, a major component of cartilage, could be detected by immunohistochemistry.

Insoluble elastin fibres were isolated from equine ligamentum nuchae. Non-elastinous tissue was removed and ligaments were pulverised and washed/treated with NaCl, organic solvents, CNBr in formic acid, urea with diluted 2-mercaptoethanol, and trypsin[32]. The purity of the elastin preparation was analysed by SDS-PAGE, TEM and SEM. Only soluble contaminations and/or elastin breakdown products will enter an SDS-PAGE gel, whereas insoluble elastin will not. SDS-PAGE of the purified elastin indicated no contaminations. SEM and TEM indicated that the purified elastin fibres were intact and free of microfibrils and no other elements could be detected in contrast to traditionally prepared elastin (Fig. 19.2B)[33,34].

The GAGs chondroitin sulfate (CS) from bovine trachea and heparan sulfate (HS) from bovine kidney were isolated using extensive papain digestion, mild alkaline borohydride treatment, diethylaminoethyl (DEAE) ion exchange chromatography, and glycosidase digestion[35]. Isolated GAGs were characterised by agarose gel electrophoresis (Fig. 19.2C)[36], and quantified using a modified Farndale-assay[37]. To study whether protein contaminations were present, the GAG preparations were evaluated using SDS-PAGE under reducing conditions. According to these methods, no contaminations with other GAGs or proteins could be detected in CS and HS preparations.

The growth factors VEGF and bFGF[38] were produced in mg quantities using recombinant DNA technology and purified using immobilised heparin affinity chromatography. The purity and structure of these components are essential for the reproducible preparation of bioactive scaffolds. The purity and bioactivity of the growth factors were assessed using SDS-PAGE. The expressed and purified recombinant rat growth factors (VEGF and bFGF) had their apparent molecular weight and no contaminated proteins could be detected (Fig. 19.2D). Under non-reducing conditions, VEGF was present as a dimer, its active form. The biological activity of growth factors was evaluated *in vitro* using human umbilical vein endothelial cells for rrVEGF-164 and human dermal fibroblasts for rrbFGF[38]. The addition of a growth factor stimulated cell proliferation threefold relative to cell cultures without growth factor.

19.4.2. Preparation of Scaffolds

Scaffold morphology is another important aspect since it influences cellular migration and tissue remodelling. Cellular migration and supply of nutrients and oxygen is more straightforward when the scaffold has a higher porosity. To prepare a porous scaffold, collagen or collagen-elastin suspensions were made by incubation in diluted acetic acid at 4°C for 16 h. The suspension was homogenised using a Potter-Elvehjem homogeniser, deaerated, poured into a mould, frozen and lyophilised, resulting in porous scaffolds. By using different freezing temperatures, the porosity of the collagen scaffold can be varied to some extent[39]. With higher freezing rates, smaller ice crystals were formed, leading to a scaffold with a smaller average pore diameter.

To strengthen the porous structure and to covalently attach GAGs to the scaffold, 1-ethyl-3-(3-dimethyl aminopropyl) carbodiimide (EDC) crosslinking was used. EDC crosslinking is generally applied to prevent rapid degradation, to suppress antigenicity, and to improve mechanical properties. EDC is a zero length crosslinker which couples biomolecules to each other by virtue of an amide (peptide) linkage, which is non-toxic and biocompatible[40]. The strength of the scaffold and the rate of biodegradation can be varied depending on the degree of crosslinking. The crosslinking of the scaffolds in the presence or absence of GAGs was performed using EDC and N-hydroxysuccinimide (NHS) in 2-morpholinoethane sulphonic acid (MES) in the presence of 40% ethanol for 4 h with or without HS or CS[5,30]. The presence of ethanol in the EDC solution preserves the porosity of the scaffold. Scaffolds were loaded with growth factors, by incubation in phosphate buffered saline (PBS) at 20°C, followed by incubation in PBS containing 7 μg growth factor/ml for 1 h at 20°C, and washing with PBS to remove unbound growth factor.

19.4.3. Characterisation of Scaffolds

The morphology of the scaffold was characterised using SEM. The air-and pan-side of the scaffold consisted of porous structures with pore diameter ranging from 20 to 200 μm (Fig. 19.3A). The inner site generally consisted of lattice like structures when scaffolds were frozen at -80°C. Collagen fibrils and elastin fibres physically interacted with each other in the collagen-elastin scaffold. Collagen and elastin were randomly distributed in the scaffold, although elastin tended to be present in small clusters (Fig. 19.3B). EDC crosslinking and GAG coupling to the scaffolds did not alter the porosity[35].

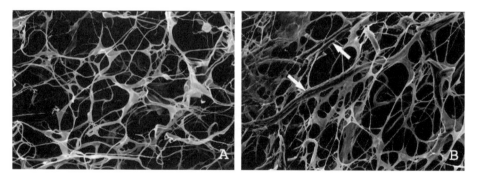

Figure 19.3. Scanning electron micrographs of a porous scaffold made of A) 100% collagen and B) 50% collagen and 50% elastin. The small fibrils consist of collagen, and the large fibres are elastin (arrows). Bar is 10 μm.

Physicochemical characteristics of various non-crosslinked and crosslinked collagen(-elastin) scaffolds, with and without GAGs, are shown in Table 19.1. The degree of scaffold crosslinking was assessed by determination of the amine group content of the scaffolds spectrophotometrically after using 2,4,6-trinitrobenzene sulfonic acid[40].

The rate of crosslinking depended on the amine group content of the non-crosslinked scaffold and the crosslinking conditions. The amine group content of collagen is higher than elastin, thus more crosslinks could be induced in collagen scaffolds than collagen-elastin scaffolds[5]. Up to 60% of the available amine groups were used in the crosslinking reaction[5,30,35]. For collagenous scaffolds, the denaturation time T_d is also indicative for the degree of crosslinking. The T_d of collagen scaffolds was determined by differential scanning calorimetry and could be increased from 62 to almost 80°C by crosslinking[30].

The amount of GAGs was determined by hexosamine analyses using p-dimethylaminobenzaldehyde[41]. The GAG amount bound to the scaffold depended on the rate of crosslinking and the type of GAG. Up to 10% of HS and 6% of CS could be incorporated in the scaffolds. Specific phage display-generated antibodies[42] were used to localise these GAGs in the scaffold[30]. Immunostaining indicated that the covalently bound GAGs were distributed throughout the whole scaffold (Fig. 19.4)[5].

Table 19.1. Biochemical, biophysical and biomechanical characteristics of various scaffolds.

Scaffold	Crosslinked with EDC/NHS	Denaturation temperature T_d [°C]	Amine group content [nmol/g]	Amount of GAG per g scaffold [mg]	Amount of bFGF per g scaffold [µg]	Water-binding capacity [# times dry weight]	Tensile strength [kPa]	E-modulus [MPa]
COL	-	62 ± 1	281 ± 7	0	0	20 ± 1	103 ± 15	0.39 ± 0.07
COL	+	79 ± 1	185 ± 3	0	0	20 ± 1	677 ± 191	1.03 ± 0.08
COL-CS	+	77 ± 1	186 ± 8	100 ± 4	0	33 ± 3	520 ± 105	0.97 ± 0.07
COL-EL 1:1	-	N.D.	147 ± 12	0	0	16 ± 1	63 ± 23	0.24 ± 0.06
COL-EL 1:1	+	N.D.	87 ± 5	0	0	16 ± 3	142 ± 8	0.42 ± 0.04
COL-EL-CS 1:1	+	N.D.	83 ± 2	58 ± 5	0	21 ± 3	128 ± 10	0.54 ± 0.11
COL	+	72 ± 1	236 ± 9	0	0	N.D.	N.D.	N.D.
COL-bFGF	+	72 ± 1	236 ± 9	0	372 ± 75	N.D.	N.D.	N.D.
COL-HS	+	69 ± 1	227 ± 17	60 ± 5	0	N.D.	N.D.	N.D.
COL-HS-bFGF	+	69 ± 1	227 ± 17	60 ± 5	1260 ± 207	N.D.	N.D.	N.D.

COL= collagen; EL= elastin; CS= chondroitin sulfate; HS= heparan sulfate; bFGF= basic fibroblast growth factor. Scaffolds above the dashed line were crosslinked with 33 mM EDC and 6 mM NHS; scaffolds below with 14 mM EDC and 8 mM NHS. Results are mean ± SD of at least 3 individual experiments. Values from [5,38].

The total amount of bFGF bound to the scaffold and its release were determined using radioactive labelling with ^{125}I. Crosslinked scaffolds, with and without HS, revealed a biphasic release profile, i.e. an initial burst of bFGF followed by a gradual and sustained release. More bFGF could be bound to a HS-containing scaffold (1.26% vs. 0.37%) compared to a scaffold without GAG[38]. Immunohistochemistry was also used to localise growth factors in the scaffold, and bFGF was mainly localised at the margins of the scaffold[38].

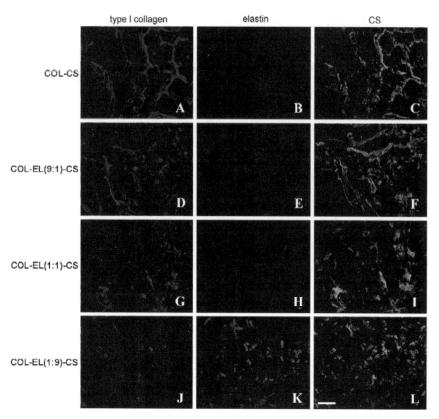

Figure 19.4 (see color insert, Figure 19.4). Immunostaining of scaffolds containing variable amounts of collagen and elastin with covalently attached chondroitin sulfate using immunostaining for type I collagen (red) and CS (green), whereas elastin was analysed by UV optics (blue). Bar is 50 μm. COL=collagen, EL=elastin, CS=chondroitin sulfate. Figure modified with permission from Daamen et al.[5].

19.5. TISSUE RESPONSE TO COLLAGENOUS SCAFFOLDS[38,43]

Before a bioactive scaffold can be applied for tissue engineering, the tissue response and biocompatibility have to be studied in animal models. To evaluate the tissue response, collagenous scaffolds were implanted subcutaneously in 3 months old male Albino Oxford rats for periods up to 10 weeks. On the back of the anaesthetised rats, subcutaneous pockets were made and scaffolds (ø 8 mm) were implanted at a distance of about 1 cm from the incisions. The implants with surrounded tissue were harvested at day 2, and at 1, 2, 4, and 10 weeks after implantation. The tissue response was evaluated by using (immuno)histological methods. Results were analysed for non-crosslinked and crosslinked scaffolds with and without GAGs and with and without growth factors.

Non-crosslinked collagen scaffolds were gradually resorbed and completely replaced by collagenous connective tissue 10 weeks after implantation. Crosslinked collagen scaffolds, however, maintained their integrity for at least 3 months and supported the formation of new ECM, i.e. deposition of type I and III collagen.

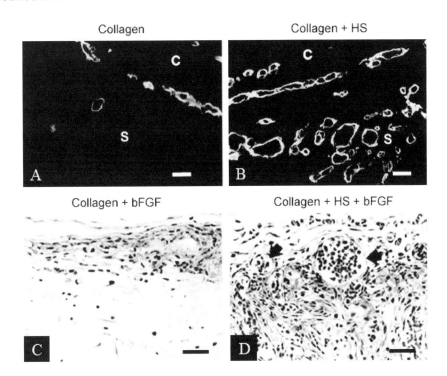

Fig. 19.5. Light-microscopy of subcutaneously implanted crosslinked collagen scaffolds. Shown are: A) collagen and B) collagen-HS scaffold immunostained for type IV collagen as a marker for blood vessels 2 weeks after implantation. Note that HS induces angiogenesis. c= capsule surrounding the implants; s= implanted scaffold. C) collagen-bFGF and D) collagen-HS-bFGF scaffold 10 weeks after implantation (HE staining). Arrows indicate blood vessels. Bar indicates 25 μm in (A, B) and 0 μm in (C, D). Figure A and B reproduced from Pieper et al. with permission[43].

To study the effect of GAGs (e.g. HS and CS), crosslinked collagen scaffolds with and without GAGs were implanted. Even after 10 weeks, the GAGs remained immobilised on the collagen scaffold as analysed by immunohistochemistry. An increased angiogenesis was found in collagen-HS relative to collagen scaffolds (Fig. 19.5A and B), indicating the angiogenesis promoting activity of HS. The presence of GAGs preserved the porous scaffold structures and delayed scaffold degradation. After 10 weeks of implantation, a minor infiltration of macrophages and giants cells was observed in both collagen-HS and collagen-CS scaffolds. It was therefore concluded that attachment of GAGs to collagenous scaffolds modulated tissue response.

The presence of GAGs promoted angiogenesis into the scaffold periphery. Angiogenesis could be further enhanced by loading the collagen-HS scaffold with bFGF. A number of growth factors, including bFGF, have a high affinity for HS and display angiogenic and mitogenic properties. Binding bFGF to collagen-HS scaffolds resulted in a major influx of cells. Collagen-HS-bFGF scaffolds became highly vascularised and remained their structural integrity throughout the implantation period (Fig. 19.5C and D). Although bFGF distribution was not homogenous, vascularisation was increased throughout the scaffold after subcutaneous implantation. bFGF loading of crosslinked collagen-GAG scaffolds is thus of additional value for tissue engineering applications that require angiogenesis.

19.6. APPLICATIONS

19.6.1. Collagen Scaffolds for Bladder Augmentation (Rabbit)[44]

Approximately 1.2 million people worldwide suffer from bladder disease. Individuals with end-stage bladder disease often require bladder replacement or repair[45]. Currently, most common techniques of bladder reconstruction with intestinal tissues are associated with various complications like mucus productions, chronic bacteria, stone formation, leakage and ruptures, electrolyte imbalance and possible development of malignancies[46-48]. Different biodegradable scaffolds have been used for pre-clinical studies. Among these, SIS (small-intestinal submucosa) is a xenogenic membrane that is harvested from porcine small intestine, which is mainly composed of a submucosal layer[49]. Complications occur when using grafts for bladder reconstruction, i.e. graft shrinkage, graft incrustation, or infection[45,50-54]. A collagen-based biocompatible and biodegradable scaffold may solve these problems.

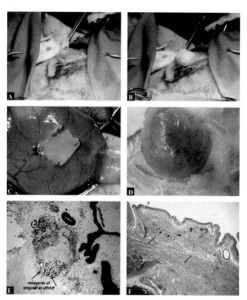

Fig. 19.6. Surgery and immunohistochemistry of an augmentation cystoplasty using a crosslinked type I collagen scaffold. Shown are: A) exposed bladder; B) collagen scaffold being sewed into the resected bladder; C) bladder with collagen scaffold filled with saline solution to examine leakage; D) collagen scaffold 3 months after implantation incorporated in the bladder wall; E) immunostaining of urothelium with cytokeratin 5 and 8 one month post-operatively; F) Masson trichrome staining of bladder wall with collagen scaffold three months post-operatively (arrows indicate muscle cells). Figure reproduced with permission from Elsevier[44].

The operation procedure was as follows: the bladder of a New Zealand white rabbit (2.5-3.5 kg) was exposed and part of the ventral surface of the detrusor (1.5 x 1.5 cm) resected (Fig. 19.6A). Collagen scaffolds were sewed into place with a running resolvable suture (6 x 0 Monocryl, Ethicon, USA) and four non-resolvable marker sutures (Fig. 19.6B). The bladder was then filled with saline solution to examine leakages (Fig.

19.6C). None of the scaffolds showed any leakage. After 1 month, the urothelium on the scaffold was multilayered and some ingrowth of smooth muscle cells was observed (Fig. 19.6E). After three months, the scaffold was fully incorporated in the bladder tissue (Fig. 19.6D) and after 9 months, the central smooth muscle cells and the periphery of the graft were further organised and the muscle layers were in a similar direction as the native bladder muscle layer (Fig. 19.6F). The collagen scaffold showed good epithelialisation and ingrowth of smooth muscle cells. However, a few rabbits developed bladder stones. A considerable amount of rabbits showed encrustation (adhesion of urate/CaO_x microcrystals) after 2 weeks, but these remarkably disappeared in time (3-9 months). Future research focuses on the introduction of HS and epidermal growth factor (EGF) on to the scaffolds in order to improve the regeneration of the bladder wall.

19.6.2. Tissue Engineering of Cartilage[55]

The extracellular matrix of articular cartilage consists mainly of type II collagen and glycosaminoglycans (GAGs). The collagen of articular cartilage is organised in a highly specific way. Most collagen bundles run from the deep mineralised layer of the cartilage to the superficial zone of the cartilage where they bent to run parallel to the surface. The cells of articular cartilage, the chondrocytes, lie more of less scattered in this matrix. In the superficial region, they are parallel to the surface, in the deeper regions they are located in columns perpendicular to the surface in-between the collagen bundles. The tissue is not innervated by nerves and is avascular, making spontaneous repair after injury or disease slow. With the increase in frequency of osteoarthritis and cartilage trauma in the population, makes cartilage a particular target for tissue engineering[56]. Various scaffolds have been reported for tissue engineering of cartilage[31,57-61].

An initial *in vivo* experiment was performed to evaluate the effect of collagenous scaffolds for cartilage regeneration. Scaffolds, made from isolated and crosslinked type I and II collagen with and without attached chondroitin sulfate (CS), were tested on their cartilage inductive properties in knees of young rabbits. Scaffolds were implanted into full-thickness articular cartilage defects. After luxation of the patella, two full-thickness defects (Ø 4 mm; 3 mm high) were made in the trochlea (Fig. 19.7A). Type I and II collagen scaffolds (Fig. 19.7B), with or without CS, were implanted and empty defects were used as controls (Fig. 19.7C). The follow-up period was 4 and 12 weeks. Empty control defects showed a considerable healing response consisting of the restoration of the original cartilage contours with cartilaginous-like tissue, and in the 12-week group, remodelling of the deeper area of the defect into bone. This unexpected good repair of the empty defects was probably related to the relatively young rabbits, which are known for their larger repair potency compared to older animals. Although differences between different scaffold types was not very large, type I and II collagen scaffolds in combination with CS showed a trend for a better defect repair as compared to the same scaffolds without CS. Scaffolds were almost completely degraded after 12 weeks and integration with the subchondral bone and adjacent cartilage was observed. In some cases, a direct connection between the graft and host cartilage was found (Fig. 19.7D). Scaffolds based on both type I and II collagen appeared to be biocompatible and biodegradable and these scaffolds favoured the maintenance of the chondrocytic phenotype in the reconstructed defect area.

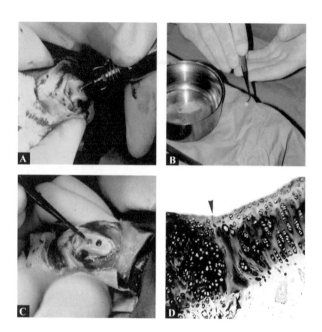

Fig. 19.7. Surgery and histology of full-thickness/subchondrial defects in the rabbit knee joint. A) Two full thickness defects were created in the trochlea using a dental high speed drill into the subchondral bone. B) Wetted collagen scaffold to be placed in the defect. C) A type II collagen-CS scaffold is applied to one defect (left); an empty defect is used as a control (right). D) Light microscopy of a defect with implanted crosslinked type II collagen-CS scaffold 12 weeks after implantation showed that the cartilage-like tissue of the implant site (right of arrowhead) is in some cases directly connected to the adjacent host tissue (left of arrowhead). Figure D reproduced from Buma et al. with permission from Elsevier[55].

19.7. CONCLUSIONS AND FUTURE OUTLOOK

The aim of our study was to construct molecularly-defined bioscaffolds which provide appropriate cues and instructions for cells to form the desired tissue/organs. Several basic tailor-made scaffolds with an appropriate porous morphology were prepared using highly purified biomaterials including fibrillar scaffold molecules (collagen, elastin), modifying molecules (glycosaminoglycans) and effector molecules (growth factors). Such scaffolds have predefined physico-chemical, biomechanical, and morphological characteristics and -especially combined with growth factors- have a great potential for tissue engineering of e.g. bladder, cartilage and skin. Organ-specific scaffolds can now be prepared mimicking the desired microenvironment. This allows the design of a specific scaffold on the drawing table, followed by its construction in the lab. As an example of such a strategy, the design of a scaffold or tissue engineering of skin is given here (Fig. 19.8).

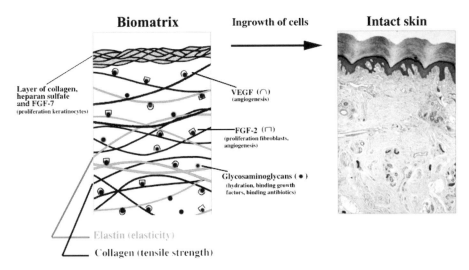

Fig. 19.8. A new acellular bilayered bioscaffold design for tissue-engineered skin.

19.8. ACKNOWLEDGMENTS

This study was financially supported by the Ministry of Economics Affairs (grants no. IIE95010 and IIE98012), the Dutch Program for Tissue Engineering (grants no. DPTE5941, DPTE6735, and DPTE6739), and European Medical Contract Manufacturing (EMCM BV).

19.9. REFERENCES

1. R.S. Langer and J.P. Vacanti. Tissue engineering: the challenges ahead. *Sci Am* **280**(4), 86-89 (1999).
2. R. Langer and J.P. Vacanti. Tissue engineering. *Science* **260**(5110), 920-926 (1993).
3. L.G. Griffith and G. Naughton. Tissue engineering--current challenges and expanding opportunities. *Science* **295**(5557), 1009-1014 (2002).
4. M.P. Lutolf and J.A. Hubbell. Synthetic biomaterials as instructive extracellular microenvironments for morphogenesis in tissue engineering. *Nat Biotechnol* **23**(1), 47-55 (2005).
5. W.F. Daamen, H.T. van Moerkerk, T. Hafmans, L. Buttafoco, A.A. Poot, J.H. Veerkamp and T.H. van Kuppevelt. Preparation and evaluation of molecularly-defined collagen-elastin-glycosaminoglycan scaffolds for tissue engineering. *Biomaterials* **24**(22), 4001-4009 (2003).
6. J.A. Hubbell. Materials as morphogenetic guides in tissue engineering. *Curr Opin Biotechnol* **14**(5), 551-558 (2003).
7. G.J. Laurent. Dynamic state of collagen: pathways of collagen degradation in vivo and their possible role in regulation of collagen mass. *Am J Physiol* **252**(1 Pt 1), C1-9 (1987).
8. D.J. Prockop and K.I. Kivirikko. Collagens: molecular biology, diseases, and potentials for therapy. *Annu Rev Biochem* **64**403-434 (1995).
9. P.H. Byers. Inherited disorders of collagen gene structure and expression. *Am J Med Genet* **34**(1), 72-80 (1989).
10. F.J. O'Brien, B.A. Harley, I.V. Yannas and L.J. Gibson. The effect of pore size on cell adhesion in collagen-GAG scaffolds. *Biomaterials* **26**(4), 433-441 (2005).
11. Y.S. Pek, M. Spector, I.V. Yannas and L.J. Gibson. Degradation of a collagen-chondroitin-6-sulfate matrix by collagenase and by chondroitinase. *Biomaterials* **25**(3), 473-482 (2004).
12. G. Marmieri, M. Pettenati, C. Cassinelli and M. Morra. Evaluation of slipperiness of catheter surfaces. *J Biomed Mater Res* **33**(1), 29-33 (1996).

13. J.A. Buckwalter and H.J. Mankin. Articular cartilage: tissue design and chondrocyte-matrix interactions. *Instr Course Lect* **47**477-486 (1998).
14. C.M. Kielty, M.J. Sherratt and C.A. Shuttleworth. Elastic fibres. *J Cell Sci* **115**(Pt 14), 2817-2828 (2002).
15. J.D. Berglund, R.M. Nerem and A. Sambanis. Incorporation of intact elastin scaffolds in tissue-engineered collagen-based vascular grafts. *Tissue Eng* **10**(9 10), 1526-1535 (2004).
16. T. Chandy, G.H. Rao, R.F. Wilson and G.S. Das. The development of porous alginate/elastin/PEG composite matrix for cardiovascular engineering. *J Biomater Appl* **17**(4), 287-301 (2003).
17. M. Li, M.J. Mondrinos, M.R. Gandhi, F.K. Ko, A.S. Weiss and P.I. Lelkes. Electrospun protein fibers as matrices for tissue engineering. *Biomaterials* **26**(30), 5999-6008 (2005).
18. C. Kielty, T. Wess, L. Haston, J. Ashworth, M. Sherratt and C. Shuttleworth. Fibrillin-rich microfibrils: elastic biopolymers of the extracellular matrix. *Journal of Muscle Research and Cell Motility* **23**(5 - 6), 581-596 (2002).
19. R. Raman, V. Sasisekharan and R. Sasisekharan. Structural insights into biological roles of protein-glycosaminoglycan interactions. *Chem Biol* **12**(3), 267-277 (2005).
20. D.R. Coombe and W.C. Kett. Heparan sulfate-protein interactions: therapeutic potential through structure-function insights. *Cell Mol Life Sci* **62**(4), 410-424 (2005).
21. S. Valla, J. Li, H. Ertesvag, T. Barbeyron and U. Lindahl. Hexuronyl C5-epimerases in alginate and glycosaminoglycan biosynthesis. *Biochimie* **83**(8), 819-830 (2001).
22. M.E. Nimni. Polypeptide growth factors: targeted delivery systems. *Biomaterials* **18**(18), 1201-1225 (1997).
23. D.G. Fernig and J.T. Gallagher. Fibroblast growth factors and their receptors: an information network controlling tissue growth, morphogenesis and repair. *Prog Growth Factor Res* **5**(4), 353-377 (1994).
24. J.E. Babensee, L.V. McIntire and A.G. Mikos. Growth factor delivery for tissue engineering. *Pharm Res* **17**(5), 497-504 (2000).
25. M. Salmivirta, K. Lidholt and U. Lindahl. Heparan sulfate: a piece of information. *Faseb J* **10**(11), 1270-1279 (1996).
26. A. Perets, Y. Baruch, F. Weisbuch, G. Shoshany, G. Neufeld and S. Cohen. Enhancing the vascularization of three-dimensional porous alginate scaffolds by incorporating controlled release basic fibroblast growth factor microspheres. *J Biomed Mater Res A* **65**(4), 489-497 (2003).
27. T. Asahara, C. Bauters, L.P. Zheng, S. Takeshita, S. Bunting, N. Ferrara, J.F. Symes and J.M. Isner. Synergistic Effect of Vascular Endothelial Growth Factor and Basic Fibroblast Growth Factor on Angiogenesis In Vivo. *Circulation* **92**(9), 365-371 (1995).
28. J.D. Zhang, L.S. Cousens, P.J. Barr and S.R. Sprang. Three-dimensional structure of human basic fibroblast growth factor, a structural homolog of interleukin 1 beta. *Proc Natl Acad Sci U S A* **88**(8), 3446-3450 (1991).
29. N. Ferrara. Role of vascular endothelial growth factor in regulation of physiological angiogenesis. *Am J Physiol Cell Physiol* **280**(6), C1358-1366 (2001).
30. J.S. Pieper, A. Oosterhof, P.J. Dijkstra, J.H. Veerkamp and T.H. van Kuppevelt. Preparation and characterization of porous crosslinked collagenous matrices containing bioavailable chondroitin sulphate. *Biomaterials* **20**(9), 847-858 (1999).
31. J.S. Pieper, P.M. van der Kraan, T. Hafmans, J. Kamp, P. Buma, J.L. van Susante, W.B. van den Berg, J.H. Veerkamp and T.H. van Kuppevelt. Crosslinked type II collagen matrices: preparation, characterization, and potential for cartilage engineering. *Biomaterials* **23**(15), 3183-3192 (2002).
32. W.F. Daamen. Isolation of intact elastin fibres devoid of microfibrils. *Tissue Eng* **11**(7/8), 1168-1176 (2005).
33. W.F. Daamen, T. Hafmans, J.H. Veerkamp and T.H. Van Kuppevelt. Comparison of five procedures for the purification of insoluble elastin. *Biomaterials* **22**(14), 1997-2005 (2001).
34. W.F. Daamen, S.T. Nillesen, T. Hafmans, J.H. Veerkamp, M.J. van Luyn and T.H. van Kuppevelt. Tissue response of defined collagen-elastin scaffolds in young and adult rats with special attention to calcification. *Biomaterials* **26**(1), 81-92 (2005).
35. J.S. Pieper, T. Hafmans, J.H. Veerkamp and T.H. van Kuppevelt. Development of tailor-made collagen-glycosaminoglycan matrices: EDC/NHS crosslinking, and ultrastructural aspects. *Biomaterials* **21**(6), 581-593 (2000).
36. C.H. van de Lest, E.M. Versteeg, J.H. Veerkamp and T.H. van Kuppevelt. Quantification and characterization of glycosaminoglycans at the nanogram level by a combined azure A-silver staining in agarose gels. *Anal Biochem* **221**(2), 356-361 (1994).
37. C.H. van de Lest, E.M. Versteeg, J.H. Veerkamp and T.H. van Kuppevelt. A spectrophotometric method for the determination of heparan sulfate. *Biochim Biophys Acta* **1201**(2), 305-311 (1994).

38. J.S. Pieper, T. Hafmans, P.B. van Wachem, M.J. van Luyn, L.A. Brouwer, J.H. Veerkamp and T.H. van Kuppevelt. Loading of collagen-heparan sulfate matrices with bFGF promotes angiogenesis and tissue generation in rats. *J Biomed Mater Res* **62**(2), 185-194 (2002).
39. F.J. O'Brien, B.A. Harley, I.V. Yannas and L. Gibson. Influence of freezing rate on pore structure in freeze-dried collagen-GAG scaffolds. *Biomaterials* **25**(6), 1077-1086 (2004).
40. L.H.H. Olde Damink, P.J. Dijkstra, M.J.A. van Luyn, P.B. van Wachem, P. Nieuwenhuis and J. Feijen. Cross-linking of dermal sheep collagen using a water-soluble carbodiimide. *Biomaterials* **17**(8), 765-773 (1996).
41. I.V. Yannas and J.F. Burke. Design of an artificial skin. I. Basic design principles. *J Biomed Mater Res* **14**(1), 65-81 (1980).
42. T.H. van Kuppevelt, M.A. Dennissen, W.J. van Venrooij, R.M. Hoet and J.H. Veerkamp. Generation and application of type-specific anti-heparan sulfate antibodies using phage display technology. Further evidence for heparan sulfate heterogeneity in the kidney. *J Biol Chem* **273**(21), 12960-12966 (1998).
43. J.S. Pieper, P.B. van Wachem, M.J.A. van Luyn, L.A. Brouwer, T. Hafmans, J.H. Veerkamp and T.H. van Kuppevelt. Attachment of glycosaminoglycans to collagenous matrices modulates the tissue response in rats. *Biomaterials* **21**(16), 1689-1699 (2000).
44. J.E. Nuininga, H. van Moerkerk, A. Hanssen, C.A. Hulsbergen, J. Oosterwijk-Wakka, E. Oosterwijk, R.P. de Gier, J.A. Schalken, T.H. van Kuppevelt and W.F. Feitz. A rabbit model to tissue engineer the bladder. *Biomaterials* **25**(9), 1657-1661 (2004).
45. F. Oberpenning, J. Meng, J.J. Yoo and A. Atala. De novo reconstitution of a functional mammalian urinary bladder by tissue engineering. **17**(2), 149-155 (1999).
46. S.V. Lima, L.A. Araujo, F.O. Vilar, C.L. Kummer and E.C. Lima. Nonsecretory sigmoid cystoplasty: experimental and clinical results. *J Urol* **153**(5), 1651-1654 (1995).
47. N. Arikan, K. Turkolmez, M. Budak and O. Gogus. Outcome of augmentation sigmoidocystoplasty in children with neurogenic bladder. *Urol Int* **64**(2), 82-85 (2000).
48. S. Herschorn and R.J. Hewitt. Patient perspective of long-term outcome of augmentation cystoplasty for neurogenic bladder. *Urology* **52**(4), 672-678 (1998).
49. A. Atala. Regenerative medicine and urology. *BJU Int* **92 Suppl 1** 58-67 (2003).
50. P.A. Merguerian, P.P. Reddy, D.J. Barrieras, G.J. Wilson, K. Woodhouse, D.J. Bagli, G.A. McLorie and A.E. Khoury. Acellular bladder matrix allografts in the regeneration of functional bladders: evaluation of large-segment (> 24 cm) substitution in a porcine model. *BJU Int* **85**(7), 894-898 (2000).
51. M. Probst, R. Dahiya, S. Carrier and E.A. Tanagho. Reproduction of functional smooth muscle tissue and partial bladder replacement. *Br J Urol* **79**(4), 505-515 (1997).
52. B.P. Kropp, B.L. Eppley, C.D. Prevel, M.K. Rippy, R.C. Harruff, S.F. Badylak, M.C. Adams, R.C. Rink and M.A. Keating. Experimental assessment of small intestinal submucosa as a bladder wall substitute. *Urology* **46**(3), 396-400 (1995).
53. B.P. Kropp. Small-intestinal submucosa for bladder augmentation: a review of preclinical studies. *World J Urol* **16**(4), 262-267 (1998).
54. P.P. Reddy, D.J. Barrieras, G. Wilson, D.J. Bagli, G.A. McLorie, A.E. Khoury and P.A. Merguerian. Regeneration of functional bladder substitutes using large segment acellular matrix allografts in a porcine model. *J Urol* **164**(3 Pt 2), 936-941 (2000).
55. P. Buma, J.S. Pieper, T. van Tienen, J.L. van Susante, P.M. van der Kraan, J.H. Veerkamp, W.B. van den Berg, R.P. Veth and T.H. van Kuppevelt. Cross-linked type I and type II collagenous matrices for the repair of full-thickness articular cartilage defects--a study in rabbits. *Biomaterials* **24**(19), 3255-3263 (2003).
56. P.M.D. Nastaran Mahmoudifar. Tissue engineering of human cartilage in bioreactors using single and composite cell-seeded scaffolds. *Biotechnology and Bioengineering* **91**(3), 338-355 (2005).
57. R. Westreich, M. Kaufman, P. Gannon and W. Lawson. Validating the subcutaneous model of injectable autologous cartilage using a fibrin glue scaffold. *Laryngoscope* **114**(12), 2154-2160 (2004).
58. S.W. Kang, O. Jeon and B.S. Kim. Poly(lactic-co-glycolic acid) microspheres as an injectable scaffold for cartilage tissue engineering. *Tissue Eng* **11**(3-4), 438-447 (2005).
59. J.S. Dounchis, W.C. Bae, A.C. Chen, R.L. Sah, R.D. Coutts and D. Amiel. Cartilage repair with autogenic perichondrium cell and polylactic acid grafts. *Clin Orthop Relat Res*(377), 248-264 (2000).
60. S.B. Cohen, C.M. Meirisch, H.A. Wilson and D.R. Diduch. The use of absorbable co-polymer pads with alginate and cells for articular cartilage repair in rabbits. *Biomaterials* **24**(15), 2653-2660 (2003).
61. H.A. Breinan, S.D. Martin, H.P. Hsu and M. Spector. Healing of canine articular cartilage defects treated with microfracture, a type-II collagen matrix, or cultured autologous chondrocytes. *J Orthop Res* **18**(5), 781-789 (2000).

20

AGE-RELATED DIFFERENCES IN ARTICULAR CARTILAGE WOUND HEALING: A POTENTIAL ROLE FOR TRANSFORMING GROWTH FACTOR β1 IN ADULT CARTILAGE REPAIR

P. K. Bos[1], J.A.N. Verhaar[2], and G.J.V.M. van Osch[3]

20.1. ABSTRACT

Objective of this study was to investigate the early wound healing reactions of immature and mature articular cartilage on experimental wound healing in the New Zealand White rabbit. The proliferation potential and glycosaminoglycan production of isolated chondrocytes of these animals was studied in an alginate culture system. A band of tissue with death chondrocytes was observed at wound edges of immature articular cartilage, whereas mature cartilage showed a significant smaller amount of dead chondrocytes. A general increase in TGFβ1, FGF2 and IGF1 was observed throughout cartilage tissue with the exception of lesion edges. The observed immunonegative area appeared to correlate with the observed cell death in lesion edges. Repair in immature cartilage was indicated by chondrocyte proliferation in clusters and a decrease in defect size. No repair response was observed in mature articular cartilage defects. The alginate culture experiment demonstrated a higher proliferation rate of immature chondrocytes. Addition of recombinant TGFβ1 increased proliferation rate and GAG production of mature chondrocytes. We were not able to further stimulate immature chondrocytes. These results indicate that TGFβ1 addition may contribute to induce cartilage repair responses in mature cartilage as observed in immature, developing cartilage.

---

[1] Department of Orthopaedic Surgery, Erasmus MC, University Medical Center Rotterdam, the Netherlands
[2] Department of Orthopaedic Surgery, Erasmus MC, University Medical Center Rotterdam, the Netherlands
[3] Departments of Orthopaedic Surgery and Otorhinolaryngology, Erasmus MC, University Medical Center Rotterdam, the Netherlands

20.2. INTRODUCTION

Articular cartilage displays a limited repair response following injury. Partial-thickness articular cartilage defects, limited to the cartilage itself, are not repaired and full thickness defects are repaired with fibrocartilage. Complete repair of partial-thickness cartilage injury has only been reported in one study on fetal lamb[1]. This repair process appears to be absent in matured animals. Current clinical and experimental treatment methods do not result in durable and predictable restoration of the articular surface in damaged joints[3,4].

An important prerequisite for durable repair of cartilage lesions is the integration of wound edges or the integration of repair tissue with the surrounding host cartilage[5]. Failure of repair caused by an impaired integration has been documented by several authors who studied the natural cartilage repair process [6-8], repair following transplantation of periosteal and perichondrial grafts[9,10], osteochondral grafts[11], natural[12] and tissue engineered grafts[13].

Knowledge of the mechanisms by which immature, developing cartilage is able to repair defects may help in developing repair strategies for mature cartilage.

Sufficient amounts of chondrocytes and extracellular matrix (ECM) production are important for new hyaline cartilage tissue formation, defect filling and possibly for integrative repair. Active proliferation and high production of ECM during development may explain the observed repair response in immature subjects[14]. Age-related differences have been shown for concentrations of proteoglycans and TGFβ1 in synovial fluid of knee joints of immature and mature New Zealand White rabbits. An increased concentration of TGFβ1 in immature joint fluid was suggested to be a reason for the observed better healing capacity[15].

Ageing has been shown to change proliferation capacity, extracellular matrix production and responsiveness to growth factor stimulation in *in vivo* studies, explant studies and in isolated chondrocyte culture studies[16-18]. However, varying results were reported in literature.

Aim of this study was to investigate the early wound healing reactions (chondrocyte survival, histological changes, and immunohistochemical expression of growth factors) of immature and mature articular cartilage on experimental cartilage injury *in vivo* and to study the potential of isolated chondrocytes from these animals to proliferate and produce ECM *in vitro*. The possibility of stimulating these chondrocytes with a potent growth factor, TGFβ1, was studied in a three dimensional alginate culture system.

20.3. MATERIALS AND METHODS

20.3.1. Surgery and Tissue Sampling

All animal experimental procedures in this study were approved by the Animal Ethics Committee (protocol no. 1169803) and carried out in accordance with the guidelines of the Erasmus University Rotterdam (The Netherlands).

Nine immature (age 6 weeks) and 9 adult (age 48-50 weeks) New Zealand White rabbits were used for these experiments (Physial growth plate closure in New Zealand White rabbits: distal femur 19-24 weeks, proximal tibia 25-32 weeks [19].) The animals were anesthetized by an intramuscular injection of 10% ketamine-hydrochloride (Ketalin, Apharma, Arnhem, the Netherlands) 0.5 ml/kg body weight and 2% xylazine-hydrochloride (Rompun, Bayer, Leverkusen, Germany) 0.5 ml/kg body weight. Both knees were shaved and disinfected with 70% alcohol prior to surgery. A midline incision was used to approach the knee, a medial arthrotomy was performed, the patella was lateralized and the knee flexed. In the weigthbearing area of the medial femoral condyle of both limbs an anterior-posterior partial-thickness cartilage defect was created using a specially designed 0.5mm wide gouge, deepness 0.3mm. Length of the defect was controlled manually and approximately 5mm. Care was taken not to penetrate the subchondral plate, no bleeding was observed in the defects. In knee cartilage of one side the subchondral bone was cut using a scalpel, thereby opening the subchondral bone. Knees were rinsed thoroughly with saline, wounds were closed in layers. Animals were allowed to move freely in their boxes. The animals were killed at 1, 3 and 7 days following surgery. Areas of the defects in articular cartilage including a small part of the calcified cartilage were harvested using a scalpel, fixed in phosphate buffered formalin 4% for 24 hours, processed and embedded in paraffin. Three to four 5µm thick sections were cut and mounted on poly-L lysine coated slides. Articular cartilage from non-operated hips served as control tissue (n=3 per age group). From the same animals, 3 mature and 3 immature, hip and shoulder cartilage was harvested aseptically and used for culture experiments.

20.3.2. Cell Cultures

Chondrocytes were isolated with pronase E (2 mg/ml saline; Sigma, St Louis, MO) followed by overnight incubation at 37 °C with collagenase B (1,5 mg/ml medium with 10%FCS; Roche diagnostics Mannheim, Germany) Cells were suspended in 1.2% low-viscosity alginate (Keltone LV, Kelco) at a density of 4×10^6 cells / ml and alginate beads were prepared as described before[20]. Beads were cultured for 14 days in 24-well plates with or without 10 ng/ml TGFβ1 (recombinant human TGFβ1, R&D systems, Oxon, UK) in DMEM/Ham's F12 medium (Life Technologies, Breda, the Netherlands) with 10% FCS, 50 µg/ml gentamicin, 1,5 µg/ml fungizone and 25 µg/ml L-ascorbic acid freshly added (n=3 animals per condition, 3 beads per animal). Medium was changed three times a week. Alginate beads were harvested directly and after 7 and 14 days of culture. Beads were snap-frozen in liquid nitrogen and stored in -80^0 until processing.

20.3.3. Histology

For histological evaluation sections were stained with Heamatoxylin & Eosin (H&E). For evaluation of proteoglycan content sections were stained in 0.04% thionin in 0.01 M aqueous sodium acetate, pH 4.5 for 5 minutes.

Proteoglycan depletion at the wound edges was measured at a 400x magnification using a grid containing 50x50µm boxes. Defect size was evaluated by measuring the maximal defect diameter at day 7 in serial sections. Chondrocyte death at wound edges was determined by measuring the distance from the wound edge until vital chondrocytes. Nuclear and cytoplasmatic changes were analyzed to judge cell viability/death:

chondrocyte death was defined as a cell with a condensed, pyknotic nucleus and either shrunken or deeply eosinophylic cytoplasm or fragmentation of the nucleus/ cytoplasm[21,22]. Cluster formation was semiquantified by counting the amount of clusters in wound edge areas at day 7. A cell-cluster was defined as 5 or more chondrocytes grouped together. The wound edge was defined as a band of 200µm of tissue bordering the lesion, both vertical and horizontal. One representative section was used to count the clusters.

20.3.4. Immunohistochemical Staining for Growth Factors

All steps were performed at room temperature. The sections were deparaffinized, preincubated for 30 minutes with normal goat serum to block non-specific antigens and incubated with antibodies against TGFβ1 (Anti Human TGFβ1 / 5µg/ml / monoclonal mouse IgG / Serotec Ltd, Oxford OX5 1JE, UK), FGF2 (Anti bovine FGF-2 / monoclonal mouse IgG / 5µg/ml / Upstate biotechnology, Campro Scientific, Veenendaal, the Netherlands) and IGF-I (Anti human IGF-I / mouse monoclonal IgG / 5µg/ml / Upstate biotechnology). The antibodies were linked with biotinylated Rabbit anti Mouse immunoglobulins and streptavidine-alkaline phosphatase (Super Sensitive Concentrated Detection Kit, Bio Genex, San Ramon 94583, USA). Alkaline phosphatase activity was demonstrated by incubation with a New Fuchsine substrate (Chroma, Kongen, Germany), resulting in a red colored signal. The slides were not counterstained with Haematoxylin and Eosin.

In control sections the primary antibody was omitted. For isotype control a mouse monoclonal negative control antibody (mouse IgG1 negative control / Dako A/S) was used.

20.3.5. Assessment of Proliferation and GAG Production

Beads were dissolved in sodium citrate and digested with papain (Sigma, St Louis, MO).

The amount of DNA in the beads was measured using Hoechst 33258 dye[23]. Calf thymus DNA (Sigma, St Louis, MO) was used as a standard. Extinction (365 nm) and emission (440 nm) were measured with a spectrofluorometer (Perkin-Elmer LS-2B).

The amount of GAG was quantified using a modified Farndale assay in microtiter plates[24]. In short, the metachromatic reaction of GAG with dimethylmethylene blue is monitored using a spectrophotometer. The ratio A_{540}/A_{595} is used to calculate the amount of GAG in the samples. Chondroitinsulfate C (Shark; Sigma, St Louis, MO) is used as a standard.

20.3.6. Statistical Analysis

Results are expressed as mean ± SD. Differences between groups were calculated using Mann-Whitney U test, $p \leq 0.05$ was considered statistically significant (*).

20.4. RESULTS

20.4.1. Wound Healing

One day after surgery, a band of tissue with avital chondrocytes was observed at wound edges of immature articular cartilage. Mature cartilage also showed chondrocyte death in lesion edges, however this band of avital tissue was significantly smaller (Figure 20.1.). In immature tissue defect size rapidly decreased during the 7 days of this study. Chondrocyte clusters were observed at lesion edges, clusters seem to grow towards the defect. Also defect walls appear to be pushed to the centre of the defect, thereby decreasing the volume of the defects. Mature defects remained significantly larger during the 7 days of this experiment as compared to immature defects (Figure 20.2). Maximum defect diameter after 7 days in mature animals was 424 +/-42µm as compared to 163 +/- 83µm in immature animals (p=0.03). Very few chondrocyte clusters were observed in mature cartilage wound edges. Wound edges of immature animals showed significant more chondrocyte clusters as compared to mature animal wound edges (6.8 +/-0.4 versus 0.3 +/-0.5; p=0.03).

Hardly any filling with new tissue was observed in partial and full-thickness defects. Small amounts of fibrous tissue were observed at the base of defects in immature tissue in 1 of 3 defects after 3 days (partial and full-thickness) and 1 of 3 defects after 7 days (full-thickness only). In mature animals in which the subchondral bone was opened, a small amount of fibrous tissue was observed in 1 of 3 defects after 7 days. In the rest of the mature defects no filling was observed at all (Figure 20.3).

A small band of tissue directly bordering the cartilage defects showed decreased proteoglycan staining in all animals. This band of proteoglycan depleted wound edges was relatively small, as compared to the zone of chondrocyte death, and remained stable during the study. No age-related or defect-related difference was observed in this early wound healing study (Figure 20.4.).

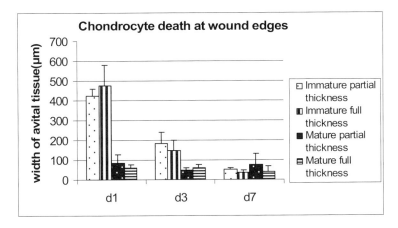

Figure 20.1. Graph representing the observed chondrocyte death in articular cartilage following experimental injury. Mean and SD of the distance between lesion edges and vital chondrocytes is shown.

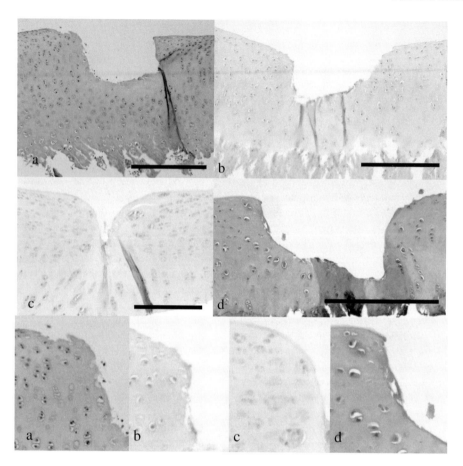

Figure 20.2. H&E stained sections from partial thickness defects are shown. Immature defects (2a) harvested 1 day after surgery show a large area of death chondrocytes. near wound edges, whereas mature defects show almost no signs of avital chondrocytes (2b) One week after surgery immature defects showed cluster formation and reduction in defect size (2c), mature defect size and shape however, was grossly unchanged (2d). Bar=500µm.

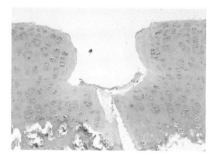

Figure 20.3. H&E stained section of an immature cartilage full-thickness defect harvested 3 days after surgery, showing a small amount of fibrous tissue at the base of the defect.

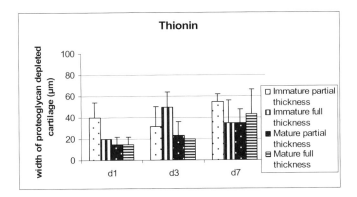

Figure 20.4. Graph representing the area of proteoglycan depletion at articular cartilage wound edges following experimental injury. Mean and SD of the distance from wound edges to normal thionin staining is shown.

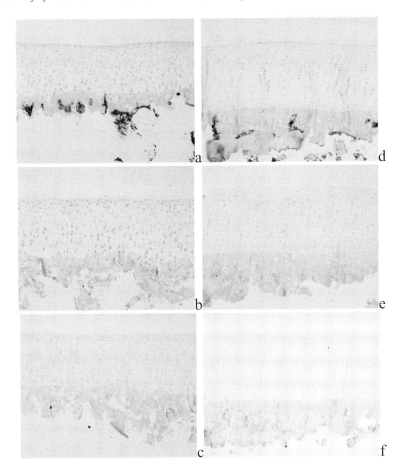

Figure 20.5. unwounded immature (a,b,c) and mature (d,e,f) hip cartilage immunostained for TGFβ1 (a and d), FGF-2 (b and e) and IGF-1 (c and f).

20.4.2. Immunohistochemistry

In unwounded articular cartilage from femoral heads immunohistochemical staining of immature cartilage showed an equally distributed weak positive signal for transforming growth factor β1 (TGFβ1) and fibroblast growth factor-2 (FGF2) and a very weak signal for insulin like growth factor-1 (IGF1). Mature tissue demonstrated merely a weak signal for TGFβ1 and FGF2 in one animal, whereas no immunoreactivity for these growth factors could be detected in the remaining 2 animals (Figure 20.5).

Following experimental injury, an intense positive immunoreactivity was observed for TGFβ1 and FGF2 behind an area immunonegative cells near lesion edges. Also throughout the cartilage tissue of the entire sections, away from the wound area, an intense positive signal for TGFβ1 and FGF2 was observed. The intensity for IGF1 staining was less, however, also stronger than in unwounded cartilage (Figure 20.6.a-f).

The absence of immunoreactivity for the growth factors in lesion edges appears to correlate with the occurrence of chondrocyte death in articular cartilage wound edges. The observed cell clusters in lesion edges were positive for the growth factors tested (Figure 20.6.e). No difference in growth factor expression was observed between sections from partial-thickness or full-thickness defects.

20.4.3. Cell Proliferation and GAG Production

Chondrocyte proliferation was observed in alginate beads containing immature cells, cultured for two weeks in medium with 10% FCS. However, no increase in DNA content was observed in alginate beads with mature chondrocytes (Figure 20.7.). GAG content gradually increased in beads with mature and immature chondrocytes, although the increase was larger with immature chondrocytes. Addition of TGFβ1 to cultures of alginate beads containing immature chondrocytes did not result in an increase in the observed proliferation and GAG production. However, addition of TGFβ1 to mature chondrocyte cultures resulted in a significant increase in DNA content in alginate beads as compared to control cultures. At the same time a significant increase in total GAG production was found (Figure 20.7).

20.5. DISCUSSION

In the present study, we have shown an early repair response in immature rabbit articular cartilage defect repair *in vivo*, and almost no repair response in mature articular cartilage defects. Immediately after wounding, chondrocyte death was induced in wound edges of both immature and mature cartilage, as is described previously in other studies[11,22,25]. Subsequent repair was initiated in immature cartilage, indicated by chondrocyte proliferation in clusters, a decrease in defect size and in some defects fibrous tissue formation. In addition to this, we observed that immature defects rapidly decreased in size during this early wound healing study, whereas mature defects remained stable in size. In a subsequent alginate culture experiment we have confirmed that immature chondrocytes possess better proliferation capacity. This is in accordance with the results of animal[26,27] and human[16,17] articular chondrocyte culture studies. The early wound reactions observed in deep wounds are in accordance with the described early observations by Shapiro et al.(1993) in their extensive study on the repair of full-thickness defects of articular cartilage in New Zealand White rabbits[6]. The observed absence of defect filling with fibrous tissue in most of our full-thickness defects may be explained by the short follow-up period of 1 week. Another explanation might be that opening the subchondral bone using a scalpel is not sufficient for ingrowth of mesenchymal stem cells.

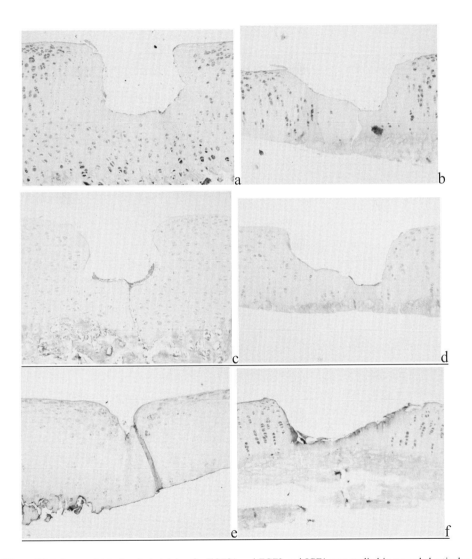

Figure 20.6. Immunohistochemical staining for TGFβ1 and FGF2 and IGF1 was studied in wounded articular cartilage. a=FGF-2, immature cartilage, day 1; b=FGF-2, mature cartilage, day 1; c=IGF-1, immature cartilage, day 3; d=IGF-1, mature cartilage, day 3; e= TGFβ1, immature cartilage, day 7; f=TGFβ1, mature cartilage, day 7. The area of tissue with immunonegative chondrocytes in wound edges correlated with the absence of immunopositive cells in wound edges. (Compare Figure 20.6.a, b. to 20.6.2a, b).

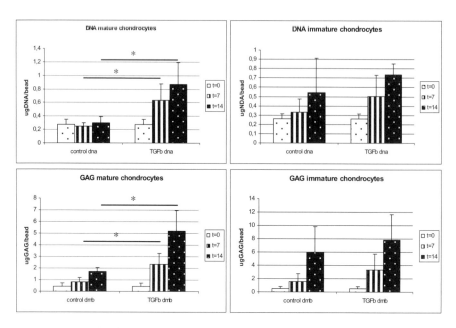

Figure 20.7. Glycosaminoglycan production and DNA content of alginate beads with immature and mature chondrocytes cultured for 14 days in medium with and without addition of 10ng/ml TGFβ1. TGFβ1 induced an increase in proliferation rate of mature chondrocytes in culture, whereas the observed proliferation rate of immature chondrocytes was not further stimulated.

Immunohistochemical staining of wounded articular cartilage showed an increased expression of TGFβ1, FGF2 and IGF1 throughout the entire cartilage sections of immature and mature cartilage, with the exception of the lesion edges. The immunonegative cartilage area appeared to correlate with chondrocyte death in wound edges. The observed increase in immunohistochemical reaction for growth factors in chondrocytes throughout cartilage tissue following experimental injury as compared to unwounded control cartilage may be explained by the occurrence of heamarthros induced by the arthrotomy. This general increase in immunoreactivity may hide a spatial or temporal difference in growth factor expression near wound edges as observed in auricular cartilage[28], osteoarthritic cartilage[29] or wound healing in other tissues[30,31].

Wei and Messner (1998) studied maturation-dependent changes of TGFβ1 and proteoglycans concentrations in rabbit synovial fluid in unwounded knees and during osteochondral defect repair. A decreased TGFβ1 concentration was demonstrated in unwounded joint synovial fluid from adult rabbits as compared to young and adolescent rabbits. Following injury, TGFβ1 levels were unchanged in young animals, whereas a minor increase was observed in adolescent and adult animals. As in our study, a better filling of defects was also observed in young and adolescent animals compared to adult animals. It was suggested that an increase in TGFβ1 levels in synovial fluid in young animals leads to a higher healing capacity. However, more cartilage degenerative signs and osteophyte formation was observed in this age group.

Barbero et al.(2004) reported that addition of a growth factor combination of TGFβ1, FGF2 and PDGF-BB to chondrocytes cultures, increased the proliferation rates of chondrocytes of all mature ages (20-91 years) and only a slight decrease with age was reported[17]. Guerne et al. showed a better response of young donor cells (ages 10-20) to recombinant PDGF-AA than to recombinant TGFβ, while the inverse pattern was observed in cells from adult donors. In this study TGFβ was the most potent stimulus in all cell preparations (compared to PDGF and FGF2), and in a large number of older donors, it was the only factor which significantly stimulated chondrocyte proliferation[16].

Fibroblast growth factor-2 was used in a partial-thickness articular cartilage defect repair study using immature and mature rabbits[32]. Defects in immature cartilage were almost completely repaired with hyaline-like cartilage following repeated intra-articular injections with FGF-2. However, no effect was observed in mature rabbits.

After having read the studies mentioned above, we have chosen to use recombinant human TGFβ1 in an attempt to stimulate proliferation and GAG production in the alginate culture system of immature and mature chondrocytes. We showed that addition of recombinant TGFβ1 to culture medium increased proliferation rate and GAG production of chondrocytes derived from mature articular cartilage. We were not able to further stimulate immature chondrocytes. These results indicate that TGFβ1 addition may contribute to induce cartilage repair responses in mature cartilage as observed in immature, developing cartilage.

In a similar experimental setup to the present study, Hunziker et al.(2001) studied the potential of various growth factors to induce chondrogenesis in a partial thickness articular cartilage defect model, using mature minipigs (age 2 to 4 years) [33]. Evaluation of defects after 6 weeks showed that TGFβ1 was able to induce chondrogenesis, although this is described to be due to synovial cells that are attracted to the defect. Possible stimulation of chondrocytes at the wound edges is not mentioned. Concentrations above 1000ng/ml however, induced side effects such as synovitis, pannus formation, cartilage erosion and joint effusion. No osteophyte formation was observed. Similar chondrogenesis, with higher cellularity without undesired side effects was observed with the use of bone morphogenetic protein 2 (BMP-2) and BMP-13.

Care must be taken to use TGFβ-superfamily proteins in high concentrations in joints. The adverse osteoarthritis-like effects of administering TGFβ-superfamily proteins into joints has been shown by many researchers (inflammatory synovitis, pannus formation, cartilage erosion and osteophyte formation)[34-36].

In summary, differences in early wound healing response of immature and mature articular cartilage are described in this study. Immature cartilage has a higher intrinsic proliferative potential and is therefore able to decrease the size of a defect. We further demonstrated that addition of TGFβ1 can restore proliferative response of mature chondrocytes in culture. Further studies need to elaborate the possibility to stimulate mature chondrocytes in explant studies and *in vivo* to proliferate, thereby increasing their ability to produce ECM needed for cartilage repair.

20.6. ACKNOWLEDGMENTS

The authors would like to thank the Animal Experimental Center of the Erasmus MC, for housing and taking care of the rabbits. Simone van der Veen is acknowledged for her help with DNA and DMB-assays, Esther de Groot for her assistance with immunohistochemical work. This project has been supported by the Foundations "De Drie Lichten" and "Vereniging Trustfonds Erasmus Universiteit Rotterdam" in The Netherlands.

20.7. REFERENCES

1. Namba, R.S., Meuli, M., Sullivan, K.M., Le, A.X. & Adzick, N.S. Spontaneous repair of superficial defects in articular cartilage in a fetal lamb model. in *J Bone Joint Surg Am*, Vol. 80 4-10 (1998).
3. Buckwalter, J.A. & Mankin, H.J. Articular cartilage repair and transplantation. in *Arthritis Rheum* Vol. 41 1331-42 (1998).
4. Buckwalter, J.A. Were the Hunter brothers wrong? Can surgical treatment repair articular cartilage? in *Iowa Orthop J* Vol. 17 1-13 (1997).
5. Ahsan, T. & Sah, R.L. Biomechanics of integrative cartilage repair. in *Osteoarthritis Cartilage* Vol. 7 29-40 (1999).
6. Shapiro, F., Koide, S. & Glimcher, M.J. Cell origin and differentiation in the repair of full-thickness defects of articular cartilage. in *J Bone Joint Surg Am* Vol. 75 532-53 (1993).
7. Messner, K. & Gillquist, J. Cartilage repair. A critical review [see comments]. in *Acta Orthop Scand* Vol. 67 523-9 (1996).
8. Verwoerd-Verhoef, H.L., ten Koppel, P.G., van Osch, G.J., Meeuwis, C.A. & Verwoerd, C.D. Wound healing of cartilage structures in the head and neck region. in *Int J Pediatr Otorhinolaryngol* Vol. 43 241-51 (1998).
9. O'Driscoll, S.W., Keeley, F.W. & Salter, R.B. Durability of regenerated articular cartilage produced by free autogenous periosteal grafts in major full-thickness defects in joint surfaces under the influence of continuous passive motion. A follow-up report at one year. in *J Bone Joint Surg [Am]* Vol. 70 595-606 (1988).
10. Amiel, D. et al. Rib perichondrial grafts for the repair of full-thickness articular- cartilage defects. A morphological and biochemical study in rabbits. in *J Bone Joint Surg [Am]* Vol. 67 911-20 (1985).
11. Tew, S.R., Kwan, A.P., Hann, A., Thomson, B.M. & Archer, C.W. The reactions of articular cartilage to experimental wounding: role of apoptosis. in *Arthritis Rheum* Vol. 43 215-25 (2000).
12. Desjardins, M.R., Hurtig, M.B. & Palmer, N.C. Heterotopic transfer of fresh and cryopreserved autogenous articular cartilage in the horse. in *Vet Surg* Vol. 20 434-45 (1991).
13. Wakitani, S. et al. Mesenchymal cell-based repair of large, full-thickness defects of articular cartilage. in *J Bone Joint Surg Am* Vol. 76 579-92 (1994).
14. Giurea, A., DiMicco, M.A., Akeson, W.H. & Sah, R.L. Development-associated differences in integrative cartilage repair: roles of biosynthesis and matrix. in *J Orthop Res* Vol. 20 1274-81 (2002).
15. Wei, X. & Messner, K. Age- and injury-dependent concentrations of transforming growth factor- beta 1 and proteoglycan fragments in rabbit knee joint fluid. in *Osteoarthritis Cartilage* Vol. 6 10-8 (1998).
16. Guerne, P.A., Blanco, F., Kaelin, A., Desgeorges, A. & Lotz, M. Growth factor responsiveness of human articular chondrocytes in aging and development. in *Arthritis Rheum* Vol. 38 960-8 (1995).
17. Barbero, A. et al. Age related changes in human articular chondrocyte yield, proliferation and post-expansion chondrogenic capacity. in *Osteoarthritis Cartilage* Vol. 12 476-84 (2004).
18. Rosen, F. et al. Differential effects of aging on human chondrocyte responses to transforming growth factor beta: increased pyrophosphate production and decreased cell proliferation. in *Arthritis Rheum* Vol. 40 1275-81 (1997).
19. Kaweblum, M. et al. Histological and radiographic determination of the age of physeal closure of the distal femur, proximal tibia, and proximal fibula of the New Zealand white rabbit. in *J Orthop Res* Vol. 12 747-9 (1994).
20. van Osch, G.J., van den Berg, W.B., Hunziker, E.B. & Hauselmann, H.J. Differential effects of IGF-1 and TGF beta-2 on the assembly of proteoglycans in pericellular and territorial matrix by cultured bovine articular chondrocytes. in *Osteoarthritis Cartilage* Vol. 6 187-95 (1998).
21. Kim, H.A. & Song, Y.W. Apoptotic chondrocyte death in rheumatoid arthritis. in *Arthritis Rheum* Vol. 42 1528-37 (1999).

22. Bos, P.K., DeGroot, J., Budde, M., Verhaar, J.A. & van Osch, G.J. Specific enzymatic treatment of bovine and human articular cartilage: implications for integrative cartilage repair. in *Arthritis Rheum* Vol. 46 976-85 (2002).
23. Kim, Y.J., Sah, R.L., Doong, J.Y. & Grodzinsky, A.J. Fluorometric assay of DNA in cartilage explants using Hoechst 33258. in *Anal Biochem* Vol. 174 168-76 (1988).
24. Farndale, R.W., Sayers, C.A. & Barrett, A.J. A direct spectrophotometric microassay for sulfated glycosaminoglycans in cartilage cultures. in *Connect Tissue Res* Vol. 9 247-8 (1982).
25. Hunziker, E.B. & Quinn, T.M. Surgical removal of articular cartilage leads to loss of chondrocytes from cartilage bordering the wound edge. in *J Bone Joint Surg Am* Vol. 85-A Suppl 2 85-92 (2003).
26. Adolphe, M. et al. Effects of donor's age on growth kinetics of rabbit articular chondrocytes in culture. in *Mech Ageing Dev* Vol. 23 191-8 (1983).
27. Evans, C.H. & Georgescu, H.I. Observations on the senescence of cells derived from articular cartilage. in *Mech Ageing Dev* Vol. 22 179-91 (1983).
28. Bos, P.K., van Osch, G.J., Frenz, D.A., Verhaar, J.A. & Verwoerd-Verhoef, H.L. Growth factor expression in cartilage wound healing: temporal and spatial immunolocalization in a rabbit auricular cartilage wound model. in *Osteoarthritis Cartilage* Vol. 9 382-9 (2001).
29. Moos, V., Fickert, S., Muller, B., Weber, U. & Sieper, J. Immunohistological analysis of cytokine expression in human osteoarthritic and healthy cartilage [In Process Citation]. in *J Rheumatol* Vol. 26 870-9 (1999).
30. Dahlgren, L.A., Mohammed, H.O. & Nixon, A.J. Temporal expression of growth factors and matrix molecules in healing tendon lesions. in *J Orthop Res* Vol. 23 84-92 (2005).
31. Komi-Kuramochi, A. et al. Expression of fibroblast growth factors and their receptors during full-thickness skin wound healing in young and aged mice. in *J Endocrinol* Vol. 186 273-89 (2005).
32. Yamamoto, T. et al. Fibroblast growth factor-2 promotes the repair of partial thickness defects of articular cartilage in immature rabbits but not in mature rabbits. in *Osteoarthritis Cartilage* Vol. 12 636-41 (2004).
33. Hunziker, E.B., Driesang, I.M. & Morris, E.A. Chondrogenesis in cartilage repair is induced by members of the transforming growth factor-beta superfamily. in *Clin Orthop Relat Res* S171-81 (2001).
34. Elford, P.R. et al. Induction of swelling, synovial hyperplasia and cartilage proteoglycan loss upon intra-articular injection of transforming growth factor beta-2 in the rabbit. in *Cytokine* Vol. 4 232-8 (1992).
35. van Beuningen, H.M., Glansbeek, H.L., van der Kraan, P.M. & van den Berg, W.B. Differential effects of local application of BMP-2 or TGF-beta 1 on both articular cartilage composition and osteophyte formation. in *Osteoarthritis Cartilage* Vol. 6 306-17 (1998).
36. van Beuningen, H.M., Glansbeek, H.L., van der Kraan, P.M. & van den Berg, W.B. Osteoarthritis-like changes in the murine knee joint resulting from intra-articular transforming growth factor-beta injections. in *Osteoarthritis Cartilage* Vol. 8 25-33 (2000).

21

INTRINSIC VERSUS EXTRINSIC VASCULARIZATION IN TISSUE ENGINEERING

Elias Polykandriotis[1], Raymund.E. Horch[1], Andreas Arkudas[1], Apostolos Labanaris[1], Kay Brune[2], Peter Greil[3], Alexander D. Bach[1], Jürgen Kopp[1], Andreas Hess[2] and Ulrich Kneser[1]

21.1. INTRODUCTION

In-vitro culture of tissues can be regulated by controlled medium administration whereas ex-vivo bioreactors are designed with the capability of providing tissue engineered devices with continuous nutrient support. When these materials or cellular constructs are transferred in vivo they have to rely on processes like interstitial fluid diffusion and blood perfusion. Here recites a core limitation for transfer of tissue engineering models from the in vitro to the in vivo environment. Diffusion is the initial process involved but it can only provide for cell support within a maximum range of 200 μm into the matrix.[1-4]

On the other hand, neovascularization from the surrounding tissues is a slow process so that constructs pre-seeded with tissue specific cells need to be sufficiently thin to ensure rapid vascularisation and cell survival.[5, 6] However, invasion of the artificial tissue with vessels is concomitant with fibrovascular ingrowth and hence scarring. Tissue-specific cell populations of the implant might both be overrun by the host inflammatory-angiogenic reaction[7] as well as be endangered by hypoxia if situated at core regions within constructs of greater dimensions.[2-4]

To tackle these issues, research has taken up on strategies for prevascularization. The authors studied the behaviour of endothelial cells in co-culture with osteoblasts for engineering of bone tissue.[8] Mooney and Mikos described an in vitro seeding of endothelial-cell-lined vessels within the structure. After implantation these vessels should be able to establish a rapid connection to the host's circulation. However, in this setting, the in-

---

[1] Dept. Plastic and Hand Surgery, University of Erlangen, Germany
[2] Institute of Pharmacology and Toxicology, University of Erlangen, Germany
[3] Institute of Materials Sciences, Dept. Glass and Ceramics, University of Erlangen, Germany

flammatory reaction along with formation of scar tissue was competing with the growth of the tissue specific cell populations.[9]

All these concepts rely on the so called "extrinsic" mode of neovascularization.[6] The neovascular bed originates from the periphery of the construct which should be implanted into a site of high vascularization potential. Subcutaneous,[10] intramuscular,[11] and intraperitoneal[12] implantation has been reported. Sufficient inflammatory-angiogenic interaction of the tissue engineered construct with the implantation site is mandatory.

Yet, plastic surgical reconstruction is most indicated for large compound defects with exposed structures like bones, joints, tendons and nerves in regions of compromised perfusion. In such cases the tissue transplant itself should bring good vascularity into the affected zone and positively affect healing in the broader sense of the nutrient flap - a concept described by Mimoun et al.[13] Bone,[14] nerves[15, 16] and tendons[17] can be harvested along with skin, muscle and fascia to achieve functional reconstruction as well as resurfacing and contour repair. Thanks to the innovative work of surgeons throughout the past decades, a plethora of free flaps are nowadays available to meet the requirements of almost any kind of tissue deficit. However, free tissue transfer is associated with donor site morbidity. Furthermore, availability is limited in quality and quantity. Tissue engineering will have to meet the core requirements of vascularization and upscaling along with the pliability in form and unlimited supply without secondary adverse effects for the patient.[18]

Hence, the extrinsic mode of vascularization may be unsuitable for this field of tissue engineering. A site of insufficient perfusion would be unable to neovascularize a cellular tissue substitute. Therefore, research is directed towards a different kind of neovascularization. In the "intrinsic" mode the construct acquires an inherent perfusion prior to implantation and does not have to rely on favourable local conditions. This is achieved by inducing angiogenesis from a centrally located vascular axis. This concept originates from the work of Erol and Spira who managed to produce a prefabricated skin flap by means of an arteriovenous vessel – loop (AV Loop).[19] In the era of tissue engineering this concept met with great interest.[20] Tanaka, Mian and Morrison augmented the model[21, 22] and utilized an isolation chamber built out of polycarbonate to enhance the vascular autonomy of the bioartificial neo-tissue. Furthermore, this system displayed a high clinical relevance since any organoid with a defined vascular axis could now be transferred by means of standard microsurgical techniques like those used in reconstructive surgery in the frame of free compound flap prefabrication.[23]

This AV Loop model has not been previously evaluated for neovascularization of a solid porous matrix suitable for bone replacement. There have been, indeed, studies with vessels inserted into constructs for tissue engineering of bone but they focused on osteogenesis rather than angiogenesis and they included vascular axis in totally different configurations.[24, 25]

In previous studies it has been confirmed that the AV Loop model is sufficient for intrinsic autonomous prevascularization of a solid biogenic hard matrix[26] suitable for bone replacement. In the present study, we tried to assess the kinetics of angiogenesis in intrinsic versus extrinsic vascularization and identify 3D micromorphological differences between the distinct groups. Micro MRI was also evaluated as a means of intravital monitoring of vascularized tissue engineered constructs.

21.2. MATERIALS AND METHODS

21.2.1. Experimental Design and Animals

Processed bovine cancellous bone (PBCB) matrices were implanted into syngeneic male Lewis rats. 28 recipients were included in the study (Table 21.1). Recipients were divided into 2 groups. In animals from group A, an arteriovenous loop was constructed between the left femoral artery and vein using a contralateral vein graft. A cylindrical PBCB (Tutobone) matrix was inserted into the AV loop. The matrix and the loop were placed in a chamber with a lid on it's top for isolation. In group B, the matrix was placed subcutaneously in the back of the animal allowing contact of the matrix with the subcutaneous tissue. Explantation intervals were 4 and 8 weeks postoperatively. 5 constructs per group and time interval were evaluated histomorphologically and another 2 per subgroup were assessed by scanning electron microscopy. Four animals from group A, 2 from each subgroup, were subjected to intravital MRI Angiography. These animals survived the investigation and were subsequently sacrificed for corrosion casting.

Table 21.1. Experimental design and groups. Recipient animals were divided in two groups. Group A : Arteriovenous loop as a vascular carrier. Group B: Subcutaneous implantation. Two explantation intervals were used per group. There were 5 animals for histomorphology and 2 animals for corrosion casting per group and explantation interval, making for 4 subgroups and 7 animals per subgroup. After MRI the animals were not immediately sacrificed, but were used for corrosion casts. Due to thrombosis, 3 additional animals had to be operated for group A

	Weeks after implantation	Histology (No. of constructs)	Corrosion Cast (No. of constructs)	MRIA (intravital)
A - AV Loop	4	5 (+1)	2	2
	8	5 (+2)	2	2
B - Subcutaneous implantation	4	5	2	0
	8	5	2	0

21.2.2. Design of Matrix and Isolation Chamber

The design of the isolation chamber and the matrix has been described previously.[27] The matrix consisted of processed bovine cancellous bone in the form of a disc 9 mm in diameter and 5 mm in height. The pore size of the matrix was 400-1000 µm with a porosity of 70-80%. Around the periphery of the disc there was a 1,5 x 2,0 mm groove accommodating the arteriovenous loop. Channels for future injection of gel-immobilized osteoblasts were included in the matrix design (Tutobone, Tutogen Medical, Neunkirchen, Germany).

The isolation chamber was essentially a cylinder with an inner diameter of 10 mm and a height of 6 mm. A base plate 12,5 mm in diameter with two perforations served for fixation of the chamber onto the adductor fascia. There was an aperture on the side for the entrance of the vessel into the matrix and a cup (diameter: 14 mm, height 2 mm) serving as an isolation lid. The chamber consisted of medical grade Teflon and was constructed by the Institute of Materials Research; Division of Glass and Ceramics, University of Erlangen.

21.2.3. Animal Model and Surgical Procedures

Imbred male Lewis rats (Charles River Laboratories, Sulzfeld, Germany) served as recipients. All experiments were approved by the animal care committee of the University of Erlangen and the Government of Mittelfranken. The animals were housed in the veterinary care facility of the University of Erlangen Medical Center and were submitted to a 12 hours dark/light cycle with standard chow (Altromin, Hamburg, Germany) and water ad libidum.

All operations were performed under inhalational anesthesia with Isoflurane (Baxter, Unterschleißheim, Germany). Prior to surgery the rats were given an injection of a 0,2 ml broad spectrum antibiotic (Tardomycel Comp III, Bayer, Leverkusen, Germany). In group A, the femoral neurovascular bundle was exposed through a 4-cm long incision at the medial thigh. Dissection of the vessels extended from the pelvic artery in the groin to the bifurcation of the femoral artery into saphenous and popliteal arteries. After dissection of the artery and vein, a femoral venous graft was harvested from the contralateral side and interposed between the femoral vessels by anastomoses using an 11-0 Nylon suture (Ethilon, Ethicon, Norderstedt, Germany). The PBCB disc was placed into the arteriovenous loop and the vascular axis was placed into the peripheral groove. The construct was placed into the Teflon chamber with the artery and vein exiting through the opening at the proximal pole. The lid was closed and the chamber with the matrix inside was fixed onto the adductor fascia at the medial thigh with a non absorbable Polypropylene suture (6-0). Interrupted vertical mattress sutures with Vicryl 4-0 were used for wound closure. In group B, the PBCB matrix was inserted into a subcutaneous pouch in the back of the animal. The surgical incision was placed laterally to the matrix and the pouch was formed by blunt dissection towards the median line.

21.2.4. India Ink Injection and Explantation of the Matrices

The aorta and inferior vena cava were exposed through a median incision from the xiphoid process to the pubic symphysis. By means of a 24G catheter the aorta was canulated and the inferior vena cava severed to allow for exsanguination and perfusion with heparinized, prewarmed saline (200 ml, 80 IU/ml, 37°C). As soon as the fluid from the inferior vena cava was clear, the animal was perfused with a 30ml mixture of 50% v/v India Ink (Rohrer, Germany), 5% Gelatine (Roth, Karlsruhe, Germany) and 4% Mannitol (Neolab, Heidelberg, Germany). The animal was stored for 30min at -20°C to allow the India ink gel to harden. After that, the constructs were explanted and left for fixation in a 3,7% formalin solution.

21.2.5. Preparation and Evaluation of Vascular Corrosion Casts

Method of corrosion casting was a modification of the one described by Lametschwandtner et al.[28] After canulation of the descending aorta, perfusion was done with pre-warmed heparinized saline (200 ml, 37°C) until the reflux from the inferior vena cava was clear. We proceeded with fixation of the vascular bed with 15 ml of Karnovsky solution (0.25% glutaraldehyde and 0.25% paraformaldehyde in 0.1 M Na-cacodylate buffer at pH = 7.2). Thereupon, 24 ml of low-viscosity resin (Mercox CL-2B, Ladd

Research; Williston; USA) mixed with 6 ml of methylmethacrylate monomer (Sigma-Aldrich Chemicals, Germany) and Benzoyl peroxide were injected into the aorta under manual pressure control. After perfusion, the cannula was removed and the aorta ligated. The rat cadaver was left in place for 30 minutes. The construct was then removed and subjected to further processing.

Complete polymerization of the resin was achieved by "tempering" in heated distilled water (50°C) for 6 hours. The construct was then subjected to three cycles of maceration in 7,5% potassium hydroxide (50°C, 12 hours) followed by 12 hours rinsing in tap water under gentle continuous flow. The macerated construct was placed into 2% hydrochloric acid at room temperature for another 24 hours for decalcification. The cast was placed in 5% formic acid for 15 minutes at room temperature for final decalcification. Drying of the specimens was carried out by means of freeze-drying.

The casts were evaluated under a dissecting microscope at a magnification of 40x. In addition, SEM was performed for investigation of the microstructure of the casts. Briefly, specimens were mounted on aluminium stubs by means of the "conductive-bridge-method" used by Lametschwandtner.[29] Measurements took place under low vacuum conditions, accelerating voltage of 10kV in an Phillips XL-30 FEG ESEM Scanning Electron Microscope (Philips, Eindhoven, Netherlands).

21.2.6. Magnetic Resonance Angiography

MRI of constructs from group A was performed on a 4.7 T Bruker Biospec scanner with a free bore of 40 cm, equipped with an actively RF-decoupled coil system. A whole-body birdcage resonator enabled homogenous excitation, and a 3 cm surface coil, located directly above the implant to maximize the signal-to-noise-ratio, was used as a receiver coil. Angiographic datasets were acquired using a non triggered 3D inflow technique (flow compensated gradient echo sequence, excited slab dimensions were 25.6x25.6x25.6 mm, measured matrix dimensions were 256x256x64, TR = 40 ms, TE = 4.9 ms, 4 averages, flip angle 40 degrees). The volume datasets were evaluated using the MRIan software for integrated analysis (www.biocom-online.de) and visualized using AMIRA software (www.mc.com/tgs). Due to the MR inflow technique high signal intensities (bright voxels) correspond to blood flow from vessels as well as perfused regions in general. These high intensity regions can be visualized using so called Maximum Intensity Projections and isosurface renderings. For MRI investigation the animals were anaesthetized using Isofluran. The measuring period was 90 minutes. The animals recovered quickly and took part in further experiments.

21.2.7. Histological and Statistic Analysis

All tissues were explanted in-toto in a standardized fashion and were fixed with 3,7% neutral buffered formalin. After fixation, tissues were decalcified using EDTA solution, embedded in paraffin and 5 µm thick histological sections were prepared by standard methods and stained with haematoxylin and eosin. Specimens were obtained from two standardized planes perpendicular to the matrix, 2,5 mm and 4 mm from the margin of the disk with a Leica microtome (Leica Microsystems, Bensheim, Germany). Microphotographs were taken using a Leica microscope and digital camera.

Digital processing of the original pictures was only performed for the purpose of morphometric analysis. The whole section was mapped by 6 sequential images under 25x magnification. After calibration to the background (ImageJ, W. Rasband, National Institutes of Health, USA) the whole specimen was reconstructed using Photomerge (Photoshop, Adobe Systems Inc.) and an image including only the cross-section of the matrix was cropped. The image was rendered bimodal (standardized threshold) (WinQ, Leica Microsystems, Bensheim, Germany) and the fractal area of the fibrovascular ingrowth was detected.

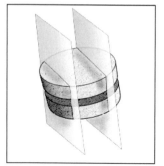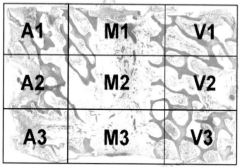

Figure 21.1. .From each construct 2 sections were prepared for evaluation. Every specimen was divided into 9 fields and inflammatory reaction was evaluated by two independent observers in every field.

Inflammatory reaction was quantified by means of a score from 0 to 5, where "0" represented absence of inflammation and "5" a very marked degree of inflammatory reaction with signs of polymorphonuclear, lymphocytic and phagocytic infiltration as well as fibrosis and stromal reaction. Each specimen was divided to 9 equal fields and three observations under 200x magnification per field were performed by two blinded independent observers. The method was a modification of the method used by Macleod et al.[30]

Values are given in average ± standard deviation. Results were statistically evaluated with the Friedman test and the Wilcoxon matched-pairs signed-ranks test. P values < 0.05 were considered as significant.

21.3. RESULTS

21.3.1. Surgeries and Macroscopic Aspects

All animals tolerated the surgical procedures well. A late postoperative wound dehiscence had to be corrected in two animals. However, in one of them thrombosis of the loop and purulent infection around the implant was observed upon explantation, so the animal was not included in the study.

INTRINSIC vs. EXTRINSIC VASCULARIZATION IN TISSUE ENGINEERING 317

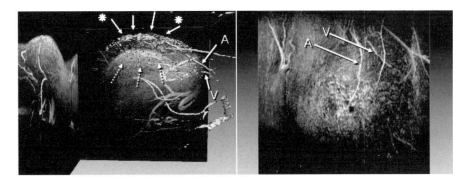

Figure 21.2. A- Artery, V- Vein, Aterisk (*) - Subdermal plexus lying directly under the coil, Interrupted arrows - Microcapillary network within the matrix. Until the 8th week the interponated vascular graft looses its significance for perfusion since a new exchange system has developed in the construct.

Upon explantation and after India ink perfusion, constructs with a patent vascular loop displayed dark coloration. Upon histology, the vessel-loop in another two constructs was found to be thrombosed. Constructs with thrombosed vascular carrier were not included in the study. So, the loop operation had to be performed in three additional animals that were included in the study with patent arteriovenous fistula. Histologically there was an overall patency rate of 82% (Table 21.1). The length of the operation was 200,9 (130-270) minutes for the AV Loop (group A) and approximately 18,2 (10-23) for the subcutaneous implantation (group B). There were no surgical complications in group B.

21.3.2. Micro MRI Evaluation

Perfusion of the matrices from group A could be verified by intravital MRI examination. Respiratory movements of the animal generated no artifacts whatsoever. However, the soft tissue elements directly over the construct produced a high intensity signal due to close proximity to the surface coil. Flow in the nutrient artery and draining vein of the loop confirmed patency (Figure 21.2.). However, on the course of the experiments, the pattern of perfusion of the construct changed from an axial pattern at the beginning to a more diffuse, organoid pattern after 8 weeks. . In other words, at later stages, the nutrient artery and the draining vein of the AV loop were readily visible whereas between them the flow was redirected within the matrix itself

21.3.3. Vascular Morphology (Corrosion Cast)

Under 25x magnification, (dissection microscope) the vascularization seemed to be the least in the graft-portion of the loop. However, all parts of the loop, including the graft segment, had given rise to new vessels.

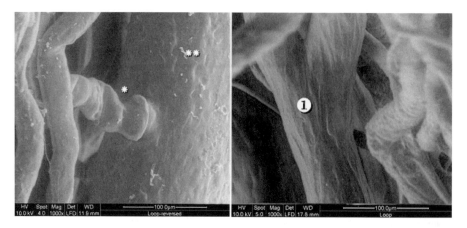

Figure 21.3. Left. At the junction of venules to larger vessels, sphincter-like structures regulate blood flow (*). Here on the venous part of the loop, the endothelial cells have not acquired the characteristic spindle-like form of the arteries (**). Right: Due to pulsatile conditions and shear stress, the endothelial cells orient themselves to the direction of blood flow. On the vascular replicas, this phenomenon is observed due to the spindle-like shape of the impressions of the nuclei of the endothelial cells on the cast (-1-).

Under 100-250x magnification, direct luminal sprouting from all areas of the loop was evident. Furthermore, there was vascular expansion with vessels of different calibres from the vasa vasorum in the arterial and venous portions. In the 4-week specimens, especially at the proximal segments (near the arterial part), the neo-vascular beds were oriented parallel to the vascular axis, as an adaptation to higher pulsatile pressure (Figure 21.3. right). On the venous side, the new vessels assumed a quite cavernous form. In the 8-week specimens, the vascular network showed an increased variability in calibre, owing to advanced remodeling and regression.

Under 500/1000x magnification, there were typical morphological characteristics of an arterialized venous graft with longitudinally oriented endothelial-cell-impressions and unruffled surface of the cast owing to the high pulsatile pressure conditions. Due to the same conditions, neo-capillaries about the arterial part of high flow, were oriented parallel to the vascular axis and resembled an expanded vasa vasorum. On the venous side, neovascularization exhibited a rather cavernous pattern (Figure 21.4.). Locally, smaller vessels became narrow in places with adhering plastic strips imitating myocytes and/or pericytes and strictures from sphincter-like regulator structures (Figure 21.3. left).

In general, the 4 week constructs displayed a higher density of angiogenetically active areas (hot spots) (Figure 21.5.left) than the constructs explanted after 8 weeks) indicating that on the latter, the vascular network was rather in the late steps of remodeling, regression and persistence as displayed by a wider variability in the diameter of capillary lumina ranging from 10 μm (capillaries) to 100 μm (arterioles).

INTRINSIC vs. EXTRINSIC VASCULARIZATION IN TISSUE ENGINEERING

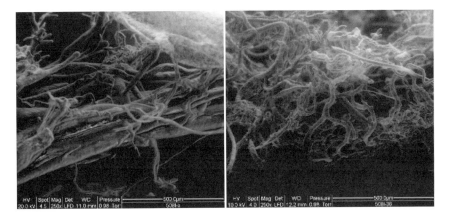

Figure 21.4. Left: On the arterial side of the loop and as an adaptation to high shear stress the neocapillaries propagate parallel to the vessel imitating an expanded vasa vasorum. Right: On the venous side the neovasculature aqcuires the form of a cavernous system.

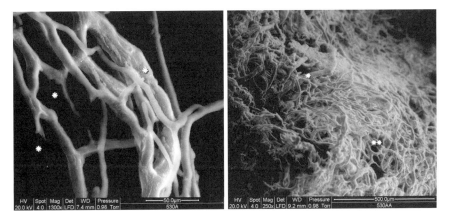

Figure 21.5. Left: New vascular sprouts are seen as sharp endings tapering off (*). "Hot" angiogenetic spots are areas with high activity of vascular growth substances. Right: Upon subcutaneous implantation angiogenesis propagates from the subdermal plexus towards the core of the matrix. Due to concomitant inflammation the interplay between intussusceptive (*) and sprouting (**) angiogenesis might be prolonged.

In the subcutaneously implanted constructs, the angiogenetic front propagated from the periphery towards the core. In these specimens we found areas of sprouting angiogenesis next to spots of intussusceptive vascular remodeling, indicating a slower propagation of the neo-capillary growth but still sufficient concentrations of angiogenic stimuli (Figure 21.5.right).

21.3.4. Microscopic Findings

Group A: In the 4-week specimens the trabeculae of the processed bovine cancellous matrix stained eosinophilic (light red) with minute hollows representing the sites where the osteocytes resided before the processing of the material. Neovascualization was demonstrated by the numerous black ink-filled lumina around the vascular axis. There was loose fibrovascular tissue emerging from the loop vessels and radiating towards the centre of the construct (Figure 21.6.). The segments of the matrix not vascularized were filled with a fibrin like substance. At the periphery there was a low degree of inflammatory response. By 8 weeks the matrix was totally filled with fibrovascular tissue replacing the fibrin substance. There was no sign of neoossification under vascularized conditions.

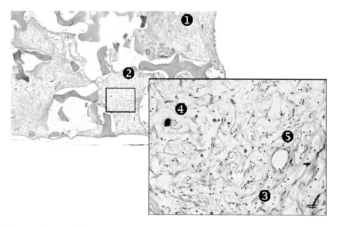

Figure 21.6.. The arteriovenous loop evokes a vivid angiogenic response with generation of loose fibrovascular tissue with almost no elements of inflammation. 1 -Loose vascularized connective tissue in the vicinity of the vein. 2 - At more distant parts, the phenomenon of "quiet" angiogenesis is more prnounced (H&E magnification x 25). 3- Proteinous matrix with few fibroblasts. 4 - A neocapillary staining black after perfusion with india ink. 5 - The void neovessel is either due to incomplete india ink perfusion or is a sign of lymphangiogenesis (H&E magnification x 200)

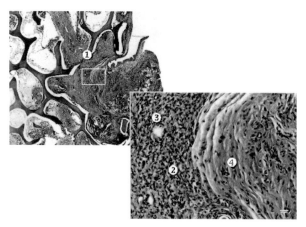

Figure 21.7. Upon subcutaneous implantation of the matrix, there is a marked basophilia with foreign body reaction (1) not only adjacent to the matrix but also throughout the substunce of the neovascularizaion.(H&E, magnification x 25). 2- Polymorphonuclear infiltration, 3- Neocapillaries. 4- Marked fibrosis (H&E, magnification x 200)

Group B: After 4 weeks there was fibrovascular tissue at the periphery of the construct. This tissue displayed a higher degree of inflammation with dense fibroblastic and granulocytic elements) (Figure 21.7.). The lumina of the capillaries were stained black by the India ink filling. The vascularized layer of the bottom regions of the construct appeared thicker than the top regions residing under the skin of the back. The central portions were filled with a loose fibrin like substance. However, the total degree of vascularization was at 4 and 8 weeks comparable to that of group A. The diameter of the neo vessels showed a lesser degree of variability with a tendency to vessels of smaller calibre.

Overall, histology displayed a propagating vascularization of the constructs in the form of fibrovascular outgrowth in group A and fibrovascular ingrowth in group B. However, there was a quite profound difference between the two groups in terms of inflammatory reaction as displayed by morphometry.

21.3.5. Image Analysis

In group A (matrix+AV Loop) there was significant rise in fibrovascular outgrowth between the 4th week (77,51%±10,06%) and the 8th week (84,20% ±4,74%) as measured by fractal area fibrovascular versus total. In group B vascularization in the form of fibrovascular ingrowth was roughly equal with (78,31% ±4,71%) at 4 weeks and (87,18% ± 3,40%). The overall score for inflammatory reaction was 1,44 ±0,79 for group A and 3,33 ±0,41 for group B (Figures 21.8. and 21.9.).

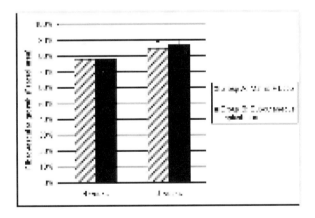

Figure 21.8. Quantification of vascularization. Vascularization is given in percent area filled with fibrovascular tissue as measured by digital image analysis in mean ± standard deviation. Each bar represents 10 specimens.

21.4. DISCUSSION

The high angiogenic capacity of the arteriovenous loop has been previously described.[31] Along with the surgical trauma and hypoxia, the configuration of the arteriovenous shunt itself seems to be enhancing angiogenesis by producing a rise in pulsatile shear stress on the venous side of the fistula. Shear stress has been known to be profoundly affecting angiogenesis and arteriogenesis on both the cellular and the molecular level by upregulation of VEGF, bFGF, PDGF and other relevant cytokines.[32-34]

The main mode of capillary growth at the early stages of angiogenesis is that of "sprouting" angiogenesis. During this process activated endothelial cells form a new sprout by proteolytic degradation of the lamina basalis of the primary vessel and proliferation into the interstitial space. Another distinct process gains significance at later stages. In this latter scheme the interstitial space forms bridges into the lumen of the preformed vessel. In this "intussusceptive" mode of angiogenesis the bridges combine and divide the primary vessel into two. At later stages of neovascular growth, there is precise spaciotemporal interplay between sprouting and intussusceptive angiogenesis leading to formation of capillary loops and further arborisation of the vascular bed.[35] Finally, some capillaries undergo "regression" whereas others persist ("persistance") and enlarge by the process of arterialization. These are the ultimate steps in remodeling leading to a mature vascular network enabling optimal flow characteristics.

The picture of the microvascular replicas in this study was in full concordance with the above mentioned phenomena. Active angiogenesis was more evident in the venous part of the shunt than from the arterial or the graft segments, as evinced by a lesser amount of direct luminal sprouting from these portions. Flow alterations on the arterial part were not as dramatic as on the venous portion, making for less shear forces and therefore less profound angiogenetic response. The neovascularization took place merely as an expansion of the vasa vasorum.

Angiogenesis was least in the segment of the interposed venous graft itself. It has been shown that Initial phenomena upon arterialization of a venous graft include denudation of the endothelium within 24 hours along with apoptotic processes in the intima. Endothelial denudation of the graft can hamper the process of angiogenesis by partially depriving the vessel from the main source of VEGF and effector of angiogenesis: the endothelial cell.[36,37] Within 4 weeks the endothelium is restored with elongated cells as an adaptation to the new flow situation.[38,39]

Coexistence of areas of sprouting angiogenesis next to spots of intussusceptive vascular remodeling in the subcutaneous constructs, might be an indication of a slower propagation of the neo-capillary growth but still sufficient concentrations of VEGF and bFGF to support remodeling and maturation of the vascular network. Alternatively, a chronic inflammatory response might be a continuous trigger to angiogenesis initiating the angiogenic cascade anew even at the presence of a preformed capillaries. The interplay between angiogenesis and inflammation is the core process in defining the pathophysiology of the "angiogenic diseases".[40]

MRI was able to provide valuable information about perfusion characteristics. Not only it could confirm patency of the vessel loop, but it could serve as a monitoring tool for anatomical conditions at the site of the construct. Furthermore, MRI micro–angiography indicated that at the AV loop constructs the exchange between the arterial and venous parts of the loop at later stages occurs through neo-capillaries of the matrix so that the interconnecting graft looses over time its significance as a shunt. New methods for cell labelling will prove invaluable for monitoring cell viability within cellular systems of tissue engineering.

Evaluation of inflammation by means of histometry indicated a significant advantage of the loop model as compared the subcutaneous implantation. A similar scoring method has been previously used by Macleod et al for subcutaneous implantation of another biomaterial.[30] These observations might have implications on tissue engineering with cell loaded matrices. Since angiogenesis and inflammation are inherently linked to each other, the process of vascularization is accompanied by fibrosis and scar formation as in wound healing. Mooney and Mikos had observed that this reaction might pose an obstacle to proliferation of the initial cell population of the matrix even if these cells were viable.[7, 9, 41]

A mode of vascularization generating a diminished inflammatory response might ensure a better environment for tisse specific growth of cells loaded onto a three dimensional matrix. Furthermore, the configuration of perfusion would allow for manipulations around the matrix without disrupting the vascularization. Hence, the intrinsic mode of angiogenesis would pose an advantageous strategy in the field of in-vivo prevascularization. An environment of good vascularity can accommodate tissue specific cells that could lead to directed tissue generation. Cell loaded constructs isolated from the surrounding tissue may open new perspectives for the study of gene manipulated cells. Organoids serving as autonomous tissue units will provide new in-vivo models.

In the clinic, upscaling of tissue engineering will bring it into the surgical theatre. Generation of "living" tissue will make reconstruction possible at sites where reconstruction is needed the most: extensive compound defects without soft tissue coverage, areas of infection and compromised perfusion as well as regions with impaired microcapillary circulation after tumor resection and radiation.

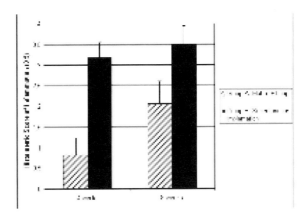

Figure 21.9. Quantification of inflammatory response. Inflammation was quantified by histomorphpometry and was evaluated by a score from 0 to 5.Two specimens from each construct (n=5) were divided into 9 equal fields and were assessed by 2 observers. Each bar represents 180 evaluations.

21.5. CONCLUSION

Intrinsic vascularization of living tissue substitutes by means of an arteriovenous vessel loop is equal to the extrinsic subcutaneous mode of vascularization in terms of neovascular bed volume and kinetics of the angiogeneic response. Accompanying inflammation and scar formation are, however, less pronounced. Another advantage of the intrinsic axial vascularization is the potential for microsurgical transfer as a free prefabricated tissue compound. Finally, from a neovascularization point of view, the construct is rendered autonomous and does not have to rely on favourable local perfusion for sufficient capillary ingrowth. This is of great significance for reconstruction in sites of high morbidity, as is the case after tumor exstirpation and radiation, after grave infections or after excessive compound tissue injury. The model also gains in clinical relevance as a strategy for neo-organ generation. Insertion of a functional vessel into a tissue construct mobilizes endogenous angiogenic affectors and initiates a profound neovascularization from within. MRI is a powerful tool for evaluation of vascularized tissue engineered constructs in vivo. To our knowledge, this is the first experimental study comparing intrinsic to extrinsic vascularization in tissue engineering. Further studies might have to be conducted on the issue of inflammatory reaction to confirm our findings.

21.6. ACKNOWLEDGMENTS

A. Lametschwandtner's instruction in the corrosion cast technique is highly appreciated. The authors thank T. Fey and A. Springer for preparation of the SEM specimens. This study was supported by research grants from the University of Erlangen (ELAN Program) and from Tutogen Medical Inc.

21.7. REFERENCES

1. Horch RE, Bannasch H, Stark GB. Transplantation of cultured autologous keratinocytes in fibrin sealant biomatrix to resurface chronic wounds. *Transplant Proc.* **33** (1-2): 642-4. (2001)
2. Goldstein AS, Juarez TM, Helmke CD, Gustin MC, Mikos AG. Effect of convection on osteoblastic cell growth and function in biodegradable polymer foam scaffolds. *Biomaterials.* **22** (11): 1279-88. (2001)
3. Greene HSN. Heterologous transplantation of mammalian tumors. *Exp. Med.* **73**: 461. (1961)
4. Folkman J, Hochberg M. Self-regulation of growth in three dimensions. *J Exp Med.* **138** (4): 745-53. (1973)
5. Eiselt P, Kim BS, Chacko B, Isenberg B, Peters MC, Greene KG, Roland WD, Loebsack AB, Burg KJ, Culberson C, Halberstadt CR, Holder WD, Mooney DJ. Development of technologies aiding large-tissue engineering. *Biotechnol Prog.* **14** (1): 134-40. (1998)
6. Cassell OC, Hofer SO, Morrison WA, Knight KR. Vascularisation of tissue-engineered grafts: the regulation of angiogenesis in reconstructive surgery and in disease states. *Br J Plast Surg.* **55** (8): 603-10. (2002)
7. Wake MC, Patrick CW, Jr., Mikos AG. Pore morphology effects on the fibrovascular tissue growth in porous polymer substrates. *Cell Transplant.* **3** (4): 339-43. (1994)
8. Wenger A, Stahl A, Weber H, Finkenzeller G, Augustin HG, Stark GB, Kneser U. Modulation of in vitro angiogenesis in a three-dimensional spheroidal coculture model for bone tissue engineering. *Tissue Eng.* **10** (9-10): 1536-47. (2004)
9. Mooney DJ, Mikos AG. Growing new organs. *Sci Am.* **280** (4): 60-5. (1999)
10. Kneser U, Voogd A, Ohnolz J, Buettner O, Stangenberg L, Zhang YH, Stark GB, Schaefer DJ. Fibrin gel-immobilized primary osteoblasts in calcium phosphate bone cement: in vivo evaluation with regard to application as injectable biological bone substitute. *Cells Tissues Organs.* **179** (4): 158-69. (2005)
11. Beier JP, Kneser U, Stern-Strater J, Stark GB, Bach AD. Y chromosome detection of three-dimensional tissue-engineered skeletal muscle constructs in a syngeneic rat animal model. *Cell Transplant.* **13** (1): 45-53. (2004)
12. Kneser U, Kaufmann PM, Fiegel HC, Pollok JM, Kluth D, Herbst H, Rogiers X. Long-term differentiated function of heterotopically transplanted hepatocytes on three-dimensional polymer matrices. *J Biomed Mater Res.* **47** (4): 494-503. (1999)
13. Mimoun M, Hilligot P, Baux S. The nutrient flap: a new concept of the role of the flap and application to the salvage of arteriosclerotic lower limbs. *Plast Reconstr Surg.* **84** (3): 458-67. (1989)

14. Bach AD, Kopp J, Stark GB, Horch RE. The versatility of the free osteocutaneous fibula flap in the reconstruction of extremities after sarcoma resection. *World J Surg Oncol*. **2** (1): 22. (2004)
15. Tamai S, Komatsu S, Sakamoto H, Sano S, Sasauchi N. Free muscle transplants in dogs, with microsurgical neurovascular anastomoses. *Plast Reconstr Surg*. **46** (3): 219-25. (1970)
16. Chuang DC. Functioning free-muscle transplantation for the upper extremity. *Hand Clin*. **13** (2): 279-89. (1997)
17. McCraw JB. On the transfer of a free dorsalis pedis sensory flap to the hand. *Plast Reconstr Surg*. **59** (5): 738-9. (1977)
18. Hillsley MV, Frangos JA. Bone tissue engineering: the role of interstitial fluid flow. *Biotechnol Bioeng*. **43** (7): 573-81. (1994)
19. Erol OO, Spira M. New capillary bed formation with a surgically constructed arteriovenous fistula. *Surg Forum*. **30**: 530-1. (1979)
20. Vacanti JP, Langer R. Tissue engineering: the design and fabrication of living replacement devices for surgical reconstruction and transplantation. *Lancet*. **354 Suppl 1**: SI32-4. (1999)
21. Mian R, Morrison WA, Hurley JV, Penington AJ, Romeo R, Tanaka Y, Knight KR. Formation of new tissue from an arteriovenous loop in the absence of added extracellular matrix. *Tissue Eng*. **6** (6): 595-603. (2000)
22. Tanaka Y, Tsutsumi A, Crowe DM, Tajima S, Morrison WA. Generation of an autologous tissue (matrix) flap by combining an arteriovenous shunt loop with artificial skin in rats: preliminary report. *Br J Plast Surg*. **53** (1): 51-7. (2000)
23. Khouri RK, Upton J, Shaw WW. Prefabrication of composite free flaps through staged microvascular transfer: an experimental and clinical study. *Plast Reconstr Surg*. **87** (1): 108-15. (1991)
24. Akita S, Tamai N, Myoui A, Nishikawa M, Kaito T, Takaoka K, Yoshikawa H. Capillary vessel network integration by inserting a vascular pedicle enhances bone formation in tissue-engineered bone using interconnected porous hydroxyapatite ceramics. *Tissue Eng*. **10** (5-6): 789-95. (2004)
25. Lee JH, Cornelius CP, Schwenzer N. Neo-osseous flaps using demineralized allogeneic bone in a rat model. *Ann Plast Surg*. **44** (2): 195-204. (2000)
26. Kneser U, Polykandriotis E, Ohnolz J, Heidner K, Grabinger L, Euler S, Amann K, Hess A, Brune K, Greil P, Stürzl M, Horch RE. Engineering of vascularized transplantable bone tissues: Induction of axial vascularization in an osteoconductive matrix using an arteriovenous loop. *Submitted to: Tissue Eng*. (2005)
27. Kneser U, Polykandriotis E, Ohnolz J, Heidner K, Bach A, Kopp J, Horch R. Vascularized bone replacement for the treatment of chronic bone defects - initial results of microsurgical hard tissue vascularization. *Zeitschr Wundheilung*. **4** (3): 62-68. (2004)
28. Lametschwandtner A, Lametschwandtner U, Weiger T. Scanning electron microscopy of vascular corrosion casts--technique and applications: updated review. *Scanning Microsc*. **4** (4): 889-940; discussion 941. (1990)
29. Lametschwandtner A, Miodonski A, Simonsberger P. On the prevention of specimen charging in scanning electron microscopy of vascular corrosion casts by attaching conductive bridges. *Mikroskopie*. **36** (9-10): 270-3. (1980)
30. Macleod TM, Williams G, Sanders R, Green CJ. Histological evaluation of Permacol as a subcutaneous implant over a 20-week period in the rat model. *Br J Plast Surg*. **58** (4): 518-32. (2005)
31. Tanaka Y, Sung KC, Tsutsumi A, Ohba S, Ueda K, Morrison WA. Tissue engineering skin flaps: which vascular carrier, arteriovenous shunt loop or arteriovenous bundle, has more potential for angiogenesis and tissue generation? *Plast Reconstr Surg*. **112** (6): 1636-44. (2003)
32. Davies PF, Remuzzi A, Gordon EJ, Dewey CF, Jr., Gimbrone MA, Jr. Turbulent fluid shear stress induces vascular endothelial cell turnover in vitro. *Proc Natl Acad Sci U S A*. **83** (7): 2114-7. (1986)
33. Westerband A, Crouse D, Richter LC, Aguirre ML, Wixon CC, James DC, Mills JL, Hunter GC, Heimark RL. Vein adaptation to arterialization in an experimental model. *J Vasc Surg*. **33** (3): 561-9. (2001)
34. Milkiewicz M, Brown MD, Egginton S, Hudlicka O. Association between shear stress, angiogenesis, and VEGF in skeletal muscles in vivo. *Microcirculation*. **8** (4): 229-41. (2001)
35. Makanya AN, Stauffer D, Ribatti D, Burri PH, Djonov V. Microvascular growth, development, and remodeling in the embryonic avian kidney: the interplay between sprouting and intussusceptive angiogenic mechanisms. *Microsc Res Tech*. **66** (6): 275-88. (2005)
36. Huang YC, Kaigler D, Rice KG, Krebsbach PH, Mooney DJ. Combined angiogenic and osteogenic factor delivery enhances bone marrow stromal cell-driven bone regeneration. *J Bone Miner Res*. **20** (5): 848-57. (2005)
37. Kirkpatrick CJ, Unger RE, Krump-Konvalinkova V, Peters K, Schmidt H, Kamp G. Experimental approaches to study vascularization in tissue engineering and biomaterial applications. *J Mater Sci Mater Med*. **14** (8): 677-81. (2003)

38. Westerband A, Gentile AT, Hunter GC, Gooden MA, Aguirre ML, Berman SS, Mills JL. Intimal growth and neovascularization in human stenotic vein grafts. *J Am Coll Surg.* **191** (3): 264-71. (2000)
39. Masuda H, Kawamura K, Nanjo H, Sho E, Komatsu M, Sugiyama T, Sugita A, Asari Y, Kobayashi M, Ebina T, Hoshi N, Singh TM, Xu C, Zarins CK. Ultrastructure of endothelial cells under flow alteration. *Microsc Res Tech.* **60** (1): 2-12. (2003)
40. Diaz-Flores L, Gutierrez R, Varela H. Angiogenesis: an update. *Histol Histopathol.* **9** (4): 807-43. (1994)
41. Patrick CW, Jr., Chauvin PB, Hobley J, Reece GP. Preadipocyte seeded PLGA scaffolds for adipose tissue engineering. *Tissue Eng.* **5** (2): 139-51. (1999)

22

PREDICTIVE VALUE OF *IN VITRO* AND *IN VIVO* ASSAYS IN BONE AND CARTILAGE REPAIR — WHAT DO THEY REALLY TELL US ABOUT THE CLINICAL PERFORMANCE?

Pamela Habibovic[1], Tim Woodfield[2], Klaas de Groot[1], and Clemens van Blitterswijk[1]

22.1. INTRODUCTION

The continuous increase of life expectancy leads to an expanding demand for repair and replacement of damaged and degraded organs and tissues. Recent completion of a first version of the human genome sequence is a great breakthrough for the field of pharmaceutics. It is conceivable that new developments in pharmaceutical research will result in a large number of novel and improved medicines. A similar development is expected in the field of biomaterials designed for bone and cartilage repair and replacement. Spinal fusions and repairs of bone defects caused by trauma, tumors, infections, biochemical disorders and abnormal skeletal development, are some examples of the frequently performed surgeries in the clinic. For most of these surgeries, there is a great need for bone graft substitutes. Similarly, the number of patients worldwide experiencing joint pain and loss of mobility through trauma or degenerative cartilage conditions is considerable, and yet, few approaches employed clinically are capable of restoring long-term function to damaged articular cartilage[1,2]. Therefore, new materials and techniques need to be developed.

This expanding number of newly developed biomaterials and techniques are accompanied by an increased need for high-throughput screening systems which are reliable in predicting the performance of the material or construct in the function it was developed for. An example of a recently developed high-throughput system is microscale screening of polymer-cell interaction by using microarrays[3].

---

[1] Institute for Biomedical Technology, University of Twente, Bilthoven, The Netherlands
[2] Centre for Bioengineering, University of Canterbury, and Department of Orthopaedic Surgery & Musculoskeletal Medicine, Christchurch School of Medicine & Health Sciences, Christchurch, New Zealand

In this review, we attempt to provide answers to two questions regarding the reliability of the existing assays used in bone and cartilage repair strategies involving biomaterials: (i) what do *in vitro* assays really tell us about the *in vivo* performance? and (ii) what do *in vivo* assays tell us about the clinical conditions?

This review consists of two parts, one regarding bone- and one regarding articular cartilage repair and regeneration.

In the first part, we focus on limitations of the existing, frequently used assays to test the performance of synthetic biomaterials for bone repair and regeneration. We provide an introduction in *in vitro* bone formation assays in general, and an overview of organs and cells which are commonly applied in the *in vitro* bone formation assays. We then give an overview of a number of *in vitro* and *in vivo* studies performed with similar materials for bone repair, in order to investigate correlation between their results. Subsequently, we address the shortcomings of the existing *in vitro* assays and give some recommendation for their improvement. Finally, we give a short overview of different *in vivo* assays used to test biological performances of biomaterials for bone repair and regeneration.

The focus of the second part of this paper is shifted from biomaterials alone to tissue-engineered hybrids for articular cartilage restoration, as in this, rather new field, the use of biomaterials alone is rare. We first give a short review of biomaterials and cells which are frequently used for development of tissue engineering hybrids for cartilage repair. We then discuss different parameters which can be of influence when combining cells and biomaterials to produce tissue engineered hybrids. We point out some drawbacks of the existing *in vitro* assays which are used to predict the *in vivo* performance of the hybrid constructs and elaborate on possible ways to improve the existing assays. Finally, we review different *in vivo* animal models, together with their advantages and shortcomings in order to shed light upon their predictive value for the clinical setting.

22.2. BACKGROUND ON *IN VITRO* BONE FORMATION ASSAYS

In research into new bone graft substitutes, two types of preclinical assays are used in general: *in vitro* assays using a cell- or an organ culture system (i.e. *in vitro* bone formation assays) and *in vivo* assays, using experimental animal models. *In vitro* assays have initially been developed to study the influence of growth factors and hormones on attachment, proliferation, differentiation and mineralization of cells for example. Subsequently, investigators started to use these *in vitro* assays in biomaterials research. Instead of studying the influence of e.g. growth factors on the differentiation of cells, the behavior of cells in the presence of the testing material is studied. However, in general, it is ignored that the *in vitro* setting may significantly be changed by the presence of a material due to e.g. material-cell culture medium interaction. If such an interaction is not expected *in vivo*, it raises the question of what the predictive value of the *in vitro* assay is for the *in vivo* performance of the material.

Besides the increasing need for reliable *in vitro* assays to test biomaterials prior to implanting them in animals and humans, investigators need tools which are helpful in unraveling mechanisms of complex *in vivo* phenomena regarding bone formation. *In vitro* assays are attractive because of their simplicity, but, at the same time, their simplicity is an important limitation. It is of course impossible to fully simulate the *in vivo* situation in a culture dish and yet in many publications, rather strong conclusions about the *in vivo* performance of biomaterials and about mechanisms of complex biological phenomena are drawn from the *in vitro* studies.

22.2.1. Cells and Cell Sources

In vitro bone formation assays have initially been developed as tools to study the effects of hormones and cytokines in a controlled environment [4]. Despite the inherent diversity in these systems, most of them share some common features. For example, the basic culture environment (e.g. medium composition, serum type and concentration, supplements, temperature and antibiotics) and methods of routine maintenance (e.g. feeding, subculturing, cloning) are very similar in all systems. Gronowicz and Raisz [4] have given an overview of the culture conditions which are generally applicable for different *in vitro* bone formation culture systems. The fact that they give a simplified reflection of the *in vivo* situation and allow for the research in a controlled environment are primary reasons for the use of *in vitro* assays. In addition, from financial and ethical point of view, *in vitro* assays are preferred above the *in vivo* ones.

The existing bone formation assays can be divided into two groups: organ culture systems and bone cell culture systems.

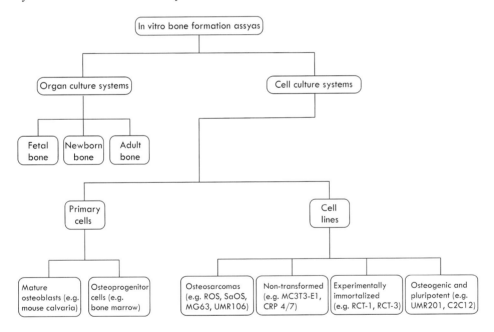

Figure 22.1. Overview of *in vitro* bone formation assays.

As reviewed by Gronowicz and Raisz [4], tissues used for bone formation assays in bone organ culture systems vary in source and age including fetal, newborn and occasionally adult bone. Chicken, mouse and rat bones are most common, although human bone fragments have also been used. Bone from calvaria and limb are the most frequently cultured tissues. Fetal calvaria are characterized by intramembraneous bone formation, while growth of long bones is mainly endochondral. However, as intra–membraneous and endochondral bone may have different responses to hormones, growth factors and environmental conditions, most *in vitro* organ culture systems have limitations and may not give a similar response as endochondral bone and adult bone cells.

In addition to organ culture systems, the *in vitro* isolation and culture of bone-derived cell populations has substantially enhanced our ability to understand factors important for the proliferation and differentiation of cells of the osteogenic lineage. As recently reviewed by Kartsogiannis and Ng [5], commonly employed model systems include either primary cultures of osteoblastic cells derived from fetal calvaria and subperiosteal fetal long bones, or established cell lines that can be divided into clonal cell lines from cells isolated from bone tumors (osteosarcomas), non-transformed cell lines, experimentally immortalized cell lines and bone marrow cultures. Figure 22.1. gives an overview of *in vitro* bone formation assays.

22.3. *IN VITRO* MODELS FOR ASSAYING BONE GRAFT SUBSTITUTES

As mentioned previously, the expanding development of (synthetic) biomaterials for support, replacement and regeneration of bone has created the need for *in vitro* systems in which the potential *in vivo* performance of these materials can be assayed. *In vitro* cell- and organ culture assays are in the first place used to investigate the "safety" of the material in terms of cytotoxicity and biocompatibility for example. In addition, *in vitro* bone formation assays are used in order to predict the performance of the material *in vivo* in its role of e.g. bone filler. In this case, the potential osteoconductivity of the material is tested. Finally, *in vitro* cell culture systems are used to study complex and not yet fully unraveled "biologically driven" phenomena such as osteoinduction. Below, we give a few examples of *in vitro* studies in which materials' cytotoxicity, osteoconductivity and osteoinductivity were assayed. In addition, the results and authors' conclusions drawn from these studies are compared to the results *in vivo*, where similar materials were tested.

22.3.1. Cytotoxicity

Hyakuna et al. investigated changes in calcium-, phosphate-, magnesium- and albumin content of cell culture medium after immersion of different biomaterials [6]. The results of this study showed that monocrystalline and polycrystalline alumina ceramics did not have any influence on the surrounding medium. Two types of apatite containing glass ceramics (apatite and wollastonite-containing glass ceramic (AW-GC) and apatite-, wollastonite- and whitlockite-containing glass ceramic (AW-CP-GC)) showed a slight decrease of phosphorus and a slight increase of calcium ion concentration in the culture medium. Hydroxyapatite (HA) ceramics sintered at 600°C and 900°C with a very high specific surface area showed a high and rapid adsorption of calcium- and phosphate ions and albumin from the medium. Changes of calcium and phosphate concentrations of the medium were suggested to be the reason for the poor attachment of V79 Chinese hamster fibroblasts, and hence for a higher apparent cytotoxicity of the HA ceramics sintered at

600 and 900°C and the two glass ceramics as compared to the tissue culture plastic and alumina ceramics.

Suzuki et al. prepared ceramics with calcium to phosphorus (Ca/P) ratios varying from 1.50 to 1.67 by mixing different amounts of HA and tricalcium phosphate (TCP) ceramics and observed variations of zeta-potentials of different surfaces after immersion in the cell culture medium [7]. Decrease of calcium- and phosphate ions in the culture medium was always observed, but its intensity depended on the Ca/P ratio of the ceramics and so did the change of the pH of the medium. Changes of the ions concentrations and pH of the medium were suggested to be of influence on the attachment of L-929 cells on the ceramic surfaces, and thus on the cytotoxicity of the material.

Knabe and coworkers performed a similar study, in which they compared attachment and proliferation of rat bone marrow cells (RBMCs) on highly resorbable calcium-phosphate (CaP) ceramics [8] and on glassy materials with different rates of resorbability [9]. Interestingly, while in the studies described previously authors observed a decrease of calcium- and phosphate ions from the medium and suggested this decrease to be the reason for poor attachment and growth of the cells, Knabe and coauthors suggested that the inhibitory effect on cellular growth on some of their materials was associated with an increased concentration of phosphorus ions released into the medium by these materials and the formation of a phosphorus-rich layer on their surface. Daily refreshment of the medium increased the osteoblast attachment on some, but not on all tested ceramics.

In later work of this group, in which highly resorbable CaP cements and CaP ceramics were compared, it was suggested that increased levels of phosphate- and potassium ions, decreased levels of calcium ions and hence elevated pH of the medium were reasons for poor attachment and proliferation of RBMCs.

The above described examples of studies in which safety of materials in terms of cytotoxicity was tested all emphasized the presence of the biomaterial-cell culture medium interaction, which seems to be responsible for, or at least of influence on the behavior of cells. Although material-medium interactions are sometimes of great influence on the behavior of cells *in vitro*, in the *in vivo* environment they might be less important if observed at all, as, unlike in a culture dish, in the body there is a continuous supply and thus refreshment of nutrients and body fluids. For the cytotoxicity tests, this probably means that the *in vitro* settings give a more "negative" reflection of *in vivo* situation.

22.3.2. Osteoconduction

Osteoconduction, defined as "spreading of bone over the surface proceeded by ordered migration of differentiating osteogenic cells" [10], is supposed to be driven by physico-chemical properties of the material, having its origin in dissolution/reprecipitation or precipitation of a CaP layer on the surface of the material [11,12]. An important aspect is thereby the direct bonding of bone to the material without fibrous tissue deposition, so-called contact or bonding osteogenesis [10]. In a few studies, these properties of the materials were tested first *in vitro* and then *in vivo*.

De Bruijn et al. used an *in vitro* RBMCs culture system to study various types of CaPs [13]. Besides the elaboration of different interfaces, mineralization occurred at a later time on slow degrading materials such as fluorapatite (FA), than on fast degrading materials such as TCP. Authors therefore suggested that a more dynamic interface is formed on degrading materials that could be favorable for bone formation to occur. This hypothesis was further tested by implanting various plasma-sprayed CaP coatings in rat femoral bone for relatively short period of time[14]. The results of this study indeed suggested that initially a greater amount of bone was formed on fast degrading amorphous HA as opposed to the slow degrading highly crystalline HA.

A recent report by Wang and coworkers described a comparison of proliferation and differentiation of SaOS-2 osteoblastic cell line on HA ceramics sintered at three different temperatures (1200°C, 1000°C and 800°C) [15]. Results of this study showed that cell proliferation rate on HA ceramic sintered at 1200°C was the greatest. In addition, Bone Sialoprotein (BSP), Osteocalcin (OC) and Osteonectin (ON) protein levels after 12-day-culture were significantly higher on HA sintered at 1200°C as compared to HA ceramics sintered at 1000°C and 800°C respectively. Authors therefore concluded that HA ceramic sintered at 1200°C, which had a significantly lower specific surface area than the other two ceramics, was the best candidate to be used as a bone graft. They suggested that the ceramic sintered at higher temperature possibly had a less reactive surface and hence a lower cytotoxicity as compared to the other two tested ceramics. These results were in accordance with the results of the *in vitro* study of Hyakuna et al.[6]. In a study by our group [16] however, biphasic calcium phosphate (BCP, consisting of HA and β-TCP) ceramics sintered at 1150°C and at 1300°C were implanted in a critical-sized iliac wing defect of goats. Significantly more bone was found in the orthotopically implanted BCP sintered at 1150°C as compared to BCP sintered at 1300°C [16]. The two materials had similar compositions and macroporosities and they only differed in their microporosities. BCP1150 with its higher microporosity and hence higher specific surface area in comparison with BCP1300 was suggested to have a higher surface reactivity, which was consequently the reason for a higher bone regenerative potential. These *in vivo* results were thus in conflict with the *in vitro* data given by Hyakuna et al.[6] and Wang et al.[15], in which ceramics sintered at higher temperatures showed a more pronounced cell proliferation and osteogenic differentiation.

The above described are only a few examples of studies in which *in vitro* bone formation assays were used to predict the performance of biomaterials *in vivo*. As can be seen, in some studies, *in vitro* results completely fit the *in vivo* results, while in the others, differences observed *in vitro* could not be found *in vivo* or were in full contrast with the *in vivo* data. In the reviewed studies, both *in vitro* and *in vivo* studies were performed with similar biomaterials. This is, however, not always the case. Sometimes, only *in vitro* results are presented, and authors use these to draw conclusions on the performance of materials *in vivo*, which makes it impossible to elaborate on the predictive value of the *in vitro* assays.

22.3.3. Osteoinduction

Osteoinduction is an even less understood phenomenon as compared to osteoconduction. In the sixties, osteoinduction was defined as "the differentiation of the undifferentiated inducible osteoprogenitor cells that are not yet committed to the osteogenic lineage to form osteoprogenitor cells"[17]. In other words, osteoinductivity is the ability of a cytokine or a material to induce bone formation ectopically. Extensive research of Urist and others led to the conclusion that a discrete protein within the demineralized bone matrix (DBM) was the sole inducer of bone formation. This finding was published in 1971 and this protein was named Bone Morphogenetic Protein (BMP)[18]. BMP was shown to be involved in the bone formation cascade of chemotaxis, mitosis, differentiation, callus formation and finally bone formation. Besides the BMP-driven osteoinduction, many investigators have shown that also some biomaterials that neither contain nor produce BMPs are also able to induce ectopic bone formation [19-25]. Despite the extensive research, the underlying mechanism of osteoinduction is still largely unknown, and reliable assays to study this mechanism are needed. Below, a few *in vitro* studies on osteoinduction are described.

Adkisson et al. [26] developed a "rapid quantitative bioassay of osteoinduction" by using SaOS-2 osteosarcomas and studied cell proliferation rates under the influence of DBM. The observed correlation between cell proliferation and osteoinduction was not strong. Osteogenic factors, like BMP are not commonly associated with mitogenic response.

Zhang et al. [27] and Wolfinbarger and Zhang [28] used human periosteal cells and human dermal fibroblasts to relate cellular ALP activity to DBM osteoinductivity. In these studies, the authors failed to show a clear correlation between *in vitro* assays and *in vivo* bone formation.

Carnes et al. used an immature osteoprogenitor cell line, 2T9 to investigate the effect of DBM on their differentiation [29]. They failed to show any effect on differentiation and concluded that there are no soluble factors being released from DBM into the culture medium.

Han et al. assayed Alkaline Phosphatase (ALP) activity of the C2C12 cells in a culture in presence of DBM, and succeeded correlating it with the *in vivo* bone formation [30]. The last study mimics the *in vivo* situation more than other described studies, although the expression of ALP is not the most sensitive marker for the osteogenic differentiation.

Regarding the mechanism of osteoinduction by biomaterials, a very limited number of studies are performed and published. In our group, an extensive number of studies have been performed *in vivo*. In addition, we have tried to perform a number of *in vitro* studies as well, however, their results were either inconclusive, or in contrast with the *in vivo* observations. A few examples of the performed studies are described below.

In an earlier published study [21], HA ceramics sintered at 1150°C and 1250°C together with biphasic calcium phosphate (BCP, consisting of HA and β-TCP) ceramics sintered at 1100°C, 1150°C and 1200°C were implanted intramuscularly in goats and we found that HA sintered at 1150°C induced bone formation intramuscularly, while no bone was induced by HA sintered at 1250°C. Furthermore, the amount of induced bone by BCP ceramics increased with decreasing sintering temperatures.

In another study [16], BCP ceramics sintered at 1150°C and at 1300°C were implanted intramuscularly in goats. Ectopic bone formation was only found in the BCP sintered at lower temperature [16]. The presence of microporosity in BCP1150 was suggested to be responsible for a higher osteoinductive potential in comparison with BCP1300 ceramic. In order to compare BCP1150 and BCP1300 *in vitro*, we cultured MC3T3-E1 osteblastic-like cells and C2C12 pluripotent mesenchymal cells (in presence and in absence of BMP-2) on BCP1150 and BCP1300 ceramics and consequently investigated the expression of various osteogenic markers using RT-PCR (e.g mRNA for ALP, Parathyroid Hormone receptor (PTH-r), OC, ON, Osteoblast-Specific Factor 2 (OSF-2) and Osterix (Osx)). For both cell types, a higher expression of most markers was observed on BCP1300 than on BCP1150 (Figure 22.2.). Furthermore, the expression of these markers was the highest in cells cultured on tissue-culture (TC) plastic.

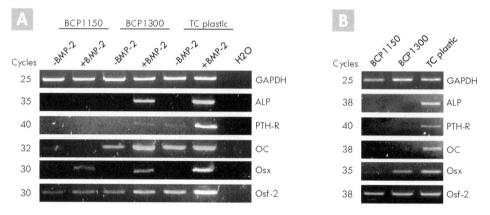

Figure 22.2. RT-PCR data showing the temporal expression of osteogenic mRNA by C2C12 cells cultured with and without BMP-2 (100ng/ml) (A) and MC3T3-E1 cells cultured without ascorbic acid (B) for 6 days on BCP1300 and BCP1150 discs (diameter 25mm, height 5 mm). The expression of most osteogenic markers by C2C12 cells (A) is increased when cells are cultured in presence of BMP-2. In both presence and absence of BMP-2, the expression of most markers is highest when the C2C12 cells are cultured on tissue culture plastic. Cells show a higher expression of osteogenic markers when cultured on BCP1300 as compared to BCP1150. Similar to C2C12 cells, the expression of all investigated osteogenic markers by MC3T3-E1 cells (B) is the highest on TC plastic, followed by BCP1300 and then BCP1150.

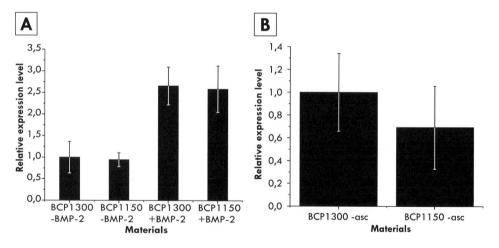

Figure 22.3. Q-PCR data (n=3) showing relative expression of Osteocalcin mRNA by C2C12 cells cultured with and without BMP-2 (100ng/ml) (A) and MC3T3-E1 cells cultured without ascorbic acid (B) for 6 days on BCP1300 and BCP1150 particles (1-2 μm). The Osteocalcin expression by C2C12 cells (A) is significantly increased when cells are cultured in presence of BMP-2 on both BCP1300 and BCP1150 ceramic. There are no significant differences in the Osteocalcin expression between cells cultured on BCP1300 and BCP1150 for neither cell type. However, the trend for both cell types is the same, namely a slight downregulation of Osteocalcin expression on BCP1150 as compared to BCP1300.

Measurements of calcium and phosphate contents of the medium after 3 hours of soaking showed a decrease of calcium concentration with 22% and a decrease of phosphate concentration with 18% in presence of BCP1300, while the decrease of calcium and phosphate concentrations in presence of BCP1150 were 62% and 60%, respectively. After 3 days of soaking, which is the normal time point at which culture medium is refreshed, calcium- and phosphate contents of the culture medium further decreased with 8% for both ceramics. No changes in calcium- and phosphate contents of the medium in the absence of ceramics were observed.

In order to decrease the change of the contents of the medium, we repeated the experiment with MC3T3-E1 and C2C12 cell lines by using considerably smaller (±100 times lower volume) amount of BCP1150 and BCP1300 scaffolds in the same volume of medium. This time, the amount of calcium decreased with 7% and the amount of phosphate with 11% in presence of BCP1300 scaffold after 3 days of soaking. Decrease of calcium concentration was 36% and that of phosphate 40% in presence of BCP1150. Although differences in the expression of OC (Figure 22.3., Q-PCR data) for MC3T3-E1 and C2C12 cells between BCP1150 and BCP1300 were smaller this time, the trend of expression remained the same. Differentiation of cells towards the osteogenic lineage was higher on BCP1300 as compared to BCP1150, while *in vivo* significantly more bone was induced by BCP1150 in comparison to BCP1300.

A similar study was performed with mouse embryonic stem cells (to be published separately), and interestingly, in this study, the expression of mRNA for OC and BSP was higher on BCP1150 as compared to BCP1300. Whether these results mean that the effect of the material is only visible in very early stages of differentiation, or simply that ESCs react differently to the changes of the medium caused by the presence of ceramics as compared to C2C12 and MC3T3-E1 cells, needs to be further investigated.

22.3.4. Limitations of *In Vitro* Models for Assaying Bone Graft Substitutes and Recommendations for Their Improvement

All examples described above suggest that the use of the existing *in vitro* assays in biomaterials research might not always be valuable. Sometimes, the *in vitro* data are completely in accordance with the *in vivo* findings, especially when rather simple physico-chemically guided processes are studied. In other studies, in which more complex, biologically driven processes are studied, *in vitro* and *in vivo* results are in full contrast with each other. The question that needs to be answered is what the cause of these inconclusive results is.

First of all it is important to note that in most cell culture and organ culture systems involving biomaterials there is, in addition to cell-biomaterial interaction, often a very important biomaterial-cell culture medium interaction which often markedly influences the outcomes of the study. In the *in vivo* environment these interactions might be less important if observed at all, as, unlike in a culture dish, in the body there is a continuous supply and thus refreshment of nutrients and body fluids.

Although most examples given above are studies performed on CaP containing biomaterials, the changes in the medium can also be caused by non-CaP materials (e.g. certain polymeric sponges [31], alumina ceramics [32], and porous titanium [33] scaffolds are capable of forming a CaP layer when immersed in a CaP-rich environment). Release of calcium, phosphate, magnesium, and other ions from highly resorbable materials, uptake of different ions from the culture medium by a high surface area of a material, changes of pH and Z-potentials on the surfaces, formation of phosphorus and/or calcium rich layers on the surfaces, adsorption of all, or selected proteins from the serum-containing cell culture media, are only a few observations from these types of studies. Obviously, all these changes of the medium differ significantly between the tested materials and raise therefore the question if such *in vitro* systems are applicable for the comparative types of experiments. Different studies focus on comparing material A with material B by studying cell attachment, proliferation, differentiation and mineralization on their surfaces. However, if the interaction between material A and the culture medium is different from the interaction between material B and the culture medium, the cells will attach, grow and differentiate in different environments and can therefore not be compared with each other when similar biomaterial-body fluid interactions are not expected *in vivo*. In addition, changes which take place in the medium due to the presence of a biomaterial will influence different cell types in a different manner, which makes comparisons between different studies difficult, if not impossible.

In addition to taking into account possible side effects of the presence of biomaterials in *in vitro* cell culture systems, the choice of cells is of great importance for the reliability of the results. For example, if one would like to compare two biomaterials and be able to draw some conclusions regarding their potential performance as bone graft substitute, would the attachment and proliferation of primary rat osteoblasts then be the right assay knowing that *in vivo* osteoblasts are not the cells which are initially in contact with biomaterial surface? The choice is probably even more difficult when one is trying to investigate a largely unknown phenomenon *in vitro*, such as osteoinduction by BMPs or even less understood osteoinduction by biomaterials. Obviously, in order to study the mechanism of osteoinduction by biomaterials, it is probably not sufficient to choose osteoblasts or osteoblast-like cells as osteoinduction is the process of differentiation of cells that are not yet committed to the osteogenic lineage to form osteoprogenitor cells. Therefore, murine pluripotent mesenchymal C2C12 cells could be better candidates than osteoblasts. However, it is well-known that ectopic bone formation by biomaterials is only very rarely found in mice [34-37], making cells of murine origin possibly an inadequate choice. In addition, it is hard to decide whether the culture of C2C12 cells on osteoinductive biomaterials should be performed in presence or in absence of e.g. BMP-2, as it is suggested, but not yet proven [22, 38], that BMPs play a role in the process of osteoinduction by biomaterials. Similar questions of the choice of cell origin and culture conditions should be answered if one would choose to use ESCs to study the phenomenon of osteoinduction by biomaterials *in vitro*.

In conclusion, in our opinion, the *in vitro* assays which are nowadays used to study the potential performance of biomaterials *in vivo*, have a largely limited predictive value. It should be emphasized again that the existing *in vitro* assays have originally been designed to test the influence of growth factors, cytokines and hormones on the behavior of cells and organs. In these *in vitro* assays, the presence of a material has never been taken into account. However, in the studies involving biomaterials, there is, in addition to the material-cell interaction, which is supposed to be studied, often a material-medium interaction, which can be of high importance for the results and should therefore not be ignored. Prior to starting an experiment, the following questions should be answered: (i) is there an interaction between the testing material and the medium?, (ii) does this interaction have a consequence for the results of the study? and (iii) is a similar interaction expected *in vivo*? If the biomaterial-cell culture medium seems to be an artifact of the system used, this effect of biomaterial-medium interaction should be removed. Knabe and coworkers suggested for example preincubation of the material in the medium prior to the start of cell culture and daily medium replenishment [8]. Although possibly successful for some biomaterials, this solution might be expensive, in particular if the cell culture is performed in presence of e.g. growth factors. Another possible solution could be the use of bioreactors in *in vitro* systems, with continuous monitoring and adjustment of the changing contents of the medium. Only if cells grow in the same medium, their interactions with different biomaterials can be compared in a useful way, and only then some careful conclusions can be drawn regarding their potential *in vivo* performance.

As mentioned previously, the choice of cells and assays can be of great importance on the outcomes of *in vitro* studies. This is important when e.g. osteoconductive potential of a biomaterial is studied. Instead of using mature osteoblasts, which are responsible for appositional bone growth rather than for *de novo* bone formation *in vivo*, the use of inducible and determined osteoprogenitor cells, as present in the bone marrow, might be more useful. When studying not yet unraveled complex biological phenomena such as osteoinduction, initially a pluripotent cell line should be used. The use of a homogeneous cell population can give an insight into processes governing osteoinduction. In the next step, adult mesenchymal stem cells from the recipient site (mostly muscle, or perivascular cells) should be used, as they are most probably involved in the process of osteoinduction.

22.4. *IN VIVO* MODELS FOR ASSAYING SYNTHETIC BONE GRAFT SUBSTITUTES

As described previously, the existing *in vitro* models used to assay safety and biological performances of synthetic bone graft substitutes are often not predictable for the *in vivo* situation, and therefore, every bone repair strategy needs to be established in an animal model before being used in human patients. Similar to the question whether *in vitro* models are predictive for the performance of biomaterials *in vivo*, it is important to investigate whether assays in animal models are predictive for the clinical setting. The number of publications in which the performance of synthetic bone graft substitutes and tissue engineered constructs for bone repair in humans is directly linked to the preclinical *in vivo* results is very limited. Therefore, this paragraph is limited to review of frequently used animal models for bone repair and regeneration. In addition, we address some limitations associated with the use of *in vivo* models.

22.4.1. Soft Tissue Models

As reviewed by Jansen [39], the first test following *in vitro* assays is *in vivo* compatibility of materials for short and prolonged periods of time. Soft tissue implantation is an attractive model to study safety of the materials in terms of e.g. toxicity and carcinogenicity, as it is rather inexpensive, readily available and yet relevant, as many materials used as bone graft substitutes come in contact with subcutaneous tissue, muscles, fasciae and tendons. The two most frequently used soft tissue models are subcutaneous and intramuscular implantation. It has been shown that biocompatibility response of implant materials can differ between the two test sites, due to differences in vascularization, regenerative capacity and intrinsic stress. The selection of a suitable animal for biocompatibility testing is another complex issue. Mice, rats and rabbits are most often used for soft tissue implantations. The advantage of these, relatively small animals is their availability and low cost. However, their metabolic and wound healing properties differ from those of large animals and humans.

In addition to testing safety of biomaterials, soft tissue models are needed to study osteoinductive potential of DBM, purified BMPs or other cytokines and growth factors, osteoinductive properties of biomaterials and osteogenic properties of e.g. cells or tissue-engineered hybrids. An and Friedman gave an overview of the frequently used soft tissue models (e.g. subcutaneous, intramuscular, intraperitoneal and mesentery) to assay osteogenicity prior to orthotopic implantation [40].

Concerning the soft tissue models used to study the mechanisms of the, still largely unknown, phenomena such as osteoinduction, a careful choice of animal model and implantation site is of large importance. For example, as mentioned earlier, bone induction by BMPs is often observed in mice and rats, so these small animals are convenient for use in models to test osteoinductive capacity of DBM for example. Osteoinduction by biomaterials is, in contrast, rarely observed in small animals, so a large animal model is needed. However, it appears that there exist differences in osteoinductive potential of the materials implanted in different large animals; the same material induced more bone in dogs than in goats and rabbits [37], and even more bone was induced in baboons [41]. The reason for this interspecies difference is not completely understood yet, but it should certainly be taken into account when designing a study and interpreting its results.

In addition to the interspecies differences, large differences between individuals within species are often observed. For example, in addition to the difference in the response to BMPs between different animals [42], there are reports of differences in the response to BMPs between the individuals of the same species, probably due to genetic factors [43]. Similar differences were also observed in humans [44]. Also osteoinduction by biomaterials in goats has been shown to significantly differ between the individuals [16, 21, 45]. In order to avoid possible intraspecies differences, paired implantations, i.e. implantations of all test materials in all test animals are recommended.

22.4.2. Bone Fracture and Bone Defect Models

As reviewed by An et al. [46], diaphyseal fractures are most commonly used model to study bone fracture healing. Frequently used animals for studying diaphyseal fracture healing are rats, rabbits, dogs and sheep. Tibial fractures in rats, sheep and dogs are examples of the models of diaphyseal fractures. In addition to diaphysael fractures, epiphysometaphyseal osteotomy in rabbits, sheep, goats and dogs and delayed union and nonunion in rats, rabbits and dogs are other models to study bone fracture healing.

In order to study healing of bone defects, e.g. in the presence of a bone graft, four types of defect are typically used: calvarial-, long bone (or mandible) segmental-, partial cortical- (e.g. cortical window, wedge defect, or transcortical drill hole) and cancellous-bone defects. The commonly used animals are rats, rabbits, sheep and dogs, while goats and primates are sometimes used as well. The calvarial (critical-sized) defect and long bone segmental defect are the most often used models for bone defect healing. Different animal models of bone defect repair are reviewed by An and Friedman [40].

22.4.3. Limitations of *In Vivo* Models for Assaying Bone Graft Substitutes and Recommendations for Their Improvement

Although animal models are used as a final test of the biomaterial performance prior to its use in the clinic, results of these preclinical studies might not be predictive for the materials performance in the clinical setting. In human patients, synthetic bone graft substitutes are used to repair and help regenerate (often large) defects caused by tumors, trauma, infections and hormonal disorders. Treatment of such diseased tissues in often elderly patients is hardly comparable with the treatment of an artificially made defect in the bone of young, healthy animals. In addition, it is conceivable that, based on frequently observed interspecies differences, results from any kind of animal are not (completely) predictive for the performance in humans. Finally, differences observed between individuals of the same species make it impossible to draw any general conclusions about the performance of a material as bone graft substitute.

Despite the fact that *in vivo* assays might not be completely predictive for the clinical performance of a material, their use can give valuable information about its biological behavior. It is, however, of great importance that *in vivo* studies are well designed and that their results are well analyzed. As already mentioned, paired implantations are important in order to exclude the effect of intraspecies variations as much as possible. In addition, more attention should be paid on finding non-invasive evaluation methods that allow for visualization of bone growth dynamics, as one of the important limitations of the classical *in vivo* studies is that only end results are visible. For example, use of fluorochrome markers is a helpful tool for the (qualitative or semi-quantitative) analysis of the bone growth dynamics [16, 47, 48]. The use of labeled cells is becoming helpful in studying the performance of bone tissue engineered hybrids [49]. Transgenic animals offer an important tool to study molecular pathways which take place in the process of bone formation in time [50]. However, so far, only transgenic mice and rats are available and therefore studying clinically relevant processes of bone formation remains a challenge.

22.5. BACKGROUND ON CARTILAGE TISSUE ENGINEERING

Tissue engineering approaches for repairing articular cartilage generally adopt two strategies; scaffold with cells, or scaffolds alone (Figure 22.4.). In general, scaffolds for cell-based strategies are intended to provide a compatible carrier for viable cells responsible for enhancing restoration of functional ECM and integration with surrounding native cartilage and subchondral bone. In strategies employing scaffolds alone, the scaffold material and geometry are designed to organize and enhance neo-tissue formation from host blood- and bone marrow-derived mesenchymal cells infiltrating the defect (i.e. osteochondral defects). The ability to further stimulate repair quality of cell-seeded scaffolds *in vitro* is possible by manipulating the culture environment via mechanical and/or bioactive stimuli, with accurate control offered via advanced bioreactor culture systems. Alternatively, scaffolds pre-seeded with genetically modified cells, or scaffolds engineered to release bioactive or gene factors can be used to promote desired repair pathways or inhibit undesired processes.

In all cases, since articular cartilage is a load bearing tissue, it is important that the scaffold contain sufficient mechanical properties to protect cells and support maturation of engineered tissue [51, 52]. Balancing these mechanical requirements, it is preferable that scaffold biodegradation rate is controlled to allow suitable function of the implant in the short- to mid-term, but be completely degradable in the long term following repair tissue maturation.

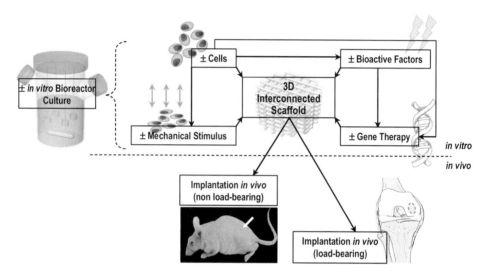

Figure 22.4. Diagram illustrating *in vitro* and *in vivo* model systems for evaluating cartilage tissue engineering strategies (adapted from Woodfield et al. [51]).

22.5.1. Scaffolds and Matrices

A full review of the various natural and synthetic biomaterials for cartilage tissue engineering strategies is beyond the scope of this chapter, and has been given previously [2, 51, 53, 54]. For the purpose of describing various *in vitro* and *in vivo* models systems and their limitations on scaffold design, it is important to introduce the common biomaterials and modern processing techniques used to develop porous 3D scaffolds for cartilage tissue engineering. These are summarized in Table 22.1.

By far the most common techniques for generating porosity include the various forms of foaming and particle leaching. Most of these techniques rely on generating porosity using porogens (*e.g.* a gas or particulate). While the size and, to a certain extent, the distribution of these porogens can be controlled during processing, their position and orientation to one another are inherently random. The control over scaffold architecture using these fabrication techniques are therefore highly *process* driven, and not *design* driven. This lack of control in pore structure, particularly with respect to the interconnectivity between pores causes considerable difficulties in designing porous scaffolds whose 3D pore architecture is critical for eliciting specific cell function and

Table 22.1. Scaffold materials and fabrication techniques for cartilage tissue engineering applications.

Biomaterial	Fabrication technique	Pore size (μm)	Application *in vitro* / *in vivo* [1]	Ref
Natural materials				
Collagen	Freeze drying, in situ cross-linked gel	-	Canine CH defect; rabbits OC defect; human OA defect	55-57
Chitosan	Thermosetting gel;	-	Chondrogenesis *in vitro* and in nude mouse; rabbit CH and OC defect	58, 59
Alginate	In situ cross-linked gel	-	Chondrogenesis *in vitro* and in nude mouse; rabbit OC defect	60-62
Agarose	In situ cross-linked gel	-	Chondrogenesis *in vitro*; rabbit CH defect.	63, 64
Hyaluronic acid (HYA)	Foaming + particulate leaching	26-83	Rabbit OC defect	65, 66
Synthetic polymers				
Polylactic acid (PLA)	Solvent casting + particulate leaching; non-woven fibre mesh	200-500	Chondrogenesis *in vitro* and in nude mouse; Rabbit OC defect	67-70
Polyglycolic acid (PGA)	Non-woven fibre mesh	<100	Chondrogenesis *in vitro* and in nude mouse; Rabbit CH defect	71-73
Polylactide-co-glycolide (PLGA)	Phase separation; solvent casting + particulate leaching	200-500	MSC Chondrogenesis in rabbit OC defect; Goat OC defect	68, 74
Polycaprolactone (PCL)	Fused deposition modelling*; nanofibre electrospinning	380-590 <10	MSC chondrogenesis *in vitro* and in subcutaneous rabbit model;	75 76
Polyehtylene glycol-terephthalate–polybutylene terephthalate (PEGT/PBT)	Compression moulding + particulate leaching; 3D plotting*	160-180 100-2000	Chondrogenesis *in vitro* and in nude mouse	77-80
Oligo-poly(ethylene glycol) fumarate (OPF)	In situ thermally cross-linked gel	-	Chondrogenesis *in vitro*	81
Poly(ethylene oxide)-dimethacrylate (PEG/DMA), polyvinyl alcohol (PVA)	In situ photo-polymerising gel	-	Chondrogenesis *in vitro* and in nude mouse	82, 83
Biphasic scaffolds (C: cartilage phase, B: bone phase)				
C: PLA B: hydroxyapatite (HA)	C: Solvent casting + particulate leaching, B: Indirect SFF (lost mould casting)*	C: 50-100 B: 300-800	Chondrogenesis, bone formation in nude mouse	84
C: OPF B: OPF	C + B: In situ thermally cross-linked gel	C: - B: -	Rabbit OC defect	85
C: PGA B: collagen/HA/tri-calcium phosphate (TCP)	C: non-woven mesh B: -	C: <100 B: -	Rabbit OC defect	86
C: PLGA/PLA B: PLGA/TCP	C + B: 3D printing* + particulate leaching	C: 250 B: > 125	Chondrogenesis *in vitro*	87
C: agarose B: devitalized bone	C: In situ cross-linked gel, B: machining of devitalized bone	C: - B: -	Chondrogenesis *in vitro* in anatomic scaffold	63

[1] CH = chondral; OC = osteochondral; * = solid free-form fabrication (SFF) technique

subsequent tissue formation. As a result, investigators have recently turned to solid free-form fabrication (SFF) techniques to produce porous scaffolds for tissue engineering applications [54, 75, 88-94]. SFF processing techniques allow highly complex and reproducible structures to be constructed one layer at a time via computer-aided design (CAD) models and computer-aided machining (CAM) processes. These techniques essentially allow researchers to *design-in* desired properties, such as porosity, interconnectivity and pore size, in a number of polymer and ceramic materials [90, 95-99].

These developments have opened the doors for more precise studies on the effects of designed pore architectures on cartilage tissue formation *in vitro* and *in vivo* [52]. The key breakthrough that these types of scaffold processing techniques offer is that they allow tissue engineers to more easily compare the influence of scaffold material, porosity and pore architecture on cartilage tissue formation *in vitro* and *in vivo*. They do so by allowing the pore geometry of the scaffold to remain fixed while maintaining a 100% interconnecting pore volume, without introducing any pores of random size or orientation, closed pores, or variation in material composition. Moreover, these techniques allow for designed scaffolds with enhanced control over mechanical properties [77, 79, 80].

22.5.2. Cells and Cell Sources

Cell types used in *in vitro* models for studying repair of both chondral and osteochondral defects have included committed chondrocytes [69, 71, 79, 100-102], cell-lines [103-108] or various progenitor, or mesenchymal stem cells (MSCs) from various sources [56, 109-113]. Articular chondrocytes are a common choice as these cells are responsible for maintenance and synthesis of essential cartilage matrix molecules. Highly promising alternative cell sources, which limit donor site morbidity associated with harvesting articular cartilage, include hyaline nasal septal cartilage [71, 114-117] and auricular cartilage [118]. Progenitor cell populations present within periosteum or perichondrium have also formed the basis for a number of *in vitro* studies [119-123]. Alternative stem cell sources receiving considerable attention for their chondrogenic potential are adipose-derived cells [124-127].

The main limitation of using committed chondrocytes is the difficulty in harvesting articular cartilage biopsies and limited number of cells that can be obtained from these small biopsies. Scaffold-based strategies to repair articular cartilage defects require large number of cells to generate sufficient volume of repair tissue, often necessitating the use of *in vitro* culture expansion techniques. One of the overriding limitations in cartilage tissue engineering is in overcoming the phenomenon of chondrocyte de-differentiation. Mature chondrocytes are well differentiated in their phenotype and are solely responsible for the maintenance of cartilage ECM components, characterized by the synthesis of predominantly type II collagen and the proteoglycan aggrecan [128]. When embedded within their native ECM, healthy chondrocytes exhibit a spherical morphology. However, when chondrocytes are released from their native ECM and cultured under conditions promoting a spread morphology, such as on 2D substrates, they progressively lose their original phenotype and display fibroblastic or pre-chondrogenic features, typically characterized by the expression of predominantly type I collagen and the proteoglycan versican [129]. This process is typically described as de-differentiation [130, 131], and can have considerable limitations for tissue engineering strategies resulting in inferior cartilage tissue (i.e. fibro-cartilage) if suitable restoration of a differentiated chondrogenic phenotype cannot be achieved.

22.6. *IN VITRO* MODELS FOR CARTILAGE TISSUE ENGINEERING

In vitro assays are the cornerstone of any tissue engineer's toolbox for evaluating articular cartilage tissue formation and repair strategies. While numerous *in vitro* models exist, they all follow the general tissue engineering paradigm; combining cells, culture media, biomaterial substrates/scaffolds and various growth factors/cytokines.

22.6.1. Factors Influencing Chondrogenesis *In Vitro*

One of the challenges in tissue engineering is the design and fabrication of biodegradable scaffolds which influence specific cellular functions, and may thus regulate cell adhesion, proliferation, expression of a specific phenotype and extracellular matrix deposition in a predictable and controlled fashion. Chondrocyte re-differentiation (i.e. the post-expansion re-expression of chondrocyte phenotype) in scaffolds can be stimulated in a number of ways and are introduced briefly below.

22.6.1.1. Growth Factors/Cell Expansion

During the expansion phase, culture media supplemented with growth factors, such as transforming growth factor-β (TGF-β), insulin-like growth factor-1 (IGF-1), basic fibroblastic growth factor (bFGF) and platelet derived growth factor (PDGF) have been shown to influence chondrocyte proliferation rate [132], whilst enhancing the ability for subsequent cell re-differentiation [133-135].

The combination of these growth factors during expansion with other potent re-differentiation factors such as insulin, TGF-β and dexamethasone during 3D culture have been shown to stimulate cartilage tissue formation in scaffolds [71]. Cell expansion on 3D microcarriers, as opposed to 2D culture plates, has also been demonstrated to influence the downstream re-differentiation potential of chondrocytes [136-138]. Alternatively, cell free strategies rely of incorporation and controlled release of GF's, such as TGF-β and rhBMP-2 from biodegradable scaffolds to stimulate MSC differentiation and cartilage tissue formation.

22.6.1.2. Pellet/Mass Culture

Culture conditions, such as high-density pellet- or mass-culture techniques, which mimic cell condensation reactions associated with embryonic chondrogenesis or the *in situ* cartilage environment have also been shown to induce re-differentiation related to cell-cell and/or cell-matrix interactions [139-141]. These culture conditions are often used in combination with growth factor stimulation [142, 143].

22.6.1.3. Bioreactors/Mechanical Stimulation

Culture conditions which place tissue-engineered constructs in a dynamic fluid environment such as those present in spinner flask [144, 145] or rotating bioreactor culture [146-150], or which simulate *in situ* joint loading conditions via dynamic hydrostatic pressure [151-156] or mechanical compression [157-162], have also been suggested to stimulate chondrocyte re-differentiation [155, 156, 160, 163]. These dynamic culture conditions also aim at optimizing nutrient and waste exchange to engineered tissues. This is not only important for maintaining cell viability, but nutrient limitations themselves may also be involved in instructing cell function. For example, a low oxygen environment, comparable to conditions in native cartilage, has been suggested to be an instructive factor in promoting chondrocyte differentiation [164].

22.6.1.4. Cell-Scaffold Interactions

It has long been known that cell behavior on biomaterial substrates is related to both the physical and chemical properties of the substratum [165]. Several properties have been suggested as potential regulators of cell behavior including wettability, surface chemistry, equilibrium water content and roughness [165-167]. Furthermore, the specific substrate properties can either directly or indirectly effect cell adhesion, morphology and subsequent cellular activity by controlling adsorption of ions, proteins and other molecules from the culture medium [165, 168]. This is the scenario when seeding and culturing cells on biomaterials in serum-containing media, thereby exposing substrates to potent cell attachment proteins such as fibronectin (FN) and vitronectin (VN).

It is this molecularly populated surface that the cells sense and respond to biochemically by means of specific cell receptors such as the integrin family (*e.g.* $\alpha_5\beta_1$, $\alpha_V\beta_3$) via Arg-Gly-Asp (RGD) sequence domains [169-171], and CD44 via GAG-binding domains [172]. Therefore, the choice of biomaterial and the influence on protein adsorption and subsequent chondrocyte phenotype play a key role in promoting chondrogenesis *in vitro*.

22.6.1.5. 3D Scaffold Architecture

It is well established that chondrocytes require a 3D environment to maintain their differentiated phenotype and synthesize necessary ECM components such as collagen type II and GAG [51, 130, 133, 173, 174]. The influence of specific surface properties of various biomaterials on chondrocyte behavior has been so far mostly investigated using 2D films [175-179]. However, little is known about the specific influence of controlled changes in 3D scaffold architecture on chondrocyte (re)differentiation.

It has been suggested that scaffold architecture may control cell function by regulating diffusion of nutrients (*e.g.,* oxygen) and waste products, as well as influencing cell–cell interactions [180,181], e.g., engineered 3D fibre scaffolds containing a large, 100% interconnecting pore network have been shown to result in enhanced chondrocyte re-differentiation capacity and homogeneous distribution of cells and ECM compared to scaffolds with randomly generated and complex pore networks [79,80,180].

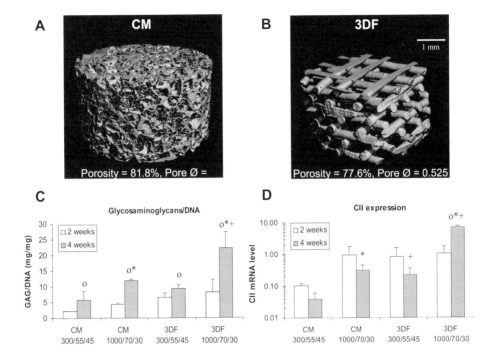

Fig 22.5. Micro-computed tomograpghy (μCT) images of porous PEGT/PBT polymer scaffolds with similar overall porosity, but varying pore architecture and average interconnecting pore diameter. (A) random pore architecture fabricated using compression molding (CM) and particle leaching techniques; (B) solid free-form fabrication (SFF) of a designed pore architecture in a layer-by-layer process via 3D fiber deposition (3DF). (C, D) The influence of PEGT/PBT scaffold composition (low PEG molecular weight 300/55/45 versus high PEG molecular weight 1000/70/30) and scaffold architecture (CM versus 3DF) on re-differentiation potential of expanded human nasal chondrocytes assessed via (C) GAG/DNA content, and (D) collagen type II mRNA expression. High PEG molecular weight composition (1000/70/30) in combination with a highly accessible pore volume and large diameter 100% interconnecting pore structure (3DF architecture) synergistically enhance restoration of human chondrocyte phenotype observed by significantly greater (GAG/DNA) and collagen type II mRNA at 4 weeks. Statistical significance (p<0.05) indicated by: ∗ = different from composition 300/55/45 for the same architecture; + = different from architecture CM for the same composition; O = different from 2 weeks of culture for the same architecture and composition (adapted from Miot et al.[77]).

Furthermore, when combining engineered 3D fiber scaffold architectures with a substrate promoting a chondrocyte phenotype, a synergistic increase in re-differentiation capacity of human expanded nasal chondrocytes in 3D fibre scaffolds has been observed [77] (Figure 22.5).

In an attempt to recreate the cartilage-bone interface and improve tissue integration in osteochondral defects, hybrid scaffolds and culture systems are being evaluated to tissue engineer both bone and cartilage layers. Such systems have been designed around a porous polymer or fibrin glue cartilage layer containing chondrocytes, anchored to a ceramic hydroxyapatite or calcium-phosphate base scaffold seeded either with or without bone progenitor cells [84, 86, 96, 182].

22.6.2. Limitations of *In Vitro* Models for Cartilage Tissue Engineering and Recommendations for Their Improvement

Pellet cultures are only useful in determining the (re)differentiation potential of chondrocytes without the influence of a biomaterial substrate [183]. While clearly advantageous for investigating the influence of various GF's and cell sources on chondrogenesis due to the small volumes of cells and culture media required, one limitation of this model is that localized chondrogenesis seen in small pellet cultures does not represent the culture environment in large 3D scaffolds of clinically relevant size, where nutrient diffusion and cell viability can vary greatly throughout the constructs [180]. Moreover, the absence of biomaterial-protein adsorption interactions from the culture medium, cell-biomaterial interactions and considerably reduced cell-cell interaction present in *in vitro* cultures on 3D scaffolds mean that to a large extent, positive results demonstrated in pellet cultures are not always directly transferable to 3D scaffolds *in vitro* [184].

Studies of chondrocytes or chondroprogenitor cells on 2D biomaterial substrates clearly offer the ability to study the influence of biomaterial-medium interaction via protein adsorption as well as cell-biomaterial and, to a certain extent, cell-cell interactions. However the influence of 3D architecture is neglected in such models. As mentioned previously, 3D architecture is vital for maintaining chondrocyte phenotype as evidenced in studies with chondrocytes maintained in 3D agarose or alginate gel culture and the prevalence for cell to typically undergo dedifferentiation when cultured on 2D substrates. The common perception is that events occurring in the 2D environment are not carried over when translated to a 3D environment. However, this may not exclusively be the case as a recent series of studies demonstrated that poly(ethylene glycol)-terephthalate – poly(butylene terephthalate) (PEGT/PBT) polymer substrates supporting maintenance of chondrocyte phenotype (i.e. a high collagen type II/I mRNA ratio) in expanded human nasal chondrocytes, also supported chondrogenic re-differentiation of these cells in identical culture conditions on 3D PEGT/PBT scaffolds produced using the same biomaterial composition [77, 185]. These data confirm that *in vitro* studies investigating controlled changes of substrate composition on chondrogenesis in 2D [185, 186] also translate to observations of substrate composition and architecture in 3D scaffolds [77].

When comparing various scaffolds for cartilage tissue engineering *in vitro*, a number of issues arise which limit the ability to draw direct comparisons between scaffolds, particularly in relation to the scaffold architecture and composition. Important constituents of a designed porous scaffold architecture include, but are not limited to, the following: porosity, pore interconnectivity (preferably 100%), accessible pore volume or permeability, pore size (i.e. size of pores and interconnection between pores), volume fraction (i.e. scaffold surface area to volume ratio), surface texture (i.e. rough microporosity or smooth), biomaterial composition, and scaffold degradation rate [51, 174]. Each of these factors together, or individually, can have an effect on cartilage tissue formation *in vitro*. For example, differences in pore architecture and volume fraction can influence the number and distribution of cells seeded within constructs [78]. Non homogeneous seeding can result in a high concentration of cells at the periphery of a scaffold, forming a fibrous capsule and preventing further cell migration and nutrient access, to the detriment of cells residing in the scaffold interior [148]. Subtle changes in scaffold composition may also influence protein adsorption and cell adhesion mechanisms resulting in altered proliferation and chondrocyte phenotype. Differences in pore interconnectivity and permeability will affect nutrient and waste diffusion, such as oxygen [164, 180, 187], throughout scaffolds which ultimately will impact cell viability. Moreover, these nutrient gradients themselves can in turn have a large impact on cartilage tissue formation [180, 188].

Development of *in vitro* bioreactor cultures which provide medium flow and control over medium composition aim to enhance nutrient exchange and cell viability in large constructs of clinically relevant size [146, 164, 189, 190]. Yet few bioreactor systems take into consideration mechanical loading of the construct. Cartilage is an avascular, load bearing tissue, relying on mechanical compression and diffusion for nutrient and waste exchange with the synovium. Therefore, constructs engineered *in vitro* must be capable of supporting significant static and dynamic compressive stress comparable to native articular cartilage. *In vitro* bioreactor culture should include dynamic loading of constructs to evaluate construct longevity, cell differentiation, but most importantly, cell viability under physiologic stress [191, 192].

One further limitation of current *in vitro* models is that very few take into account the highly organized zonal structure of native articular cartilage in terms of cell distribution, GAG content and collagen type II orientation throughout the depth of the articular cartilage layer [51]. Recent *in vitro* studies have been aimed at recreating the zonal cartilage architecture by combining individual layers of chondrocytes isolated from superficial, middle and deep zone chondrocytes embedded in alginate or agarose gels [193, 194]. Other studies have engineered pore-size gradients into 3D scaffolds from which a heterogenous population of cells from all zones were seeded. These scaffolds promoted an inhomogeneous cell and ECM distribution similar to that seen in native cartilage [78]. However, it is unclear from studies to date, if it is possible to control the synthesis and zonal organization of collagen type II *in vitro*.

Each of these factors relating to scaffold architecture ultimately results in an altered differentiation state of the cell (e.g. GAG/DNA content) and the ability for it to synthesize cartilage ECM (e.g. collagen II) in the same quality and quantity as native articular cartilage. Many *in vitro* studies to date have compared various scaffolds *in vitro* where many of these factors are inherently different. While the conclusion may be that one scaffold performs better than another, it is often impossible to deduce if it was the influence of scaffold composition, accessible pore volume, or total cell content and distribution for example, without having precise control over the processing of scaffold architecture. Current efforts using SFF to produce designed scaffold architectures in which only one of the number of these factors is varied at a time are helping to unfold some of the key criteria that are necessary to engineer articular cartilage *in vitro* that can then be taken to the *in vivo* level [52, 77, 96, 97, 195].

22.7. *IN VIVO* MODELS FOR CARTILAGE TISSUE ENGINEERING

The ultimate success of any cartilage repair strategy must be established in animal models prior to clinical application. Such studies serve to highlight some of the existing problems confounding scaffold-based tissue engineering strategies in articular cartilage, as well as reveal some inherent limitations of the animal models themselves in relation to the clinical setting.

22.7.1. Non Load-Bearing Animal Models

As a first step in evaluating chondrogenic potential in an *in vivo* model, subcutaneous implantation of tissue engineered constructs in immuno-deficient mice can provide useful information in a non load-bearing environment, and help bridge the gap between *in vitro* and *in vivo* load-bearing models in larger animals [79, 80, 138, 196, 197]. Subcutaneous implantation of tissue engineered cartilage constructs typically results in enhanced tissue formation compared with constructs cultured *in vitro*, even in a controlled bioreactor environment. For example, Malda et al. [79, 180] demonstrated significantly higher GAG/DNA content and collagen type II staining in scaffolds subcutaneously implanted in nude mice after 4 weeks compared to constructs that remained in spinner flask culture *in vitro* over the same period [79, 180]. Implantation in subcutaneous pockets exposes constructs to host vasculature and local systemic growth hormones and the relatively inhospitable non-load bearing environment, however, there is the potential for host cells to infiltrate the scaffold and contribute to the repair process. Unless cells are tracked [198], limitations arise when evaluating MSC strategies for cartilage repair where it becomes unclear if the engineered construct and/or host MSC infiltration are responsible for the observed responses.

22.7.2. Load-Bearing Animal Models

Numerous animal models have been used to assess scaffold-based repair strategies in load bearing joints including rats, dogs, sheep and horses, however, most common small and large animal studies are carried out using rabbit [61, 64, 67, 68, 101, 199] and goat models [74, 200-204] respectively. While large animal models may more closely represent the human joint compared with small animal models, no animal model exists that is directly applicable to the human. Careful selection of animal age, chondral or osteochondral defect, partial or full load-bearing post surgery and uniform methods to assess outcome is necessary [205]. Immature animals (i.e. <6 months is the rabbit) may not be skeletally mature and have an increased spontaneous repair capacity which may override any repair strategy under evaluation.

22.7.3. Limitations of *In Vivo* Animal Models for Cartilage Tissue Engineering

As outlined recently by Hunziker [206], limitations in anatomical scale between osteochondral components in animals and humans are considerable, and relate to overall joint size, joint loading and thickness of and cell distribution within the cartilage layer itself. For example, the cartilage layer in the rabbit is only 200-300 μm thick compared to 3-5 mm thick in human cartilage [207].

The catabolic joint environment present in advanced degenerative diseases (e.g. in osteoarthritis, OA) as well as joint loading can also have significant consequences for scaffold-based repair with respect to the fate of implanted neo-tissue and scaffold degradation issues. These events are overlooked in *in vitro* studies and are difficult to assess *in vivo* in healthy animals. However, studies demonstrating clear differences in scaffold-based repair tissue between "freshly created" defects and "old" defects created 2 months prior to scaffold implantation, suggest the potential for future studies to incorporate a degenerative joint environment for evaluating cartilage repair [201].

The inexorable inconsistencies between animal models and the clinical setting make drawing definitive conclusions on various scaffold designs and repair strategies difficult. For example, recent studies have demonstrated the species variability in expansion and re-differentiation potential of human, dog and sheep chondrocytes [197]. It is clear from these studies that expansion and culture conditions optimized in animal models can by no means be directly translated to the clinical setting in humans. In addition, with the large variation in scaffold materials, cell types and culture conditions used, comparisons between *in vivo* studies are almost impossible. Standardized evaluation methods are necessary to not only compare different scaffold-based repair strategies, but also compare if such strategies are more favorable than traditional repair strategies, rather than just empty defects. Assessment criteria and histological grading scales such as that established by the International Cartilage Repair Society (ICRS) for example should become commonly adopted [208].

22.7.3.1. Scaffold Architecture

Many of the limitations discussed previously relating to the influence of scaffold architecture on *in vitro* culture also hold true for the *in vivo* environment. Issues of scaffold mechanical stability become more prevalent in the load bearing *in vivo* environment where a delicate balance between scaffold integrity and biodegradation rate is needed. In the case of osteochondral defects, scaffold architectures need to be designed to support integration with the subchondral bone and surrounding native cartilage. A range of biphasic constructs have been evaluated for this purpose and SFF techniques are leading the way in developing constructs based on polymeric and/or ceramic scaffolds with optimized architectures for cartilage and bone layers respectively [52, 84, 195]. Cell free strategies in which MSC's are recruited *in vivo* from the underlying subchondral bone spaces also require similar attention to scaffold architecture, as well as incorporating the controlled release of GFs (e.g. rhBMP-2) [209] or gene therapy products (e.g. cells over-expressing insulin-like growth factor) [61] necessary to stimulate both osteo- and chrondro-genic differentiation in various regions.

22.7.3.2. Cell Viability and Retention

Additional concern regarding scaffold-based repair strategies is the lack of knowledge with respect to the location, retention and viability of reparative cells once implanted *in vivo*. The large variation in repair results and limited success of tissue-engineered scaffold constructs to date may be, in part, related to the loss of cell viability and/or the inability to retain a critical number of chondrogenic cells in the proper region of the defect with time. For example, Ostrander et al. [210] seeded rabbit perichondral cells in PLA constructs into osteochondral defects in rabbits. Repair tissue was harvested at various intervals from 0-28 days after implantation, and the number of donor cells determined via gender-specific gene tracking. Average cell viability was found to be 87% or more, with donor cells present in repair tissue for 28 days after implantation. However, the number of donor cells declined from approximately 1 million at time zero to approximately 140,000 at day 28. This decline in donor cells was accompanied by a significant influx of host cells into the repair tissue. This is also significant for repair strategies that incorporate MSCs into osteochondral defects, as it cannot been excluded that enhanced tissue repair is derived from host cells recruited to the defect in response to the implant, rather than the repopulation of the tissue by the implanted MSCs. In this regard, Quintavalla et al. [202] implanted fluorescently labeled MSC/gelatin constructs into osteochondral defects in goats. The cells retained the dye up to 1 month and were detected by histology and flow cytometry. At intervals spanning 2 weeks post-implantation, gradual loss of implanted cells in the defect as well as fragments of gelatin sponge containing labelled MSCs in deep marrow spaces were observed. Although longer assessment times are necessary, the authors suggested that by determining the fate of implanted cells in short-term *in vivo* models, scaffold designs could be more rapidly optimized with respect to cell retention needed for successful, long-term cartilage regeneration. This was confirmed in a recent study where the length of pre-culture positively correlated with increased perichondral cell retention in tissue engineered PLA constructs following implantation in osteochondral defects in rabbits [67]. These results, however, act in direct contrast to other studies investigating the integration between the tissue engineered construct and the native surrounding tissue. Obradovic et al. [211] showed that integration in immature (1 week-old) *in vitro* cultured constructs with articular cartilage explants was enhanced due to cell proliferation and progressive matrix remodelling at the tissue interface, as opposed to mature (8 week-old) constructs. Obradovic et al., stated that while integration of immature tissue improved integration, the bulk mechanical properties of the tissue were low compared with mature constructs. This suggests that future scaffold designs which support rapid cartilage ECM synthesis and cell proliferation to enhance integration, but on the other hand, have sufficient mechanical stability to protect this newly-formed tissue from *in vivo* joint loads, could offer significant promise.

Unfortunately, since long-term functional stability of repair tissue *in vivo* is critical, the length of time needed to assess new treatment options, even at the pre-clinical stage, limits rapid innovation and development of scaffold-based repair strategies. Better *in vitro* models and more rapid *in situ* evaluation techniques, such as high resolution MRI [212] or imaging of luciferase markers in transgenic mice [213-215], that are capable of providing biochemical data (*e.g.* GAG) as well as structural and morphological images in real-time are necessary.

22.8. CONCLUSIONS

Today's *in vitro* assays in which biomaterials and tissue-engineered constructs for bone and cartilage repair and regeneration are tested often give inconclusive results and their predictive value for the *in vivo* performance is limited. One of the reasons for the limited predictive value on *in vitro* models is the undesired biomaterial-cell culture interaction. In addition, *in vitro* systems are often not representative for the *in vivo* situation in terms of cell population, nutrients supply, 3D environment and mechanical loading. Similarly, although they are a good source of valuable information about the biological performance of biomaterials and tissue engineered constructs, the results obtained from studies in *in vivo* models cannot directly be extrapolated to their performance clinically. The increasing number of new materials and technologies for bone and cartilage regeneration requires fast and reliable *in vitro* and *in vivo* assays. However, the existing assays need improvements in order to be predictive for the final, clinical application of bone and cartilage repair strategies.

22.9. ACKNOWLEDGMENTS

The authors would like to thank Gilles Bluteau and Jerôme Guicheux (INSERM UMRS 9903, Faculty of Dental Surgery, Nantes, France) for their help with cell culture and RT-PCR analysis and Sanne Both (University of Twente, Institute for Biomedical Technology, Bilthoven, The Netherlands) for performing the QPCR analysis.

22.10. REFERENCES

1. A. Abbott, Cell culture: biology's new dimension, *Nature* **424**(6951), 870-2 (2003).
2. E. B. Hunziker, Articular cartilage repair: basic science and clinical progress. A review of the current status and prospects., *Osteoarthritis Cartilage* **10**(6), 432-63 (2002).
3. D. G. Anderson, D. Putnam, E. B. Lavik, T. A. Mahmood, and R. Langer, Biomaterial microarrays: rapid, microscale screening of polymer-cell interaction, *Biomaterials* **26**(23), 4892-7 (2005).
4. G. Gronowicz and L. G. Raisz, Bone formation assays, in Principles of bone biology, J. P. Bilezikian, L. G. Raisz, and G. A. Rodan, Editors. Academic Press, San Diego, USA. 1253-1265 (1996).
5. V. Kartsogiannis and K. W. Ng, Cell lines and primary cell cultures in the study of bone cell biology, *Mol Cell Endocrinol* **228**(1-2), 79-102 (2004).
6. K. Hyakuna, T. Yamamuro, Y. Kotoura, Y. Kakutani, T. Kitsugi, H. Takagi, M. Oka, and T. Kokubo, The influence of calcium phosphate ceramics and glass-ceramics on cultured cells and their surrounding media, *J Biomed Mater Res* **23**(9), 1049-66 (1989).
7. T. Suzuki, T. Yamamoto, M. Toriyama, K. Nishizawa, Y. Yokogawa, M. R. Mucalo, Y. Kawamoto, F. Nagata, and T. Kameyama, Surface instability of calcium phosphate ceramics in tissue culture medium and the effect on adhesion and growth of anchorage-dependent animal cells, *J Biomed Mater Res* **34**(4), 507-17 (1997).
8. C. Knabe, R. Gildenhaar, G. Berger, W. Ostapowicz, R. Fitzner, R. J. Radlanski, and U. Gross, Morphological evaluation of osteoblasts cultured on different calcium phosphate ceramics, *Biomaterials* **18**(20), 1339-47 (1997).
9. C. Knabe, W. Ostapowicz, R. J. Radlanski, R. Gildenhaar, G. Berger, R. Fitzner, and U. Gross, In vitro investigation of novel calcium phosphates using osteogenic cultures, *J Mater Sci Mater Med* **9**(6), 337-45 (1998).
10. J. E. Davies, Mechanisms of endosseous integration, *Int J Prosthodont* **11**(5), 391-401 (1998).
11. R. G. Geesink, K. de Groot, and C. P. Klein, Bonding of bone to apatite-coated implants, *J Bone Joint Surg Br* **70**(1), 17-22 (1988).
12. T. Hanawa, Y. Kamiura, S. Yamamoto, T. Kohgo, A. Amemiya, H. Ukai, K. Murakami, and K. Asaoka, Early bone formation around calcium-ion-implanted titanium inserted into rat tibia, *J Biomed Mater Res* **36**(1), 131-6 (1997).
13. J. D. de Bruijn, C. P. A. T. Klein, K. de Groot, and C. A. van Blitterswijk, Influence of crystal structure on the establishment of the bone-calcium phosphate interface in vitro, *Cells and materials* **3**, 407-17 (1993).
14. J. D. de Bruijn, Y. P. Bovell, and C. A. van Blitterswijk, Structural arrangements at the interface between plasma sprayed calcium phosphates and bone, *Biomaterials* **15**(7), 543-50 (1994).
15. C. Wang, Y. Duan, B. Markovic, J. Barbara, R. C. Howlett, X. Zhang, and H. Zreiqat, Proliferation and bone-related gene expression of osteoblasts grown on hydroxyapatite ceramics sintered at different temperature, *Biomaterials* **25**(15), 2949-56 (2004).
16. P. Habibovic, H. Yuan, M. van den Doel, T. M. Sees, C. A. van Blitterswijk, and K. de Groot, Relevance of osteoinductive biomaterials in a critical-sized orthotopic defect, *J Orthop Res* ***in press*** (2006).
17. A. Y. Friedenstein, Induction of bone tissue by transitional epithelium, *Clin Orthop Relat Res* **59**, 21-37 (1968).
18. M. R. Urist and B. S. Strates, Bone morphogenetic protein, *J Dent Res* **50**(6), 1392-406 (1971).

19. A. K. Gosain, L. Song, P. Riordan, M. T. Amarante, P. G. Nagy, C. R. Wilson, J. M. Toth, and J. L. Ricci, A 1-year study of osteoinduction in hydroxyapatite-derived biomaterials in an adult sheep model: part I, *Plast Reconstr Surg* **109**(2), 619-30 (2002).
20. P. Habibovic, C. M. van der Valk, G. Meijer, C. A. van Blitterswijk, and K. de Groot, Influence of octacalcium phosphate coating on osteoinductive properties of biomaterials, *J Mater Sci Mater Med* **15**(4), 373-380 (2004).
21. P. Habibovic, H. Yuan, C. M. van der Valk, G. Meijer, C. A. van Blitterswijk, and K. de Groot, 3D microenvironment as essential element for osteoinduction by biomaterials, *Biomaterials* **26**(17), 3565-75 (2005).
22. U. Ripamonti, J. Crooks, and A. N. Kirkbride, Sintered porous hydroxyapatites with intrinsic osteoinductive activity: geometric induction of bone formation, *South African J Sci* **95**, 335-343 (1999).
23. S. Fujibayashi, M. Neo, H. M. Kim, T. Kokubo, and T. Nakamura, Osteoinduction of porous bioactive titanium metal, *Biomaterials* **25**(3), 443-50 (2004).
24. H. Yuan, J. D. de Bruijn, Y. Li, Z. Feng, K. Yang, K. de Groot, and X. Zhang, Bone formation induced by calcium phosphate ceramics in soft tissue of dogs: a comparative study between alpha-TCP and beta-TCP, *J Mater Sci Mater Med* **12**, 7-13 (2001).
25. H. Yuan, M. van den Doel, S. H. Li, C. A. van Blitterswijk, K. de Groot, and J. D. de Bruijn, A comparison of the osteoinductive potential of two calcium phosphate ceramics implanted intramuscularly in goats, *J Mater Sci Mater Med* **13**, 1271-5 (2002).
26. H. D. Adkisson, Strauss-Schoenberger, J., Gillis, M., Wilkins, R., Jackson, M. and Hruska, K. A., Rapid quantitative bioassay of osteoinduction, *J Orthop Res* **18**(3), 503-11 (2000).
27. M. Zhang, R. M. Powers, Jr., and L. Wolfinbarger, Jr., A quantitative assessment of osteoinductivity of human demineralized bone matrix, *J Periodontol* **68**(11), 1076-84 (1997).
28. L. Wolfinbarger, Jr. and Y. Zheng, An in vitro bioassay to assess biological activity in demineralized bone, *In Vitro Cell Dev Biol Anim* **29A**(12), 914-6 (1993).
29. D. L. Carnes, Jr., J. De La Fontaine, D. L. Cochran, J. T. Mellonig, B. Keogh, S. E. Harris, N. Ghosh-Choudhury, D. D. Dean, B. D. Boyan, and Z. Schwartz, Evaluation of 2 novel approaches for assessing the ability of demineralized freeze-dried bone allograft to induce new bone formation, *J Periodontol* **70**(4), 353-63 (1999).
30. B. Han, B. Tang, and M. E. Nimni, Quantitative and sensitive in vitro assay for osteoinductive activity of demineralized bone matrix, *J Orthop Res* **21**(4), 648-54 (2003).
31. G. D. Winter and B. J. Simpson, Heterotopic bone formed in a synthetic sponge in the skin of young pigs, *Nature* **223**(201), 88-90 (1969).
32. H. Yuan, J. D. de Bruijn, X. Zhang, C. A. van Blitterswijk, and K. de Groot, Osteoinduction by porous alumina ceramic, *Trans European Conference on Biomaterials*, 209 (2001).
33. M. Takemoto, S. Fujibayashi, T. Matsushita, J. Suzuki, T. Kokubo, and T. Nakamura, Osteoinductive ability of porous titanium implants following three types of surface treatment, *Trans 51st Annual Meeting of the Orthopaedic Research Society*, Poster No: 0992 (2005).
34. J. Goshima, V. M. Goldberg, and A. I. Caplan, The osteogenic potential of culture-expanded rat marrow mesenchymal cells assayed in vivo in calcium phosphate ceramic blocks, *Clin Orthop Relat Res* **262**, 298-311 (1991).
35. H. Ohgushi, Y. Dohi, S. Tamai, and S. Tabata, Osteogenic differentiation of marrow stromal stem cells in porous hydroxyapatite ceramics, *J Biomed Mater Res* **27**(11), 1401-7 (1993).
36. H. Ohgushi, V. M. Goldberg, and A. I. Caplan, Heterotopic osteogenesis in porous ceramics induced by marrow cells, *J Orthop Res* **7**(4), 568-78 (1989).
37. Z. Yang, H. Yuan, W. Tong, P. Zou, W. Chen, and X. Zhang, Osteogenesis in extraskeletally implanted porous calcium phosphate ceramics: variability among different kinds of animals, *Biomaterials* **17**(22), 2131-7 (1996).
38. U. Ripamonti, Smart biomaterials with intrinsic osteoinductivity: geometric control of bone differentiation, in Bone engineering, J. M. Davies, Editor. em squared Corporation, Toronto, Canada. 215-221 (2000).
39. J. A. Jansen, Animal models for studying soft tissue biocompatibiliyu of biomaterials, in Animal models in orthopaedic research, Y. H. An and R. J. Friedman, Editors. CRC Press, Boca Raton, USA. 393-405 (1999).
40. Y. H. An and R. J. Friedman, Animal models of bone defect repair, in Animals models in orthopaedic research, Y. H. An and R. J. Friedman, Editors. CRC Press LLC, Boca Raton, USA. 241-60 (1999).
41. U. Ripamonti, Osteoinduction in porous hydroxyapatite implanted in heterotopic sites of different animal models, *Biomaterials* **17**(1), 31-5 (1996).
42. E. Solheim, Osteoinduction by demineralised bone, *Int Orthop* **22**(5), 335-42 (1998).

43. A. Marusic, V. Katavic, D. Grcevic, and I. K. Lukic, Genetic variability of new bone induction in mice, *Bone* **25**(1), 25-32 (1999).
44. R. G. Geesink, N. H. Hoefnagels, and S. K. Bulstra, Osteogenic activity of OP-1 bone morphogenetic protein (BMP-7) in a human fibular defect, *J Bone Joint Surg Br* **81**(4), 710-8 (1999).
45. P. Habibovic, J. Li, C. M. van der Valk, G. Meijer, P. Layrolle, C. A. van Blitterswijk, and K. de Groot, Biological performance of uncoated and octacalcium phosphate-coated Ti6Al4V, *Biomaterials* **26**(1), 23-36 (2005).
46. Y. An, R. Friedman, and R. Draughn, Animal models of bone fracture or osteotomy, in Animal models in orthopaedic research, Y. H. An and R. J. Friedman, Editors. CRC Press LLC, Boca Raton, USA. 197-217 (1999).
47. M. C. Kruyt, J. D. de Bruijn, C. E. Wilson, F. C. Oner, C. A. van Blitterswijk, A. J. Verbout, and W. J. Dhert, Viable osteogenic cells are obligatory for tissue-engineered ectopic bone formation in goats, *Tissue Eng* **9**(2), 327-36 (2003).
48. M. C. Kruyt, W. J. Dhert, H. Yuan, C. E. Wilson, C. A. van Blitterswijk, A. J. Verbout, and J. D. de Bruijn, Bone tissue engineering in a critical size defect compared to ectopic implantations in the goat, *J Orthop Res* **22**(3), 544-51 (2004).
49. M. C. Kruyt, J. De Bruijn, M. Veenhof, F. C. Oner, C. A. Van Blitterswijk, A. J. Verbout, and W. J. Dhert, Application and limitations of chloromethyl-benzamidodialkylcarbocyanine for tracing cells used in bone Tissue engineering, *Tissue Eng* **9**(1), 105-15 (2003).
50. S. Clark and D. W. Rowe, Transgenic animals, in Principles of bone biology, J. P. Bilezikian, L. G. Raisz, and G. A. Rodan, Editors. Academic Press, San Diego, USA. 1161-1172 (1996).
51. T. B. F. Woodfield, J. M. Bezemer, J. S. Pieper, C. A. van Blitterswijk, and J. Riesle, Scaffolds for tissue engineering of cartilage, *Crit Rev Eukaryot Gene Expr* **12**(3), 209-36 (2002), with permission from Begell House.
52. S. J. Hollister, Porous scaffold design for tissue engineering, *Nat Mater* **4**(7), 518-24 (2005).
53. S. N. Redman, S. F. Oldfield, and C. W. Archer, Current strategies for articular cartilage repair, *Eur Cell Mater* **9**, 23-32; discussion 23-32 (2005).
54. D. W. Hutmacher, Scaffolds in tissue engineering bone and cartilage, *Biomaterials* **21**(24), 2529-43 (2000).
55. S. Nehrer, H. A. Breinan, A. Ramappa, H. P. Hsu, T. Minas, S. Shortkroff, C. B. Sledge, I. V. Yannas, and M. Spector, Chondrocyte-seeded collagen matrices implanted in a chondral defect in a canine model, *Biomaterials* **19**(24), 2313-28 (1998).
56. S. Wakitani, K. Imoto, T. Yamamoto, M. Saito, N. Murata, and M. Yoneda, Human autologous culture expanded bone marrow mesenchymal cell transplantation for repair of cartilage defects in osteoarthritic knees, *Osteo Cart* **10**(3), 199-206 (2002).
57. S. Wakitani, T. Goto, R. Young, J. Mansour, V. Goldberg, and A. Caplan, Repair of large full-thickness articular cartilage defects with allograft articular chondrocytes embedded in a collagen gel., *Tissue Eng* **4**(4), 429-44 (1998).
58. C. D. Hoemann, J. Sun, A. Legare, M. D. McKee, and M. D. Buschmann, Tissue engineering of cartilage using an injectable and adhesive chitosan-based cell-delivery vehicle, *Osteoarthritis Cartilage* **13**(4), 318-29 (2005).
59. A. Chenite, C. Chaput, D. Wang, C. Combes, M. D. Buschmann, C. D. Hoemann, J. C. Leroux, B. L. Atkinson, F. Binette, and A. Selmani, Novel injectable neutral solutions of chitosan form biodegradable gels in situ, *Biomaterials* **21**(21), 2155-61 (2000).
60. K. Paige, L. Cima, M. Yaremchuk, J. Vacanti, and C. Vacanti, Injectable cartilage., *Plast Reconstr Surg* **96**(6), 1390-8; discussion 1399-400 (1995).
61. H. Madry, G. Kaul, M. Cucchiarini, U. Stein, D. Zurakowski, K. Remberger, M. D. Menger, D. Kohn, and S. B. Trippel, Enhanced repair of articular cartilage defects in vivo by transplanted chondrocytes overexpressing insulin-like growth factor I (IGF-I), *Gene Ther* **12**(15), 1171-9 (2005).
62. D. R. Diduch, L. C. Jordan, C. M. Mierisch, and G. Balian, Marrow stromal cells embedded in alginate for repair of osteochondral defects, *Arthroscopy* **16**(6), 571-7 (2000).
63. C. T. Hung, E. G. Lima, R. L. Mauck, E. Taki, M. A. LeRoux, H. H. Lu, R. G. Stark, X. E. Guo, and G. A. Ateshian, Anatomically shaped osteochondral constructs for articular cartilage repair, *J Biomech* **36**(12), 1853-64 (2003).
64. B. Rahfoth, J. Weisser, F. Sternkopf, T. Aigner, d. M. K. von, and R. Brauer, Transplantation of allograft chondrocytes embedded in agarose gel into cartilage defects of rabbits., *Osteo Cart* **6**(1), 50-65 (1998).
65. L. A. Solchaga, J. S. Temenoff, J. Gao, A. G. Mikos, A. I. Caplan, and V. M. Goldberg, Repair of osteochondral defects with hyaluronan- and polyester-based scaffolds, *Osteoarthritis Cartilage* **13**(4), 297-309 (2005).

66. L. Solchaga, J. Yoo, M. Lundberg, J. Dennis, B. Huibregtse, V. Goldberg, and A. Caplan, Hyaluronan-based polymers in the treatment of osteochondral defects., *J Orthop Res* **18**(5), 773-80 (2000).
67. S. T. Ball, R. S. Goomer, R. V. Ostrander, W. L. Tontz, Jr., S. K. Williams, and D. Amiel, Preincubation of tissue engineered constructs enhances donor cell retention, *Clin Orthop Relat Res* **420**, 276-85 (2004).
68. K. Uematsu, K. Hattori, Y. Ishimoto, J. Yamauchi, T. Habata, Y. Takakura, H. Ohgushi, T. Fukuchi, and M. Sato, Cartilage regeneration using mesenchymal stem cells and a three-dimensional poly-lactic-glycolic acid (PLGA) scaffold, *Biomaterials* **26**(20), 4273-9 (2005).
69. L. Freed, J. Marquis, A. Nohria, J. Emmanual, A. Mikos, and R. Langer, Neocartilage formation in vitro and in vivo using cells cultured on synthetic biodegradable polymers., *J Biomed Mater Res* **27**(1), 11-23 (1993).
70. C. R. Chu, R. D. Coutts, M. Yoshioka, F. L. Harwood, A. Z. Monosov, and D. Amiel, Articular cartilage repair using allogeneic perichondrocyte-seeded biodegradable porous polylactic acid (PLA): a tissue-engineering study, *J Biomed Mater Res* **29**(9), 1147-54 (1995).
71. W. Kafienah, M. Jakob, O. Demarteau, A. Frazer, M. Barker, I. Martin, and A. Hollander, Three-dimensional tissue engineering of hyaline cartilage: comparison of adult nasal and articular chondrocytes., *Tissue Eng* **8**(5), 817-26 (2002).
72. N. Mahmoudifar and P. M. Doran, Tissue engineering of human cartilage in bioreactors using single and composite cell-seeded scaffolds, *Biotechnol Bioeng* **91**(3), 338-355 (2005).
73. L. Freed, D. Grande, Z. Lingbin, J. Emmanual, J. Marquis, and R. Langer, Joint resurfacing using allograft chondrocytes and synthetic biodegradable polymer scaffolds., *J Biomed Mater Res* **28**(8), 891-9 (1994).
74. G. G. Niederauer, M. A. Slivka, N. C. Leatherbury, D. L. Korvick, H. H. Harroff, W. C. Ehler, C. J. Dunn, and K. Kieswetter, Evaluation of multiphase implants for repair of focal osteochondral defects in goats, *Biomaterials* **21**(24), 2561-74 (2000).
75. Q. Huang, J. Goh, D. Hutmacher, and E. Lee, In Vivo Mesenchymal Cell Recruitment by a Scaffold Loaded with Transforming Growth Factor beta1 and the Potential for in Situ Chondrogenesis, *Tissue Eng* **8**(3), 469-82 (2002).
76. W. J. Li, R. Tuli, C. Okafor, A. Derfoul, K. G. Danielson, D. J. Hall, and R. S. Tuan, A three-dimensional nanofibrous scaffold for cartilage tissue engineering using human mesenchymal stem cells, *Biomaterials* **26**(6), 599-609 (2005).
77. S. Miot, T. B. F. Woodfield, A. U. Daniels, R. Suetterlin, I. Peterschmitt, M. Heberer, C. A. van Blitterswijk, J. Riesle, and I. Martin, Effects of scaffold composition and architecture on human nasal chondrocyte redifferentiation and cartilaginous matrix deposition, *Biomaterials* **26**(15), 2479-89 (2005), with permission from Elsevier.
78. T. B. F. Woodfield, C. A. van Blitterswijk, J. de Wijn, T. J. Sims, A. P. Hollander, and J. Riesle, Polymer scaffolds fabricated with pore-size gradients as a model for studying the zonal organization within tissue-engineered cartilage constructs, *Tissue Engineering* **11**(9-10) (2005).
79. J. Malda, T. B. F. Woodfield, F. van der Vloodt, C. Wilson, D. E. Martens, J. Tramper, C. A. van Blitterswijk, and J. Riesle, The effect of PEGT/PBT scaffold architecture on the composition of tissue engineered cartilage, *Biomaterials* **26**(1), 63-72 (2005).
80. T. B. F. Woodfield, J. Malda, J. de Wijn, F. Péters, J. Riesle, and C. A. van Blitterswijk, Design of porous scaffolds for cartilage tissue engineering using a three-dimensional fiber-deposition technique, *Biomaterials* **25**(18), 4149-4161 (2004).
81. H. Park, J. S. Temenoff, T. A. Holland, Y. Tabata, and A. G. Mikos, Delivery of TGF-beta1 and chondrocytes via injectable, biodegradable hydrogels for cartilage tissue engineering applications, *Biomaterials* **26**(34), 7095-103 (2005).
82. K. Anseth, A. Metters, S. Bryant, P. Martens, J. Elisseeff, and C. Bowman, In situ forming degradable networks and their application in tissue engineering and drug delivery., *J Controlled Release* **78**(1-3), 199-209 (2002).
83. J. Elisseeff, K. Anseth, D. Sims, W. McIntosh, M. Randolph, M. Yaremchuk, and R. Langer, Transdermal photopolymerization of poly(ethylene oxide)-based injectable hydrogels for tissue-engineered cartilage., *Plast Reconstr Surg* **104**(4), 1014-22 (1999).
84. R. M. Schek, J. M. Taboas, S. J. Segvich, S. J. Hollister, and P. H. Krebsbach, Engineered osteochondral grafts using biphasic composite solid free-form fabricated scaffolds, *Tissue Eng* **10**(9-10), 1376-85 (2004).
85. T. A. Holland, E. W. Bodde, L. S. Baggett, Y. Tabata, A. G. Mikos, and J. A. Jansen, Osteochondral repair in the rabbit model utilizing bilayered, degradable oligo(poly(ethylene glycol) fumarate) hydrogel scaffolds, *J Biomed Mater Res A* **75**(1), 156-67 (2005).

86. D. Schaefer, I. Martin, G. Jundt, J. Seidel, M. Heberer, A. Grodzinsky, I. Bergin, G. Vunjak-Novakovic, and L. Freed, Tissue-engineered composites for the repair of large osteochondral defects., *Arthritis Rheum* **46**(9), 2524-34 (2002).
87. J. K. Sherwood, S. L. Riley, R. Palazzolo, S. C. Brown, D. C. Monkhouse, M. Coates, L. G. Griffith, L. K. Landeen, and A. Ratcliffe, A three-dimensional osteochondral composite scaffold for articular cartilage repair, *Biomaterials* **23**(24), 4739-51 (2002).
88. I. Zein, D. W. Hutmacher, K. C. Tan, and S. H. Teoh, Fused deposition modeling of novel scaffold architectures for tissue engineering applications, *Biomaterials* **23**(4), 1169-85 (2002).
89. C. E. Wilson, J. D. de Bruijn, C. A. van Blitterswijk, A. J. Verbout, and W. J. Dhert, Design and fabrication of standardized hydroxyapatite scaffolds with a defined macro-architecture by rapid prototyping for bone-tissue-engineering research, *J Biomed Mater Res* **68A**(1), 123-32 (2004).
90. K. F. Leong, C. M. Cheah, and C. K. Chua, Solid freeform fabrication of three-dimensional scaffolds for engineering replacement tissues and organs, *Biomaterials* **24**(13), 2363-78 (2003).
91. W. Sun and P. Lal, Recent development on computer aided tissue engineering - a review, *Comput Methods Programs Biomed* **67**(2), 85-103 (2002).
92. R. Landers, U. Hubner, R. Schmelzeisen, and R. Mulhaupt, Rapid prototyping of scaffolds derived from thermoreversible hydrogels and tailored for applications in tissue engineering, *Biomaterials* **23**(23), 4437-47 (2002).
93. S. Yang, K. Leong, Z. Du, and C. Chua, The design of scaffolds for use in tissue engineering. Part II. Rapid prototyping techniques., *Tissue Eng* **8**(1), 1-11 (2002).
94. D. W. Hutmacher, T. Schantz, I. Zein, K. W. Ng, S. H. Teoh, and K. C. Tan, Mechanical properties and cell cultural response of polycaprolactone scaffolds designed and fabricated via fused deposition modeling, *J Biomed Mater Res* **55**(2), 203-16 (2001).
95. W. Sun, B. Starly, A. Darling, and C. Gomez, Computer-aided tissue engineering: application to biomimetic modelling and design of tissue scaffolds, *Biotechnol Appl Biochem* **39**(Pt 1), 49-58 (2004).
96. J. Taboas, R. Maddox, P. Krebsbach, and S. Hollister, Indirect solid free form fabrication of local and global porous, biomimetic and composite 3D polymer-ceramic scaffolds, *Biomaterials* **24**(1), 181-94 (2003).
97. S. Hollister, R. Maddox, and J. Taboas, Optimal design and fabrication of scaffolds to mimic tissue properties and satisfy biological constraints, *Biomaterials* **23**(20), 4095-103 (2002).
98. N. Porter, R. Pilliar, and M. Grynpas, Fabrication of porous calcium polyphosphate implants by solid freeform fabrication: a study of processing parameters and in vitro degradation characteristics., *J Biomed Mater Res* **56**(4), 504-15 (2001).
99. S. J. Hollister, R. A. Levy, T. M. Chu, J. W. Halloran, and S. E. Feinberg, An image-based approach for designing and manufacturing craniofacial scaffolds, *Int J Oral Maxillofac Surg* **29**(1), 67-71 (2000).
100. E. Tognana, R. F. Padera, F. Chen, G. Vunjak-Novakovic, and L. E. Freed, Development and remodeling of engineered cartilage-explant composites in vitro and in vivo, *Osteoarthritis Cartilage* **13**(10), 896-905 (2005).
101. B. Grigolo, L. Roseti, M. Fiorini, M. Fini, G. Giavaresi, N. Aldini, R. Giardino, and A. Facchini, Transplantation of chondrocytes seeded on a hyaluronan derivative (HYAff-11) into cartilage defects in rabbits., *Biomaterials* **22**(17), 2417-24 (2001).
102. S. Nehrer, H. A. Breinan, A. Ramappa, S. Shortkroff, G. Young, T. Minas, C. B. Sledge, I. V. Yannas, and M. Spector, Canine chondrocytes seeded in type I and type II collagen implants investigated in vitro, *J Biomed Mater Res* **38**(2), 95-104 (1997).
103. Y. Hatakeyama, J. Nguyen, X. Wang, G. H. Nuckolls, and L. Shum, Smad signaling in mesenchymal and chondroprogenitor cells, *J Bone Joint Surg Am* **85-A Suppl 3**, 13-8 (2003).
104. R. S. Tare, D. Howard, J. C. Pound, H. I. Roach, and R. O. Oreffo, Tissue engineering strategies for cartilage generation-Micromass and three dimensional cultures using human chondrocytes and a continuous cell line, *Biochem Biophys Res Commun* **333**(2), 609-21 (2005).
105. L. Yeh, F. Mallein-Gerin, and J. Lee, Differential effects of osteogenic protein-1 (BMP-7) on gene expression of BMP and GDF family members during differentiation of the mouse MC615 chondrocyte cells., *J Cell Physiol* **191**(3), 298-309 (2002).
106. B. Thomas, S. Thirion, L. Humbert, L. Tan, M. Goldring, G. Bereziat, and F. Berenbaum, Differentiation regulates interleukin-1beta-induced cyclo-oxygenase-2 in human articular chondrocytes: role of p38 mitogen-activated protein kinase., *Biochem J* **362**(Pt 2), 367-73 (2002).
107. N. Kamiya, A. Jikko, K. Kimata, C. Damsky, K. Shimizu, and H. Watanabe, Establishment of a novel chondrocytic cell line N1511 derived from p53-null mice, *J Bone Miner Res* **17**(10), 1832-42 (2002).
108. W. Chang, C. Tu, S. Pratt, T. Chen, and D. Shoback, Extracellular Ca(2+)-sensing receptors modulate matrix production and mineralization in chondrogenic RCJ3.1C5.18 cells., *Endocrinology* **143**(4), 1467-74 (2002).

109. A. Caplan, Mesenchymal stem cells., *J Orthop Res* **9**(5), 641-50 (1991).
110. D. A. Grande, A. S. Breitbart, J. Mason, C. Paulino, J. Laser, and R. E. Schwartz, Cartilage tissue engineering: current limitations and solutions, *Clin Orthop* **367**(Suppl), S176-85 (1999).
111. B. Johnstone and J. Yoo, Mesenchymal cell transfer for articular cartilage repair, *Expert Opin Biol Ther* **1**(6), 915-21 (2001).
112. M. Radice, P. Brun, R. Cortivo, R. Scapinelli, C. Battaliard, and G. Abatangelo, Hyaluronan-based biopolymers as delivery vehicles for bone-marrow-derived mesenchymal progenitors, *J Biomed Mater Res* **50**(2), 101-9 (2000).
113. S. Wakitani, T. Goto, S. Pineda, R. Young, J. Mansour, A. Caplan, and V. Goldberg, Mesenchymal cell-based repair of large, full-thickness defects of articular cartilage., *J Bone Joint Surg Am* **76**(4), 579-92 (1994).
114. N. Rotter, L. J. Bonassar, G. Tobias, M. Lebl, A. K. Roy, and C. A. Vacanti, Age dependence of cellular properties of human septal cartilage: implications for tissue engineering, *Arch Otolaryngol Head Neck Surg* **127**(10), 1248-52 (2001).
115. G. van Osch, S. van der Veen, and H. Verwoerd-Verhoef, In vitro redifferentiation of culture-expanded rabbit and human auricular chondrocytes for cartilage reconstruction., *Plast Reconstr Surg* **107**(2), 433-40 (2001).
116. N. Rotter, J. Aigner, A. Naumann, H. Planck, C. Hammer, G. Burmester, and M. Sittinger, Cartilage reconstruction in head and neck surgery: comparison of resorbable polymer scaffolds for tissue engineering of human septal cartilage, *J Biomed Mater Res* **42**(3), 347-56 (1998).
117. A. G. Tay, J. Farhadi, R. Suetterlin, G. Pierer, M. Heberer, and I. Martin, Cell yield, proliferation, and postexpansion differentiation capacity of human ear, nasal, and rib chondrocytes, *Tissue Eng* **10**(5-6), 762-70 (2004).
118. E. Mandl, S. van der Veen, J. Verhaar, and G. van Osch, Serum-free medium supplemented with high concentration of FGF-2 for cell expansion culture of human ear chondrocytes promotes redifferentiation capacity, *Tissue Eng* **8**(4), 573-580 (2002).
119. M. M. Stevens, R. P. Marini, I. Martin, R. Langer, and V. Prasad Shastri, FGF-2 enhances TGF-beta1-induced periosteal chondrogenesis, *J Orthop Res* **22**(5), 1114-9 (2004).
120. S. W. O'Driscoll and J. S. Fitzsimmons, The role of periosteum in cartilage repair, *Clin Orthop* **391**(Suppl), S190-207 (2001).
121. Y. Miura and S. W. O'Driscoll, Culturing periosteum in vitro: the influence of different sizes of explants, *Cell Transplant* **7**(5), 453-7 (1998).
122. J. Mason, D. Grande, M. Barcia, R. Grant, R. Pergolizzi, and A. Breitbart, Expression of human bone morphogenic protein 7 in primary rabbit periosteal cells: potential utility in gene therapy for osteochondral repair., *Gene Ther* **5**(8), 1098-104 (1998).
123. H. Nakahara, S. Bruder, S. Haynesworth, J. Holecek, M. Baber, V. Goldberg, and A. Caplan, Bone and cartilage formation in diffusion chambers by subcultured cells derived from the periosteum., *Bone* **11**(3), 181-8 (1990).
124. P. A. Zuk, M. Zhu, H. Mizuno, J. Huang, J. W. Futrell, A. J. Katz, P. Benhaim, H. P. Lorenz, and M. H. Hedrick, Multilineage cells from human adipose tissue: implications for cell-based therapies, *Tissue Eng* **7**(2), 211-28 (2001).
125. A. Winter, S. Breit, D. Parsch, K. Benz, E. Steck, H. Hauner, R. Weber, V. Ewerbeck, and W. Richter, Cartilage-like gene expression in differentiated human stem cell spheroids: A comparison of bone marrow-derived and adipose tissue-derived stromal cells, *Arthritis Rheum* **48**(2), 418-29 (2003).
126. J. L. Dragoo, B. Samimi, M. Zhu, S. L. Hame, B. J. Thomas, J. R. Lieberman, M. H. Hedrick, and P. Benhaim, Tissue-engineered cartilage and bone using stem cells from human infrapatellar fat pads, *J Bone Joint Surg Br* **85**(5), 740-7 (2003).
127. G. R. Erickson, J. M. Gimble, D. M. Franklin, H. E. Rice, H. Awad, and F. Guilak, Chondrogenic potential of adipose tissue-derived stromal cells in vitro and in vivo, *Biochem Biophys Res Commun* **290**(2), 763-9 (2002).
128. K. E. Kuettner, Biochemistry of articular cartilage in health and disease, *Clin Biochem* **25**(3), 155-63 (1992).
129. A. Aulthouse, M. Beck, and E. Griffey, Expression of the human chondrocyte phenotype in vitro, *In Vitro Cell Dev Biol Anim* **25**, 659-668 (1989).
130. P. Benya and J. Shaffer, Dedifferentiated chondrocytes re-express the differentiated collagen phenotype when cultured in agarose gels., *Cell* **30**, 215-224 (1982).
131. F. Binette, D. McQuaid, D. Haudenschild, P. Yaeger, J. McPherson, and R. Tubo, Expression of a stable articular cartilage phenotype without evidence of hypertrophy by adult human articular chondrocytes in vitro., *J Orthop Res* **16**(2), 207-16 (1998).

132. B. Dunham and R. Koch, Basic fibroblast growth factor and insulinlike growth factor I support the growth of human septal chondrocytes in a serum-free environment., *Arch Otolaryngol Head Neck Surg* **124**(12), 1325-30 (1998).
133. I. Martin, G. Vunjak-Novakovic, J. Yang, R. Langer, and L. E. Freed, Mammalian chondrocytes expanded in the presence of fibroblast growth factor 2 maintain the ability to differentiate and regenerate three-dimensional cartilaginous tissue, *Exp Cell Res* **253**(2), 681-8 (1999).
134. M. Jakob, O. Demarteau, D. Schafer, B. Hintermann, W. Dick, M. Heberer, and I. Martin, Specific growth factors during the expansion and redifferentiation of adult human articular chondrocytes enhance chondrogenesis and cartilaginous tissue formation in vitro., *J Cell Biochem* **81**(2), 368-77 (2001).
135. M. Pei, J. Seidel, G. Vunjak-Novakovic, and L. Freed, Growth factors for sequential cellular de- and re-differentiation in tissue engineering, *Biochem Biophys Res Commun* **294**(1), 149-54 (2002).
136. C. Frondoza, A. Sohrabi, and D. Hungerford, Human chondrocytes proliferate and produce matrix components in microcarrier suspension culture., *Biomaterials* **17**(9), 879-88 (1996).
137. J. Malda, C. A. van Blitterswijk, M. Grojec, D. E. Martens, J. Tramper, and J. Riesle, Expansion of bovine chondrocytes on microcarriers enhances redifferentiation, *Tissue Eng* **9**(5), 939-48 (2003).
138. J. Malda, E. Kreijveld, J. S. Temenoff, C. A. van Blitterswijk, and J. Riesle, Expansion of human nasal chondrocytes on macroporous microcarriers enhances redifferentiation, *Biomaterials* **24**(28), 5153-61 (2003).
139. G. Schulze-Tanzil, S. P. De, C. H. Villegas, T. John, H. Merker, A. Scheid, and M. Shakibaei, Redifferentiation of dedifferentiated human chondrocytes in high-density cultures, *Cell Tissue Res* **308**(3), 371-9 (2002).
140. M. Solursh and S. Meier, Effects of cell density on the expresion of differentiation by chick embryo chondrocytes., *J Exp Zool* **187**, 311-322 (1974).
141. C. Xu, B. Oyajobi, A. Frazer, L. Kozaci, R. Russell, and A. Hollander, Effects of growth factors and interleukin-1 alpha on proteoglycan and type II collagen turnover in bovine nasal and articular chondrocyte pellet cultures., *Endocrinology* **137**(8), 3557-65 (1996).
142. T. Blunk, A. Sieminski, K. Gooch, D. Courter, A. Hollander, A. Nahir, R. Langer, G. Vunjak-Novakovic, and L. Freed, Differential effects of growth factors on tissue-engineered cartilage., *Tissue Eng* **8**(1), 73-84 (2002).
143. P. Yaeger, T. Masi, J. de Ortiz, F. Binette, R. Tubo, and J. McPherson, Synergistic action of transforming growth factor-beta and insulin-like growth factor-I induces expression of type II collagen and aggrecan genes in adult human articular chondrocytes., *Exp Cell Res* **237**(2), 318-25 (1997).
144. K. Gooch, J. Kwon, T. Blunk, R. Langer, L. Freed, and G. Vunjak-Novakovic, Effects of mixing intensity on tissue-engineered cartilage., *Biotechnol Bioeng* **72**(4), 402-7 (2001).
145. G. Vunjak-Novakovic, B. Obradovic, I. Martin, P. Bursac, R. Langer, and L. Freed, Dynamic cell seeding of polymer scaffolds for cartilage tissue engineering., *Biotechnol Prog* **14**(2), 193-202 (1998).
146. G. Vunjak-Novakovic, B. Obradovic, I. Martin, and L. Freed, Bioreactor studies of native and tissue engineered cartilage, *Biorheology* **39**(1,2), 259-268 (2002).
147. M. Pei, L. Solchaga, J. Seidel, L. Zeng, G. Vunjak-Novakovic, A. Caplan, and L. Freed, Bioreactors mediate the effectiveness of tissue engineering scaffolds., *FASEB J* **16**(12), 1691-4 (2002).
148. I. Martin, B. Obradovic, S. Treppo, A. J. Grodzinsky, R. Langer, L. E. Freed, and G. Vunjak-Novakovic, Modulation of the mechanical properties of tissue engineered cartilage, *Biorheology* **37**(1-2), 141-7 (2000).
149. L. E. Freed, A. P. Hollander, I. Martin, J. R. Barry, R. Langer, and G. Vunjak-Novakovic, Chondrogenesis in a cell-polymer-bioreactor system, *Exp Cell Res* **240**(1), 58-65 (1998).
150. L. E. Freed and G. Vunjak-Novakovic, Cultivation of Cell-Polymer Tissue Constructs in Simulated Microgravity, *Biotechnology and Bioengineering* **46**(4), 306-313 (1995).
151. U. Hansen, M. Schunke, C. Domm, N. Ioannidis, J. Hassenpflug, T. Gehrke, and B. Kurz, Combination of reduced oxygen tension and intermittent hydrostatic pressure: a useful tool in articular cartilage tissue engineering, *J Biomech* **34**(7), 941-9 (2001).
152. R. Wilkins, J. Browning, and J. Urban, Chondrocyte regulation by mechanical load., *Biorheology* **37**(1-2), 67-74 (2000).
153. J. K. Suh, G. H. Baek, A. Aroen, C. M. Malin, C. Niyibizi, C. H. Evans, and A. Westerhausen-Larson, Intermittent sub-ambient interstitial hydrostatic pressure as a potential mechanical stimulator for chondrocyte metabolism, *Osteo Cart* **7**(1), 71-80 (1999).
154. S. E. Carver and C. A. Heath, Semi-continuous perfusion system for delivering intermittent physiological pressure to regenerating cartilage, *Tissue Eng* **5**(1), 1-11 (1999).
155. S. E. Carver and C. A. Heath, Increasing extracellular matrix production in regenerating cartilage with intermittent physiological pressure, *Biotechnol Bioeng* **62**(2), 166-74 (1999).

156. S. E. Carver and C. A. Heath, Influence of intermittent pressure, fluid flow, and mixing on the regenerative properties of articular chondrocytes, *Biotechnol Bioeng* **65**(3), 274-81 (1999).
157. O. Demarteau, M. Jakob, D. Schafer, M. Heberer, and I. Martin, Development and validation of a bioreactor for physical stimulation of engineered cartilage., *Biorheology* **40**(1-3), 331-6 (2003).
158. L. J. Bonassar, A. J. Grodzinsky, E. H. Frank, S. G. Davila, N. R. Bhaktav, and S. B. Trippel, The effect of dynamic compression on the response of articular cartilage to insulin-like growth factor-I, *J Orthop Res* **19**(1), 11-7 (2001).
159. D. A. Lee, T. Noguchi, S. P. Frean, P. Lees, and D. L. Bader, The influence of mechanical loading on isolated chondrocytes seeded in agarose constructs, *Biorheology* **37**(1-2), 149-61 (2000).
160. T. M. Quinn, A. J. Grodzinsky, M. D. Buschmann, Y. J. Kim, and E. B. Hunziker, Mechanical compression alters proteoglycan deposition and matrix deformation around individual cells in cartilage explants, *J Cell Sci* **111**(Pt 5), 573-83 (1998).
161. M. D. Buschmann, Y. A. Gluzband, A. J. Grodzinsky, and E. B. Hunziker, Mechanical compression modulates matrix biosynthesis in chondrocyte/agarose culture, *J Cell Sci* **108 (Pt 4)**, 1497-508 (1995).
162. Y. J. Kim, R. L. Sah, A. J. Grodzinsky, A. H. Plaas, and J. D. Sandy, Mechanical regulation of cartilage biosynthetic behavior: physical stimuli, *Arch Biochem Biophys* **311**(1), 1-12 (1994).
163. F. Guilak, B. C. Meyer, A. Ratcliffe, and V. C. Mow, The effects of matrix compression on proteoglycan metabolism in articular cartilage explants, *Osteo Cart* **2**(2), 91-101 (1994).
164. J. Malda, D. E. Martens, J. Tramper, C. A. van Blitterswijk, and J. Riesle, Cartilage tissue engineering: controversy in the effect of oxygen, *Crit Rev Biotechnol* **23**(3), 175-94 (2003).
165. M. J. Lydon, T. W. Minett, and B. J. Tighe, Cellular interactions with synthetic polymer surfaces in culture, *Biomaterials* **6**(6), 396-402 (1985).
166. B. D. Boyan, T. W. Hummert, D. D. Dean, and Z. Schwartz, Role of material surfaces in regulating bone and cartilage cell response, *Biomaterials* **17**(2), 137-46 (1996).
167. Z. Schwartz, J. Martin, D. Dean, J. Simpson, D. Cochran, and B. Boyan, Effect of titanium surface roughness on chondrocyte proliferation, matrix production, and differentiation depends on the state of cell maturation., *J Biomed Mater Res* **30**(2), 145-55 (1996).
168. R. Singhvi, A. Kumar, G. P. Lopez, G. N. Stephanopoulos, D. I. Wang, G. M. Whitesides, and D. E. Ingber, Engineering cell shape and function, *Science* **264**(5159), 696-8 (1994).
169. R. F. Loeser, Integrins and cell signaling in chondrocytes, *Biorheology* **39**(1-2), 119-24 (2002).
170. R. F. Loeser, Chondrocyte integrin expression and function, *Biorheology* **37**(1-2), 109-16 (2000).
171. R. F. Loeser, Integrin-mediated attachment of articular chondrocytes to extracellular matrix proteins, *Arthritis Rheum* **36**(8), 1103-10 (1993).
172. W. Knudson and R. Loeser, CD44 and integrin matrix receptors participate in cartilage homeostasis., *Cell Mol Life Sci* **59**(1), 36-44 (2002).
173. B. Grigolo, G. Lisignoli, A. Piacentini, M. Fiorini, P. Gobbi, G. Mazzotti, M. Duca, A. Pavesio, and A. Facchini, Evidence for redifferentiation of human chondrocytes grown on a hyaluronan-based biomaterial (HYAff 11): molecular, immunohistochemical and ultrastructural analysis, *Biomaterials* **23**(4), 1187-95 (2002).
174. L. Lu, X. Zhu, R. G. Valenzuela, B. L. Currier, and M. J. Yaszemski, Biodegradable polymer scaffolds for cartilage tissue engineering, *Clin Orthop* **391**(Suppl), S251-70 (2001).
175. J. Hambleton, Z. Schwartz, A. Khare, S. W. Windeler, M. Luna, B. P. Brooks, D. D. Dean, and B. D. Boyan, Culture surfaces coated with various implant materials affect chondrocyte growth and metabolism, *J Orthop Res* **12**(4), 542-52 (1994).
176. S. L. Ishaug-Riley, L. E. Okun, G. Prado, M. A. Applegate, and A. Ratcliffe, Human articular chondrocyte adhesion and proliferation on synthetic biodegradable polymer films., *Biomaterials* **20**(23-24), 2245-56 (1999).
177. A. Lahiji, A. Sohrabi, D. Hungerford, and C. Frondoza, Chitosan supports the expression of extracellular matrix proteins in human osteoblasts and chondrocytes., *J Biomed Mater Res* **51**(4), 586-95 (2000).
178. S. Lee, G. Khang, Y. Lee, and H. Lee, Interaction of human chondrocytes and NIH/3T3 fibroblasts on chloric acid-treated biodegradable polymer surfaces, *J Biomater Sci Polym Ed* **13**(2), 197-212 (2002).
179. M. Papadaki, T. Mahmood, P. Gupta, M. B. Claase, D. W. Grijpma, J. Riesle, C. A. van Blitterswijk, and R. Langer, The different behaviors of skeletal muscle cells and chondrocytes on PEGT/PBT block copolymers are related to the surface properties of the substrate., *J Biomed Mater Res* **54**(1), 47-58 (2001).
180. J. Malda, T. B. F. Woodfield, F. van der Vloodt, F. K. Kooy, D. E. Martens, J. Tramper, C. A. van Blitterswijk, and J. Riesle, The effect of PEGT/PBT scaffold architecture on oxygen gradients in tissue engineered cartilaginous constructs, *Biomaterials* **25**(26), 5773-80 (2004).
181. J. Zeltinger, J. Sherwood, D. Graham, R. Mueller, and L. Griffith, Effect of pore size and void fraction on cellular adhesion, proliferation, and matrix deposition., *Tissue Eng* **7**(5), 557-72 (2001).

182. B. Kreklau, M. Sittinger, M. B. Mensing, C. Voigt, G. Berger, G. R. Burmester, R. Rahmanzadeh, and U. Gross, Tissue engineering of biphasic joint cartilage transplants, *Biomaterials* **20**(18), 1743-9 (1999).
183. Z. Zhang, J. M. McCaffery, R. G. Spencer, and C. A. Francomano, Hyaline cartilage engineered by chondrocytes in pellet culture: histological, immunohistochemical and ultrastructural analysis in comparison with cartilage explants, *J Anat* **205**(3), 229-37 (2004).
184. T. Tallheden, C. Bengtsson, C. Brantsing, E. Sjogren-Jansson, L. Carlsson, L. Peterson, M. Brittberg, and A. Lindahl, Proliferation and differentiation potential of chondrocytes from osteoarthritic patients, *Arthritis Res Ther* **7**(3), R560-8 (2005).
185. T. B. F. Woodfield, S. Miot, I. Martin, C. A. van Blitterswijk, and J. Riesle, The regulation of expanded human nasal chondrocyte re-differentiation capacity by substrate composition and gas plasma surface modification, *Biomaterials* **in press** (2006).
186. T. A. Mahmood, S. Miot, O. Frank, I. Martin, J. Riesle, R. Langer, and C. A. van Blitterswijk, Cell and tissue engineering by material-directed molecular response, submitted for publication (2005).
187. J. Malda, J. Rouwkema, D. E. Martens, E. P. Le Comte, F. K. Kooy, J. Tramper, C. A. van Blitterswijk, and J. Riesle, Oxygen gradients in tissue-engineered PEGT/PBT cartilaginous constructs: Measurement and modeling, *Biotechnol Bioeng* **86**(1), 9-18 (2004).
188. J. Malda, Cartilage Tissue Engineering: The Relevance of Oxygen, PhD Thesis - University of Twente, Enschede, The Netherlands. **2003**; 224.
189. G. Vunjak-Novakovic, L. Meinel, G. Altman, and D. Kaplan, Bioreactor cultivation of osteochondral grafts, *Orthod Craniofac Res* **8**(3), 209-18 (2005).
190. E. M. Darling and K. A. Athanasiou, Articular cartilage bioreactors and bioprocesses, *Tissue Eng* **9**(1), 9-26 (2003).
191. O. Démarteau, D. Schäfer, M. Jacob, M. Heberer, and I. Martin, Dynamic compression increases expression of cartilage-specific genes by adult human chondrocytes seeded into hyaluronic acid-based scaffolds, *Trans Orthop Res Soc*, 254 (2002).
192. R. L. Mauck, M. A. Soltz, C. C. Wang, D. D. Wong, P. H. Chao, W. B. Valhmu, C. T. Hung, and G. A. Ateshian, Functional tissue engineering of articular cartilage through dynamic loading of chondrocyte-seeded agarose gels, *J Biomech Eng* **122**(3), 252-60 (2000).
193. T. K. Kim, B. Sharma, C. G. Williams, M. A. Ruffner, A. Malik, E. G. McFarland, and J. H. Elisseeff, Experimental model for cartilage tissue engineering to regenerate the zonal organization of articular cartilage., *Osteoarthritis Cartilage* **11**(9), 653-64 (2003).
194. K. Ng, C. C. Wang, X. E. Guo, G. A. Ateshian, and C. T. Hung, Characterization of inhomogeneous bi-layered chondrocyte-seeded agarose constructs of differing agarose concentrations, *Trans Orthop Res Soc*, 960 (2003).
195. D. W. Hutmacher, M. Sittinger, and M. V. Risbud, Scaffold-based tissue engineering: rationale for computer-aided design and solid free-form fabrication systems, *Trends Biotechnol* **22**(7), 354-62 (2004).
196. L. Solchaga, J. Dennis, V. Goldberg, and A. Caplan, Hyaluronic acid-based polymers as cell carriers for tissue-engineered repair of bone and cartilage., *J Orthop Res* **17**(2), 205-13 (1999).
197. P. Giannoni, A. Crovace, M. Malpeli, E. Maggi, R. Arbico, R. Cancedda, and B. Dozin, Species variability in the differentiation potential of in vitro-expanded articular chondrocytes restricts predictive studies on cartilage repair using animal models, *Tissue Eng* **11**(1-2), 237-48 (2005).
198. M. Oyama, A. Tatlock, S. Fukuta, K. Kavalkovich, K. Nishimura, B. Johnstone, P. D. Robbins, C. H. Evans, and C. Niyibizi, Retrovirally transduced bone marrow stromal cells isolated from a mouse model of human osteogenesis imperfecta (oim) persist in bone and retain the ability to form cartilage and bone after extended passaging, *Gene Ther* **6**(3), 321-9 (1999).
199. P. G. ten Koppel, G. J. van Osch, C. D. Verwoerd, and H. L. Verwoerd-Verhoef, A new in vivo model for testing cartilage grafts and biomaterials: the 'rabbit pinna punch-hole' model, *Biomaterials* **22**(11), 1407-14 (2001).
200. E. B. Hunziker, Tissue engineering of bone and cartilage. From the preclinical model to the patient, *Novartis Found Symp* **249**, 70-8; discussion 78-85, 170-4, 239-41 (2003).
201. D. B. Saris, W. J. Dhert, and A. J. Verbout, Joint homeostasis. The discrepancy between old and fresh defects in cartilage repair, *J Bone Joint Surg Br* **85**(7), 1067-76 (2003).
202. J. Quintavalla, S. Uziel-Fusi, J. Yin, E. Boehnlein, G. Pastor, V. Blancuzzi, H. Singh, K. Kraus, E. O'Byrne, and T. Pellas, Fluorescently labeled mesenchymal stem cells (MSCs) maintain multilineage potential and can be detected following implantation into articular cartilage defects, *Biomaterials* **23**(1), 109-19 (2002).
203. J. van Susante, P. Buma, L. Schuman, G. Homminga, W. van den Berg, and R. Veth, Resurfacing potential of heterologous chondrocytes suspended in fibrin glue in large full-thickness defects of femoral articular cartilage: an experimental study in the goat., *Biomaterials* **20**(13), 1167-75 (1999).

204. J. van Susante, P. Buma, G. Homminga, W. van den Berg, and R. Veth, Chondrocyte-seeded hydroxyapatite for repair of large articular cartilage defects. A pilot study in the goat., *Biomaterials* **19**(24), 2367-74 (1998).
205. G. G. Reinholz, L. Lu, D. B. Saris, M. J. Yaszemski, and S. W. O'Driscoll, Animal models for cartilage reconstruction, *Biomaterials* **25**(9), 1511-21 (2004).
206. E. B. Hunziker, Biologic repair of articular cartilage. Defect models in experimental animals and matrix requirements, *Clin Orthop* **367**(Suppl), S135-46 (1999).
207. B. Kladny, P. Martus, K. Schiwy-Bochat, G. Weseloh, and B. Swoboda, Measurement of cartilage thickness in the human knee joint by magnetic resonance imaging using a three-dimensional gradient echo sequence, *Int Orthop* **23**, 264-267 (1999).
208. S. W. O'Driscoll, Preclinical cartilage repair: current status and future perspectives, *Clin Orthop* **391**(Suppl), S397-401 (2001).
209. N. Tamai, A. Myoui, M. Hirao, T. Kaito, T. Ochi, J. Tanaka, K. Takaoka, and H. Yoshikawa, A new biotechnology for articular cartilage repair: subchondral implantation of a composite of interconnected porous hydroxyapatite, synthetic polymer (PLA-PEG), and bone morphogenetic protein-2 (rhBMP-2), *Osteoarthritis Cartilage* **13**(5), 405-17 (2005).
210. R. Ostrander, R. Goomer, W. Tontz, M. Khatod, F. Harwood, T. Maris, and D. Amiel, Donor cell fate in tissue engineering for articular cartilage repair., *Clin Orthop* **389**, 228-37 (2001).
211. B. Obradovic, I. Martin, R. F. Padera, S. Treppo, L. E. Freed, and G. Vunjak-Novakovic, Integration of engineered cartilage, *J Orthop Res* **19**(6), 1089-97 (2001).
212. K. Potter, J. Butler, W. Horton, and R. Spencer, Response of engineered cartilage tissue to biochemical agents as studied by proton magnetic resonance microscopy., *Arthritis Rheum* **43**(7), 1580-90 (2000).
213. T. L. Clemens, H. Tang, S. Maeda, R. A. Kesterson, F. Demayo, J. W. Pike, and C. M. Gundberg, Analysis of osteocalcin expression in transgenic mice reveals a species difference in vitamin D regulation of mouse and human osteocalcin genes, *J Bone Miner Res* **12**(10), 1570-6 (1997).
214. H. R. Herschman, Molecular imaging: looking at problems, seeing solutions, *Science* **302**(5645), 605-8 (2003).
215. T. Grant, J. Cho, K. Ariail, N. Weksler, R. Smith, and W. Horton, Col2-GFP reporter marks chondrocyte lineage and chondrogenesis during mouse skeletal development., *Dev Dyn* **218**(2), 394-400 (2000).

SECTION 6

SCIENCE, REGULATION, AND THE PUBLIC

23

ENGINEERED TISSUES: THE REGULATORY PATH FROM CONCEPT TO MARKET

Kiki B. Hellman, PhD.[1]

23.1. INTRODUCTION

Therapeutic approaches for replacement, repair, or regeneration of diseased or damaged human organs or tissues have evolved over the last several years from human donor organ and tissue transplants and implants of synthetic materials to *in vitro* engineered tissue constructs composed of autologous, allogeneic, or xenogeneic cells coupled with synthetic or natural matrix materials, and/or pharmacological agents for either *in vivo* implantation or *ex vivo* use and cell therapies using either native, stem, or progenitor autologous, or allogeneic cells for *in vivo* delivery. While organ/tissue transplantation and synthetic material implants continue as the standard of care, donor organ shortages and indications where such approaches may not be feasible have led to a search for alternatives utilizing living tissue, which, in turn, have provided the impetus for engineered tissue solutions.

Engineered tissues can provide either a structural/mechanical or metabolic function[1,2]. Examples, published in the scientific literature, include, among others: artificial skin constructs; musculoskeletal applications, such as autologous cells for cartilage regeneration, engineered ligament and tendon, and bone graft substitutes; approaches for repair and regeneration of the cardiovascular system including the myocardium, valves, and vessels; periodontal tissue repair; engineered cornea and lens; spinal cord repair and nerve regeneration; repair of the urogenital system; and approaches for functional restoration of vital, metabolic organs such as the pancreas, liver, and kidney through either biohybrid organ implants or *ex vivo* support systems.

The promise of engineered tissue therapies has been realized.[3,4] Skin and musculoskeletal substitutes have been approved for use in the US by the FDA. Others cited are under either preclinical investigation or regulatory evaluation. Recent advances in stem cell and cytokine biology, materials science, engineering, and computer

---

[1] The Hellman Group, LLC, Clarksburg, Maryland, USA

modeling, among others, are contributing to development of second-generation engineered tissue therapies.

In addition to therapeutic applications, *in vitro* engineered tissue constructs are being applied as biosensors in diagnostic systems and as test models for toxicity assessment of pharmacological and other agents. Development of enabling technologies provides promising avenues for establishment of a service industry, e.g., cell banks/repositories, scaffold/matrix materials and reference material libraries, and customized tissue-specific bioreactors.

Integrity of the science, together with other critical determinants, is basic to the successful translation of tissue engineering research into applications for the clinic and marketplace.[5] Of these determinants, understanding the strategies developed by government entities for providing appropriate product regulatory oversight is key. Since a primary goal is the establishment of a global industry enabling companies to market products across national boundaries, a harmonized international regulatory approach, such as the International Conference on Harmonization for pharmaceutical products, would be ideal. While groups work toward that goal, and recognizing that the public's perception and subsequent market acceptance can be influenced by local social, political, legal, and ethical concerns, it is important to understand the approaches of regulatory entities where the research has moved successfully thorough product development to the marketplace[4]. Although the science is now worldwide and regulatory approaches are being developed in Europe and the Far East, among others, this discussion will be limited to the regulatory strategies and evolving initiatives in the US.

The FDA has recognized that an important segment of the products that it regulates results from application of novel technology such as tissue engineering, and that product applications often pose new and complex issues. Thus, the Agency has worked since the early 1990's on developing appropriate strategies for the regulatory oversight of human cells, tissues, and cellular- and tissue-based products. Most, if not all, engineered tissues fall into these categories.

23.2. LEGISLATIVE AUTHORITY

23.2.1. Laws

Since approaches for organ and tissue replacement, repair, and regeneration and their source materials span a broad spectrum of potential clinical applications, the responsibility for overseeing their development and commercialization within the US federal government has been divided among different regulatory agencies, centers, and offices. The Health Resources Services Administration (HRSA) oversees the National Organ Transplant Program and the National Marrow Donor Program. The remaining products are regulated by the FDA.

The FDA is a science-based regulatory agency in the US Public Health Service (PHS). The agency's legislative authority for product oversight, premarket approval, and post market surveillance and enforcement is derived principally from the Federal Food, Drug, and Cosmetic (FD&C) Act and the Public Health Service (PHS) Act. Under these authorities, the FDA evaluates and approves products for the marketplace, inspects manufacturing facilities sometimes before and routinely during commercial distribution, and takes corrective action to remove products form commerce when they are unsafe, misbranded, or adulterated.

23.2.2. FDA Mission and Organization

The FDA's mission is to promote and protect the public health through regulation of a broad range of products by assuring the safety of foods, cosmetics, and radiation-emitting electronic products, as well as assuring the safety and effectiveness of human and veterinary pharmaceuticals, biologicals, and medical devices. The FDA's six centers are staffed with individuals expert in the science and regulations(s) appropriate to a center's mission. The centers with regulatory oversight for human medical products are the: Center for Drug Evaluation and Research (CDER) which regulates drugs; Center for Biologics Evaluation and Research (CBER) which regulates biological products; and the Center for Devices and Radiological Health (CDRH) which regulates medical devices and radiation-emitting electronic products. However, each center can apply any of the statutory authorities to regulate its products. For example, many products reviewed by CBER are regulated under the medical device authority. In addition to the centers, other offices such as the Office of Regulatory Affairs (ORA) and Office of Orphan Products (OOP), provide assistance to the centers on regulatory procedures and facility inspections, when necessary. The Office of Combination Products (OCP) is responsible for the regulatory oversight of combination products. While the office does not perform product reviews for market approval or clearance, it assigns the combination product to the appropriate FDA center, ensures timely and effective premarket review and appropriate post market regulation, and serves as a resource to industry and the FDA centers' review staff.[3,4] The OCP serves a very important function for regulation of engineered tissue products, since many are combination products.

23.3. PRODUCT REGULATORY PROCESS

23.3.1. Classification of Products

Under federal law, a human medical product is classified as either a drug, biological drug (biologic), device, or combination product, e.g. a combination of a drug, biologic, and/or device. The product's classification determines the premarket review and approval process for demonstration of safety and effectiveness utilized by FDA, and the FDA center with lead responsibility and jurisdiction for the product. For example, a drug is an article intended for use in the diagnosis, cure, mitigation, treatment, or prevention of disease in humans or other animals, and an article (other than food) and other articles intended to affect the structure or any function of the body of humans or other animals [21USC321(g)]. A biologic is defined as a virus, therapeutic serum, toxin, antitoxin, vaccine, blood, blood component or derivative, allergenic product or analogous product, . . . applicable to the prevention, treatment, or cure of diseases or injuries of man [42USC262(a)]. A device is an instrument, apparatus, . . . implant, in vitro reagent or other similar or related article which is intended for use in diagnosis of disease or conditions, or in the cure, mitigation, treatment or prevention of disease, in humans or other animals, or intended to affect the structure or any function of the body . . . and which does not achieve any of its principal intended purposes through chemical action within or on the body . . ., and which is not dependent on being metabolized for the achievement of any of its principal intended purposes [21USC201(h)].

23.3.1.1. Combination Products

Advances in biomedical technology have generated products not readily classifiable as drugs, biologics, or devices as these terms are defined by federal law. To provide for the expanding varieties of products expressing features of more than one of these classifications, the FDA has been authorized to recognize combination products. These products constitute a growing category of innovative medical products. Examples include a drug with an implantable delivery device and autologous cells coupled with a scaffold for orthopedic use. While these products contribute to advancing medical care, they also pose a challenge for the FDA, since they straddle existing statutory classifications of regulated products, complicating the determination of the appropriate regulatory process[4].

Congress recognized the existence of combination products when it enacted the Safe Medical Device Act of 1990 and established that the FDA shall classify a combination product according to its primary mode of action [Section 503(g) of the FD&C Act [21USC 353(g)]. From its determination of the product's primary mode of action, the Agency could assign jurisdiction over the product to one of its established centers. For example, if the primary mode of action is that of a drug, the product is assigned to CDER, if that of a device to CDRH, and biologics to CBER. The FDA issued a final rule in 1991 establishing the process, i.e., Request for Designation (RFD), by which a product sponsor could petition the agency to make such an assignment [21CFR3.7].

The Medical Device User Free and Modernization Act of 2002 (MDUFMA) modified Section 503(g) of the FD&C Act to require the FDA to establish an office with the primary responsibility for providing regulatory oversight of combination products. The Office of Combination Products in the Office of the Commissioner assigns the product to the appropriate FDA center; resolves any disputes over a product's regulation, and is the focal point for both the FDA staff and industry regarding combination products.

There has been much progress since the office was established in making this somewhat complex regulatory area more efficient, transparent, and better understood. Because of its role, the office has become the focus and, often, the primary point of entry for sponsors of combination products. The office encourages informal as well as formal interactions, i.e., through the RFD process, with sponsors regarding product jurisdictional questions.

While the FDA has traditionally required sponsors of a RFD to identify the product's primary mode of action and recommend the lead center for product premarket review and regulation, there is no statutory definition of what constitutes primary mode of action. To address concerns that, without a statutory codified definition, the assignment process has appeared arbitrary at times, the office published a proposed rule to amend the regulations and to define and codify both mode of action and primary mode of action, "Definition of Primary Mode of Action of a Combination Product: Proposed Rule" (69FR25527, May 7, 2004) (the PMOA Proposed Rule). Mode of action is defined as the means by which a product achieves a therapeutic effect, i.e., drug, biologic, or device mode of action. Since combination products have more than one identifiable mode of action, the primary mode of action is the single mode that provides the most important therapeutic effect. The PMOA Proposed Rule also describes an algorithm that the agency would use to assign a product to a center when it cannot determine with reasonable certainty which mode of action provides the most important therapeutic effect. The Proposed Rule would require a sponsor to base its recommendation of the center with primary jurisdiction for its product by using the definition and, if appropriate, the assignment algorithm. This framework is based on an assessment of the product as a whole; its intended use and effect; consistency with assignment of similarly situated products; and safety and effectiveness issues.[6] Of note is that most, if not all, engineered tissue products are combination products.

23.3.2. Product Premarket Submissions

23.3.2.1. Investigational Studies

The FD&C Act requires demonstration of safety and effectiveness for new drugs and devices prior to introduction into interstate commerce. The PHS Act requires demonstration of safety, purity, and potency for biological products before introduction into interstate commerce. Consequently, premarket clinical studies must be performed under exemptions from these laws. For drugs and biologics, which are considered drugs under the FD&C Act, the application for the exemption is an Investigational New Drug (IND) application, (21CFR312). The application for exemption of a device is an Investigational Device Exemption (IDE) (21CFR812).

The contents of IND and IDE applications are similar[2]. Applications will include a description of the product and manufacturing processes sufficient for an evaluation of product safety, and preclinical studies that have been designed to assess risks and potential benefits of the product. The IND and IDE applications contain a proposal for a clinical protocol, which describes the indication being treated, proposed patient population, patient inclusion and exclusion criteria, treatment regimen, study end points, patient follow-up methods, and clinical trial stopping rules. Both IND and IDE investigations require Institutional Review Board (IRB) approval before they may commence. Although IND and IDE requirements are somewhat different (e.g., in cost recovery and device risk assessment areas), the FDA applies comparable standards of safety and effectiveness for either type of application. When the FDA determines that there is sufficient information to allow a clinical investigation to proceed, the IND or IDE exemptions are approved.

The first clinical studies conducted under the IND or IDE applications are often clinical trials involving a small number of individuals (e.g., phase 1/feasibility studies) designed primarily to assess product safety. If these earlier studies indicate reasonable safety, phase 2/studies may be developed to investigate proper and safe dosing and potential efficacy. Phase 3/pivotal studies utilize well-controlled clinical trial designs that support a determination of safety and effectiveness and lead to an application to the FDA for premarket approval of the product.

There may be situations in which the first study under an IND or IDE will not be a phase1/feasibility study[2]. For example, this may occur when there is sufficient clinical experience to establish the safety of a product after use outside the US or in a different patient population. The FDA may review data from clinical studies performed outside the US in the IND/IDE process and/or in an application for marketing approval. The agency strongly recommends that the sponsor meets with FDA staff to discuss the clinical protocol, study results, statistical analyses, and applicability of the data to a US population before submitting the premarket submission, i.e. Biologics License or Premarket Approval application (BLA/PMA).

23.3.2.2. Premarket Submissions

According to the laws and regulations governing commercial distribution of human medical products, there are several different types of product premarket submissions determined by the product's FDA classification. In general, the type of submission will depend on the type of product; i.e., drug, biologic or device.

Engineered tissue products regulated as biologics will require review and approval of a BLA that demonstrates the safety and effectiveness of the product before it may be marketed commercially. If it is regulated as a device, a PMA demonstrating safety and effectiveness must be approved, or a premarket notification [510(k)] must receive clearance. In order to obtain 510(k) premarket clearance, the sponsor must demonstrate substantial equivalence of the device to a legally marketed predicate device.

23.3.2.3. Special Product Designations and Submissions

The FD&C Act recognized that there may be situations where the demand for new medical products may be such that the cost of obtaining marketing approval for a product may be prohibitive in view of the small size of the intended population[4]. To reduce the possibility that a cost-benefit analysis applied to product development for rare diseases will result in no available therapy, the FDA is authorized to grant special consideration and exceptions to reduce the economic burdens on product developers of products under such conditions. As a result, the FDA may be petitioned to grant a Humanitarian Device Exemption (HDE) for certain devices (FD&C Act, 520m) or to recognize certain drugs or biologics as orphan drugs (FD&C Act, 525, et.seq.)

A Humanitarian Use Device (HUD) is a product that may be marketed under an exemption for treatment or diagnosis of a disease or condition that affects fewer than 4,000 individuals per year in the US. A HDE exempts a HUD from the effectiveness requirements for devices if certain criteria are met (FD&C Act, 529(m)(1), as amended February 1998). Several engineered skin constructs have been approved for market under the HUD designation.

Orphan drugs are those intended to treat a disease or condition affecting fewer than 200,000 individuals in the US for which there is little likelihood that the cost of developing and distributing it in the US will be recovered from sales of the drug in the US. The orphan drug designation was established through an amendment of the FD&C Act by the 1982 Orphan Drug Act. An orphan drug is defined to include biologics licensed under Section 351 of the PHS Act. Under certain conditions, the FDA has authority to grant marketing exclusivity for an orphan drug in the US for a period of seven years from the date the drug is approved for clinical use. Other benefits to sponsors include grant support for clinical trials; tax credits for clinical research expenses; and waiver of the prescription drug filing fee[4]. A sponsor must file a petition for orphan drug designation before any application for marketing approval.

23.3.3. Post-Market Surveillance

Post-market surveillance for therapeutic engineered tissue products is an important area of consideration. Manufacturers, user facilities, and health care professionals should report adverse events through the FDA MedWatch process. Post marketing studies may be necessary when a sponsor seeks a change in product labeling; studies are a condition of the FDA approval; or such studies are necessary to protect the public health or to provide safety and effectiveness data[2]. Additionally, post market surveillance of a device introduced into interstate commerce after January 1, 1991, may be required if it is: intended for use in supporting or sustaining human life; presents a potential risk to human health; or is a permanent implant, whose failure may cause serious, adverse health consequences or death (Section 522, FD&C Act).

23.4. REVIEW OF PRODUCT PREMARKET SUBMISSIONS

Advances in tissue engineering research have led to potential therapeutic products for many different medical conditions characterized by organ and/or tissue damage. As indicated previously, the products may provide either a structural/mechanical or metabolic function. To date, products have been developed either as *in vitro* engineered tissue constructs for implantation, cell therapies for *in vivo* delivery, or *ex vivo* systems. Representatives of these products are in different stages of development; first generation products have been approved for use in the US (Table 23.1), while many others are under either preclinical investigation or regulatory evaluation.

Since many of the products may consist of more than one component, i.e., biomolecule, cell/tissue, and/or biomaterial, they are considered combination products. A determination of the product's primary mode of action dictates the jurisdictional authority for the product and the primary reviewing center, i.e., CDER, CBER, or CDRH. However, regardless of the product's designation, review of any regulated product considers four basic elements, i.e., product manufacture, preclinical (laboratory and animal model) testing, clinical performance, and product labeling in order to determine safety and effectiveness in support of the manufacturer's claim of intended use.

Regulatory evaluation is conducted on a case-by-case basis and, the manufacturer/sponsor is responsible for providing evidence of the product's safety and effectiveness. As indicated, product safety and effectiveness are evaluated with respect to the product's manufacture and clinical performance, as applicable, as well as the manufacturer's claim of intended use, i.e., the patient population to be treated and the product's role in the diagnosis, prevention, monitoring, treatment, or cure of a disease or condition. For engineered tissue products as well as other human medical products, issues of product manufacture include, among others: cell/tissue, biomaterial, and/or biomolecule sourcing, processing, and characterization; detection and avoidance of

Table 23.1. FDA-Approved Human Cellular- and Tissue-Based Products (HCT/Ps)

Skin Applications			
Product	**Sponsor**	**Intended Use**	**Approval**
Carticel (Autologous Cultured Chondrocytes)	Genzyme Corporation	Repair of femoral condyle caused by acute or repetitive fracture	1997-Biologic (BLA)
Apligraf (Viable Allogeneic Fibroblasts/ Keratinocytes On Type-1 Bovine Collagen)	Organogenesis Inc.	Standard therapeutic compression for treatment of non-infected partial and full-thickness skin ulcers	1998-Device (PMA)
Dermagraft (Cryopreserved Dermal Substitute: Allogeneic Fibroblasts; Extracellular Matrix; Bioabsorbable Scaffold)	Advanced Tissue Sciences, Inc.	Treatment of full-thickness diabetic foot ulcers	2001-Device (PMA)
Composite Cultured Skin (Viable Allogeneic Fibroblasts/ Keratinocytes On Collagen Matrix	Ortec International, Inc.	Adjunct to standard autograft procedures for covering wounds and donor sites after surgical release of hand contractions in Recessive Dystrophic Epidermolysis Bullosa patients	2001-Device (HDE)
Dermagraft (Cryopreserved Dermal Substitute: Allogeneic Fibroblasts; Extracellular Matrix; Bioabsorbable Scaffold)	Smith and Nephew Wound Management	Treatment of wounds related to Dystrophic Epidermolysis Bullosa	2003-Device (HDE)
Musculoskeletal Applications			
Product	**Sponsor**	**Intended Use**	**Approval**
OP-1 Implant (Recombinant Human Osteogenic Protein (rh OP-1), Type-1 Bovine Bone Collagen Matrix)	Stryker Biotech	Alternative to autograft in recalcitrant long bone non-unions	2002-Device (PMA)
InFUSE Bone Graft/ LT-Cage Lumbar Tapered Fusion Device (Recombinant Human Bone Morphogenetic Protein-2, Type-1 Bovine Bone Collagen, Titanium Alloy Cage)	Medtronic	Spinal fusion for degenerative disc disease	2002-Device (PMA)
OP-1 Putty (Recombinant Human Osteogenic Protein (rh OP-1), Type-1 Bovine Bone Collagen Matrix, Putty Additive – Carboxymethyl Cellulose Sodium)	Stryker Biotech	Alternative to autograft in compromised patients requiring revision posterolateral lumbar spinal fusion for whom autologous bone and bone marrow-harvest are not feasible or expected to promote fusion	2004-Device (HDE)

adventitious agents; product consistency and stability; as well as quality control/quality assurance procedures. Other important considerations include evaluation of the preclinical data, e.g., toxicity and immunogenicity testing for local/systemic and acute/chronic responses, as well as assessment of *in vivo* remodeling. Collecting data on product performance in humans requires insight into clinical trial design, e.g., patient entry criteria and study endpoints, study conduct, and subsequent data analyses.

At the request of the sponsor of a new drug, the FDA will facilitate the development and expedite the review of such a drug if it is intended for the treatment of a serious or life-threatening condition and it demonstrates the potential to address unmet medical needs for such a condition. The development program for such a drug or biologic may be designated a fast-track development program and may apply special procedures such as accelerated approval based on surrogate end points, submission and review of portions of an application, and priority review to facilitate its development and expedite its review[2].

For devices, PMAs, PMA Supplements, and 510(k) applications may also undergo expedited review[2]. In general, applications dealing with the treatment or diagnosis of life-threatening or irreversibly debilitating diseases or conditions may be candidates for expedited review if: the device represents a clear, clinically meaningful advantage over existing technology; the device is a diagnostic or therapeutic modality for which no approved alternative exists; the device offers a significant advantage over existing approved alternatives or; availability of the device is in the best interests of patients. Granted expedited review status means that the marketing application will receive priority review before other applications. When multiple applications for the same type of device have also been granted expedited review, the applications will be reviewed with the priority according to their respective submission due dates.

23.5. HUMAN CELLS, TISSUES, AND CELLULAR- AND TISSUE-BASED PRODUCTS

With the recognition that an important segment of the products that it regulates often arises from applications of new technology, such as tissue engineering, and that the product applications may pose unique and complex questions, the FDA has devoted considerable resources since the early 1990's to the regulatory considerations of what have been termed human cellular-and tissue-based products (HCT/Ps). In February 1997, the FDA proposed a comprehensive tier-based approach for regulation of these products with the level of product review proportional to the degree of risk. On May 25, 2005, the final piece of this regulatory framework was put in place when the Current Good Tissue Practice for Human Cell, Tissues, and Cellular-and Tissue-Based Product Establishments: Final Rule (the CGTP Rule) became effective.[7] Two earlier final rules, one providing for establishment registration and the other establishing processes for donor screening had already set out significant portions of this framework. Publication of the CGTP Rule completes the set of regulations proposed in 1997 and issued in proposed or interim form since 2001 to implement the FDA's framework for regulation of HCT/Ps.

Defined as articles containing or consisting of human cells or tissues that are intended for implantation, transplantation, infusion, or transfer into a human recipient, HCT/Ps include skin; musculoskeletal tissue (bone and ligaments); ocular tissue (especially cornea); heart valve allografts; dura mater; hematopoietic stem and progenitor cells derived from peripheral and cord blood; reproductive tissue; cellular therapies; and combination products consisting of cells/tissue with a device and/or drug (such as cells on a natural or synthetic matrix).

The agency recognized the need for regulatory oversight of these products in the late 1980s and early 1990's because of a number of concerns. First, documented evidence of communicable disease transmission to recipients from infected donor tissue presented a primary public health concern. Second, the rapid growth of the industry with development of new applications and technologies for processing human cells and tissues, coupled with increased demand and international commerce presented different issues. Finally, voluntary standards established by certain organizations had not been followed uniformly, as they are not legally enforceable. These factors, together with public demand for safe products compelled the agency to effect appropriate solutions.

The tenets of the tiered risk-based approach initially outlined by the agency have been maintained in the CGTP Rule. Essentially, products meeting certain criteria, so-called "kick-down" factors, would be regulated solely under provisions of Section 361 of the US PHS Act (361 Products) and would not be required to undergo premarket review. All others not meeting the kick-down factors would be regulated under existing drug, biologics, and device regulations, in addition to the new regulations addressing the incorporation of living biological materials into the finished product (Figure 23.1).

FDA Regulatory Oversight for Cells, Tissues, and Human Cellular and Tissue-Based Products (HCT/Ps)

Tiered Approach

- Regulated solely under Section 361 (PHS Act) if all "kick down" criteria apply:

    - Minimally manipulated
    - Homologous use only
    - Not combined with another article (except: sterilizing, preserving, or storage agent, water, crystalloids)
    - Does not have systemic effect and is not dependent on metabolic activity of living cells (except: autologous/reproductive use, use in 1°/2° blood relatives)

    - Examples: "Banked Human Tissue" - cornea, skin, umbilical cord blood stem cells, cartilage, bone
    - **Premarket application not required**
- Regulated under Section 361 AND biologic (IND/BLA) or device (IDE/PMA) regulations if HCT/P does not meet all "kick down" criteria.

* Current Good Tissue Practice Final Rule, Published 1/24/2004; Effective 5/25/05; www.fda.gov/cber/rules/gtp.htm

Figure 23.1. FDA Regulatory Oversight for Cells, Tissues, and Human Cellular and Tissue-Based Products (HCT/Ps): Tiered Approach

The kick-down factors include: minimal manipulation of the source tissue through the processing stage; homologous use; freedom from combination with another article, except a sterilizing, preserving, or storage agent, water, and crystalloids; absence of intended systemic effect or dependence upon the metabolic activity of living cells (except in cases of autologous use; use in first or second degree blood relatives; or reproductive use). Those HCT/Ps not meeting these criteria would be regulated under the FD&C Act as drugs, biologics, or devices. The risk-based approach is tiered, i.e., stratified, to provide the appropriate type and level of regulation, based on a product's characteristics with a platform of minimal requirements for all cells and tissues and additional requirements when necessary for product safety and effectiveness.

The CGTP requirements cover all aspects of production, including: cell and tissue recovery; donor screening and testing; processing and process controls; supplies and reagents; equipment and facilities; environmental and labeling controls; storage conditions; product receipt; predistribution shipment and distribution; advertisement and deviation reporting; and tracking form donor to product consignee. Each establishment of the affected industry must develop and maintain a quality program covering all these requirements and take measures to report and track any product-related adverse event. The CGTP Rule also grants additional provisions to the FDA, including inspection authority, control of imports, and enforcement authority.

Thus, predictable regulatory requirements serve to support innovation in technology and the industry and to minimize elements of uncertainty in the product development process. Since many, if not all, engineered tissues are human cell or tissue-based and/or combination products, the CGTP Rule and PMOA Proposed Rule serve to clarify the regulatory requirements for such products and to demonstrate the FDA's commitment for facilitating the development process for these products while, at the same time, maintaining the public confidence in safe, effective medical products for the marketplace.

23.6. SCIENCE AND PRODUCT DEVELOPMENT

Federal investment in basic biomedical research is expected to lead to an overall improvement in public health. However, as observed and reported by the FDA in its March 2004 report, "Challenges and Opportunity on the Critical Path to New Medical Products" (Critical Path Report) (www.fda.gov/oc/initiatives/critialpath), that expectation is not being fulfilled, and there is a discontinuity form basic research to application.[8]

Data, based on ten-year trends show that, while there has been an increase in research spending by federal government agencies, such as the National Institutes of Health, and industry, there has been a concomitant decrease in major drug and biological product submissions to the FDA. This is also true for devices, although not to as great an extent.

The FDA's analysis of this pipeline problem has led to the conclusion that the current medical product development path is becoming increasingly challenging, inefficient, and costly. To address these concerns, the FDA launched the Critical Path Initiative to identify the most pressing obstacles in the path and in technology translation. With publication of the Critical Path Report, the FDA framed the challenge as the shortage of modern tools to enable effective and efficient assessment of the safety and effectiveness of new medical products. Since then, the FDA has worked with FDA staff and external stakeholders to identify the most important challenges and to create the Critical Path Opportunities List as an outline of its strategy to overcome them.

While a number of issues and opportunities have been identified, certain common themes have emerged. The primary concerns are clinical trials and surrogate endpoints. There is a need to improve clinical trials and outcomes assessment generally. Accelerating the development and regulatory acceptance of biomarkers is perceived as an approach for their use in characterizing the product as well as in measuring outcome(s) for both preclinical and clinical studies. Other areas identified include manufacturing and scale-up generally, i.e., moving from laboratory bench studies to a manufacturing process with appropriate system design controls to assure a consistently reproducible, stable product, and progress in evaluating products developed through tissue engineering approaches. The FDA has projected publication of the Critical Path Opportunities List, which will identify product development areas for late 2005.

The initiative will continue as a formal process for continued input from all stakeholders and will be helpful to those engaged in engineered tissues research and product development.

23.7. CONCLUSIONS AND FUTURE PERSPECTIVES

Strategic investment in science, engineering, and allied disciplines is a critical determinant for advancing both basic and translational research in organ/tissue replacement, repair, and regeneration towards products for the clinic and marketplace. However, to achieve successful product commercialization and market penetration, research strategies must be based on sound market analysis and demonstrated clinical need and with a product development plan in place to attract the needed funding support from the financial communities and approval from product regulatory and reimbursement authorities. Understanding the product regulatory process and specific points to consider for engineered human cellular- and tissue-based products will help companies in development of their overall commercialization strategy. Moreover, since low reimbursement rates can often be the single greatest impediment to product acceptance by end users in the healthcare environment, attention to cost recovery issues and their relationship to clinical and economic outcomes is equally important.[9] All these determinants are interdependent and must be considered by companies in developing a sound business plan, since uncertainties in any one determinant can have a profound effect on the entire commercialization pathway.

The FDA's approach to regulation of human cellular- and tissue-based products and combination products as well as other evolving initiatives are indicative of the agency's commitment to providing the appropriate regulatory oversight for products generated from novel technology, such as tissue engineering. It is expected that the FDA will continue to build on these initiatives and on the cooperative approaches across the appropriate FDA Centers and the Office of the Commissioner in its regulatory oversight for engineered tissues so that: questions from manufacturers/sponsors are addressed early on in product development; product regulatory jurisdiction questions are addressed in a timely manner and; the product premarket review process becomes more transparent and simplified. This is especially important since the pursuit of new and different research directions focused on tissue and organ regeneration, such as the apparent shift toward the use of stem cell technology,[10] will lead to the development of new and different products, posing unique product-specific issues (Figure 23.2).

The challenges for the tissue engineering community are similarly multifold. For example, sponsors should consider the important determinants in the product regulatory path such as: the nature of the product; its manufacture and classification, i.e., tissue or product; its mode of action or primary mode of action if a combination product and overall therapeutic approach; and preclinical (animal models) and clinical strategies to assess safety and effectiveness, such as selection of appropriate outcome measures and assessment tools/methods. The sponsor's claim of intended use and whether the product will provide incremental or substantive therapeutic benefit compared to the standard of care will be important for end-user and market acceptance, and, ultimately, cost reimbursement. The time to clinic and market will be dependent on the product's classification and subsequent submission and review of sponsor-generated data. For example, an orphan drug or humanitarian use device will have a relatively shorter regulatory timeline than a product regulated under existing authorities as a drug, biologic, or device.

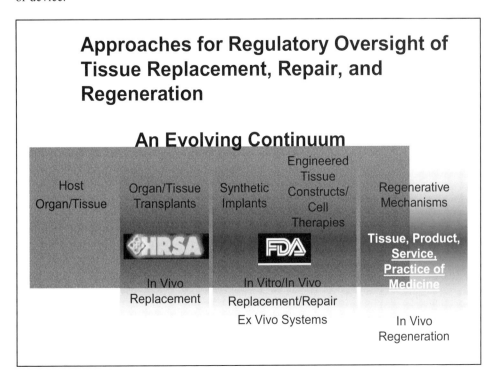

Figure 23.2. Approaches for Regulatory Oversight of Tissue Replacement, Repair, and Regeneration: An Evolving Continuum

To advance the science and minimize the variables in engineered tissue systems, understanding the mechanisms and control processes in normal as well as diseased or damaged human organs and tissues will continue to be a necessary prerequisite for design of novel research strategies focused on applications for tissue repair, replacement, or regeneration. In this context and to advance the science the following should continue to be examined: operative mechanisms in cell and developmental biology; interactions of engineered tissue constructs with the host and remodeling by the *in vivo* environment; and acute/chronic as well as local/systemic sequelae of either reparative or regenerative approaches through appropriate preclinical large animal and clinical monitoring studies. Progress in biomaterials science such as: the development of matrix materials customized for the cell(s) and application of interest; advances in manufacturing and scale-up techniques such as development of tissue-customized bioreactors and process system design; and outcomes assessment tools such as non-invasive *in vivo* monitoring of implanted engineered tissues will be important for translating research to applications.

Ultimately, the challenge for the tissue engineering community is to continue advances in the science while maintaining awareness of the product regulatory environment in the US and abroad and to be an active voice for articulating the important issues in order to maintain a productive dialogue with the regulatory agencies and consumers so that engineered tissues find their proper place in the clinic and market.

23.8. REFERENCES

1. Kiki B. Hellman, Emma Knight, and Charles N. Durfor, Tissue Engineering: Product Applications and Regulatory Issues, *Frontiers in Tissue Engineering*, pp. 341-366, 1998.
2. Kiki B. Hellman, Ruth R. Solomon, Claudia Gaffey, Charles N. Durfor, and John G. Bishop, III, Regulatory Considerations, *Principles of Tissue Engineering, Second Edition*, pp. 915-928 (2000).
3. David S. Smith and Kiki B. Hellman, Regulatory Oversight and Product Development: Charting the Path, Regulatory Page, *Tissue Engineering*, 9(5), 1057-1058 (2003).
4. Kiki B. Hellman and David S. Smith, The Regulation of Engineered Tissues: Emerging Approaches, The Biomedical Engineering Handbook, *Tissue Engineering Section, Fourth Edition* (in press).
5. Kiki B. Hellman, Introduction, presentation at Inaugural Engineering Tissue Growth Executive Forum, Seattle, Washington (June 2004).
6. Kiki B. Hellman, and David S. Smith, FDA Regulation of Combination Products: Evolving Initiatives, *Genetic Engineering News*, 25(10) (May 15, 2005).
7. Kiki B. Hellman and David S. Smith, FDA Final 'Current Good Tissue Practice' Rule, *Genetic Engineering News,* 25(6) (March 15, 2005).
8. Kiki B. Hellman and David S. Smith, Taking a Look at the FDA's Critical Path Initiative, *Genetic Engineering News,* 25(2) (January 15, 2005).
9. Kim Norton, Regulation Reimbursement – Efficacy vs. Effectiveness: What Determines Coverage, presentation at Inaugural Engineering Tissue Growth Executive Forum, Seattle, Washington (June 9, 2004).
10. Michael J. Lysaght and A.L. Hazelhurst, Tissue Engineering: The End of the Beginning, *Tissue Engineering,* 10, 309-321 (2004).

SECTION 7

TISSUE ENGINEERING STRATEGIES

24

FIBRIN IN TISSUE ENGINEERING

Daniela Eyrich[1], Achim Göpferich[1], and Torsten Blunk[1]

24.1. INTRODUCTION

Every year, millions of people suffer loss or failure of tissue or organs due to an accident or clinical condition. A revolutionary strategy to treat these patients is the engineering of the lacking organ or tissue with autologous cells in combination with polymeric matrices[1]. For several years there has been enormous interest in hydrogels as a soft scaffold for tissue engineering[2-4]. In nearly every intact native tissue, cells are held within an extracellular matrix that modulates tissue development, homeostasis and regeneration. Many hydrogels are structurally similar to the extracellular matrix of various tissues and many are considered to be biocompatible. They have a variety of potential functions in the field of tissue engineering and, thus, must fulfill many different requirements to promote new tissue growth, depending on their application. Hydrogels act as a space filling agent and three-dimensional structure to organize the expanded cells, to maintain a specific shape and structural integrity, and to direct growth and formation for adequate new tissue development. In general, hydrogels can be processed under relatively mild conditions suitable for many cell types. Furthermore, the liquid components of hydrogels may be easily delivered into the patient's defect in a minimally invasive manner.

One of the most widely used hydrogels is fibrin. Fibrin glue is a commonly used surgical haemostatic agent and has been commercially available for over 20 years in surgery and clinical practice. The hydrogel fibrin is a polypeptide consisting of the plasma components fibrinogen and thrombin. Physiologically, fibrin formation occurs as the final step in the natural blood coagulation cascade, producing a clot that assists wound healing. After activation with calcium ions, thrombin cleaves small peptides from the fibrinogen chain to produce soluble fibrin monomers[5]. These monomers are covalently cross-linked through the action of factor XIII to form an insoluble, polymerized fibrin clot[6] (Fig. 24.1). In recent years, fibrin has been utilized for different applications in the field of tissue engineering with specific physical and biological

---

[1] Department of Pharmaceutical Technology, University of Regensburg, 93040 Regensburg, Germany

requirements. The current use of fibrin for each of these categories of request will be subsequently reviewed.

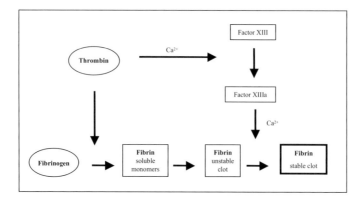

Figure 24.1. Scheme of fibrin gel formation.

24.2. FIBRIN GLUE IN SURGERY AND CLINICAL PRACTICE

Several reviews published in recent years have focused on uses of fibrin glue, also referred to as fibrin tissue adhesive or fibrin sealant, in clinical and surgical practice[7-11]. In the literature, fibrin was first mentioned more than 90 years ago. It has been documented that fibrinogen combined with thrombin was used to improve the adhesion of skin grafts of soldiers with burn injuries during the Second World War[7].

A commercial product has been available in Europe and Japan since the 80s, whereas fibrin glue was not FDA approved until 1998 because of possible viral contamination. At the moment, fibrin sealant is considered the most effective physiological tissue adhesive available.

There are a number of commercially available fibrin products with different amounts and origins of the components[7, 9]. The concentration of fibrinogen, varying between 40 and 125 mg/ml, is directly correlated to the tensile strength of the fibrin clot, whereas the concentration of thrombin influences the degree and speed of clotting. The latter proves useful for quick haemostasis to prevent blood loss (e.g., in suturing of vessels) or in surgical procedures involving careful glue adjustment to fit a tissue or organ[9]. Within 3 days of application, a preliminary granulation tissue with a large number of wound healing cells is present and is subsequently replaced with collagen fibers one to two weeks later. During normal wound healing the fibrin glue is absorbed within days to weeks depending on the type of sealant and location of application[12]. The majority of glues contain an anti-fibrinolytic component to reduce the degradation rate. A common agent is the protease inhibitor aprotinin, which inhibits human trypsin and plasmin by blocking the active sites of the enzymes. Due to the fact that fibrin is a physiological blood component, it is considered to be biocompatible and biodegradable. However, despite a number of rigorous national and international guidelines during manufacturing to assure the high quality of commercial fibrin components, the risk of viral infection or foreign body response, especially due to bovine components, still exists[7]. Additionally, the development of antibodies against coagulation plasma proteins has been documented after application of bovine thrombin resulting in significant anticoagulation[10]. Although most of the commercial products now contain human fibrinogen and thrombin, the majority still contain bovine aprotinin, which was shown to cause hypersensitivity, especially after repeated administration[10]. Autologous preparation methods have been described[13-16] to prevent these foreign body reactions, however, the composition, resulting appearance, and mechanical strength of these gels depend on the patient's physique and constitution. Therefore, there is a great interest in optimizing these methods leading to standardization and validation in clinical practice.

The most prevalent application of fibrin in clinical practice is its use as a haemostatic agent, especially in heparinized or coagulopathic patients, to reduce operative bleeding, e.g., in cardiovascular surgery. The application is most effective when polymerized prior to the onset of bleeding, for example in surgery of a vascular anastomosis[8]. When using fibrin sealants or sprays as adjunct to sutures, a better wound healing and optimal wound integrity results in operative locations where the use of conventional sutures is not feasible or would result in intense bleedings[8, 10].

Fibrin polymers play a key role in tissue and organ sealing, particularly in plastic and reconstructive surgery, including skin grafting[8]. Exact adjustment is possible, bleeding is reduced, fewer sutures are necessary, the length of the operation time is shortened, and fewer post-operative infections occur.

Fibrin glue applications are common in other important fields of clinical practice, including thoracic, orthopedic, neuro-, and oral surgery[7, 8, 12]. Since the recent approval of fibrin glues by the FDA, the number of clinical applications has increased dramatically and companies have started to investigate and improve the use of the sealant in more diverse surgical settings.

24.3. PRINCIPLES AND METHODS OF FIBRIN APPLICATION IN TISSUE ENGINEERING

In order for fibrin gels to be utilized as a tissue scaffold, the material must provide an environment enabling adequate cellular function, e.g., cell migration, proliferation, and differentiation, and must allow for tissue development. For example, it has been shown that chondrocytes in fibrin gel retain their round and vital morphology, do not dedifferentiate, and produce extracellular matrix[17, 18]. The glue components fibrinogen and thrombin are thought to modulate the attachment, migration, and proliferation of different cell types, e.g., chondrocytes, fibroblasts, smooth muscle cells, or keratinocytes[19-23]. Fibrinogen possesses a specific peptide chain, also referred to as a heptide, that contributes to cell attachment and binding primarily of mesenchymal cells, e.g., fibroblasts, endothelial cells, and smooth muscle cells[24]. This data is consistent with a study published by Brown, who investigated the effect of cross-linking various fibrin chains on fibroblast migration[25]. An important factor modulating fibroblast movement into a fibrin gel has been shown to be factor XIII which mediates the cross-linking of the fibrin α-chains[26].

The variation of fibrin parameters can generate gels with different mechanical stiffnesses. These mechanical properties potentially influence the gene expression of different growth factors and cytokines, e.g., of human dermal fibroblasts[27]. Important parameters affecting fibrin characteristics are thrombin, fibrinogen, and calcium concentration, ionic strength, and pH, resulting in either more rigid and stable or more soft and soluble gels[28-30], although the exact contributions of each parameter are still not fully understood. Nevertheless, it may be possible to tailor specific structural fibrin features for specific cell types and for a particular application to modulate individual cell proliferation, migration and differentiation[31].

Another fibrin glue characteristic is an increasing instability and solubility over time, due to fibrinolysis[28]. Commercially available fibrin sealants tend to shrink and disintegrate in vitro and in vivo after a few days and almost completely dissolve within 4 weeks[17, 32-35]. While this could be an advantage in wound sealing or other surgical applications in which dissolution is desired after closure of the defect[7, 9, 12], this can represent a major problem for use as a shape-specific scaffold in tissue engineering. Here, long-term stability is necessary to provide enough time for cell proliferation and matrix production. Therefore, fibrinolysis inhibitors, mostly protease inhibitors, e.g., aprotinin, ε-amino caproic acid or tranexamic acid, are used within the fibrin gel and/or as a supplement to the cell culture medium; they can help slow down degradation and, thus, stabilize the fibrin gel shape[32, 36, 37]. As a result, degradation of the temporary matrix may be controlled for specific purposes.

The application of fibrin in tissue engineering can be grouped into three main areas: fibrin as cell matrix material alone, fibrin as a cell matrix material combined with a polymeric scaffold, and as delivery system for growth factors or other therapeutic agents.

A simple method for the use of fibrin as a scaffold material involves suspending primary or expanded cells in a liquid component of the fibrin glue with subsequent polymerization in suitable cell culture plates. The resulting three-dimensional construct may be cultivated in vitro to obtain an adequate tissue for re-implantation. In addition to the application as scaffold in vitro, the fibrin system can also be used as cell delivery vehicle in vivo. Cells suspended in fibrin glue can be directly injected into a defect in a minimally invasive procedure with little stress for the patient; the fibrin gel can be polymerized in vivo in the desired three-dimensional shape, at the same time ensuring the retention of the cells at the injection site[22, 36].

An alternative strategy for tissue engineering is the combination of hydrogels with polymeric scaffolds. Highly porous solid scaffolds can provide sufficient load-bearing capacity for the process of implantation and for structural integrity in vivo. However, many scaffold systems lack adequate cell seeding efficiency, sufficient cell distribution and subsequent sufficient extracellular matrix synthesis and deposition. In contrast, fibrin gels generally incorporate all of the applied cells and enable a good cell distribution providing the requirements for a coherent tissue development, but often lack adequate biomechanical strength and volume stability[34, 38-40]. Therefore, the advantages of fibrin glue combined with favorable characteristics of synthetic or naturally derived polymeric scaffolds can be utilized to develop a simple, stable composite for implantation. This way tissue development in the desired three-dimensional shape can be achieved; furthermore the time for tissue development may be reduced as compared to the use of either system alone[41]. This strategy has been successfully applied in tissue engineering of urothelium[42], cartilage[43-45], and cardiovascular engineering[41].

Fibrin can also be applied as delivery system for the release of growth factors, cytokines or other bioactive molecules to control cell adhesion, proliferation, migration, differentiation, and matrix production. Many growth factors bind to fibrin, bFGF and VEGF are even supposed to bind specifically. Alternatively, such proteins can be incorporated into the gel during polymerization[46-48]. Fibrin is known to protect growth factors against denaturation and proteolysis in vitro and in vivo[49]. Furthermore, when applied in vivo the presence of the growth factor in the defect is maintained over a long time. Additionally, the kinetics of growth factor release can be controlled by varying fibrinogen and thrombin concentration as well as by the addition of degradation inhibitors. Factors released from fibrin gels used for tissue regeneration include bFGF, VEGF, NTF, ECGF, GDNF and NGF[48, 50-62]. Hubbell et al. developed an innovative technology for growth factor delivery on the basis of a combination of fibrin and heparin, utilizing the ability of heparin to stabilize the bioactivity of growth factors and control their release[49]. A fibrin gel was modified by covalently binding exogenous bi-domain peptides with a heparin-binding domain using the transglutaminase activity of factor XIIIa during coagulation. These peptides can bind heparin and subsequently heparin-binding growth factors (Fig. 24.2). This approach was successfully applied in the controlled release of different growth factors[53, 54, 62-67] either by passive release or facilitated by enzymatic factors secreted by migrating cells.

Andree et al. established a method to deliver EGF expression plasmids from a fibrin matrix to a human keratinocyte culture system. These plasmids can enhance keratinocyte proliferation during expansion in vitro as well as directly after transplantation of the cells in combination with a fibrin matrix into a skin defect in vivo[68].

Besides release of growth factors, the local delivery of antibiotics and chemotherapeutic agents from a fibrin gel could be beneficial in clinical applications[69, 70]. Skin replacement therapies, a common application in tissue engineering, carries a high risk of infection during the implantation procedure that could be moderated by the release of antibiotics from the tissue replacement itself. Unfortunately, the time span of release from fibrin hydrogels is rather short due to the fast diffusion of the small molecules. Release may be prolonged, however, by varying drug concentration or by use of fibrin insoluble antibiotics[71]; these drugs dissolve slowly inside the defect due to low hydrophilicity.

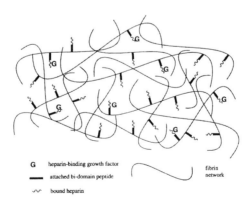

Figure 24.2. Fibrin matrix as gel for delivery system utilizing the growth factor binding properties of heparin. A bi-domain peptide, containing a factor XIIIa substrate and a heparin-binding domain, is covalently cross-linked to the fibrin matrix during coagulation. Heparin is immobilized to the heparin-binding domain of the peptide by electrostatic interactions. Heparin-binding growth factors are immobilized by binding to the immobilized heparin within the fibrin matrix (with permission of Elsevier; Ref: 63).

24.4. FIBRIN IN THE ENGINEERING OF SPECIFIC TISSUES

24.4.1. Skin Tissue

Numerous authors have investigated fibrin glue for skin tissue engineering during the last years. Not only can fibrin be used as a graft sealant as well as a haemostatic and antibacterial agent[72], fibrin is a functional scaffold material for engineering of skin tissue. It has been shown that fibrinogen stimulates the migration of epidermal cells and keratinocytes[73-75]. Fibronectin, a specific glycoprotein in fibrin glue, enhances cellular migration during wound healing[76, 77]. A common clinical application consists of a single cell suspension of in vitro expanded autologous human keratinocytes in fibrin sealant and delivery directly into the skin defect. The cell-glue system adheres and spreads over the defect resulting in re-epithelialization within a few weeks[76, 78, 79]. Additionally, cultivation of keratinocytes onto a fibrin layer in vitro maintains the status of differentiation[80].

An alternative therapy for chronic wounds and severe burns includes isolation of a small biopsy of the patient's skin, expansion of the resultant single keratinocytes in vitro onto a supportive 3T3 feeder layer and transfer of the developed epidermal sheet directly to the wound. However, this is an expensive and time-consuming process and careful enzymatic detachment and handling of the cell sheet is critical. The application of fibrin as culture bed during expansion and transfer of the cell-fibrin construct facilitates and accelerates the operative procedure[81]. Meana et al. investigated a fibrin gel either with or without human fibroblasts as a base for a dermal equivalent. Only in the group with fibroblasts, cultivation of even low cell numbers of primary keratinocytes on this gel system resulted in a newly developed epithelium within 10-14 days (Fig. 24.3). The cell layer was manually detached from the culture flask without enzymatic treatment and could be easily transplanted into the skin defect[82]. Gorodetsky et al. developed an innovative technology to deliver cells from fibrin-derived microbeads instead of conventional fibrin gel systems[83]. These biodegradable microbeads, 50-200μm in diameter, represent a simple provisional matrix and cell carrier with good attachment properties for different cell types. Fibroblasts seeded at low density can proliferate in vitro on the fibrin particles and may be easily transferred from the culture plate into specific defects for wound healing. The cell-seeded microbeads showed improved formation of granulation tissue in pig wound healing as compared to fibrin-derived microbeads alone. This strategy may be transferable to the engineering of other tissues as well.

24.4.2. Vascular Tissue

There is a tremendous demand for blood vessel repair, especially in cardiovascular surgery due to the high number of patients with arteriosclerosis. The investigation of fibrin gel parameters and the effects of exogenous factors added to fibrin scaffolds on inducing cells to form vascular tissue within these gels are important first steps towards a clinical solution[84, 85]. Koolwijk et al. used in vitro experiments to analyze the effect of TNFα, bFGF and VEGF on human microvascular endothelial cells seeded on fibrin gels to form capillary-like tubular structures for angiogenesis[84]. The data showed that the inflammatory mediator TNFα is necessary in addition to bFGF and/or VEGF for development of capillary-like structures by endothelial cells.

Moreover, fibrin gels can serve as a three-dimensional matrix molded to the exact structure of vessels. Jockenhoevel et al. developed a method towards the engineering of valve conduits[86]. Fibroblasts were suspended in a fibrin gel that was polymerized in silicone-coated aluminium molds. 2mm thick constructs were cultivated in vitro and cells subsequently produced collagen bundles, an element of valve conduits. In another study, the same group investigated methods to prevent the shrinkage of fibrin gels so they could be used in cardiovascular engineering. In addition to supplementing protease inhibitors to the culture medium, the mechanical and chemical fixation of gels onto culture plates was tested[40]. Matrix analysis and histology showed the best collagen synthesis and tissue development using a chemical border fixation onto culture plates. In contrast, Mol et al. discussed the possible advantage of shrinking fibrin gels for vascular engineering leading to higher mechanical forces inside the construct and thereby potentially enhancing collagen production[41].

Furthermore, fibrin gels were tested as a scaffold for cardiovascular tissue engineering using myofibroblasts. Ye et al. suspended human myofibroblasts in a fibrin matrix[39]. Microscopy showed homogenous cell growth and collagen synthesis. Additionally, a higher concentration of aprotinin supplemented to the medium resulted in improved gel stability and enhanced tissue development. Cummings et al. investigated the morphological and mechanical properties of fibrin gel, collagen type I gel, and a combination of both for vascular engineering using rat aortic smooth muscle cells. A combination of rigid, less elastic collagen with a weaker, more instable fibrin gel resulted in higher ultimate tensile stress, increased toughness, and increased gel compaction compared to each system alone[87]. As an alternative, the variation in fibrin parameters resulting in more stable and rigid gels may be a means to avoid the more complex combinations with another gel system for this kind of application.

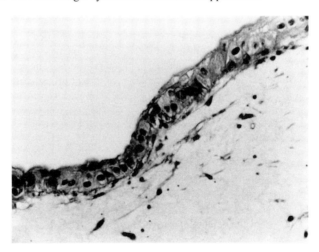

Figure 24.3. Fibrin as an approach to generate a dermal equivalent: keratinocytes were cultured on a fibroblast-containing fibrin gel. Histological appearance after 15 days of culture (H&E staining, x 250) (with permission of Elsevier; Ref: 82).

24.4.3. Bone Tissue

Another potential field of application of fibrin is the healing of critical size defects of bone, although there are only a few papers published on the topic so far. One strategy, again, is the delivery of cells suspended in a fibrin gel directly into the bone defect. Isogai et al. injected a periosteal cell-fibrin mixture into the dorsum of athymic mice. Histology showed new bone development and western blot assay demonstrated production of osteopontin, a specific protein in bone tissue[88]. Ng et al. investigated the potential of suspending cells derived from four different sites of the body in fibrin glue for three-dimensional bone constructs in vivo[89]. Osteoprogenitor cells isolated from periosteum showed best results, whereas using cells derived from cancellous and cortical bone as well as bone marrow resulted in less bone-forming activity.

Bensaid et al. tested the potential of fibrin a as scaffolding structure for mesenchmal stem cells in bone tissue engineering in vitro[22]. They varied fibrinogen concentration and thrombin activity and analysed the effect on cell spreading and proliferation in vitro. Perka et al. compared the cultivation of periosteal cells on PLGA polymer fleece and on fibrin beads. Both groups were cultivated in vitro for 14 days and subsequently implanted into metadiaphyseal ulna defects of white rabbits[90]. Histological and radiological analysis showed intense bone formation in both groups.

Karp et al. combined fibrin glues containing different thrombin concentrations with interconnecting, macroporous PLGA scaffolds for use in bone engineering[91]. However, no difference was seen between the control group (only PLGA scaffold, no fibrin) and the group with low thrombin concentration, whereas scaffolds filled with fibrin gel containing high thrombin concentrations showed less bone formation. Fibrin parameters may be optimized for this kind of application to obtain improved cell migration and matrix production.

Finally, Haisch et al. investigated a method to induce transdifferentiation of articular chondrocytes into bone-forming cells with addition of corticosteroids[92]. Auricular rabbit chondrocytes were suspended in fibrin or agarose and the mixture was injected into polymer fleeces. Constructs were subsequently implanted subcutaneously into the ridge of New Zealand rabbits with and without methylprednisolone treatment. Histology showed that the simple injection of corticosteroids prevented fibrous tissue formation and enhanced bone development.

24.4.4. Cartilage Tissue

Fibrin is widely used in approaches to tissue engineering of cartilage. Fortier et al. tested fibrin as a matrix for engineering articular cartilage in vitro using equine chondrocytes. Positive effects of exogenously applied IGF-I and TGF-β on chondrocyte matrix synthesis was shown[93, 94]. In another study, autologous fibrinogen was demonstrated to better maintain differentiation of chondrocytes compared to commercially available fibrinogen[18]. To further enhance cartilage development, Hunter et al. tested the influence of oscillatory compression on development of chondrocyte-fibrin constructs[95]. Though dynamic compression has frequently been shown to stimulate matrix production and gene expression in tissue, mechanical stimulus of the fibrin constructs resulted in the inhibition of cartilage matrix production. The effect of

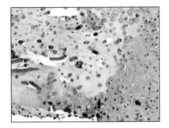 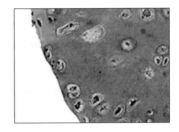

Figure 24.4. Fibrin combined with a PGA non-woven mesh for cartilage engineering employing swine chondrocytes. Distributions of sulphated GAG, assessed with safranin-O staining within a composite cell construct after 7 days (left) and after 28 days (right) of in vitro culture. Dark segmented lines (left) are polymer fibers (with permission of Elsevier; Ref: 43).

mechanical stimulation may depend on the structure and mechanical properties of the fibrin gel itself, which in turn depends on the concentration of the individual components and has to be tested for specific applications.

Several studies were published showing tissue engineering of cartilage after subcutaneous implantation in mice. Silverman et al. suspended swine chondrocytes in fibrin gel, injected the cell-fibrin mixture directly into the back of nude mice and determined the optimal fibrinogen and cell concentration required for adequate tissue development[38]. Sims et al. were the first who reported about the successful tissue engineering of cartilage in the back of nude mice after construct preparation in vitro[96]. Bovine chondrocytes were isolated and suspended in fibrinogen; after polymerization with bovine thrombin, the constructs were implanted subcutaneously into mice. Quantitative analysis and histology demonstrated that differentiated cells were producing cartilaginous extracellular matrix after 6 and 12 weeks. Using the same method, the growth and development of swine chondrocytes from different sites of the body as well as the volume stability of the constructs were explored[97]. Cultivation of articular chondrocytes resulted in decreased construct volume, whereas auricular chondrocytes produced high amounts of extracellular matrix resulting in construct overgrowth. These results indicate the importance of cell source.

Furthermore, the cultivation of chondrocytes in fibrin gels with expanded highly porous polytetrafluoroethylene as a stabilizing pseudoperichondrial layer was suggested as an intelligent functional composite for repair of craniofacial defects by Xu et al. The pseudoperichondrium was either placed in the center of the construct with the cell-fibrin mixture on both sides or on both surfaces with the cell-fibrin mixture in the middle. Implantation of these constructs without pre-cultivation in vitro into the dorsal subcutaneous pocket of nude mice for 8 months resulted in good infiltration of the transplanted chondrocytes into the microporous structure of the polymer, the creation of a stable connection to the pseudoperichondrium and the development of an elastic construct for cartilage engineering[98, 99].

Cartilage is still the most important application of fibrin in tissue engineering. However, several publications complain about fast fibrin shrinkage and disintegration during chondrocyte cultivation. To overcome these problems, protease inhibitors or higher fibrinogen concentrations were employed as mentioned before[32, 36]. Other strategies include combinations with other hydrogels and polymeric scaffolds, respectively. Perka et al. mixed fibrin with stabilizing alginate, which can be easily removed prior to implantation[100]. Histology of human chondrocytes cultivated in this mixture for 30 days in vitro showed differentiated cells and formation of cartilaginous matrix. In an approach using a combination of fibrin and a polymeric scaffold, a high number of swine chondrocytes were suspended in fibrin gel and added to a PGA mesh[43]. It was reported that this combination already resulted in more mechanically stable constructs directly after cell seeding, i.e., the gel injected into the scaffold was more stable than the scaffold alone. After 4 weeks of cultivation in vitro, the combination of fibrin and polymeric scaffold resulted in a higher amount of glycosaminoglycans, an effect that was partially attributed to increased matrix retention in the fibrin gel, and advanced mechanical stability of constructs for implantation compared to polymeric scaffold alone (Fig. 24.4).

24.5. CONCLUSIONS

We have summarized a wide range of fibrin applications in tissue engineering approaches to date. Fibrin glue can serve as a scaffold material alone, in combination with other hydrogels or porous polymeric scaffolds, and as delivery system for growth factors. However, fibrin gels have a complex composition. Their appearance and mechanical strength varies enormously due to different components and concentrations. Therefore, it is extremely important to determine the exact matrix parameters necessary for a specific application. A soft gel is necessary for easy migration of cells inside the scaffold. The fast degradation of fibrin may be useful in sealants or for cell or growth factor delivery. In contrast, a strong and long-term stable gel is often beneficial in tissue engineering in vitro, where cells need enough time and sufficient mechanical integrity to produce their tissue-specific matrix. Also for an earlier implantation after cell-fibrin construct preparation, i.e. to shorten the in vitro culture period, mechanically stronger gels appear desirable. By varying the fibrin composition, cell number, and cultivation time, fibrin gels with different properties can be developed that are suitable for many different applications in clinical practice and the engineering of tissues. Such manipulations of fibrin properties may even eliminate the need for the more complex combinations with polymeric scaffolds or other hydrogels and supplements like protease inhibitors, in turn minimizing the risk of undesired side effects.

24.6. ACKNOWLEDGMENTS

This work is part of the "Bayerischer Forschungsverbund für Tissue Engineering und Rapid Prototyping" and is supported by the "Bayerische Forschungsstiftung", Germany.

24.7. REFERENCES

1. R.Langer and J.P.Vacanti, Tissue engineering, Science 260(5110), 920-926 (1993).
2. K.Y.Lee and D.J.Mooney, Hydrogels for tissue engineering, Chem.Rev. 101(7), 1869-1879 (2001).
3. H.Shin, S.Jo, and A.G.Mikos, Biomimetic materials for tissue engineering, Biomaterials 24(24), 4353-4364 (2003).
4. J.L.Drury and D.J.Mooney, Hydrogels for tissue engineering: Scaffold design variables and applications, Biomaterials 24(24), 4337-4351 (2003).

5. B.Blomback, Fibrinogen and fibrin-proteins with complex roles in hemostasis and thrombosis, Thromb.Res. 83(1), 1-75 (1996).
6. B.Blomback, B.Hessel, and M.Tomikawa, Fibrinogen: structure, function and interaction with proteins and cells, Z.Ges.Inn.Med.Ihre Grenzgeb. 33(17), 610-612 (1978).
7. M.R.Jackson, Fibrin sealants in surgical practice: An overview, Am.J.Surg. 182(2), 1S-7S (2001).
8. W.D.Spotnitz, Commercial fibrin sealants in surgical care, Am.J.Surg. 182(2), 8S-14S (2001).
9. D.M.Albala, Fibrin sealants in clinical practice, Cardiovasc.Surg. 11(Supplement 1), 5-11 (2003).
10. T.E.MacGillivray, Fibrin sealants and glues, J.Card.Surg. 18(6), 480-485 (2003).
11. T.Fattahi, M.Mohan, and G.T.Caldwell, Clinical applications of fibrin sealants, J.Oral Pathol.Med. 62(2), 218-224 (2004).
12. C.J.Dunn and K.L.Goa, Fibrin sealant: a review of its use in surgery and endoscopy, Drugs 58(5), 863-886 (1999).
13. R.L.Quigley, J.A.Perkins, R.J.Gottner, R.D.Curran, B.E.Kuehn, W.J.Hoff, M.E.Wallock, C.E.Arentzen, and J.C.Alexander, Intraoperative procurement of autologous fibrin glue, Ann.Thorac.Surg. 56(2), 387-389 (1993).
14. H.K.Kjaergard, U.S.Weis-Fogh, and J.J.Thiis, Preparation of autologous fibrin glue from pericardial blood, Ann.Thorac.Surg. 55(2), 543-544 (1993).
15. A.Haisch, A.Loch, J.David, A.Pruss, R.Hansen, and M.Sittinger, Preparation of a pure autologous biodegradable fibrin matrix for tissue engineering, Med.Bio.Eng.Comput. 38(6), 686-689 (2000).
16. B.H.I.Ruszymah, Autologous human fibrin as the biomaterial for tissue engineering, Med.J.Malaysia 59(Supplement B), 30-31 (2004).
17. G.N.Homminga, P.Buma, H.W.Koot, P.M.van der Kraan, and W.B.van den Berg, Chondrocyte behavior in fibrin glue in vitro, Acta Orthop.Scand. 64(4), 441-445 (1993).
18. L.A.Fortier, P.J.Brofman, A.J.Nixon, and H.Mohammed, Disparate chondrocyte metabolism in three-dimensional fibrin cultures derived from autogenous or commercially manufactured fibrinogen, Am.J.Vet.Res. 59(4), 514-520 (1998).
19. R.Gorodetsky, A.Vexler, J.An, X.Mou, and G.Marx, Haptotactic and growth stimulatory effects of fibrin(ogen) and thrombin on cultured fibroblasts, J.Lab.Clin.Med. 131(3), 269-280 (1998).
20. L.A.Sporn, L.A.Bunce, and C.W.Francis, Cell proliferation on fibrin: modulation by fibrinopeptide cleavage, Blood 86(5), 1802-1810 (1995).
21. J.Gille, U.Meisner, E.M.Ehlers, A.Muller, M.Russlies, and P.Behrens, Migration pattern, morphology and viability of cells suspended in or sealed with fibrin glue: A histomorphologic study, Tissue Cell 37(5), 339-348 (2005).
22. W.Bensaid, J.T.Triffitt, C.Blanchat, K.Oudina, L.Sedel, and H.Petite, A biodegradable fibrin scaffold for mesenchymal stem cell transplantation, Biomaterials 24(14), 2497-2502 (2003).
23. P.S.Ciano, R.B.Colvin, A.M.Dvorak, J.McDonagh, and H.F.Dvorak, Macrophage migration in fibrin gel matrices, Lab.Invest. 54(1), 62-70 (1986).
24. R.Gorodetsky, A.Vexler, M.Shamir, J.An, L.Levdansky, I.Shimeliovich, and G.Marx, New cell attachment peptide sequences from conserved epitopes in the carboxy termini of fibrinogen, Exp.Cell Res. 287(1), 116-129 (2003).
25. L.F.Brown, N.Lanir, J.McDonagh, K.Tognazzi, A.M.Dvorak, and H.F.Dvorak, Fibroblast migration in fibrin gel matrices, Am.J.Pathol. 142(1), 273-283 (1993).
26. E.A.Ryan, L.F.Mockros, A.M.Stern, and L.Lorand, Influence of a Natural and a Synthetic Inhibitor of Factor XIIIa on Fibrin Clot Rheology, Biophys.J. 77(5), 2827-2836 (1999).
27. S.Cox, M.Cole, and B.Tawil, Behavior of human dermal fibroblasts in three-dimensional fibrin clots: dependence on fibrinogen and thrombin concentration, Tissue Eng. 10(5-6), 942-954 (2004).
28. J.J.Sidelmann, J.Gram, J.Jespersen, and C.Kluft, Fibrin clot formation and lysis: basic mechanisms, Semin.Thromb.Hemost. 26(6), 605-618 (2000).
29. V.Nehls and R.Herrmann, The configuration of fibrin clots determines capillary morphogenesis and endothelial cell migration, Microvasc.Res. 51(3), 347-364 (2001).
30. H.K.Kjaergard and U.S.Weis-Fogh, Important factors influencing the strength of autologous fibrin glue; the fibrin concentration and reaction time--comparison of strength with commercial fibrin glue, Eur.Surg.Res. 26(5), 273-276 (1994).
31. C.B.Herbert, C.Nagaswami, G.D.Bittner, J.A.Hubbell, and J.W.Weisel, Effects of fibrin micromorphology on neurite growth from dorsal root ganglia cultured in three-dimensional fibrin gels, J.Biomed.Mater.Res.A 40(4), 551-559 (1998).
32. J.Meinhart, M.Fussenegger, and W.Hobling, Stabilization of fibrin-chondrocyte constructs for cartilage reconstruction, Ann.Plast.Surg. 42(6), 673-678 (1999).

33. V.Ting, C.D.Sims, L.E.Brecht, J.G.McCarthy, A.K.Kasabian, P.R.Connelly, J.Elisseeff, G.K.Gittes, and M.T.Longaker, In vitro prefabrication of human cartilage shapes using fibrin glue and human chondrocytes, Ann.Plast.Surg. 40(4), 413-420 (1998).
34. G.M.Peretti, M.A.Randolph, M.T.Villa, M.S.Buragas, and M.J.Yaremchuk, Cell-based tissue-engineered allogeneic implant for cartilage repair, Tissue Eng. 6(5), 567-576 (2000).
35. J.L.van Susante, P.Buma, L.Schuman, G.N.Homminga, W.B.van den Berg, and R.P.Veth, Resurfacing potential of heterologous chondrocytes suspended in fibrin glue in large full-thickness defects of femoral articular cartilage: an experimental study in the goat, Biomaterials 20(13), 1167-1175 (2001).
36. M.Fussenegger, J.Meinhart, W.Hobling, W.Kullich, S.Funk, and G.Bernatzky, Stabilized Autologous Fibrin-Chondrocyte Constructs for Cartilage Repair in Vivo, Ann.Plast.Surg. 51(5), 493-498 (2003).
37. L.K.Krishnan, A.Vijayan Lal, P.R.Uma Shankar, and M.Mohanty, Fibrinolysis inhibitors adversely affect remodeling of tissues sealed with fibrin glue, Biomaterials 24(2), 321-327 (2003).
38. R.P.Silverman, D.Passaretti, W.Huang, M.A.Randolph, and M.J.Yaremchuk, Injectable tissue-engineered cartilage using a fibrin glue polymer, Plast.Reconstr.Surg. 103(7), 1809-1818 (1999).
39. Q.Ye, G.Zund, P.Benedikt, S.Jockenhoevel, S.P.Hoerstrup, S.E.Sakiyama, J.A.Hubbell, and M.Turina, Fibrin gel as a three dimensional matrix in cardiovascular tissue engineering, Eur.J.Cardiothorac.Surg. 17(5), 587-591 (2000).
40. S.Jockenhoevel, G.Zund, S.P.Hoerstrup, K.Chalabi, J.S.Sachweh, L.Demircan, B.J.Messmer, and M.Turina, Fibrin gel -- advantages of a new scaffold in cardiovascular tissue engineering, Eur.J.Cardiothorac.Surg. 19(4), 424-430 (2001).
41. A.Mol, M.I.van Lieshout, C.G.Dam-de Veen, S.Neuenschwander, S.P.Hoerstrup, F.P.T.Baaijens, and C.V.C.Bouten, Fibrin as a cell carrier in cardiovascular tissue engineering applications, Biomaterials 26(16), 3113-3121 (2005).
42. G.Wechselberger, T.Schoeller, A.Stenzl, M.Ninkovic, S.Lille, and R.C.Russell, Fibrin glue as a delivery vehicle for autologous urothelial cell transplantation onto a prefabricated pouch, J.Urol. 160(2), 583-586 (1998).
43. G.A.Ameer, T.A.Mahmood, and R.Langer, A biodegradable composite scaffold for cell transplantation, J.Orthop.Res. 20(1), 16-19 (2002).
44. A.Haisch, O.Schultz, C.Perka, V.Jahnke, G.R.Burmester, and M.Sittinger, Tissue engineering of human cartilage tissue for reconstructive surgery using biocompatible resorbable fibrin gel and polymer carriers, HNO 44(11), 624-629 (2001).
45. X.Fei, B.K.Tan, S.T.Lee, C.L.Foo, D.F.Sun, and S.E.Aw, Effect of fibrin glue coating on the formation of new cartilage, Transplant.Proc. 32(1), 210-217 (2000).
46. S.L.Helgerson, T.Seelich, J.DiOrio, B.Tawil, K.M.Bittner, and R.Spaethe, Fibrin, Encyc.Biomat.Biomed.Eng. 603-610 (2004).
47. C.Wong, E.Inman, R.Spaethe, and S.L.Helgerson, Fibrin-based biomaterials to deliver human growth factors, Thromb.Haemost. 89(3), 573-582 (2003).
48. A.Sahni, T.Odrljin, and C.W.Francis, Binding of basic fibroblast growth factor to fibrinogen and fibrin, J.Biol.Chem. 273(13), 7554-7559 (1998).
49. J.Oju, H.R.Soo, H.C.Ji, and B.S.Kim, Control of basic fibroblast growth factor release from fibrin gel with heparin and concentrations of fibrinogen and thrombin, J.Control.Release 105(3), 249-459 (2005).
50. A.Sahni, L.A.Sporn, and C.W.Francis, Potentiation of endothelial cell proliferation by fibrin(ogen)-bound fibroblast growth factor-2, J.Biol.Chem. 274(21), 14936-14941 (1999).
51. A.Quirinia and A.Viidik, The effect of recombinant basic fibroblast growth factor (bFGF) in fibrin adhesive vehicle on the healing of ischaemic and normal incisional skin wounds, Scand.J.Plast.Reconstr.Surg.Hand Surg. 32(1), 9-18 (1998).
52. A.Sahni and C.W.Francis, Vascular endothelial growth factor binds to fibrinogen and fibrin and stimulates endothelial cell proliferation, Blood 96(12), 3772-3778 (2000).
53. M.Ehrbar, A.Metters, P.Zammaretti, J.A.Hubbell, and A.H.Zisch, Endothelial cell proliferation and progenitor maturation by fibrin-bound VEGF variants with differential susceptibilities to local cellular activity, J.Control.Release 101(1-3), 93-109 (2005).
54. A.H.Zisch, U.Schenk, J.C.Schense, S.E.Sakiyama-Elbert, and J.A.Hubbell, Covalently conjugated VEGF--fibrin matrices for endothelialization, J.Control.Release 72(1-3), 101-113 (2001).
55. P.K.Shireman and H.P.Greisler, Mitogenicity and release of vascular endothelial growth factor with and without heparin from fibrin glue, J.Vasc.Surg. 31(5), 936-943 (2000).
56. K.Iwaya, K.Mizoi, A.Tessler, and Y.Itoh, Neurotrophic agents in fibrin glue mediate adult dorsal root regeneration into spinal cord, Neurosurgery 44(3), 589-595 (1999).
57. T.R.Santhosh Kumar and L.K.Krishnan, Endothelial cell growth factor (ECGF) enmeshed with fibrin matrix enhances proliferation of EC in vitro, Biomaterials 22(20), 2769-2776 (2001).

58. R.Fasol, B.Schumacher, K.Schlaudraff, K.H.Hauenstein, and R.Seitelberger, Experimental use of a modified fibrin glue to induce site-directed angiogenesis from the aorta to the heart, J.Thorac.Cardiovasc.Surg. 107(6), 1432-1439 (1994).
59. H.Cheng, B.Hoffer, I.Stromberg, D.Russell, and L.Olson, The effect of glial cell line-derived neurotrophic factor in fibrin glue on developing dopamine neurons, Exp.Brain Res. 104(2), 199-206 (1995).
60. H.Cheng, M.Fraidakis, B.Blomback, P.Lapchak, B.Hoffer, and L.Olson, Characterization of a fibrin glue-GDNF slow-release preparation, Cell Transplantation 7(1), 53-61 (1998).
61. A.C.Lee, V.M.Yu, J.B.Lowe III, M.J.Brenner, D.A.Hunter, S.E.Mackinnon, and S.E.Sakiyama-Elbert, Controlled release of nerve growth factor enhances sciatic nerve regeneration, Exp.Neurol. 184(1), 295-303 (2003).
62. S.E.Sakiyama-Elbert and J.A.Hubbell, Controlled release of nerve growth factor from a heparin-containing fibrin-based cell ingrowth matrix, J.Control.Release 69(1), 149-158 (2000).
63. S.E.Sakiyama-Elbert and J.A.Hubbell, Development of fibrin derivatives for controlled release of heparin-binding growth factors, J.Control.Release 65(3), 389-402 (2000).
64. S.E.Sakiyama, J.C.Schense, and J.A.Hubbell, Incorporation of heparin-binding peptides into fibrin gels enhances neurite extension: an example of designer matrices in tissue engineering, FASEB J. 13(15), 2214-2224 (1999).
65. J.C.Schense, J.Bloch, P.Aebischer, and J.A.Hubbell, Enzymatic incorporation of bioactive peptides into fibrin matrices enhances neurite extension, Nat.Biotechnol. 18(4), 415-419 (2000).
66. A.H.Zisch, S.M.Zeisberger, M.Ehrbar, V.Djonov, C.C.Weber, A.Ziemiecki, E.B.Pasquale, and J.A.Hubbell, Engineered fibrin matrices for functional display of cell membrane-bound growth factor-like activities: Study of angiogenic signaling by ephrin-B2, Biomaterials 25(16), 3245-3257 (2004).
67. J.C.Schense and J.A.Hubbell, Cross-linking exogenous bifunctional peptides into fibrin gels with factor XIIIa, Bioconjugate Chem. 10(1), 75-81 (2000).
68. C.Andree, M.Voigt, A.Wenger, T.Erichsen, K.M.Bittner, D.Schaefer, K.J.Walgenbach, J.Borges, R.E.Horch, and Eriksson, Plasmid gene delivery to human keratinocytes through a fibrin-mediated transfection system, Tissue Eng. 7(6), 757-766 (2001).
69. M.J.MacPee, M.P.Singh, R.Brady, N.Akhyani, G.Liau, C.Lasa, C.Hue, A.Best, and W.Drohan, Fibrin sealant: a versatile delivery vehicle for drugs and biologics, in: "Surgical adhesives and sealants: current technology and application", D.H.Sierra and R.Saltz, eds., Technomic Publishing AG, Basel (1996).
70. M.J.MacPee, A.Campagna, A.Best, R.Kidd, and W.Drohan, Fibrin sealant as a delivery vehicle for sustained and controlled release of chemotherapy agents, in: "Surgical adhesives and sealants: current technology and applications", D.H.Sierra and R.Saltz, eds., Technomic Publishing AG, Basel (1996).
71. M.P.Singh, R.Brady, W.Drohan, and M.J.MacPee, Sustained release of antibiotics from fibrin sealant, in: "Surgical adhesives and sealants: current technology and applications", D.H.Sierra and R.Saltz, eds., Technomic Publishing AG, Basel (1996).
72. L.J.Currie, J.R.Sharpe, and R.Martin, The use of fibrin glue in skin grafts and tissue-engineered skin replacements: a review, Plast.Reconstr.Surg. 108(6), 1713-1726 (2001).
73. D.J.Donaldson, J.T.Mahan, D.Amrani, and J.Hawiger, Fibrinogen-mediated epidermal cell migration: structural correlates for fibrinogen function, J.Cell Sci. 94 101-108 (1989).
74. D.J.Donaldson, J.T.Mahan, D.L.Amrani, D.H.Farrell, and J.H.Sobel, Further studies on the interaction of migrating keratinocytes with fibrinogen, Cell Commun.Adhes. 2(4), 299-308 (1994).
75. M.Krasna, F.Planinsek, M.Knezevic, Z.M.Arnez, and M.Jeras, Evaluation of a fibrin-based skin substitute prepared in a defined keratinocyte medium, Int.J.Pharm. 291(1-2), 31-37 (2005).
76. R.E.Horch, H.Bannasch, J.Kopp, C.Andree, and G.B.Stark, Single-cell suspensions of cultured human keratinocytes in fibrin-glue reconstitute the epidermis, Cell Transplant. 7(3), 309-317 (1998).
77. R.A.F.Clark, J.M.Lanigan, P.DellaPelle, E.Manseau, H.F.Dvorak, and R.B.Colvin, Fibronectin and Fibrin Provide a Provisional Matrix for Epidermal Cell Migration During Wound Reepithelialization, J.Invest.Dermatol. 79(5), 264-269 (1982).
78. J.Kopp, M.G.Jeschke, A.D.Bach, U.Kneser, and R.E.Horch, Applied tissue engineering in the closure of severe burns and chronic wounds using cultured human autologous keratinocytes in a natural fibrin matrix, Cell Tissue Bank. 5(2), 89-96 (2004).
79. R.E.Horch, H.Bannasch, and G.B.Stark, Transplantation of cultured autologous keratinocytes in fibrin sealant biomatrix to resurface chronic wounds, Transplant.Proc. 33(1-2), 642-644 (2001).
80. G.Pellegrini, R.Ranno, G.Stracuzzi, S.Bondanza, L.Guerra, G.Zambruno, G.Micali, and M.De Luca, The control of epidermal stem cells (holoclones) in the treatment of massive full-thickness burns with autologous keratinocytes cultured on fibrin, Transplantation 68(6), 868-879 (1999).
81. V.Ronfard, H.Broly, V.Mitchell, J.P.Galizia, D.Hochart, E.Chambon, P.Pellerin, and J.J.Huart, Use of human keratinocytes cultured on fibrin glue in the treatment of burn wounds, Burns 17(3), 181-184 (1991).

82. A.Meana, J.Iglesias, M.Del Rio, F.Larcher, B.Madrigal, M.F.Fresno, C.Martin, F.San Roman, and F.Tevar, Large surface of cultured human epithelium obtained on a dermal matrix based on live fibroblast-containing fibrin gels, Burns 24(7), 621-630 (1998).
83. R.Gorodetsky, R.A.F.Clark, J.An, J.Gailit, L.Levdansky, A.Vexler, E.Berman, and G.Marx, Fibrin Microbeads (FMB) as Biodegradable Carriers for Culturing Cells and for Accelerating Wound Healing1, J.Invest.Dermatol. 112(6), 866-872 (1999).
84. P.Koolwijk, M.G.van Erck, W.J.de Vree, M.A.Vermeer, H.A.Weich, R.Hanemaaijer, and V.W.van Hinsbergh, Cooperative effect of TNFalpha, bFGF, and VEGF on the formation of tubular structures of human microvascular endothelial cells in a fibrin matrix. Role of urokinase activity, J.Cell Biol. 132(6), 1177-1188 (1996).
85. D.A.Weatherford, J.E.Sackman, T.T.Reddick, M.B.Freeman, S.L.Stevens, and M.H.Goldman, Vascular endothelial growth factor and heparin in a biologic glue promotes human aortic endothelial cell proliferation with aortic smooth muscle cell inhibition, Surgery 120(2), 433-439 (1996).
86. S.Jockenhoevel, K.Chalabi, J.S.Sachweh, H.V.Groesdonk, L.Demircan, M.Grossmann, G.Zund, and B.J.Messmer, Tissue engineering: complete autologous valve conduit--a new moulding technique, Thorac.Cardiovasc.Surg. 49(5), 287-290 (2001).
87. C.L.C.Cummings, D.Gawlitte, R.M.R.Nerem, and J.P.J.Stegemann, Properties of engineered vascular constructs made from collagen, fibrin, and collagen-fibrin mixtures, Biomaterials 25(17), 3699-3706 (2004).
88. N.Isogai, W.J.Landis, R.Mori, Y.Gotoh, L.C.Gerstenfeld, J.Upton, and J.P.Vacanti, Experimental use of fibrin glue to induce site-directed osteogenesis from cultured periosteal cells, Plastic And Reconstructive Surgery 105(3), 953-963 (2000).
89. A.M.-H.Ng, A.B.Saim, K.K.Tan, G.H.Tan, S.A.Mokhtar, I.M.Rose, F.Othman, and R.B.H.Idrus, Comparison of bioengineered human bone construct from four sources of osteogenic cells, J.Orthop.Sci. 10(2), 192-199 (2005).
90. C.Perka, O.Schultz, R.S.Spitzer, K.Lindenhayn, G.R.Burmester, and M.Sittinger, Segmental bone repair by tissue-engineered periosteal cell transplants with bioresorbable fleece and fibrin scaffolds in rabbits, Biomaterials 21(11), 1145-1153 (2000).
91. J.M.Karp, F.Sarraf, M.S.Shoichet, and J.E.Davies, Fibrin-filled scaffolds for bone-tissue engineering: An in vivo study, J.Biomed.Mater.Res.A 71(1), 162-171 (2004).
92. A.Haisch, F.Wanjura, C.Radke, K.Leder-Johrens, A.Groger, M.Endres, S.Klaering, A.Loch, and M.Sittinger, Immunomodulation of tissue-engineered transplants: In vivo bone generation from methylprednisolone-stimulated chondrocytes, Eur.Arch.Otorhinolaryngol. 261(4), 216-224 (2004).
93. L.A.Fortier, A.J.Nixon, H.Mohammed, and G.Lust, Altered biological activity of equine chondrocytes cultured in a three-dimensional fibrin matrix and supplemented with transforming growth factor beta-1, Am.J.Vet.Res. 58(1), 66-70 (1997).
94. L.A.Fortier, G.Lust, H.Mohammed, and A.J.Nixon, Coordinate upregulation of cartilage matrix synthesis in fibrin cultures supplemented with exogenous insulin-like growth factor-I, J.Orthop.Res. 17(4), 467-474 (1999).
95. C.J.Hunter, J.K.Mouw, and M.E.Levenston, Dynamic compression of chondrocyte-seeded fibrin gels: effects on matrix accumulation and mechanical stiffness, Osteoarthritis Cartilage 12(2), 117-130 (2004).
96. C.D.Sims, P.E.Butler, Y.L.Cao, R.Casanova, M.A.Randolph, A.Black, C.A.Vacanti, and M.J.Yaremchuk, Tissue engineered neocartilage using plasma derived polymer substrates and chondrocytes, Plast.Reconstr.Surg. 101(6), 1580-1585 (1998).
97. J.W.Xu, V.Zaporojan, G.M.Peretti, R.E.Roses, K.B.Morse, A.K.Roy, J.M.Mesa, M.A.Randolph, L.J.Bonassar, and M.J.Yaremchuk, Injectable tissue-engineered cartilage with different chondrocyte sources, Plast.Reconstr.Surg. 113(5), 1361-1371 (2004).
98. J.W.Xu, J.Nazzal, G.M.Peretti, C.H.Kirchhoff, M.A.Randolph, and M.J.Yaremchuk, Tissue-engineered cartilage composite with expanded polytetrafluoroethylene membrane, Ann.Plast.Surg. 46(5), 527-532 (2001).
99. J.Xu, G.M.Peretti, J.Nazzal, R.E.Roses, K.R.Morse, and M.J.Yaremchuk, Producing a flexible tissue-engineered cartilage framework using expanded polytetrafluoroethylene membrane as a pseudoperichondrium, Plast Reconstr Surg 116(2), 577-589 (2005).
100. C.Perka, R.S.Spitzer, K.Lindenhayn, M.Sittinger, and O.Schultz, Matrix-mixed culture: new methodology for chondrocyte culture and preparation of cartilage transplants, J.Biomed.Mater.Res.A 49(3), 305-311 (2002).

25

ECTOPIC BONE INDUCTION BY EQUINE BONE PROTEIN EXTRACT

Haisheng Li[1], Marco Springer[2], Xuenong Zou[1], Arne Briest[2], Cody Bünger[1]

25.1. ABSTRACT

Demineralized bone matrix from horse has been reported to be osteoinductive. However, its performance was inferior to autogenous bone graft in terms of new bone formation. In the present experiment, an equine bone protein extract-COLLOSS E was investigated for its osteoinductivity in a rat model. At the mean time, carboxymethylcellulose (CMC) was tested as a potential carrier for the protein extract.

18 male Wistar rats (8 weeks) were employed in the experiment. Each rat was implanted randomly with the 2 of the following implants, one on each side of the abdominal muscle. 1) COLLOSS E lyophilisate. 2) PEEK ring holder. 3) 3% or 10% CMC .in gel or lyophilized form 4) COLLOSS E lyophilisate with 3% CMC, implanted as gel or in lyophilized form. 5) COLLOSS E suspension with 10% CMC, implanted as gel or in lyophilized form. The rats were followed up for 21 days. After termination, samples were subjected to macroscopic examination, plain radiograph, micro-CT and histological evaluations.

The results showed that PEEK ring or CMC alone could not induce ectopic bone formation. COLLOSS E lyophilisate has a slightly higher (6 out of 7) positive bone formation rate over COLLOSS E/3% CMC (3 out of 5, both gel and lyophilized form), however, the difference is non-significant (p=0.36, Fisher's exact test). 10% CMC with COLLOSS E did not show ectopic bone formation when implanted as gel form (0/8), while 1 positive bone formation was found when implanted as the lyophilized form (1/4). Bone tissue volume ranged from 0 mm^3 to 23.1mm^3 for COLLOSS-E lyophilisate alone and 0 to 29.7mm^3 for COLLOSS E/3%CMC (gel or lyophilized form).

We concluded that equine bone protein extract has the ability to induce ectopic bone formation in the rat model. CMC could be a potential carrier, however, further studies are needed to verify the proportion and efficacy.

---

[1] Orthopedic Research Laboratory, Aarhus University Hospital, 8000 Aarhus C, Denmark.
[2] Ossacur AG, D-71720 Oberstenfeld, Germany.

25.2. INTRODUCTION

A significant part of orthopedic surgery involves attempts to stimulate bone healing. While autogenous iliac crest bone is the 'gold standard' of bone graft materials to promote bone mineralization and facilitate bone healing, various bone graft alternatives have been developed because of the morbidities related to autogenous bone graft harvesting and the limited quantity available. Purified bovine protein extract has been proved to be osteoinductive and successful spine fusion results have been reported in animal studies and pilot clinical trials[1;2]. The present authors have also reported a bovine collagen extract achieved the same fusion rate and new bone formation as that of autograft bone in a porcine spinal fusion model [3]. However, osteoinductive potential of protein extract and collagen from equine bone has not been well characterized. Vail TB et al reported that demineralized equine bone matrix was osteoinductive in the horse muscle pouch after an allogenic implantation[4]. Like the bovine bone, equine bone protein extract has a rich source and could be a cost-effective alternative as bone graft material. In this study, we investigated the ectopic osteoinductive ability of an equine bone collagen extract and the role of carboxymethylcellulose (CMC) as a potential carrier in a rat model.

25.3. MATERIALS AND METHODS

25.3.1. Implant

Equine bone collagen extract (COLLOSS E, OSSACUR AG, Oberstenfeld, Germany) is processed from the cortical diaphyseal equine bone. It is lyophilized in collagenous matrix form, and according to the manufacture, it consists mostly type I collagen with other insoluble proteins. COLLOSS E was provided in two forms for the experiment: protein suspension and lyophilisate.

A PEEK (Polyetheretherketone, Invibio Ltd., EPPK-OPTIMA LT1R12) ring was used as holder for the samples to be implanted into the rat. The size of the ring: 10mm in inner diameter and 5mm in height.

CMC (Aqualon, division of Hercules Incorporated, Dusseldorf, Germany) was mixed with COLLOSS E to function as a carrier and bulking agent. It was used in the experiment in two concentrations: 3% and 10% (W/V). COLLOSS E and CMC were mixed to comprise the following groups:

Group 1) 50mg COLLOSS E lyophilisate was dissolved in 0.5ml saline (isotonic solution of sodium chloride), which resulted in a viscous solution, and then 0.25ml CMC (3%) was added. This mixing procedure decreased the apparent viscosity of the 3% CMC stock solution only slightly. The mixed gel was either directly filled into the PEEK ring or re-lyophilized in a sterile syringe for 48 hours and then filled as a dry solid sponge into the PEEK ring.

Group 2) Unconcentrated COLLOSS E suspension (dry weight/weight of COLLOSS E suspension is 1.56 mg/g) was used to mix CMC powder (10% w/v). Mixed gel was again filled into the PEEK ring in gel form (1ml).

Group 3) COLLOSS E suspension was concentrated by centrifugation at 10000rpm for 20 minutes (dry weight/weight of concentrated COLLOSS E suspension is 12.26 mg/g), after discarding the supernatant, 10% CMC powder (w/v) was added to the viscous COLLOSS E pellet. The mixed gel was again filled into the PEEK ring in gel form (1ml).

Group 4) COLLOSS E suspension (1.56 mg/g) was concentrated by centrifugation at 10000rpm for 20 minutes, after discarding the supernatant, 2.5 % CMC powder (w/v) was added to 4g of the viscous COLLOSS E pellet (12.26mg/g) after centrifugation (12.26mg/g * 4g = app. 50mg). The mixed gel was filled into a syringe and re-lyophilized for 48 hours and then a much higher concentration pressed to 1/4 of its original volume could be put as a pressed dry solid sponge into the PEEK ring, which then contained app. 50mg of COLLOSS E and now 10% CMC (w/v).

25.3.2. Animals

18 male Wistar rats (8 weeks old) weighing around 220g were employed in the study. The animals were anesthetized by the mixture of ketamine and xylazine, and then two muscle pouches were made on each side of the abdominal muscle. Implants of COLLOSS-E with or without CMC were randomly inserted into the muscle pouches. After incision was closed, the rats were followed up to 21 days. The rats were terminated by CO_2 asphyxiation followed by exanguination. The muscle pouches were dissected, examined macroscopically and preserved in neutral buffered 8% formaldehyde solution.

25.3.3. Evaluation Methods

First a normal X-ray was taken of all the samples to screening the possible bone formation. Micro CT and histology evaluations were employed later to quantify the ectopic bone formation. As for micro-CT scanning (μ-CT 40, Scanco Medical AG., Zürich, Switzerland), the samples were put into a holder and subjected to a high-resolution scanning. The scanned images have a three-dimensional (3-D) reconstruction of cubic voxel sizes $31\times31\times31$ μm^3. Each 3-D image dataset consisted of approximately 200 to 300 micro-CT slide images (1024 × 1024 pixels) with 16-bit-gray-levels. From accurate 3-D datasets, bone volume (BV) could be calculated based on unbiased, assumption-free 3-D methods.

After scanning, the samples were dehydrated in graded ethanol (70-99%) and embedded in methylmethacrylate. 3 to 4 histological sections were cut through each sample. Sections without PEEK ring were cut to the thickness of 7 to 10μm. Samples with PEEK ring were sectioned with a special diamond saw to the thickness of 40 μm. They were stained with toluidine blue or basic fuchsin and light green to demonstrate both cellular content and bone formation.

25.3.4. Statistics

Data were processed in statistic software SPSS 13.0 (SPSS Inc. IL, USA). The rates of positive bone formation were compared between groups by Fisher's Exact Test. The difference was considered significant when $p<0.05$.

25.4. RESULTS

25.4.1. General Findings

All the rats appeared to be in good health throughout the observation period. There were no signs of haematoma, severe inflammation, or other complications around the implantation sites. At the time of explantation, large tissue mass could be palpated on both side of the abdomen. The consistency of the explants range from soft to moderate hard, and the sizes range from 1.5cm to 3cm in diameter. General results are summarized in Table 25.1.

25.4.2. Plain Radiograph

Patches of moderate density could be seen with COLLOSS E, but not with PEEK ring or with CMC gel alone. PEEK ring could be clearly visualized from the radiograph.

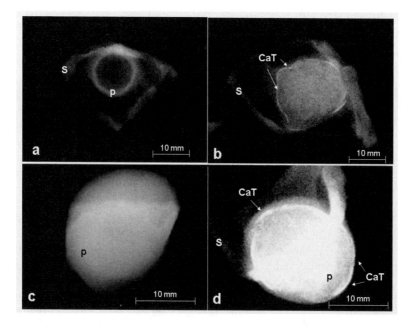

Figure 25.1. Images show plain radiograph evaluation of tissue explants. PEEK ring (a) and 3%CMC (c) alone did not show any high density patches, while COLLOSS E alone without PEEK ring holder (b) and COLLOSS E/3%CMC gel (d) demonstrated irregular patches with moderate to high density. **P**=PEEK ring, **S**=skin, **CaT**=calcified tissue.

When COLLOSS E was mixed with 3% or 10% CMC gel, moderate density patches that is representative of calcified tissue could also be noted (Figure 25.1).

25.4.3. Micro-CT

Empty PEEK rings or CMC gel alone (both 3% and 10%) did show no bone formation with micro-CT scanning. When COLLOSS E (50mg) was inserted into the muscle pouches alone without PEEK ring, bone-like calcified tissue formation was seen from the images. A thin layer of bone-like calcified tissue was formed outside the PEEK ring when COLLOSS E was loaded in the ring. Mixing the 3%CMC with COLLOSS E also resulted in bone-like tissue formation. However when 10% CMC gel was utilized, no bone-like tissue could be detected (Figure 25.2). Bone-like tissue volume varied from 0 mm^3 to 23.1mm^3 for COLLOSS-E (50mg) alone, 0 to 29.7mm^3 for COLLOSS E/3%CMC gel, and 0 mm^3 to 7.9 mm^3 for COLLOSS E/10% CMC.

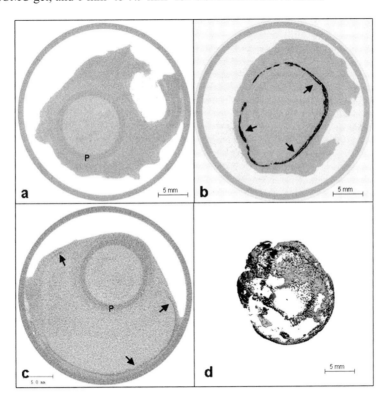

Figure 25. 2. Micro-CT images showing empty PEEK ring with no sign of bone formation (a). When COLLOSS E was packed inside the ring, a bone like shell was formed outside (arrows in b). Higher concentration of CMC (10%) with COLLOSS E (group 3) resulted in a large cyst (arrows indicate cyst wall) with no sign of bone tissue (c). 3D image demonstrate that spherical newly formed bone like tissue around the ring holder (d). P= PEEK ring.

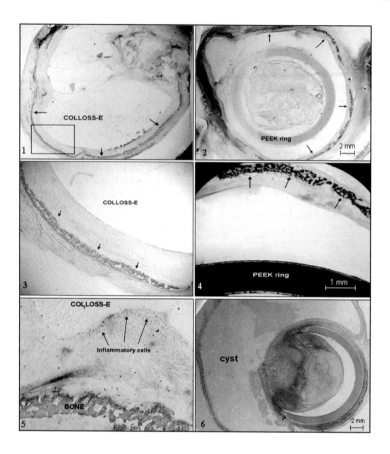

Figure 25.3. Histological micrographs: 1) Overview of COLLOSS E implanted into the muscle pouch alone. Large areas of COLLOSS E appeared as white mass presented inside a bony rim (arrows). Magnification of the newly formed bone (square) is shown in image 3 where the thin shell of bone tissue is clearly noted (arrows). 2) Overview of COLLOSS E/3% CMC gel (group 1) implanted with a PEEK ring holder. New bone tissue (arrows) formed between the ring and the muscle tissue. The relation of new bone tissue and PEEK ring is better viewed in image 4. 5) Infiltration of inflammatory cells presented in the loose connective tissue near COLLOSS E region. 6) The COLLOSS E/10%CMC combination did not yield any new bone (group3). A large cyst encapsulated by a fibrous wall can be seen around the PEEK ring, which was probably resulted from high concentration of CMC gel. Staining methods: toluidine blue (image 1,3,5); basic fuchsin and light green (image 2,4,6).

25.4.4. Histology

Histological sections confirmed the micro-CT results. No ectopic bone formation could be seen when PEEK ring or CMC gel alone was implanted. New bone tissue was induced by COLLOSS E alone or together with 3% CMC gel. Bone tissue formed in the shape of round shell in between the PEEK ring and the muscle layer. Bone tissue was never seen inside the PEEK ring, instead, loose connective tissue with unabsorbed COLLOSS E mass filled up the ring. Inflammatory cells could be seen around the unabsorbed COLLOSS E area. When higher concentration of CMC (10%) was mixed with COLLOSS E suspension and implanted in the form of liquid gel (group 3), large cyst around the PEEK ring was noted. New bone tissue was only found in one out of 4 samples when the same mixture was implanted in lyophilized form (group 4). Results are depicted in Figure 25.3. There is no statistical difference between the COLLOSS E alone and the mixture of COLLOSS E/3% CMC (group 1) in terms of positive bone formation rates ($p=0.36$). However, the differences are significant between the COLLOSS E and PEEK ring ($p=0.03$) or CMC alone ($p=0.001$) when tested by Fisher's Exact test. Positive number of bone tissue formation appeared higher with 3%CMC/COLLOSS E (group 1) than that with COLLOSS E/10% CMC (group 4), however, the difference is not significant ($p=0.36$).

25.5. DISCUSSION

Banked allograft bone and demineralized bone matrix (DBM) are among the most commonly used osteoinductive graft materials. However, allograft is immunogenic and holds the risk of infectious disease transmission despite different processing and preservation methods used[5]. DBM offer another source for bone substitute. They can be available in reasonable quantities and have been shown to induce new bone formation in animals as well as in a number of clinical observations[6-9]. DBM from horse has previous been shown to be osteoinductive and particle size was an influential factor of its osteoinductive capacity[4]. When compared with autogenous bone graft in a rib defect horse model, DBM produced less bone and lower percent of ash and calcium[10]. The present experiment demonstrates that an equine bone protein extract – COLLOSS E could induce ectopic bone formation in rat abdominal muscle pouches. COLLOSS E was extracted from equine cortical bone and consist mostly collagen type I and other non-collagenous proteins. The exact mechanism of this bone inductivity is yet unclear, however, experiments from the bovine COLLOSS, which is processed by the same way as COLLOSS E, indicated that bone morphogenetic proteins (BMPs) may exist as non-collagenous proteins[11,12]. The collagen matrix, though not osteoinductive, could also play an important role in chemotaxis of mesenchymal stem cells, adhesion and formation of complexes with growth factors [13;14], which may also add up to the overall osteoinductive effect. The reason why ectopic bone tissue formed outside the implant in the shape of a spherical could not be clarified by the study. Possible explanations could be that a haematoma was formed around the implant right after the surgery, and ectopic bone tissue could only be formed later in the outer surface of the haematoma where there was rich blood supply and mesenchymal cells from the muscle. In the present rat model, 50mg COLLOSS E could produce an average amount of 7.29 ± 9.94 mm^3 ectopic bone tissue when implanted alone or inside the PEEK ring. The bone tissue volume increased to 16.77 ± 18.3 mm^3 when COLLOSS E was mixed with 3% CMC gel. Due to the fixed observation time, we do not know if the bone volume would increase over time. On the other hand, caution need to be taken when extrapolating the results from ectopic site to orthopedic site regard to the dosage, the amount of bone formed and the time to achieve bone formation.

The extracted equine protein matrix has a poor space-keeping property. A carrier could not only help to define the shape of the implant, but also retain the proteins in the specific area for an adequate time period. Moreover, a carrier may serve as a scaffold and bear certain mechanical load. Among the different carrier scaffolds we have screened,

Table 25.1. Experimental setup and overall results

Implant composition	Physical property	Number of samples	X-ray	Micro-CT (M±SD) mm^3	Histology
COLLOSS E lyophilisate 50mg (control)	Lyophilized, no PEEK ring	2	Faint to moderate density patch in 2/2	8.01± 10.89	New bone formation in 2/2
	Lyophilized, with PEEK ring	5	Moderate density patch in 4/5	6.48± 11.07	New bone formation in 4/5
PEEK ring (control)	Solid ring	3	No visible patch	0	No bone formation
3% CMC gel (control)	Gel, with PEEK ring	1	No visible patch	0	No bone formation
	Lyophilized, with PEEK ring	2	No visible patch	0	No bone formation
10% CMC gel (control)	Gel, with PEEK ring	2	No visible patch	0	No bone formation
	Lyophilized, with PEEK ring	4	No visible patch	0	No bone formation
50mg COLLOSS E lyophilisate dissolved in saline +3% CMC gel	Gel, with PEEK ring. Group 1	3	High density patch in 1/3	3.83± 6.63	Good bone formation in 1/3
	Lyophilized, with PEEK ring. Group 1	2	Moderate to high density patch in 2/2	16.77± 18.3	New bone formation in 2/2
COLLOSS E suspension (unconcentrated or concentrated) + 10% CMC gel	Group 2. Gel (unconcentrated COLLOSS E suspension), with PEEK ring	4	Faint to moderate density patch in 4/4	0	No bone formation
	Group 3. Gel (concentrated COLLOSS E suspension), with PEEK ring	4	No visible signal (1/4) to moderate density patch (3/4)	0	No bone formation
50mg COLLOSS E suspension +10%CMC gel	Group 4 Lyophilized, with PEEK ring	4	Faint to moderate density patch	2.64± 4.58	Bone formation in 1/4

Group 1 to 4 refers to the experimental group design in the Materials and Methods part. Different numbers of samples were due to the table is a summary of several screening animal experiments.

such as tricalcium phosphate and collagen sponge, CMC gel was employed in the present experiment. As a biocompatible material, CMC has been successfully used as carrier for OP-1 and rhBMP-2 deliveries [15;16]. CMC alone has been found to raise the alkaline phosphatase activity of fibroblast and even encourage bone growth[15;17]. In the present experiment, 3% CMC gel carrying 50mg of COLLOSS E performed just as good as COLLOSS E alone. CMC alone, either 3% or 10%, could not induce ectopic bone formation in this rat model. Even though no additional bone stimulation effect was introduced, CMC gave the COLLOSS E physical properties of either a gel or a lyophilized sponge, which made it much easy to handle during implantation. Higher percent CMC in liquid gel form somewhat inhibited the osteoinductivity of COLLOSS E. None out of the 8 samples gave raise to new bone formation. When the same mixture was implanted in lyophilized form, 1 out the 4 samples showed new bone tissue. The reason may be that higher concentration of CMC isolated COLLOSS E from direct interaction with the surrounding muscle tissue and provide no surface for early cell attachment due to its high viscosity, while lyophilized form could help this interaction during the rehydration process right after implantation. Another reason could be that the COLLOSS E used with 3% CMC was resuspended from the lyophilized form, which is different from the COLLOSS E suspension used with 10% CMC. Some bioactive proteins may be discarded with the supernatant when preparing the COLLOSS E suspension. Future approaches would be the addition of higher concentrations of collagen or related materials to facilitate the attachment and migration of cells attracted by COLLOSS E into the highly viscous gel.

Inflammatory cell infiltration was noted on histological sections. They appeared mostly around the unabsorbed COLLOSS E material. Being a xenograft material, COLLOSS E could trigger minor immune reactions due to remodeling. Autoantibodies have been reported on treatment with bovine collagen implants in human, while neither adverse reactions to the bovine collagen implant nor any other clinical symptoms were observed[18]. In the present experiment, we did not monitor the antibody formation because of our primary focus of osteoinductivity. We did not find any noticeable systemic or local reactions related to the implant.

In conclusion, COLLOSS E has the ability to induce ectopic bone formation in the rat muscle pouch. 3% CMC gel could act as carrier or bulking agent either in gel or in lyophilized form. However, the optimal concentrations of different combinations need further investigation with multiple time points.

25.6. ACKNOWLEDGMENTS

OSSACUR AG, Oberstenfeld, Germany provided the support for the study. Anette Milton and Lisa Feng are thanked for their excellent technical assistance in histological preparation.

25.7. REFERENCES

1. S.D. Boden. Ne-Osteo Bone Growth Factor for Posterolateral Lumbar Spine Fusion: Results From a Nonhuman Primate Study and a Prospective Human Clinical Pilot Study. *Spine* 29[5], 504-514.(2004).

3. H. Li, X. Zou, C. Woo, M. Ding, M. Lind, and C. Bunger, Experimental anterior lumbar interbody fusion with an osteoinductive bovine bone collagen extract, *Spine* 30:890 (2005).
4. T.B. Vail, G.W. Trotter, and B.E. Powers, Equine demineralized bone matrix: relationship between particle size and osteoinduction, *Vet.Surg.* 23:386 (1994).
5. B.E. Buck, T.I. Malinin, and M.D. Brown, Bone transplantation and human immunodeficiency virus. An estimate of risk of acquired immunodeficiency syndrome (AIDS), *Clin.Orthop.*129 (1989).
6. T.A. Einhorn, J.M. Lane, A.H. Burstein, C.R. Kopman, and V.J. Vigorita, The healing of segmental bone defects induced by demineralized bone matrix. A radiographic and biomechanical study, *J Bone Joint Surg Am.* 66:274 (1984).
7. R. Gepstein, R.E. Weiss, and T. Hallel, Bridging large defects in bone by demineralized bone matrix in the form of a powder. A radiographic, histological, and radioisotope-uptake study in rats, *J Bone Joint Surg Am.* 69:984 (1987).
8. J.L. Russell and J.E. Block, Clinical utility of demineralized bone matrix for osseous defects, arthrodesis, and reconstruction: impact of processing techniques and study methodology, *Orthopedics* 22:524 (1999).
9. P. Ragni and T.S. Lindholm, Interaction of allogeneic demineralized bone matrix and porous hydroxy-apatite bioceramics in lumbar interbody fusion in rabbits, *Clin.Orthop.*292 (1991).
10. C.E. Kawcak, G.W. Trotter, B.E. Powers, R.D. Park, and A.S. Turner, Comparison of bone healing by demineralized bone matrix and autogenous cancellous bone in horses, *Vet.Surg.* 29:218 (2000).
11. J. Wiltfang, F.R. Kloss, P. Kessler, E. Nkenke, S. Schultze-Mosgau, R. Zimmermann, and K.A. Schlegel, Effects of platelet-rich plasma on bone healing in combination with autogenous bone and bone substitutes in critical-size defects. An animal experiment, *Clin.Oral Implants.Res.* 15:187 (2004).
12. K.A. Schlegel, K. Donath, S. Rupprecht, S. Falk, R. Zimmermann, E. Felszeghy, and J. Wiltfang, De novo bone formation using bovine collagen and platelet-rich plasma, *Biomaterials* 25:5387 (2004).
13. M. Mizuno, R. Fujisawa, and Y. Kuboki, Type I collagen-induced osteoblastic differentiation of bone-marrow cells mediated by collagen-alpha2beta1 integrin interaction, *J.Cell Physiol* 184:207 (2000).
14. Mundy GR. Osteoblasts, bone formation and mineralization. In: Fogelman I, editor. Bone remodeling and its disorders. London: Maetin Dunitz; 1995. p 17-38.
15. A. Santa-Comba, A. Pereira, R. Lemos, D. Santos, J. Amarante, M. Pinto, P. Tavares, and F. Bahia, Evaluation of carboxymethylcellulose, hydroxypropylmethylcellulose, and aluminum hydroxide as potential carriers for rhBMP-2, *J.Biomed.Mater.Res.* 55:396 (2001).
16. H. Wang, I.N. Springer, H. Schildberg, Y. Acil, K. Ludwig, D.R. Rueger, and H. Terheyden, Carboxy-methylcellulose-stabilized collagenous rhOP-1 device-a novel carrier biomaterial for the repair of mandibular continuity defects, *J.Biomed.Mater.Res.A* 68:219 (2004).
17. J.B. Rodgers, H.C. Vasconez, M.D. Wells, P.P. DeLuca, M.C. Faugere, B.F. Fink, and D. Hamilton, Two lyophilized polymer matrix recombinant human bone morphogenetic protein-2 carriers in rabbit calvarial defects, *J.Craniofac.Surg.* 9:147 (1998).
18. F. Trautinger, E.M. Kokoschka, and E.J. Menzel, Antibody formation against human collagen and C1q in response to a bovine collagen implant, *Arch.Dermatol.Res.* 283:395 (1991).

26

ADIPOSE TISSUE INDUCTION *IN VIVO*

Filip B.J.L. Stillaert[1,2], Phillip Blondeel[1], Moustapha Hamdi[1], Keren Abberton[2], Erik Thompson[2,3] and Wayne A. Morrison[2,3]

26.1. ABSTRACT

Engineering adipogenic tissue *in vivo* requires the concomitant induction of angiogenesis to generate a stable long-term three-dimensional construct. Histioconductive tissue engineering strategies have been used. The disadvantage of using biodegradable scaffolds is a delayed angiogenic induction resulting in ischemic necrosis of the central cell population in the scaffold. We evaluated an histioinductive approach for adipose tissue engineering by combining essential key components for adipogenic induction: (1) a precursor cell source, (2) a vascular pedicle, (3) a supportive matrix, and (4) a chamber to preserve space for the new tissue to develop. We observed concomitant adipogenic and angiogenic induction after 6 weeks in three-dimensional adipose tissue constructs.

26.2. INTRODUCTION

Adipose tissue is a dynamic, easily manipulated tissue which makes it practical for tissue augmentation or contour repair for soft tissue defects of any etiology. Treatment of soft tissue defects is not just a matter of "filling the gap" but of generating a long-term, stable tissue which interacts with adjacent tissue. Problems associated with fat flap transfer, such as resorption at the recipient site and donor site morbidity, are an issue but no ideal surgical alternative or substitutive tissue currently exists.

---

[1]Department of Plastic and Reconstructive Surgery, University Hospital Ghent, Belgium
[2]Bernard O'Brien Institute of Microsurgery, Melbourne, Australia
[3]University of Melbourne, Department of Surgery, St Vincent's Hospital, Melbourne, Australia

Identification of the intrinsic cellular and molecular characteristics of adipose tissue could identify new pathways in tissue engineering research for enhancing fat survival or inducing *de novo* adipogenesis at the recipient site, using either conductive or inductive strategies. Both types of strategies require several key components for a successful construct: progenitor cells, growth factors and cytokines to induce differentiation, an extracellular matrix, a vascular supply and space for the new tissue to develop. Several theories on adipose tissue generation using free fat grafts have been proposed, such as the host replacement theory and the cell survival theory. In the host replacement theory, host derived histiocytes would invade the graft taking on lipid material and replacing all adipose tissue of the graft [1]. In the cell survival theory, histiocytes would act as scavengers of lipid but would not replace the graft adipose tissue. Only part of the graft tissue would survive and be present in the tissue construct after the host reaction subsides.

The extracellular matrix (ECM) plays a number of essential roles in tissue engineering by providing a scaffold for cells to attach and migrate to, as a microenvironment of differentiation, and a preserver of space.

26.3. TISSUE ENGINEERING STRATEGIES

Histioconductive approaches use *ex vivo* biodegradable scaffolds for replacement of missing tissue. Cultured or isolated cells can be seeded onto those scaffolds and implanted *in vivo* [2,3,4]. The substrate dependence of specific cells for proliferation and differentiation will be an essential factor to take into account in this method. On the other hand, the disadvantage here is that pre-cultured tissue constructs, which must become vascularized once implanted within the recipient, may not be as successful in the long-term as methods which foster a primary neovascularisation of a biological matrix scaffold. This is followed by secondary recruitment and migration of native cells with stem cell characteristics for the production of the wanted tissue in an inductive manner. The central cell population of these pre-cultured constructs will be at risk of ischemia before any appropriate vascularisation of the graft occurs.

Growth of any tissue requires *a fortiori* the formation of a functional and mature vasculature. Histioinductive approaches will facilitate self-repair or tissue generation *de novo* at the recipient site. Kawaguchi [5] obtained vascularized plugs of newly formed adipose tissue by injecting Matrigel® supplemented with bFGF into the subcutaneous fat pads of mice. Matrigel® is an extracellular matrix hydrogel derived from the murine EHS sarcoma, and contains basement membrane proteins such as laminin, collagen IV and heparan sulfate proteoglycans as well as several growth factors, such as bFGF, TGF-β, IGF-1, PDGF, NGF and EGF [6]. They further demonstrated that subcutaneous injection of Matrigel® enriched with bFGF, induced neo-adipogenesis in mice [5]. Neovascularisation at the site of injection, together with the basement membrane-rich Matrigel® matrix, apparently creates a suitable micro-environment for endogenous precursor cells to migrate, proliferate and differentiate into mature, vascularized adipocyte clusters [7]. In this *in vivo* model, access to fat is constitutive and adipogenesis is *de facto* host-derived. They suggest that the endogenous progenitor cells penetrated the Matrigel® matrix, in addition to the migration of endothelial cells, from the surrounding host tissue.

In our studies (Cronin et al., 2004; Kelly et al., 2005, Tissue Engineering, on press; Stillaert et al., 2005, in preparation) we used a sealed tissue engineering chamber based on a vascular pedicle (Figure 26.1.) and supplied with an instructive matrix (BD Matrigel®) and access to adipose tissue. Chambers without a fat xenograft did not generate adipogenic tissue. The rationale of transplanting a fat tissue graft in a suitable ECM was that early studies using the closed chamber showed that access to preexisting adipose tissue was essential (Kelly et al., 2005) to generate adipogenic tissue. The cell-cell or cell-matrix interactions could be temporarily better preserved and cells in whole tissue biopsies could resist hypoxic conditions longer when placed in Matrigel®. We initially hypothesized that the vascularized fat tissue generated in the chamber (Figure 26.2.) originated from the adipose tissue graft, more specifically from its stromal-vascular fraction located precursor cell population. However, careful immunohistochemical analysis of human xenografted fat biopsies in SCID-mice revealed the generated fat tissue was predominantly host-derived. An alternative hypothesis was that those isolated fat sources may be providing stimuli for the recruitment of mesenchymal stem cells directly from perivascular cell populations within the chamber or from the systemic circulation via the newly developed vascular network (Figure 26.2.).

These studies have considerable bearing on the growing number of approaches to adipose tissue engineering, such as use of inductive fat with autografted "preadipocytes" or preadipocyte conferring components such as processed-lipoaspirate (PLA). It may also shed further light on the question of whether it is graft survival ("cell survival theory") or *de novo* adipogenesis ("host replacement theory") or a combination of both which occurs during autologous fat transplantation, with significance for trying to understand why such variable results are obtained with this widely utilized technique.

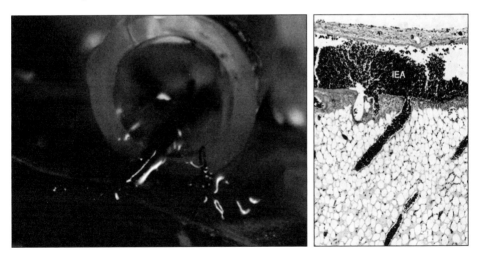

Figure 26.1. Left. Silicon tissue engineering chamber positioned around the inferior epigastric artery ("IEA") in the mouse groin. **Right.** Angiogenesis sprouting from the main vascular pedicle (IEA) with concomitant adipogenesis (magnification × 20).

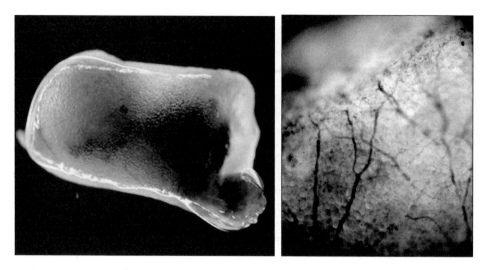

Figure 26.2 Left. In vivo generated 3D fat construct after 6 weeks. **Right.** Angiogenesis at the surface of the generated fat construct resulting in a 3D vascular framework supporting further adipogenic tissue development.

26.4. POTENTIAL PROGENITOR CELLS FOR ADIPOSE TISSUE ENGINEERING

Within the connective tissue matrices of most adult organs there are lineage-committed and lineage-uncommitted progenitor cells able to differentiate towards different cell lineages under appropriate differentiation conditions [8]. Adipose tissue is derived from the embryonic mesoderm, and contains a heterogeneous stromal–vascular fraction (SVF) which includes such progenitor cells.

Isolated lineage-uncommitted stromal cells from subcutaneous fat have been shown to be capable of differentiating *in vitro* into adipocytes and other cell types when cultured in the presence of established differentiation factors [8]. Others have used exogenous SV fraction/preadipocytes to induce fat, usually subcutaneously [9]. This population in the SVF is phenotypically similar to mesenchymal stem cells (MSCs), they express some of the CD antigens observed on bone marrow MSCs but they also exhibit an unique CD marker profile and gene expression, distinct from those seen in MSCs [10]. Adipose precursor cells in developing fat pads arise from multipotential MSCs, whose origins are unknown. These stem cells develop into unipotential adipoblasts, which become committed to the adipocyte lineage under the influence of various factors such as hormones, growth factors, cell-cell and cell-matrix interactions which have not yet been fully elucidated, developing into preadipocytes with a fibroblast-like morphology. Although adipoblasts are assumed to appear primarily during embryonic development, it is not clear whether some remain postnatally or whether only preadipocytes are present in the latter stages of development.

Preadipocytes express early differentiation markers such as Pref-1 (Sul et al., 1989) but have not accumulated intracellular triglyceride droplets. Preadipocytes have been estimated to represent 0.02% of the total cell population in the SVF of subcutaneous fat pads in adults [11] and considerable expansion of this population would be desirable for use in tissue engineering applications. The precursor population within the SVF is heterogeneous, composed of preadipocytes at various stages of differentiation (early, late and very late), and adipoblasts [12]. In our *in vivo* experiment we have included some tissue engineering chambers in which muscle xenografts were implanted. Adult skeletal muscle also contains progenitor cells, known as satellite cells that have been shown to be pluripotent (Asukara et al., 2001; Shefer et al., 2004). A second population of potential progenitor cells in muscle is the muscle derived stem cells which are distinct from satellite cells. The prevailing hypothesis is that both populations co-exist as distinct stem cell tiers in a state of equilibrium within adult muscle, with both cell types having the potential to be used as progenitor cells for adipocytes and adipose tissue engineering. The signaling interaction between myogenic cells and adipocytes has been implicated as playing a significant role in the rate and extent of adipogenesis, myogenesis, and lipogenesis/lipolysis. Key factors in these processes include leptin, insulin-growth factors, and adiponectin [13]. The skeletal muscle-containing tissue engineering chambers did generate a vascularized adipose tissue construct after 6 weeks. In some harvested tissue constructs we observed additional myogenesis *de novo* and this phenomenon was dependant on the presence of a healthy fraction of interstitial tissue within the implanted muscle xenograft (Figure 26.3.).

There is also potential for the recruitment of bone marrow-derived mesenchymal stem cells to our *in vivo* engineered construct. However, little evidence exists so far to support a functional role for circulating cells in mesenchymal tissue repair [14]. The idea is that undifferentiated MSCs, following delivery and migration to the engineered environment, will differentiate into adipocytes under the influence of local signals. The local factors directing this multi-step process are not yet fully determined although several candidates exist, such as leptin (Aprath-Husmann et al., 2001), adiponectin (Farmer, 2005), plasminogen activation inhibitor-1 (PAI-1) [15,16], CCAAT/enhancer binding protein-β (C/EBPβ) (Loftus et al., 1997), PPARγ (Cowherd et al., 1999; Farmer, 2005), hypoxia and insulin.

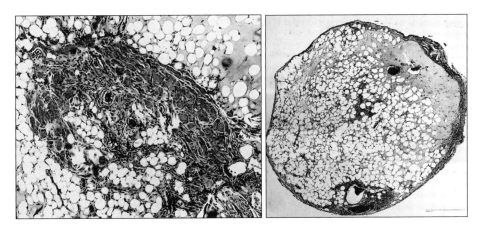

Figure 26.3. Skeletal muscle xenograft implanted in the in vivo tissue engineering chamber. Adipogenic and myogenic induction after 6 weeks (magnification ×20). **Right** Cross section through harvested specimen after 6 weeks containing muscle xenograft in the center. Abundant adipogenesis is observed (magnification ×10)

26.5. EXTRACELLULAR INDUCING SIGNALS

Preadipocytes are capable of synthesizing PAI-1, a key factor in angiogenesis, cell migration differentiation and proteolysis [15,16]. PAI-1 synthesis is increased during preadipocyte migration towards adipose tissue development, and the levels decrease *in vitro* when a confluent preadipocyte layer is attained and active migration ceases. Other key regulatory events in fat cell differentiation include the induction of CCAAT/enhancer binding proteins -β (C/EBPβ) and -δ (C/EBPδ) followed by induction of PPARγ and C/EBPα, which upregulate adipose functional genes. PPARγ appears to be crucial for adipocyte differentiation, with studies showing that blocking the PPARγ pathway in preadipocytes not only inhibits their differentiation into mature adipocytes, but can also inhibits angiogenesis *in vivo* [17].

Preadipocytes have the unique ability to enhance *in vivo* angiogenesis and cause the remodeling of vessels into an efficient network with a mature, stable architecture [18]. Hypoxia is known to be one of the strongest stimuli that boosts capillary angiogenesis and exerts its effect through an upregulation of vascular endothelial growth factor (VEGF). As the PPARγ gene expression is inhibited by hypoxia, angiogenic vessel remodeling may accelerate adipogenesis by increasing hypoxia inducible factor 1 (HIF-1) degradation, thus potentiating PPARγ activation. VEGF is an endothelial mitogen and chemokine, and is highly expressed in adipose tissue, increasing during adipocyte differentiation [19,20,21]. Adipose stromal cells, isolated from human subcutaneous fat tissue, were found to secrete 5-fold more VEGF when cultured in hypoxic conditions. Conditioned media derived from hypoxic adipose stromal cells significantly increased endothelial cell growth with reduced endothelial cell apoptosis. Established preadipocytes in the stromal compartment of white adipose tissue are less vulnerable to hypoxemia. Hypoxia is known to occur in our tissue engineering chambers, transiently (Lokmic et al., in preparation), and this could help drive the adipogenic result..

26.6. EXTRACELLULAR MATRICES AND SCAFFOLDS

The ECM is a non cellular substance, made up of protein and long-chain sugars (polysaccharides) in which cells are embedded. This "biological glue", in which growth factors can be released from matrix storage, functions as a framework for physical cell support, coordinates cell development via cell-cell and cell-matrix interactions, and in turn stimulates cells to produce the ECM components [22,23]. ECM substrates not only provide mechanical support for cells, but also orientate and constrain cells during regeneration. They provide extra space for the coordination of growth factor and cell derived signals between the ECM and cells, effect intercellular communication, and mediate cellular growth, differentiation and ultrastructural stability [24]. This suggests that binding and storage of growth factors by the matrix are important determinants in regulating cellular metabolism. ECM proteins coordinate cell migration, proliferation and tissue homeostasis by binding to specific integrin cell surface receptors. Binding to those receptors activates intracellular signaling pathways, causing cytoskeletal reorganization and alteration of cell morphology [24]. Cell migration and tissue remodeling events are regulated by different proteolytic systems. For example, degradation of the basement membranes surrounding the capillary is necessary for sprouting angiogenesis to proceed.

Cellular differentiation of new tissues is induced by cues in the microenvironment immediately surrounding cells. Salasznyk et al. (2004) indicates that ECM stimuli also play an important role in inducing osteogenesis of human MSC.

The differentiation of fat precursor cells will depend on spatially and temporally controlled expression of multifunctional adhesive glycoproteins and their cellular receptors, and on a tight regulation of different proteolytic enzyme families. Human preadipocytes accumulate lipid droplets in their cytoplasm and express positive immunoreactivity for collagen type IV and laminin from the 6th week of gestation onward [23]. Culture dishes coated with Matrigel® promote attachment and spreading of preadipocytes whereas spreading of nonpreadipocytes was antagonized. Components, such as laminin which also enhance selective proliferation of preadipocytes [22], play active roles which extend to developmental as well as regenerative processes. This selective spreading of preadipocytes on Matrigel® coated wells has been observed in our *in vitro* experiment with ongoing proliferation of fibroblast-like cells from adult fat biopsies (Figure 26.4.).

Multifunctional glycoproteins are present in the ECM which regulate adhesive processes, coordinating proteolytic degradation and influencing cell migration, proliferation and differentiation. One of those glycoproteins is vitronectin which has been discovered only recently in the SVF of white adipose tissue. It is well-known to play a leading role in cell migration with subsequent differentiation [25], and may well be important in adipogenic tissue engineering.

26.7. VASCULATURE

There is convincing evidence of autocrine/paracrine or developmental relationship between capillaries/endothelial cells and preadipocytes, with vascular cells expressing receptors for most adipocyte-derived factors [26,27]. Adipose tissue and vasculature reside in a steady-state balance with each other and the complex relationship between adipose tissue formation, angiogenesis, and vessel remodeling may explain why isolated fat graft transplantation results in poor and unpredictable results.

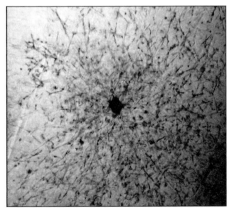 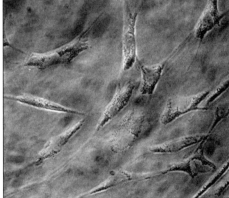

Figure 26.4. Human fat biopsy seeded on Matrigel® coated tissue culture wells. Selective spreading of preadipocytes is observed from the biopsy.

Preadipocytes produce PAI-1 which would ensure coordination of adipogenesis and angiogenesis at the local level [19]. Studies have shown that human preadipocytes and endothelial cells express $\alpha_V\beta_3$ integrin and express and secrete PAI-1, which regulates preadipocyte and endothelial cell migration *in vivo* [19]. Microvascular endothelial cells secrete factors and ECM components which induce proliferation with subsequent differentiation of preadipocytes and neovascularisation will not be triggered without adipocyte differentiation. The established adipose tissue mass in adult life can be regulated through its vasculature, as a wide range of vasoactive signals are secreted by adipose tissue, specifically from the SVF. The expression of factors such as angiopoietins and PAI-1 have been reported, depending on the state of cell differentiation, site of growth, and external stimuli [18]. The molecular mechanisms underlying blood vessel maturation during *de novo* adipose formation are yet to be determined. The close relationship between developing adipocytes and neocapillaries could be observed in our specimens harvested from the sealed tissue engineering after 6 weeks (Figure 26.5.).

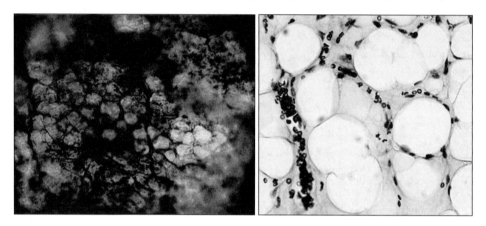

Figure 26.5. Left. Angiogenesis observed at the surface of the harvested fat construct. Adipocytes are surrounded by capillaries. **Right.** Histological section showing adipogenesis and concomitant angiogenesis in the Matrigel® matrix after 6 weeks in vivo (magnification × 60).

26.8. CONCLUSIONS

Engineering fat tissue *in vivo* is a challenging research area as several key factors need to be considered. Not only potential precursor cells but the ECM will play a crucial role as this extracellular compartment will coordinate and regulate ongoing cellular processes. Histioconductive methods with the use of biodegradable rigid scaffolds will be difficult to extrapolate in a clinical setting as the induction of angiogenesis *de novo* will be necessary for further (precursor) cell support and the differentiation into mature adipocytes. Adipose tissue is a densely vascularized tissue and the relationship between those two compartments is fundamental for further stabilization of the generated adipose tissue construct within adjacent anatomical structures.

In this respect, histioinductive methods are preferable as they could foster a complementary and harmonious development of angiogenesis and adipogenesis. The interaction between those two cellular events will depend on the availability of an appropriate supporting ECM. A human derived supporting ECM is not yet available but our work with the murine derived Matrigel®, a basement membrane substrate, could direct future work in the field of adipose tissue engineering. We observed that xenografts where a considerable fraction of SVF was included generated considerable adipogenesis *de novo* and *in vivo* in our tissue engineering chamber, however the resultant adipogenic induction seemed to be host-derived. The host-derived nature of the adipose tissue construct was rather surprisingly as we observed ongoing proliferation of fibroblast-like cells out of fat biopsies seeded on Matrigel® coated wells *in vitro*. The hypothesis is that signals or cytokines present in the SVF of the implanted xenografts could direct the adipogenic processes in the tissue engineering chamber and this particular fraction will be the subject of future research in order to identify those cytokines responsible for inducing adipogenesis at the recipient site. Subsequently, this could enhance the development of a human ECM suitable for supporting adipogenesis *in vivo* in a clinical setting.

26.9. REFERENCES

1. E. Billings Jr., and J.W. May Jr., Historical review and present status on free fat graft autotransplantation in plastic and reconstructive surgery, *Plast Reconstr Surg.* **83** (2), 368-381 (1989 Feb).
2. M. Knight, G. Evans, Tissue engineering: progress and challenges, *Plast Reconstr Surg* **114**(2), 26E-37E (2004).
3. C.W. Patrick Jr, P.B. Chauvin, J. Hobley, and G.P. Reece, Preadipocytes seeded PLGA scaffolds for adipose tissue engineering, . *Tissue Eng* **5** (2), 139-151 (1999 Apr).
4. D. von Heimburg, S. Zachariah, I. Heschel, H. Kühling, H. Schoof, B. Hafemann, N. Pallua, Human preadipocytes seeded on freeze-dried collagen scaffolds investigated in vitro and in vivo, *Biomaterials* **22** (5), 429-438 (2001 Mar).
5. N. Kawaguchi, K. Toriyama, E. Nicodemou-Lena, K. Inou, S. Torii, and Y. Kitagawa, De novo adipogenesis in mice at the site of injection of basement membrane and basic fibroblast growth factor, (1998). *Proc. Natl. Acad. Sci. USA* 95(3): 1062-1066.
6. BD Biosciences 2003 Product Catalog Discovery Labware. Extracellular Matrices, BD Matrigel™, pp.120-121.
7. K. Toriyama, N. Kawaguchi, J. Kitoh, R. Tajima, K. Inou, Y. Kitagawa, S. Torii, Endogenous adipocyte precursor cells for regenerative soft-tissue engineering, *Tissue Eng* **8**(1), 157-165 (2002 Feb).
8. P. Zuk, M. Zhu, H. Mizuno, J. Huang, J. Futrell, A. Katz, P. Benhaim, H. Lorenz, and M. Hedrick, Multilineage cells from human adipose tissue: implications for cell-based therapies, *Tissue Eng* **7**(2), 211-228 (2001 Apr).
9. H. Green, and O. Kehinde, Formation of normally differentiated subcutaneous fat pads by an established preadipocyte cell line, *J Cell Physiol*, **101**(1), 169-171 (1979 Oct).
10. P. Zuk, M. Zhu, P. Ashjian, D. De Ugarte, J. Huang, H. Mizuno, Z. Alfonso, J. Fraser, P. Benhaim, and M. Hedrick, Human adipose tissue is a source of multipotent stem cells.. *Mol Biol Cell* **13** (12), 4279-4295 (2002 Dec).
11. P. Pettersson, M. Cigolini, L. Sjostrom, U. Smith, and P. Bjorntorp, Cells in human adipose tissue developing into adipocytes, *Acta Med Scand* **215**(5): 447-451 (1984).
12. F. Gregoire, G. Todoroff, N. Hauser, C. Remacle, The stromal-vascular fraction of rat inguinal and epididymal adipose tissue and the adipoconversion of fat cell precursors in primary culture, *Biol Cell* **69**(3), 215-222 (1990).
13. M. Delaigle, J. Jonas, I. Bauche, O. Cornu, S. Brichard, Induction of adiponectin in skeletal muscle by inflammatory cytokines: in vivo and in vitro studies, *Endocrinology* **145**(12), 5589-5597 (2004 Dec)
14. H. Hauner, T. Skurk, M. Wabitsch, Cultures of human adipose precursor cells. *Methods Mol Biol* 155, 239-247 (2001).
15. D. Crandall, D. Busler, B. McHendry-Rinde, T. Groeling, and J. Kral, Autocrine regulation of human preadipocyte migration by plasminogen activator inhibitor-1, *J Clin Endocrinol Metab* **85**(7), 2609-2614 (2000).

16. D. Crandall, E. Quinet, G. Morgan, D. Busler, B. McHendry-Rinde, J. Kral, Synthesis and secretion of plasminogen activator inhibitor-1 by human preadipocytes, *J Clin Endocrinol Metab* **84**(9), 3222-3227 (1999).
17. J. Rehman, D. Traktuev, J. Li, S. Merfeld-Clauss, C. Temm-Grove, J. Bovenkerk, C. Pell, B. Johnstone, R. Considine, K. March, Secretion of angiogenic and antiapoptotic factors by human adipose stromal cells, *Circulation* **109**(10), 1292-1298 (2004 March 16).
18. M. Rupnick, D. Panigraphy, C. Zhang, S. Dallabrida, B. Lowell, R. Langer, M. Folkman, Adipose tissue mass can be regulated through the vasculature, Proc Natl Acad Sci USA **99**(16), 10730-10735 (2002 Aug).
19. D. Fukumura, A. Ushiyama, D. Duda, L. Xu, J. Tam, V. Krishna, K. Chatterjee, I. Garkavtsev, R. Jain, Paracrine regulation of angiogenesis and adipocyte differentiation during in vivo adipogenesis, *Circ Res* **93**(9), e88-97 (2003 Oct).
20. K. Claffey, W. Wilkison, B. Spiegelman, Vascular endothelial growth factor: regulation by cell differentiation and activated second messenger pathways, *J Biol Chem* **267**(23), 16317-16322 (1992).
21. A. Cucina, V. Borrelli, B. Randone, P. Coluccia, P. Sapienza, and Cavallero, Vascular endothelial growth factor increases the migration and proliferation of smooth cells through the mediation of growth factors released by endothelial cells, *J Surg Res* **109**(1), 16-23 (2003).
22. J. Hausman, J. Wright, R. Richardson, The influence of extracellular matrix substrata on preadipocyte development in serum-free cultures of stromal-vascular cells, *J Animal Sci* **74**(9), 2117-2128 (1996 Sep)
23. P. Atanassova, Formation of basal lamina in human embryonal adipose cells – immunohistochemical and ultrastructural evidence, *Folia Med. (Plovdiv)* **45**(4), 31-5 (2003).
24. N. Boudreau, and P. Jones, Extracellular matrix and integrin signalling: the shape of things to come, *Biochem J* **339**(Pt3), 481-488 (1999).
25. R. Salasznyk, W. Williams, A. Boskey, A. Batorsky, G. Plopper, Adhesion to vitronectin and collagen I promotes osteogenic differentiation of human mesenchymal stem cells, *J Biomed Biotechnol* 2004(1), 24-34 (2004).
26. G. Fruhbeck, The Adipose Tissue as a Source of Vasoactive Factors, *Curr Med Chem Cardiovasc Hematol Agents* **2**(3):197-208 (2004 Jul).

27

OCULAR TISSUE ENGINEERING

Florian Sommer[1], Ferdinand Brandl[1], and Achim Göpferich[1]

27.1. INTRODUCTION

In the early 1990s, tissue engineering emerged as a new concept to overcome the problem of tissue and organ failure. It proposed to supply engineered, yet biological, organ and tissue substitutes. It was anticipated that this technology would soon allow us to overcome donor shortages and graft rejection, the major limitations of tissue and organ transplantation. Tissue engineering approaches that were developed on the basis of this paradigm relied on the use of cells and stem cells, preferably of autologous origin, the application of growth factors and cytokines, the design of biodegradable scaffolds and bioreactor technology[1,2].

Over the past decades, there has been tremendous progress towards the regeneration of tissues such as bone[3], heart valves[4], myocardial tissue[5] and cartilage[6]. While these examples impressively show that tissue engineering technology holds great promise for the manufacture of tissue grafts, even more diverse applications have emerged in recent years. Tissue constructs have been used to investigate cellular and molecular mechanisms[7], are used for in vitro drug screening and can be expected to reduce the number of time and cost intensive in vivo experiments in drug development[8]. Despite this success, one may still question, why tissue engineering has not progressed even faster and further.

Obviously, we underestimated some of the obstacles on the way towards the development of functional tissue-engineered grafts. Frequently, the host tissue fails to support the integration of engineered tissue. In many cases wound healing processes leading to scar formation dominate over the intended tissue repair and biodegradable scaffolds frequently raise concerns due to the risk of inflammatory responses[9]. With increasing size, engineered tissues also suffer from insufficient nutrient availability and limited metabolic waste removal by passive diffusion, resulting in cell death and necrosis. A rapid and adequate vascularization of an implanted tissue has, therefore, been identified as an essential prerequisite for its survival and integration. Induction of

---

[1] Department of Pharmaceutical Technology, University of Regensburg, Regensburg, Germany

angiogenesis is recognized as one of the most critical factors to the success of tissue engineering[10, 11]. Although growth factors, such as vascular endothelial growth factor (VEGF) or basic fibroblast growth factor (bFGF), are potent angiogenic factors, their use is associated with problems spanning from limited in vivo stability to an abnormal growth of blood vessels resembling the vascularization of tumor tissue[12, 13].

For the reasons outlined above, it would be advantageous to focus our tissue engineering efforts on systems that display less complexity. With these role models, it would be possible to gather experience that helps in the future to solve problems related to the regeneration of more complex tissues. Ocular tissues seem an ideal candidate for this strategy. Most of them, such as the corneal epithelium or the retinal pigment epithelium (RPE), are not vascularized and resemble more sheet-like than three-dimensional structures. Nutrients and oxygen are sufficiently supplied by diffusion from adjacent tissues and, finally, parts of the eye enjoy an immune privilege that adds additional degrees of freedom with respect to the choice of materials and cells.

Altogether, ocular tissues seem to be predestined for regeneration using tissue engineering approaches. But besides the scientific and strategic incentive for reconstructing ocular tissues, there is also a tremendous need for novel therapeutic options for treating numerous eye diseases related to tissue failure. Age-related macular degeneration (ARMD), glaucoma and diabetic retinopathy (DR) are leading causes of blindness. The prevalence of these diseases among persons aged over 50 is between 3 and 10 %[14], illustrating the significance of the problem. Despite the tremendous medical progress made in recent years, especially in ophthalmology, the prevalence of age-related blindness is still increasing, spurred by demographic trends[15, 16], outlining the need for alternative treatments.

This article will review the state of the art in ocular tissue engineering. The goal is to illustrate the progress already made and the strides still necessary to create clinically relevant tissue substitutes.

27.2. CORNEAL TISSUE ENGINEERING

The cornea is the transparent barrier between the eye and the environment, protecting the eye from pathogenic microbes and dryness. The cornea is comprised of three major cellular layers: an outermost stratified squamous epithelium, a stroma with corneal fibroblasts (keratocytes), and an innermost monolayer of specialized endothelial cells[17] (Figure 27.1). In severe diseases of the cornea, their transparency is no longer maintained, usually due to a malfunction of only one of the three parts of the cornea. Therefore, tissue engineering developments focus on the reconstruction of the damaged part to restore transparency of the whole cornea. These strategies, especially the regeneration of the corneal epithelium, will probably be clinically approved in the near future.

27.2.1. Corneal Epithelium

The corneal epithelium consists of five cell layers in the tissue center and about ten layers on its periphery. It shows a distinct physiological turnover; the cells are constantly renewed by proliferating cells of the basal epithelium, often termed transient amplifying cells[18, 19]. These cells can divide only a limited number of times[20] and are themselves replaced by slowly proliferating stem cells of the limbus[21]. The limbus is surrounding the cornea; it was demonstrated to be a reservoir of corneal epithelial stem cells, cells that are, therefore, also termed limbal stem cells. If these corneal epithelial stem cells are completely absent due to limbal disorders from severe trauma (for example thermal or chemical burns) or eye diseases (for example Stevens-Johnson syndrome), the source of corneal epithelial cells is exhausted, resulting in opacification of the cornea and severe visual impairment[22]. Therefore, in patients with unilateral limbal stem-cell deficiency, an autologous limbal transplantation is performed to restore the corneal epithelium[23]. However, there is an associated risk of inducing limbal stem cell deficiency in the healthy eye[24]. In patients with bilateral lesions, autologous limbal transplantation is rarely possible, due to the large number of cells necessary for transplantation. Limbal or corneal allograft transplantation, however, is limited by the number of organ donors and requires long-term immunosupression associated with severe side effects[25]. To overcome these limitations, strategies to cultivate autologous corneal epithelium in vitro based on tissue engineering concepts have been developed. The general idea is to cultivate physiological corneal epithelium including a sufficient number of stem cells for physiological regeneration in a culture dish, starting with a small sample of cells[26]. Corneal epithelial stem cells seemed to be an optimal cell source, as the corneal epithelial cells are physiologically renewed by these stem cells.

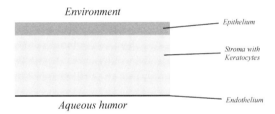

Figure 27.1. Schematic survey of the three major cellular layers of the cornea: an outermost stratified epithelium, a stroma with corneal fibroblasts (keratocytes) and an innermost monolayer of endothelial cells.

In 1997, Pellegrini et al. reported the first clinical success in two patients with complete loss of corneal-limbal epithelium of one eye using cultivated limbal stem cells[27]. After isolation and propagation of cells from a small biopsy of the limbus of the healthy eye, they cultured a sheet of cells for 19 days to prepare the epithelial graft. According to the authors, the resulting graft was microscopically similar to the cornea, stained positive for cytokeratin 3, a specific marker of the corneal lineage[20] and, therefore, represented an authentic in vitro cultured corneal epithelium. After release of the sheet from the culture plastic using the protease Dispase II, they transplanted the cultured cornea onto the patient's prepared eye and patched it tightly for three days. After grafting of the cultured epithelium, both patients developed a stable and transparent corneal epithelium without vascularization. More than two years after grafting, the patients were clinically stable and the authors strongly suggest that this was due to a successful engraftment of the stem cells.

In the following years, attempts were made to optimize this encouraging new therapy. The use of biomaterials was investigated to improve the handling and manipulability of the epithelial constructs, as well as their integration onto the corneal stroma[26]. Furthermore, as the use of proteolytic enzymes is associated with the destruction of cell-cell junctions and extracellular matrix, both critical to sheet integrity and function, new culture techniques were studied that allowed for the removal of the epithelial sheets from the culture plastic without using enzymes[28].

Searching for suitable biomaterials, amniotic membrane (AM) seemed suitable as a first cell carrier. AM is the inner layer of the fetal membranes and consists of a single layer of columnar cells firmly attached to an underlying basement membrane. It is known to suppress inflammation and scarring and serves as an anti-microbial barrier[29]. The successful transplantation of human AM to severely damaged rabbit cornea[30] has been reported. In 2000, Tsai et al. took a small limbal-biopsy specimen from the healthy eyes of six patients suffering from unilateral limbal epithelial cell deficiency and expanded them on AM to form an epithelial-cell sheet[31]. After about three weeks of culture, they transplanted the resulting epithelial-cell sheet, together with the membrane, to the damaged eyes of the same patient. Complete reepithelialization of the corneal surface occurred within two to four days in all of the patients, followed by improved clarification of the cornea after one month. No patient had recurrent neovascularization or inflammation in the transplanted area during the follow-up period of about 15 months and all patients demonstrated improved vision. The authors concluded that the use of autologous limbal epithelial cells grown on AM had all the benefits of AM transplantation, including the facilitation of epithelialization, reduction of inflammation and scarring, and replacement of substrate when the underlying stromal tissue is destroyed. Furthermore, in contrast to the report of Pellegrini et al.[27], the handling and suturing had been simplified.

In contrast to the work of Tsai et al.[31], Rama et al. used a fibrin glue for the preparation of epithelial cell sheets[32]. After transplantation of these sheets, all of these patients showed complete reepithelialization within the first week, similarly to the previous report.

The introduction of biomaterials as a cell carrier showed several advantages, as for example improved handling of the constructs, however, post-transplant effects from the carrier were expected to influence the clinical outcome. This was confirmed by the observation of eye-threatening complications in a patient after AM transplantation[33]. Therefore, Nishida et al. focused again on the culture of epithelial sheets without a carrier. As temperature-responsive culture surfaces, established by Yamada et al. in 1990[34], were shown to allow the harvest of intact multilayered keratinocyte sheets without the use of proteolytic enzymes[35], this technology was used for the culture of corneal epithelial sheet grafts[36]. This method enabled them to obtain a well-structured, compact multilayered cell sheet architecture with the expected native cell microstructure, such as tight junctions, desmosomes and basement membrane, comparable to those in native corneal tissue. The resulting convenient and robust tissues could be transplanted onto the cornea of rabbits and adhered strongly to the corneal stroma within minutes, making sutures unnecessary. According to the authors, the grafts remained stable at the initial placement, exhibited a normal appearance and expressed the typical corneal marker cytokeratin 3.

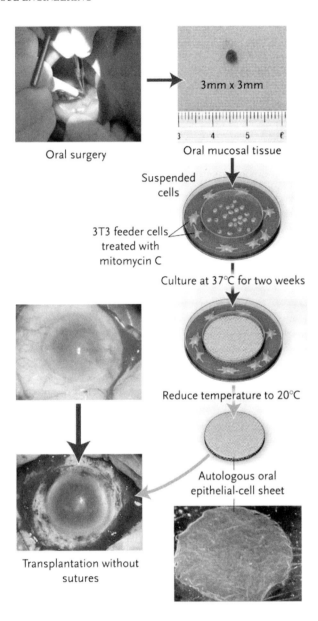

Figure 27.2. In vitro culture of a corneal epithelial transplant using mucosal epithelial cells. After isolation of autologous oral mucosal epithelial cells, the cells were cultured in the presence of a feeder layer onto temperature-responsive culture surfaces at 37°C. Reduction of the temperature to 20°C leads to the removal of the cell sheet, which can subsequently be transplanted to the patient without the need for suturing. Reprinted from Nishida et al.[37] Copyright © 2004 Massachusetts Medical Society. All rights reserved.

This approach overcame a number of problems associated with other related techniques, however, there was still the need for autologous limbal stem cells for the culture of the corneal epithelium. To overcome this need, Konoshita et al. demonstrated the feasibility of using autologous mucosal epithelial cells for reconstruction of the ocular surface[38, 39]. Nishida et al. combined the culture of mucosal epithelial cells with the technique using temperature-responsive surfaces and established an alternative replacement strategy for damaged corneal epithelium[37] (Figure 27.2). According to the authors, the cultured sheets showed transparency equal to that of sheets originating from limbal stem cells and were microscopically similar to native corneal epithelium. The sheets could be transplanted onto the patients' corneas without suturing. During the follow-up period of 14 months, corneal transparency was maintained, visual acuity was improved and complications could not be observed. Therefore, the sheets of tissue engineered epithelial cells fabricated ex vivo from autologous oral mucosal epithelium seemed effective for reconstruction of the ocular surface, providing a possible therapy even for patients with bilateral total stem-cell deficiencies. However, it is still unclear whether stem cells of the mucosa can differentiate into corneal epithelium. It is also possible that the therapeutic success in this study was due to a stimulation and re-proliferation of a small number of still remaining autologous epithelial stem cells in the recipient's cornea[40]. Long-term studies and a larger number of patients will, therefore, be necessary to assess the benefits and risks of this therapy.

27.2.2. Corneal Stroma

The corneal stroma is the largest part of the cornea, underlying the epithelium and consisting of fibroblasts, also called keratocytes, embedded in a matrix of collagens and glycosaminoglycans. Blood vessels are absent in the central cornea in contrast to the limbus and conjunctiva, which are highly vascularized. Transparency of the tissue is caused by a small diameter and a distinct orientation of the collagen fibrils within the tissue[41]. Culture of corneal stroma, in combination with epithelium, seems useful for clinical therapy of deep corneal lesions and failures in keratomileusis (the carving of the cornea to reshape it), furthermore the stroma displays the "backbone" of completely engineered cornea. Stroma engineering, however, could become a great challenge, as transparency of the stroma is essential because of the thickness of this corneal layer.

The successful cultivation of corneal stroma, even in combination with corneal epithelium and endothelium, has been reported[42, 43]. However, in many of the reports immortalized cell lines were used, cells that seem unsuitable for a clinical therapy. In 1999, Germain et al. reported the successful engineering of human cornea cultured with primary keratocytes and epithelial cells[44]. They reconstructed the corneal stroma by culturing keratocytes within collagen and cultured them for four days. After this cultivation, they seeded the gels with epithelial cells and cultured them for three more days. The resulting corneas were histologically similar to native cornea and expressed components of the epithelial basement membrane at the epithelium-stroma junction, but data about the transparency of the systems are missing. In 2004, Hu et al. reported the in vitro cultivation of corneal stroma for one week using rabbit keratocytes mixed with polyglycolic acid and the subsequent transplantation in vivo[45]. According to them, the tissue became transparent within eight weeks of transplantation of the cultured stroma and no differences in the diameters of native and engineered cornea could be observed. They confirmed that the cornea was formed by the cultured cells by transfecting them with GFP and detecting a green fluorescence within the whole stroma. Although the results for corneal stroma culture are encouraging, long-term in vivo data and clinical trials are still lacking.

27.2.3. Corneal Endothelium

The corneal endothelium consists centrally of a monolayer of endothelial cells underlying the corneal stroma and represents, from a medical point of view, the most important part of the cornea, as only an intact endothelium with a sufficient cell density can function properly and maintain clarity of the cornea by its dehydrating pump function[46]. In cases of intraocular surgery or inherited diseases, a drastic decrease in the number of cells can be observed. As the proliferative capacity of the endothelial cells is restricted[47], transplantation of isolated and cultured corneal endothelial cells (CEC) has been studied, however, the success of these experiments was limited[48] due to insufficient cell numbers or a lack of adherence. The first in vivo report of the transplantation of human CEC was published in 1991 by Insler and Lopez[49], who seeded human neonatal CEC on human corneas that were denuded of their native epithelium. After implantation of the cultured corneas into African green monkeys, 75 % of the corneas cleared up and showed a clear decrease in diameter (large diameter indicates edema of the cornea) for up to twelve months. Ishino et al. reported the first in vivo study using adult cultured human CEC[50]. After propagation of the cells, they transplanted the endothelial cells onto amniotic membrane; they reached a sufficient cell density on the membrane by gently centrifugating the cells onto the membrane. After cultivation of these endothelial sheets for two weeks, they transplanted the sheets into rabbits' eyes and observed excellent transparency with little edema for at least seven days. Long-term consequences, however, could not be determined, as the corneal endothelium of rabbits proliferates in vivo, in contrast to human endothelium, and, therefore, this animal model seems not suitable for long-term evaluation. Similar results were reported by Mimura et al.[51] using adult human corneal endothelial cells in a rat model. Again, transparency of the cornea was restored by CEC after seeding them onto the excised cornea and subsequent transplantation of the cornea. In contrast to Ishino et al., no carrier membrane was used. Furthermore, Mimura et al. demonstrated that the corneal transparency was maintained for one month after transplantation.

Mimura et al. also evaluated a novel approach for corneal endothelial regeneration[52]. They exposed cultured CEC to iron powder and injected the cells after endocytosis of the iron into the anterior chamber of rabbits' eyes, subsequent to cryo-injury of the corneal endothelium. By fixing a magnet on the lid of animals, the injected CEC were attracted to the cornea for 24 h. They could demonstrate that the cells adhered to the Descemet's membrane, the native location of the CEC, resulting in decreased corneal edema over the whole investigation period of eight weeks. As this method could have several drawbacks associated with the iron powder, long-term observations have been performed. According to Mimura[53], the iron powder was not detectable after twelve months, however, in contrast to a negative control, sufficient numbers of CEC could be detected in the study group, resulting in a decreased edema score. Drawbacks, such as increased intraocular pressure or other ocular complications, could not be detected. Therefore, the authors conclude, the magnetic attachment of iron-endocytosing CEC can be an effective and safe method for corneal endothelial repair. This therapeutic option was the first to effectively restore corneal endothelium simply by injecting cells into the anterior chamber of the patient, however, no reports on human studies are published yet.

Besides the direct treatment of the patients' cornea, there is another interesting application of CEC transplantation: the improvement of corneas from organ donors. About 40 % of the corneas could not be transplanted, because they failed the quality criteria of the cornea banks, mostly due to their low endothelial cell density. To overcome this problem, several approaches were performed to increase the cell density by transplanting CEC onto the corneas. These strategies, such as suitable isolation and cultivation conditions for human CEC, the use of growth factors or the transfection of endothelial cells with viral genes to enhance the cell proliferation, are discussed in detail by Engelmann et al.[54]

27.2.4. Summary

To conclude, the tissue engineering of the cornea is a promising field. Especially the reconstruction of the corneal epithelium seems to be a promising therapeutic option for the treatment of patients suffering from limbal stem cell deficiencies. To completely substitute corneal transplants, the culture of all three corneal layers, including epithelium, stroma and corneal endothelium is necessary. This will probably remain a challenging task, as optimal culture conditions for all three layers have to be established. Furthermore, for clinical approval, the use of serum or feeder layers of cells likely becomes problematic.

A future challenge will also be the innervation of the cultured cornea, as the cornea is one of the most innervated tissues and missing innervation could lead for example to the clinical syndrome of the "dry eye"[55]. Innervation of the cornea was already studied within biosynthetic tissue templates[56]; the control of complex interaction between materials, different corneal cell types and nerve conduits, however, remains a challenge ahead.

27.3. RETINAL PIGMENT EPITHELIUM ENGINEERING

The retinal pigment epithelium (RPE) consists of a monolayer of cuboidal cells located between the choroidal layer of the eye and the neurosensory retina. It is part of the blood-retinal barrier and responsible for the attachment of the retina to the choroidal layer by a net transport of ions and water in an apical to basal direction. Further functions of the RPE are the absorption of stray light, the uptake, processing and transport of retinoids, and the phagocytosis of rod and cone outer segment fragments. Once differentiated, the RPE is not able to regenerate itself by cell division[57].

Disorders of the RPE are implicated in the pathogenesis of age-related macular degeneration (ARMD), the leading cause of blindness in people aged over 55[58], and other degenerative and hereditary ocular diseases. In "dry" (non-exudative) ARMD, which is the most common form, vision is impaired due to progressive atrophy of the RPE with subsequent loss of the choriocapillaris and photoreceptors within the macula. In contrast, loss of vision in "wet" (exudative) ARMD is associated with bleeding from abnormal blood vessels grown from the choriocapillaris beneath the RPE and macula (choroidal neovascularization, CNV). Currently, there are no treatments for "dry" ARMD and the available therapies for "wet" ARMD, such as laser photocoagulation, are still controversially discussed because of their only moderate efficacy in preventing blindness[59].

As a potentially curative therapy, the concept of transplanting healthy RPE in the subretinal space has been extensively investigated in the past decades. Due to immune reactions, however, patients receiving transplants of homologous RPE had no visual benefit[60, 61]. Thus, the interest has been focused on autologous cells. The first prospective trials demonstrated that CNV membrane surgery combined with simultaneous transplantation of freshly isolated RPE cells resulted in clinically relevant improvements of vision compared to other surgical procedures. Potential drawbacks of this approach are the limited number of healthy cells that can be harvested from patients with degenerative eye diseases and the delivery of the cells in suspension[62, 63]. Since RPE cells are polar with distinct apical/basal characteristics and well established intracellular relationships[64], the implantation of an organized sheet of RPE cells with appropriate orientation is thought to be an important factor for a successful graft.

The concept of tissue engineering offers the chance to cope with the above mentioned problems: 1) Autologous cells are harvested from the patient and expanded in vitro to a sufficient number. 2) Dysfunctional donor cells can be manipulated to perform the required function in the retina by ex vivo gene manipulation[65]. 3) Culturing the cells under suitable conditions allows for the maintenance of a differentiated and epithelial phenotype of RPE. 4) Organized patches of tissue engineered RPE can be transplanted into the subretinal space of the patient in a proper orientation.

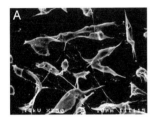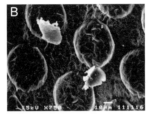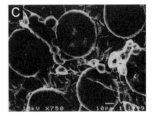

Figure 27.3. Scanning electron micrographs of RPE cells adhering to plain PLGA films (adhesive) (A), PLGA surfaces modified with PEG/PLA (continuous region, non-adhesive) (B) and reversed patterns of PEG/PLA modified with PLGA (continuous region) after 8 h of cell seeding at 15 000 cells/cm2. Cells on the micropatterned surfaces (B, C) exhibited typical round RPE cell morphology. Scale bars are 10 μm. Reprinted from Lu et al.[66] Copyright © 2001 with permission from Elsevier.

In accordance with this concept, the group headed by A. G. Mikos proposed the use of biodegradable polymer films as temporary substrates for RPE cell culture and the subsequent transplantation of these polymer-cell complexes into the subretinal space. However, RPE cells cultured on thin films made of poly(lactic-co-glycolic acid) (PLGA) lost their characteristic cuboidal morphology during a 7-day culture period[66-71]. To retain normal RPE cell morphology and function in vitro, Lu et al., therefore, developed novel degradable micropatterned substrates from PLGA and block copolymers of poly(ethylene glycol) (PEG) and poly(lactic acid) (PLA) using a microcontact printing technique. The film surfaces consisting of adhesive (PLGA) and non-adhesive (PEG/PLGA) domains affected cell attachment and spreading, and allowed the maintenance of differentiated cell phenotype throughout the 8-h period of the study (Figure 27.3). The polymer substrate was thought to facilitate the handling during transplantation and to ensure the correct orientation of the graft in the subretinal space. During a period of several weeks, the matrix will be degraded into non-toxic products, which can be removed from the body by metabolic pathways[66, 70, 71].

Although PLA and PLGA have been shown to be biocompatible, their degradation products (lactic acid and glycolic acid) arouse concern due to their acidic nature. To meet these concerns, several research groups investigated the use of amniotic membrane (AM) as an alternative matrix substrate that modulates proliferation and differentiation of RPE cells in culture[72, 73]. Transplanted AM act as a suitable substrate for proper epithelialization and are widely used in ophthalmology for the treatment of persisting epithelial defects[74]. Stanzel et al. demonstrated that epithelially denuded AM promotes the formation of a RPE monolayer with tight junctions and, therefore, recommended its use as basement membrane-containing matrix to facilitate the clinical transplantation of RPE in treating ARMD[73].

Attempts to use RPE cell sheets without any supportive matrix are associated with various drawbacks. First, it is more difficult to handle the patches during transplantation[66]. In addition, the non-specific enzymatic detachment (using trypsin/EDTA, for example) of cultured RPE sheets leads to a substantial decrease in the retinoid metabolism[75]. A novel type of detachable tissue culture substrate, developed in the group of T. Okano, holds the potential to overcome the latter problem. Those surfaces are grafted with thermally responsive polymers, such as poly(N-isopropylacrylamide-co-cinnamoylcarbamidemethylstyrene) and allow the detachment of cells as a continuous sheet by simply lowering the temperature to 20 °C[76]. As von Recum et al. published later, the initial isolation of RPE cells using specific enzymes (such as collagenase type 3/ hyaluronidase) and the subsequent passaging on thermally responsive surfaces is an appropriate method to preserve metabolic activity in cultured RPE cells suitable for transplantation[75].

As an alternative approach, Ito et al. applied a novel methodology, termed "magnetic force-based tissue engineering", that also aims at the construction and delivery of RPE cell sheets. Briefly, ARPE-19 cells, a human RPE cell line, were magnetically labeled using magnetic cationic liposomes and seeded on ultra-low-attachment plates. In the presence of a magnetic force perpendicular to the culture plate, ARPE-19 cells formed multilayered sheet-like constructs that could be easily transferred into another tissue culture dish by a magnetic iron wire[77]. Even if this methodology provides various opportunities, especially for the delivery of tissue-engineered grafts, one should keep in mind that the multilayered structure of the constructed RPE sheets does not resemble the physiologic situation. It is quite questionable, whether the function of an epithelial monolayer, such as RPE, will be restored after the transplantation of multilayered RPE cell patches. As it is known from animal experiments that thickening of the RPE graft due to folding may reduce the width of the overlaying photoreceptor layer[78], further investigations using animal models will be necessary in order to evaluate the benefit of this recent approach.

Despite many advances in the past decades, especially in the field of cell culturing and material sciences, guaranteeing the long-term survival of an RPE graft still poses a big challenge. As epithelial cells generally fail to survive in suspension, RPE cells must reattach to a substrate to avoid apoptosis[79]. Unfortunately, age-related alterations, pathological processes during ARMD, or surgical treatments may inhibit the repopulation of Bruch's membrane (BM), the extracellular environment of RPE cells in the eye[80, 81]. To avoid graft failure and to enhance the medical benefit of RPE cell transplantation, Del

Priore's group investigated ways to reengineering BM. They suggest the transplantation of extracellular matrix (ECM) prior to the transplantation of RPE[82] or the cleaning of BM with nonionic detergents and the subsequent coating with ECM proteins such as collagen, fibronectin, laminin and vitronectin[80]. However, the biological tolerability and the clinical applicability of these techniques have yet to be proven.

Against this background, it remains unclear, whether the transplantation of RPE sheets without any supportive matrix is superior to the injection of cell suspensions or not. Along with the RPE patches themselves, the utility of biodegradable polymers and amniotic membrane as temporary substrates must be evaluated after implantation in the subretinal space. Therefore, in order to determine the medical benefit of these promising strategies, in vivo examinations using animal models are mandatory.

27.4. RETINA REGENERATION

The neural retina is the key tissue of the eye, responsible for the conversion of light into electric signals that can be processed by the brain. The retina represents a highly specialized part of the central nervous system that is frequently subject to both traumatic and genetic conditions. Retinitis pigmentosa[83] for example, the group of hereditary conditions involving death of retinal photoreceptors, is a common cause of blindness worldwide and effective therapeutic options are still lacking. As yet, only one report using tissue engineering strategies applied to retina regeneration has been published, however, the potential for retina tissue engineering will be addressed shortly in the following paragraph.

The discovery of neural stem cells in adult mammals[84], even in the eye[85, 86], raised the possibility for the development of powerful new therapeutic strategies, as the existence of these cells indicated a potential regenerative capacity of the retina. First evidence for the potential of neural stem cell transplantation to replace lost retinal cells emerged with the observation that adult hippocampus derived neural stem cells survived and integrated into the host retina after injection in the vitreous cavity of rats[87]. The cells, however, failed to express any retina-specific markers. Progenitor cells, isolated from rat embryonic retina, were demonstrated to express photoreceptor-specific markers after transplantation[88], but they did not show migration and integration into the host retina comparable to that of the hippocampus-derived stem cells. Therefore, conditions must be defined that promote structural as well as functional integration of the transplanted cells into the retina[89]. Injury-induced cues, for example, were demonstrated to play a significant role in promoting the incorporation of ocular stem cells/progenitors regardless of their origin or their differentiation along specific retinal sub-lineage[90]. By optimization of isolation, expansion and transplantation procedures of retinal progenitor cells, Qiu et al. were able to reach extensive rhodopsin expression as well as apparent integration of the cells within the host retina following subretinal transplantation into retina degeneration models[91]. The functional connections between grafted cells and the host retina, however, were not evaluated. These few examples can only give an indication of the large field of neural stem cell transplantation and its potential for retina regeneration; for more detailed information, we recommend the reviews by Klassen et al.[92] and Ahmad et al.[93]

The simple cell injection of retinal progenitor cells into the subretinal space or the vitreous is the most prominent experimental approach at the moment. A first report using retinal progenitor cells seeded on a highly porous scaffold was published by Lavik et al.[94]

They could demonstrate that cells up-regulate markers of differentiation after seeding onto a scaffold with pores oriented normally to the plane of the scaffold. Therefore, they conclude that the scaffold likely provides a useful system for delivering retinal progenitor cells and may assist in the formation of photoreceptors. These first data suggest that further advances in tissue engineering could play an important role in the development of strategies to treat complex retinal pathologies in the future. Towards a clinical application, the isolation of human retinal progenitor cells from fetal[95] as well as post mortem retina[96] were important steps. In our opinion, further characterization of these cells, using for example reaggregated neurospheres[97, 98] or 3D retina-like structures created in a bioreactor[99], combined with the improvements in the field of biomaterials research and scaffold technologies could result in retinal grafts that are able to restore vision.

27.5. REGENERATION OF THE LENS

The bulk of the human lens is composed of lens fibers. These fibers are derived from an epithelial monolayer, which covers the anterior face of the lens. Opacification of the lens, termed cataract, is the most common cause of visual impairment world-wide[100]. In addition to genetic disposition, cataracts are induced as a result of aging. At present, cataracts are only treatable by surgical removal of the opacified lens and the subsequent replacement by an artificial substitute, which is held in place by the remaining lens capsule[101]. The major complication of cataract surgery is posterior capsule opacification (PCO). PCO is usually secondary to the proliferation and migration of remaining lens epithelial cells and often necessitates another surgery[102]. If lens regeneration were to be successful in humans, there would be no need for such an operation[103].

Among vertebrates, however, only some urodeles and fish can regenerate their lens into their adult life. After lensectomy, lens regeneration in the adult newt, for example, begins with the dedifferentiation and proliferation of dorsal iris pigment epithelial (PE) cells. Then these cells differentiate into lenticular cells and produce a new lens. The whole process of dedifferentiation and differentiation into another cell type has been called transdifferentiation[104]. In mammals, lens regeneration has been observed in rabbits, cats and mice, but only if the lens capsule is left behind. Obviously, lens regeneration is not achieved by transdifferentiation as in newts, but by differentiation of lens epithelial cells that remain attached to the lens capsule[105]. However, the potential of PE cells to transdifferentiate is not restricted to urodeles and corresponding culture systems using PE cells from embryonic chick retina have been well established (see the reviews by Eguchi et al. for further information)[106, 107].

In 2001, Tsonis et al. first reported on the differentiation of a human dedifferentiated retinal PE cell line (H80HrPE-6) into lentoids and lens-like structures. H80HrPE-6 cells cultured in MATRIGEL®, a commercially available basement membrane preparation extracted from a murine tumor, were induced to synthesize crystallins and to form transparent structures resembling lentoids in vitro[108]. According to the authors, this cell line might provide an useful system for investigating the regeneration of the lens by human PE cells. Nevertheless, therapies based on these fascinating findings are still far away and one may question, if we will succeed in reconstructing the human lens with its outstanding abilities in the foreseeable future. Furthermore, with respect to the excellent outcomes achievable by the implantation of synthetic intraocular lenses, developing new therapeutic strategies in order to supersede cataract surgery may not be the urgent aim of the current research.

27.6. CONCLUDING REMARKS

The specific characteristics of the human eye, such as the sheet-like structure of many tissues and their diffusion-based nutrient supply, make it an ideal candidate for regeneration of diseased tissues using tissue engineering strategies. Consequently, significant progress has been made especially towards the regeneration of corneal epithelium. It seems feasible that engineered corneal grafts may be introduced into clinical therapy in the near future. Another promising field is the reconstruction of dysfunctional RPE. This could provide a curative therapy for degenerative diseases, such as ARMD. Long-term studies using animal models are currently under way.

Surprisingly, there are only few initiatives towards the regeneration of the vitreous body. Consisting mainly of collagens and glycosaminoglycans, this avascular gel-like system would be an ideal tissue to be regenerated using tissue engineering strategies. Elucidating the role of hyalocytes, the only cell-type lining the cortex of this tissue, which is currently investigated by our group, will be a first step towards that goal[109].

However, despite of these fascinating perspectives, we should still be aware of the numerous obstacles to be overcome in bringing this technology to the clinics. Minimally invasive techniques that require clever approaches to properly place delicate tissues or persisting disease-related factors that may also damage the regenerated tissue are just two examples of the numerous obstacles that have to be overcome.

27.7. ACKNOWLEDGEMENTS

This work was supported by the "Bayerische Forschungsstiftung", Germany.

27.8. REFERENCES

1. R. Langer and J. P. Vacanti, Tissue engineering, *Science* **260**(5110), 920–926 (1993).
2. T. Blunk, A. Goepferich, and J. Tessmar, Special issue Biomimetic Polymers, *Biomaterials* **24**(24), 4335–4335 (2003).
3. W. C. Puelacher, J. P. Vacanti, N. F. Ferraro, B. Schloo, and C. A. Vacanti, Femoral shaft reconstruction using tissue-engineered growth of bone, *Int.J.Oral Maxillofac.Surg.* **25**(3), 223–228 (1996).
4. T. Shinoka, C. K. Breuer, R. E. Tanel, G. Zund, T. Miura, P. X. Ma, R. Langer, J. P. Vacanti, and J. E. Mayer, Jr., Tissue engineering heart valves: valve leaflet replacement study in a lamb model, *Ann.Thorac.Surg.* **60**(6 Suppl), S513–S516 (1995).
5. J. Leor, Y. Amsalem, and S. Cohen, Cells, scaffolds, and molecules for myocardial tissue engineering, *Pharmacol.Ther.* **105**(2), 151–163 (2005).
6. C. A. Vacanti, R. Langer, B. Schloo, and J. P. Vacanti, Synthetic polymers seeded with chondrocytes provide a template for new cartilage formation, *Plast.Reconstr.Surg.* **88**(5), 753–759 (1991).
7. C. Fischbach, J. Seufert, H. Staiger, M. Hacker, M. Neubauer, A. Goepferich, and T. Blunk, Three-dimensional in vitro model of adipogenesis: comparison of culture conditions, *Tissue Eng.* **10**(1-2), 215–229 (2004).
8. S. Reichl, J. Bednarz, and C. C. Mueller-Goymann, Human corneal equivalent as cell culture model for in vitro drug permeation studies, *Br.J.Ophthalmol.* **88**(4), 560–565 (2004).
9. J. Yang, M. Yamato, C. Kohno, A. Nishimoto, H. Sekine, F. Fukai, and T. Okano, Cell sheet engineering: Recreating tissues without biodegradable scaffolds, *Biomaterials* **26**(33), 6415–6422 (2005).
10. K. H. Bouhadir and D. J. Mooney, Promoting angiogenesis in engineered tissues, *J.Drug Target.* **9**(6), 397–406 (2001).
11. Z. S. Patel and A. G. Mikos, Angiogenesis with biomaterial-based drug- and cell-delivery systems, *J.Biomater.Sci.Polym.Ed.* **15**(6), 701–726 (2004).
12. M. Nomi, A. Atala, P. D. Coppi, and S. Soker, Principals of neovascularization for tissue engineering, *Mol.Aspects Med.* **23**(6), 463–483 (2002).
13. A. H. Zisch, M. P. Lutolf, and J. A. Hubbell, Biopolymeric delivery matrices for angiogenic growth factors, *Cardiovasc.Pathol.* **12**(6), 295–310 (2003).

14. U. S. Centers for Disease Control and Prevention (CDC), Prevalence of visual impairment and selected eye diseases among persons aged >/=50 years with and without diabetes, *MMWR Morb.Mortal Wkly.Rep.* **53**(45), 1069–1071 (2004).
15. S. Resnikoff, D. Pascolini, D. Etya'ale, I. Kocur, R. Pararajasegaram, G. P. Pokharel, and S. P. Mariotti, Global data on visual impairment in the year 2002, *Bull.World Health Organ.* **82**(11), 844–851 (2004).
16. K. D. Frick and A. Foster, The magnitude and cost of global blindness: an increasing problem that can be alleviated, *Am.J.Ophthalmol.* **135**(4), 471–476 (2003).
17. D. G. Pitts and R. N. Kleinstein, *Environmental Vision* (Butterworth-Heinemann, Boston, 1993).
18. R. A. Thoft and J. Friend, The X, Y, Z hypothesis of corneal epithelial maintenance, *Invest.Ophthalmol.Vis.Sci.* **24**(10), 1442–1443 (1983).
19. R. M. Lavker, G. Dong, S. Z. Cheng, K. Kudoh, G. Cotsarelis, and T. T. Sun, Relative proliferative rates of limbal and corneal epithelia. Implications of corneal epithelial migration, circadian rhythm, and suprabasally located DNA-synthesizing keratinocytes, *Invest.Ophthalmol.Vis.Sci.* **32**(6), 1864–1875 (1991).
20. A. Schermer, S. Galvin, and T. T. Sun, Differentiation-related expression of a major 64K corneal keratin in vivo and in culture suggests limbal location of corneal epithelial stem cells, *J.Cell Biol.* **103**(1), 49–62 (1986).
21. G. Cotsarelis, S. Z. Cheng, G. Dong, T. T. Sun, and R. M. Lavker, Existence of slow-cycling limbal epithelial basal cells that can be preferentially stimulated to proliferate: implications on epithelial stem cells, *Cell* **57**(2), 201–209 (1989).
22. H. S. Dua and J. V. Forrester, The corneoscleral limbus in human corneal epithelial wound healing, *Am.J.Ophthalmol.* **110**(6), 646–656 (1990).
23. K. R. Kenyon and S. C. Tseng, Limbal autograft transplantation for ocular surface disorders, *Ophthalmology* **96**(5), 709–722 (1989).
24. J. J. Chen and S. C. Tseng, Corneal epithelial wound healing in partial limbal deficiency, *Invest.Ophthalmol.Vis.Sci.* **31**(7), 1301–1314 (1990).
25. K. Tsubota, Y. Satake, M. Kaido, N. Shinozaki, S. Shimmura, H. Bissen-Miyajima, and J. Shimazaki, Treatment of severe ocular-surface disorders with corneal epithelial stem-cell transplantation, *N.Engl.J.Med.* **340**(22), 1697–1703 (1999).
26. L. Germain, P. Carrier, F. A. Auger, C. Salesse, and S. L. Guerin, Can we produce a human corneal equivalent by tissue engineering?, *Prog.Retin.Eye Res.* **19**(5), 497–527 (2000).
27. G. Pellegrini, C. E. Traverso, A. T. Franzi, M. Zingirian, R. Cancedda, and M. De Luca, Long-term restoration of damaged corneal surfaces with autologous cultivated corneal epithelium, *Lancet* **349**(9057), 990–993 (1997).
28. K. Nishida, Tissue engineering of the cornea, *Cornea* **22**(7 Suppl), S28–S34 (2003).
29. G. M. Tosi, M. Massaro-Giordano, A. Caporossi, and P. Toti, Amniotic membrane transplantation in ocular surface disorders, *J.Cell.Physiol.* **202**(3), 849–851 (2005).
30. J. C. Kim and S. C. Tseng, Transplantation of preserved human amniotic membrane for surface reconstruction in severely damaged rabbit corneas, *Cornea* **14**(5), 473–484 (1995).
31. R. J. Tsai, L. M. Li, and J. K. Chen, Reconstruction of damaged corneas by transplantation of autologous limbal epithelial cells, *N.Engl.J.Med.* **343**(2), 86–93 (2000).
32. P. Rama, S. Bonini, A. Lambiase, O. Golisano, P. Paterna, M. De Luca, and G. Pellegrini, Autologous fibrin-cultured limbal stem cells permanently restore the corneal surface of patients with total limbal stem cell deficiency, *Transplantation* **72**(9), 1478–1485 (2001).
33. B. A. Schechter, W. J. Rand, R. S. Nagler, I. Estrin, S. S. Arnold, N. Villate, and G. E. Velazquez, Corneal melt after amniotic membrane transplant, *Cornea* **24**(1), 106–107 (2005).
34. N. Yamada, T. Okano, H. Sakai, F. Karikusa, Y. Sawasaki, and Y. Sakurai, Thermo-responsive polymeric surfaces; control of attachment and detachment of cultured cells, *Makromolekulare Chemie, Rapid Communications* **11**(11), 571–576 (1990).
35. M. Yamato, M. Utsumi, A. Kushida, C. Konno, A. Kikuchi, and T. Okano, Thermo-responsive culture dishes allow the intact harvest of multilayered keratinocyte sheets without dispase by reducing temperature, *Tissue Eng.* **7**(4), 473–480 (2001).
36. K. Nishida, M. Yamato, Y. Hayashida, K. Watanabe, N. Maeda, H. Watanabe, K. Yamamoto, S. Nagai, A. Kikuchi, Y. Tano, and T. Okano, Functional bioengineered corneal epithelial sheet grafts from corneal stem cells expanded ex vivo on a temperature-responsive cell culture surface, *Transplantation* **77**(3), 379–385 (2004).
37. K. Nishida, M. Yamato, Y. Hayashida, K. Watanabe, K. Yamamoto, E. Adachi, S. Nagai, A. Kikuchi, N. Maeda, H. Watanabe, T. Okano, and Y. Tano, Corneal reconstruction with tissue-engineered cell sheets composed of autologous oral mucosal epithelium, *N.Engl.J.Med.* **351**(12), 1187–1196 (2004).

38. S. Kinoshita and T. Nakamura, Development of cultivated mucosal epithelial sheet transplantation for ocular surface reconstruction, *Artif.Organs* **28**(1), 22–27 (2004).
39. S. Kinoshita, N. Koizumi, and T. Nakamura, Transplantable cultivated mucosal epithelial sheet for ocular surface reconstruction, *Exp.Eye Res.* **78**(3), 483–491 (2004).
40. G. Pellegrini, Changing the cell source in cell therapy?, *N.Engl.J.Med.* **351**(12), 1170–1172 (2004).
41. M. J. Doughty and J. P. G. Bergmanson, Resolution and reproducibility of measures of the diameter of small collagen fibrils by transmission electron microscopy--application to the rabbit corneal stroma, *Micron* **36**(4), 331–343 (2005).
42. C. J. Doillon, M. A. Watsky, M. Hakim, J. Wang, R. Munger, N. Laycock, R. Osborne, and M. Griffith, A collagen-based scaffold for a tissue engineered human cornea: physical and physiological properties, *Int.J.Artif.Organs* **26**(8), 764–773 (2003).
43. M. Griffith, R. Osborne, R. Munger, X. Xiong, C. J. Doillon, N. L. Laycock, M. Hakim, Y. Song, and M. A. Watsky, Functional human corneal equivalents constructed from cell lines, *Science* **286**(5447), 2169–2172 (1999).
44. L. Germain, F. A. Auger, E. Grandbois, R. Guignard, M. Giasson, H. Boisjoly, and S. L. Guerin, Reconstructed human cornea produced in vitro by tissue engineering, *Pathobiology* **67**(3), 140–147 (1999).
45. X. Hu, M. Wang, G. Chai, Y. Zhang, W. Li, W. Liu, and Y. Cao, Reconstruction of rabbit corneal stroma using tissue engineering technique, *Zhonghua Yan Ke Za Zhi* **40**(8), 517–521 (2004).
46. D. M. Maurice, The location of the fluid pump in the cornea, *J.Physiol.* **221**(1), 43–54 (1972).
47. G. O. Waring, III, W. M. Bourne, H. F. Edelhauser, and K. R. Kenyon, The corneal endothelium. Normal and pathologic structure and function, *Ophthalmology* **89**(6), 531–590 (1982).
48. J. P. McCulley, D. M. Maurice, and B. D. Schwartz, Corneal endothelial transplantation, *Ophthalmology* **87**(3), 194–201 (1980).
49. M. S. Insler and J. G. Lopez, Extended incubation times improve corneal endothelial cell transplantation success, *Invest.Ophthalmol.Vis.Sci.* **32**(6), 1828–1836 (1991).
50. Y. Ishino, Y. Sano, T. Nakamura, C. J. Connon, H. Rigby, N. J. Fullwood, and S. Kinoshita, Amniotic membrane as a carrier for cultivated human corneal endothelial cell transplantation, *Invest.Ophthalmol.Vis.Sci.* **45**(3), 800–806 (2004).
51. T. Mimura, S. Amano, T. Usui, M. Araie, K. Ono, H. Akihiro, S. Yokoo, and S. Yamagami, Transplantation of corneas reconstructed with cultured adult human corneal endothelial cells in nude rats, *Exp.Eye Res.* **79**(2), 231–237 (2004).
52. T. Mimura, N. Shimomura, T. Usui, Y. Noda, Y. Kaji, S. Yamgami, S. Amano, K. Miyata, and M. Araie, Magnetic attraction of iron-endocytosed corneal endothelial cells to Descemet's membrane, *Exp.Eye Res.* **76**(6), 745–751 (2003).
53. T. Mimura, S. Yamagami, T. Usui, Y. Ishii, K. Ono, S. Yokoo, H. Funatsu, M. Araie, and S. Amano, Long-term outcome of iron-endocytosing cultured corneal endothelial cell transplantation with magnetic attraction, *Exp.Eye Res.* **80**(2), 149–157 (2005).
54. K. Engelmann, J. Bednarz, and M. Valtink, Prospects for endothelial transplantation, *Exp.Eye Res.* **78**(3), 573–578 (2004).
55. M. E. Stern, R. W. Beuerman, R. I. Fox, J. Gao, A. K. Mircheff, and S. C. Pflugfelder, A unified theory of the role of the ocular surface in dry eye, *Adv.Exp.Med.Biol.* **438**, 643–651 (1998).
56. F. Li, D. Carlsson, C. Lohmann, E. Suuronen, A. Vascotto, K. Kobuch, H. Sheardown, R. Munger, M. Nakamura, and M. Griffith, Cellular and nerve regeneration within a biosynthetic extracellular matrix for corneal transplantation, *Proc.Natl.Acad.Sci.U.S.A.* **100**(26), 15346–15351 (2003).
57. D. Bok, The retinal pigment epithelium: a versatile partner in vision, *J.Cell Sci.Suppl.* **17**, 189–195 (1993).
58. B. S. Hawkins, A. Bird, R. Klein, and S. K. West, Epidemiology of age-related macular degeneration, *Mol.Vis.* **5**, 26 (1999).
59. T. H. Tezel, N. S. Bora, and H. J. Kaplan, Pathogenesis of age-related macular degeneration, *Trends Mol.Med.* **10**(9), 417–420 (2004).
60. P. V. Algvere, L. Berglin, P. Gouras, Y. Sheng, and E. D. Kopp, Transplantation of RPE in age-related macular degeneration: observations in disciform lesions and dry RPE atrophy, *Graefes Arch.Clin.Exp.Ophthalmol.* **235**(3), 149–158 (1997).
61. P. V. Algvere, P. Gouras, and K. E. Dafgard, Long-term outcome of RPE allografts in non-immunosuppressed patients with AMD, *Eur.J.Ophthalmol.* **9**(3), 217–230 (1999).
62. S. Binder, I. Krebs, R. D. Hilgers, A. Abri, U. Stolba, A. Assadoulina, I. Kellner, B. V. Stanzel, C. Jahn, and H. Feichtinger, Outcome of transplantation of autologous retinal pigment epithelium in age-related macular degeneration: a prospective trial, *Invest.Ophthalmol.Vis.Sci.* **45**(11), 4151–4160 (2004).
63. S. Binder, U. Stolba, I. Krebs, L. Kellner, C. Jahn, H. Feichtinger, M. Povelka, U. Frohner, A. Kruger, R. D. Hilgers, and W. Krugluger, Transplantation of autologous retinal pigment epithelium in eyes with

foveal neovascularization resulting from age-related macular degeneration: a pilot study, *Am.J.Ophthalmol.* **133**(2), 215–225 (2002).
64. P. Gouras, H. Cao, Y. Sheng, T. Tanabe, Y. Efremova, and H. Kjeldbye, Patch culturing and transfer of human fetal retinal epithelium, *Graefes Arch.Clin.Exp.Ophthalmol.* **232**(10), 599–607 (1994).
65. G. M. Acland, G. D. Aguirre, J. Ray, Q. Zhang, T. S. Aleman, A. V. Cideciyan, S. E. Pearce-Kelling, V. Anand, Y. Zeng, A. M. Maguire, S. G. Jacobson, W. W. Hauswirth, and J. Bennett, Gene therapy restores vision in a canine model of childhood blindness, *Nat.Genet.* **28**(1), 92–95 (2001).
66. L. Lu, K. Nyalakonda, L. Kam, R. Bizios, A. Goepferich, and A. G. Mikos, Retinal pigment epithelial cell adhesion on novel micropatterned surfaces fabricated from synthetic biodegradable polymers, *Biomaterials* **22**(3), 291–297 (2001).
67. R. C. Thomson, G. G. Giordano, J. H. Collier, S. L. Ishaug, A. G. Mikos, D. Lahiri-Munir, and C. A. Garcia, Manufacture and characterization of poly(alpha-hydroxy ester) thin films as temporary substrates for retinal pigment epithelium cells, *Biomaterials* **17**(3), 321–327 (1996).
68. L. Lu, C. A. Garcia, and A. G. Mikos, Retinal pigment epithelium cell culture on thin biodegradable poly(DL-lactic-co-glycolic acid) films, *J.Biomater.Sci.Polym.Ed.* **9**(11), 1187–1205 (1998).
69. G. G. Giordano, R. C. Thomson, S. L. Ishaug, A. G. Mikos, S. Cumber, C. A. Garcia, and D. Lahiri-Munir, Retinal pigment epithelium cells cultured on synthetic biodegradable polymers, *J.Biomed.Mater.Res.* **34**(1), 87–93 (1997).
70. L. Lu, L. Kam, M. Hasenbein, K. Nyalakonda, R. Bizios, A. Goepferich, J. F. Young, and A. G. Mikos, Retinal pigment epithelial cell function on substrates with chemically micropatterned surfaces, *Biomaterials* **20**(23-24), 2351–2361 (1999).
71. L. Lu, M. J. Yaszemski, and A. G. Mikos, Retinal pigment epithelium engineering using synthetic biodegradable polymers, *Biomaterials* **22**(24), 3345–3355 (2001).
72. K. Ohno-Matsui, S. Ichinose, K. Nakahama, T. Yoshida, A. Kojima, M. Mochizuki, and I. Morita, The effects of amniotic membrane on retinal pigment epithelial cell differentiation, *Mol.Vis.* **11**, 1–10 (2005).
73. B. V. Stanzel, E. M. Espana, M. Grueterich, T. Kawakita, J. M. Parel, S. C. Tseng, and S. Binder, Amniotic membrane maintains the phenotype of rabbit retinal pigment epithelial cells in culture, *Exp.Eye Res.* **80**(1), 103–112 (2005).
74. H. S. Dua, Amniotic membrane transplantation, *Br.J.Ophthalmol.* **83**(6), 748–752 (1999).
75. H. A. von Recum, T. Okano, S. W. Kim, and P. S. Bernstein, Maintenance of retinoid metabolism in human retinal pigment epithelium cell culture, *Exp.Eye Res.* **69**(1), 97–107 (1999).
76. H. von Recum, A. Kikuchi, M. Okuhara, Y. Sakurai, T. Okano, and S. W. Kim, Retinal pigmented epithelium cultures on thermally responsive polymer porous substrates, *J.Biomater.Sci.Polym.Ed.* **9**(11), 1241–1253 (1998).
77. A. Ito, E. Hibino, C. Kobayashi, H. Terasaki, H. Kagami, M. Ueda, T. Kobayashi, and H. Honda, Construction and delivery of tissue-engineered human retinal pigment epithelial cell sheets, using magnetite nanoparticles and magnetic force, *Tissue Eng.* **11**(3-4), 489–496 (2005).
78. P. Gouras and P. Algvere, Retinal cell transplantation in the macula: new techniques, *Vision Res.* **36**(24), 4121–4125 (1996).
79. T. H. Tezel and L. V. Del Priore, Reattachment to a substrate prevents apoptosis of human retinal pigment epithelium, *Graefes Arch.Clin.Exp.Ophthalmol.* **235**(1), 41–47 (1997).
80. T. H. Tezel, L. V. Del Priore, and H. J. Kaplan, Reengineering of aged Bruch's membrane to enhance retinal pigment epithelium repopulation, *Invest.Ophthalmol.Vis.Sci.* **45**(9), 3337–3348 (2004).
81. V. K. Gullapalli, I. K. Sugino, Y. Van Patten, S. Shah, and M. A. Zarbin, Impaired RPE survival on aged submacular human Bruch's membrane, *Exp.Eye Res.* **80**(2), 235–248 (2005).
82. T. C. Ho, L. V. Del Priore, and H. J. Kaplan, En bloc transfer of extracellular matrix in vitro, *Curr.Eye Res.* **15**(9), 991–997 (1996).
83. G. J. Farrar, P. F. Kenna, and P. Humphries, On the genetics of retinitis pigmentosa and on mutation-independent approaches to therapeutic intervention, *EMBO J.* **21**(5), 857–864 (2002).
84. F. H. Gage, Mammalian neural stem cells, *Science* **287**(5457), 1433–1438 (2000).
85. I. Ahmad, L. Tang, and H. Pham, Identification of Neural Progenitors in the Adult Mammalian Eye, *Biochem.Biophys.Res.Commun.* **270**(2), 517–521 (2000).
86. V. Tropepe, B. L. Coles, B. J. Chiasson, D. J. Horsford, A. J. Elia, R. R. McInnes, and D. van der Kooy, Retinal stem cells in the adult mammalian eye, *Science* **287**(5460), 2032–2036 (2000).
87. M. Takahashi, T. D. Palmer, J. Takahashi, and F. H. Gage, Widespread integration and survival of adult-derived neural progenitor cells in the developing optic retina, *Mol.Cell.Neurosci.* **12**(6), 340–348 (1998).
88. D. M. Chacko, J. A. Rogers, J. E. Turner, and I. Ahmad, Survival and differentiation of cultured retinal progenitors transplanted in the subretinal space of the rat, *Biochem.Biophys.Res.Commun.* **268**(3), 842–846 (2000).

89. I. Ahmad, Stem cells: new opportunities to treat eye diseases, *Invest.Ophthalmol.Vis.Sci.* **42**(12), 2743–2748 (2001).
90. D. M. Chacko, A. V. Das, X. Zhao, J. James, S. Bhattacharya, and I. Ahmad, Transplantation of ocular stem cells: the role of injury in incorporation and differentiation of grafted cells in the retina, *Vision Res.* **43**(8), 937–946 (2003).
91. G. Qiu, M. J. Seiler, C. Mui, S. Arai, R. B. Aramant, J. Juan, and S. Sadda, Photoreceptor differentiation and integration of retinal progenitor cells transplanted into transgenic rats, *Exp.Eye Res.* **80**(4), 515–525 (2005).
92. H. Klassen, D. S. Sakaguchi, and M. J. Young, Stem cells and retinal repair, *Prog.Retin.Eye Res.* **23**(2), 149–181 (2004).
93. I. Ahmad, A. V. Das, J. James, S. Bhattacharya, and X. Zhao, Neural stem cells in the mammalian eye: types and regulation, *Semin.Cell Dev.Biol.* **15**(1), 53–62 (2004).
94. E. B. Lavik, H. Klassen, K. Warfvinge, R. Langer, and M. J. Young, Fabrication of degradable polymer scaffolds to direct the integration and differentiation of retinal progenitors, *Biomaterials* **26**(16), 3187–3196 (2005).
95. P. Yang, M. J. Seiler, R. B. Aramant, and S. R. Whittemore, In Vitro Isolation and Expansion of Human Retinal Progenitor Cells, *Exp.Neurol.* **177**(1), 326–331 (2002).
96. H. Klassen, B. Ziaeian, I. I. Kirov, M. J. Young, and P. H. Schwartz, Isolation of retinal progenitor cells from post-mortem human tissue and comparison with autologous brain progenitors, *J.Neurosci.Res.* **77**(3), 334–343 (2004).
97. P. G. Layer, A. Robitzki, A. Rothermel, and E. Willbold, Of layers and spheres: the reaggregate approach in tissue engineering, *Trends Neurosci.* **25**(3), 131–134 (2002).
98. D. M. Gamm, A. D. Nelson, and C. N. Svendsen, Human retinal progenitor cells grown as neurospheres demonstrate time-dependent changes in neuronal and glial cell fate potential, *Ann.N.Y.Acad.Sci.* **1049**, 107–117 (2005).
99. K. Dutt, S. Harris-Hooker, D. Ellerson, D. Layne, R. Kumar, and R. Hunt, Generation of 3D retina-like structures from a human retinal cell line in a NASA bioreactor, *Cell Transplant.* **12**(7), 717–731 (2003).
100. I. Kocur and S. Resnikoff, Visual impairment and blindness in Europe and their prevention, *British Journal of Ophthalmology* **86**(7), 716–722 (2002).
101. P. J. Francis, V. Berry, A. T. Moore, and S. Bhattacharya, Lens biology: development and human cataractogenesis, *Trends Genet.* **15**(5), 191–196 (1999).
102. D. J. Apple, K. D. Solomon, M. R. Tetz, E. I. Assia, E. Y. Holland, U. F. Legler, J. C. Tsai, V. E. Castaneda, J. P. Hoggatt, and A. M. Kostick, Posterior capsule opacification, *Surv.Ophthalmol.* **37**(2), 73–116 (1992).
103. P. A. Tsonis and K. Rio-Tsonis, Lens and retina regeneration: transdifferentiation, stem cells and clinical applications, *Exp.Eye Res.* **78**(2), 161–172 (2004).
104. P. A. Tsonis, M. Madhavan, E. E. Tancous, and K. Rio-Tsonis, A newt's eye view of lens regeneration, *Int.J.Dev.Biol.* **48**(8-9), 975–980 (2004).
105. M. K. Call, M. W. Grogg, K. Rio-Tsonis, and P. A. Tsonis, Lens regeneration in mice: implications in cataracts, *Exp.Eye Res.* **78**(2), 297–299 (2004).
106. G. Eguchi, Lens transdifferentiation in the vertebrate retinal pigmented epithelial cell, *Progress in Retinal Research* **12**, 205–230 (1993).
107. G. Eguchi, in: *Cellular and Molecular Basis of Regeneration. From Invertebrates to Humans*, edited by P.Ferretti and J.Geraudie (John Wiley & Sons, Chichester, 1998).
108. P. A. Tsonis, W. Jang, K. Rio-Tsonis, and G. Eguchi, A unique aged human retinal pigmented epithelial cell line useful for studying lens differentiation in vitro, *Int.J.Dev.Biol.* **45**(5-6), 753–758 (2001).
109. F. Sommer, K. Kobuch, F. Brandl, B. Wild, B. Weiser, V.-P. Gabel, T. Blunk, and A. Goepferich, Ascorbic acid for in vitro hyalocyte culture - an important factor towards a cellular vitreous substitute, in: *Aegean Conferences Series* **16**, 124-125, 2nd International Conference on Tissue Engineering, Crete, Greece, May 22-27, (2005).

28

MOLECULAR MECHANISM OF OSTEOCHONDROPROGENITOR FATE DETERMINATION DURING BONE FORMATION

Lijin Zou[1,2], Xuenong Zou[1,3,*], Haisheng Li[1], Tina Mygind[1], Yuanlin Zeng[2], Nonghua Lü[2], and Cody Bünger[1]

28.1. ABSTRACT

Osteoblasts and chondrocytes, which derive from a common mesenchymal precursor (osteochondroprogenitor), are involved in bone formation and remodeling in vivo. Determination of osteochondroprogenitor fate is under the control of complex hormonal and local factors converging onto a series of temporospatial dependent transcription regulators. Sox9, together with L-Sox5 and Sox6, of the Sox family is required for chondrogenic differentiation commitment, while Runx2/Cbfa1, a member of runt family and Osterix/Osx, a novel zinc finger-containing transcription factor play a pivotal role in osteoblast differentiation decision and hypertrophic chondrocyte maturation. Recent in vitro and in vivo evidence suggests β-catenin, a transcriptional activator in the canonical Wnt pathway, can act as a determinant factor for controlling chondrocyte and osteoblast differentiation. Here we focus on several intensively studied transcription factors and Wnt/β-catenin signal molecules to illustrate the regulatory mechanism in directing commitment between osteoblast and chondrocyte, which will eventually allow us to properly manipulate the mesenchymal progenitor cell differentiation on bone and regeneration of cartilage tissue engineering.

---

[1] Orthopaedic Research Laboratory, Aarhus University Hospital, 8000 Aarhus C, Denmark
[2] The First Affiliated Hospital of Nanchang University, 330006 Nanchang, Jiangxi, China
[3] Department of Orthopaedics, the 5th Affiliated Hospital of Sun Yat-sen University, Zhuhai, Guangdong, China
[*] Correspondence and reprint requests: zxnong@hotmail.com (X. Zou)

28.2. INTRODUCTION

Bone formation starts from mesenchymal progenitor condensation. The subsequent progress involves either intramembranous ossification or endochondral ossification. The former is characterized by osteoblast differentiation directly from mesenchymal progenitor without chondrogenesis. The progress takes place in most part of the skull formation. Whereas, in the latter, both chondrocyte and osteoblast form and chondrocytes at various stages of differentiation including resting, proliferating, prehypertrophic and hypertrophic chondrocytes formation precedes endochondral bone formation. The progress occurs in most skeleton formation and repair. It is generally believed, however, in both processes, that osteochondroprogenitor is a common origin of osteoblast and chondrocyte[1]. Interestingly, cultured embryonic calvarial cell can form chondrocyte in conditions that are permissive for chondrogenesis in vitro, although not normally observed due to intramembranous ossification[2,3]. This indicates that there is a competitive mechanism at the molecular level that contributes in determining the fate of the common mesenchymal progenitor cell to osteoblast or chondrocyte differentiation, regardless of ossification pathways.

Sox9 and Runx2, Oxterix are mutually exclusive transcription factors, which are necessary in cell fate decision. In general, Sox9, a high-mobility-group (HMG box) transcription factor induces overt chondrogenesis and inhibits the transition of chondrocyte into hypertrophic chondrocyte[4]. As has already been suggested, Runx2 plays a role in the commitment step for preosteoblast decision, while Osterix plays a role in the final differentiation step in osteogenesis. Overexpression of either Sox9 or Runx2 can enhance chondrogenesis or osteogenesis and vice versa. New advance has shown that β-catenin, a transcriptional activator in the canonical Wnt pathway can act as a determinant factor for controlling chondrocyte and osteoblast differentiation. In this review, we discuss these master factors and mutual relationship to illustrate molecular regulation of cell fate decision.

28.3. SOX9 IS REQUIRED FOR DETERMINATION OF THE CHONDROGENIC CELL LINEAGE

Normally, Sox9 is expressed predominantly in mesenchymal progenitor cells and in proliferating chondrocytes, but not in hypertrophic chondrocytes and osteoblasts[5]. The vital role of Sox9 in chondrocyte commitment has been demonstrated by loss- and gain-of-function studies in vivo or in vitro. Previous in vitro studies revealed that Sox9 can upregulate expression of chondrocyte-specific markers such as Collagen2α1 (Col2α1)[6], Col11α1[7], or aggrecan genes[8] by binding to their enhancer sequences. In addition, L-Sox5 and Sox6, which are present after cell condensation[9,14], together with Sox9 activate Col2 and aggrecan genes[10,11]. Sox9 transfecting into mouse bone marrow-derived mesenchymal stem cells by lipofection, could enhance chondrogenesis in vitro and in vivo[12]. In vivo mutants over expression of Sox9 in chondrocytes of mouse embryos, display a phenotype with decreased chondrocyte proliferation, delayed hypertrophic chondrocyte differentiation and endochondral bone formation[13]. Conversely, a loss of Sox9 markedly inhibits overt chondrocyte differentiation, similar to that in Sox5 and Sox6 double knock-out mice[9]. Inactivation of Sox9 in mouse limb buds by using the Cre recombinase/loxP (Cre/loxP) recombination system results in a complete absence of expression of Sox5, Sox6 and Runx2, and eventually cartilage and bone formation as well[14]; Intramembranous ossification, however, occurred normally in Sox9 mutant embryos[15]. Thus, Sox9 is required for the specification of an osteochondroprogenitor, both chondrocyte and osteoblast lineages, during endochondral bone formation, but it is not needed for osteoblast in intramembranous skeletal elements[15]. Interestingly, however, the cells of the osteoblast lineage that are destined for intramembranous bone formation also have the potential to become chondrocytes when Sox9 is present[2,3].

28.4. RUNX2 AND OSTERIX IN OSTEOGENESIS AND CHONDROCYTE MATURATION

28.4.1. Runx2 is a Key Regulator of Osteoblast Differentiation and Is Involved in Chondrocyte Maturation

Runx2 (previously called Cbfa1/AML3/Osf2/PEBP2αA) is a member of the Runt family. Mouse models can enhance our understanding of the basic functions of Runx2. Runx2$^{-/-}$ null mice die immediately after birth[16]. They are devoid of expression of osteoblast-specific genes such as osteocalcin (OC) and also exhibit disturbance of chondrocyte maturation. Likewise, ΔRunx2-expressing mouse, which has no transcription activity, has a normal skeleton at birth but develops an osteopenic phenotype postnatally due to lack of osteoblast function not number, indicating that Runx2 can also control gene expression of differentiated osteoblasts in postnatal life[17]. Calvarial cells are mesenchymal cells involved in intramembranous ossification. In vitro Runx2 deficient mouse calvarial cells do not acquire osteoblast phenotype, but differentiate into chondrocytes and further to terminal hypertrophic chondrocytes in culture with BMP2, indicating that Runx2-deficient calvarial cells completely lack the ability to differentiate into mature osteoblasts[18]. Based on these loss-of-function investigations, it is clear that Runx2 is essential for differentiation of precursor into osteoblasts and may have a role during chondrocyte maturation as well. However, over expression of Runx2 in mice embryos using an osteoblast-specific promotor, inhibits osteoblast differentiation and causes fractures[19]. In chicken embryos transduced the cloned chicken's Runx2, there is neither any ectopic site of calcification nor an alteration in the amount or quality of bone[20]. This shows that Runx2, albeit essential, is not sufficient to induce the differentiation of mesenchymal cells to osteoblasts.

Runx2 can increase gene markers expression of osteoblasts by binding to the cis-acting sequence which is present in the promoter of Collagen1 (Col1), osteopontin (OP), OC, and bone sialoprotein (BSP)[17,21,22]. In addition, the promoter of Osterix (Osx), acting as a downstream of Runx2, also contains Runx2 potential cis-regulatory sites[23].

Furthermore, Runx2 gene produces two major isoforms: Runx2-I, for which expression predominately occurs in prehypertrophic chondrocyte[24,25] and Runx2-II, which is expressed in hypertrophic chondrocyte and osteoblast[26]. A combination of Runx2-I and -II null newborn mice completely lack a mineralized skeleton, the selective Runx2-II knockout mice form an intact mineralized skeleton and improve survival; however, they do display a greater impairment of endochondral bone development compared to intramembranous bone formation[27]. In addition, compared to non-selective Runx2$^{+/-}$ mice and Runx2-II$^{+/-}$ mice, Runx2-II$^{-/-}$ adult mice have more severe skeletal phenotype, which suggests the possibility of Runx2-I and Runx2-II having distinct functions imparted by their different N-termini [27].

Although in Runx2$^{-/-}$ null mice chondrocyte maturation is delayed, the terminal stage of maturation does eventually occur, indicating Runx2 as not sufficient for chondrocyte maturation. Another two members of the Runt family, Runx1 and Runx3, can cooperate with Runx2[28,29] in this process.

28.4.2. Twist and Downstream Mediator of Runx2: Osterix

Runx2 expression is detected as early as embryonic day 10 (E10) during mouse development, yet osteoblasts will not appear before E13. This delay, between Runx2 expression and osteoblast differentiation, implies that other regulatory proteins involved in this process exist. The regulators could in the upstream of Runx2 act as inhibitors of Runx2 function, which would be expressed transiently in osteoblast progenitors and negatively regulate osteoblast differentiation. Twist, a basic helix-loop-helix (bHLH)-containing transcription factor, is such a molecule. Alternatively, they could be mediate activators of Runx2 downstream such as Osterix.

28.4.2.1. Twist Is a Negative Regulator that Controls Runx2 Transcription Function

Molecular and genetic evidence demonstrate that the interaction between Twist proteins and Runx2 inhibits osteoblast differentiation. Firstly, a physical binding between Twist-box in Twist and the Runx domain of Runx2 exists. Secondly, Twist-1 and Twist-2 are expressed in precursor cells, and osteoblast-specific gene expression occurs just when their expression decreases with maturity. Moreover, Runx2$^{+/-}$Twist-1$^{+/-}$ mice have no skull abnormalities. Twist-1 or Twist-2 deficiency leads to premature osteoblast differentiation[30-32]. In general, Twist is a negative regulator which determinates osteoblast differentiation of mesenchymal cells. In addition, it is known that Id (inhibitor of DNA binding, an inhibitory bHLH) can decrease Twist activity and then increase osteoblast differentiation[33, 34].

28.4.2.2. Osterix (OSX/SP7): A More Specific Transcription Factor than Runx2 in Osteoblast Differentiation Commitment

Osx is originally described by Nakashima[35]. It belongs to the Sp subgroup of the Krüppel-like family of transcription factors (XKLF) characterized by a three zinc-finger DNA-binding domain.

The role of Osx in osteogenesis is demonstrated by the Osx knockout experiment. Osx null mice show a complete lack of osteoblast differentiation and therefore no signs of either endochondral or intramembranous bone formation similar to Runx2 mutants. Furthermore, visual evidence using Osx-GFP fusion protein[36] shows that Osx regulates and commits precursor cells to the osteoblast lineage, preventing them from adopting a chondrocyte phenotype.

There are important differences in Runx2- and Osx- null mice that may be due to inhibition of hypertrophic chondrocyte differentiation in Runx2 mice. The cellular organization of the cartilage growth plate is normal in Osx-null mice. In endochondral bone elements of Runx2 mutants, markers of hypertrophic chondrocytes are not expressed and a mineralization defect exists. Thus, Osx is capable of inducing osteoblast differentiation, while Runx2 has two distinct roles in bone formation. One is to induce differentiation of progenitor into osteoblast. The other is to stimulate chondrocyte maturation.

In Osx null mice, Runx2 is expressed to a wide-type osteoblast level, whereas there is no Osx expression in Runx2 knockout mice, suggesting Osx acts as downstream of Runx2[35]. However, Runx2 seems to not induce Osx directly since Runx2-overexpression in C2C12 cells can not induce Osx expression[37] and additional signal components may be necessary to regulate Osx[38]. Dlx5, a bone-inducing transcription factor induces Osx independent of Runx2[37]. Overexpression of Osx increases Runx2 expression, suggesting there may be feedback from Osx to Runx2[39].

Osx as opposed to Runx2, is regarded as the more specific transcription factor for osteoblast differentiation than Runx2 and can determinate progenitor cell fate. In Osx-null mice, Runx2 is still normally expressed. Runx2 positive preosteoblasts do not deposit bone matrix and show the potent to differentiation into either chondrocyte or osteoblast. Furthermore, Osx is not expressed in hypertrophic chondrocytes despite expression of Runx2 in these cells.

Taken together, it is possible that osteochondrogenitor cell fate is determinated by synergy of Runx2 with Osx. Firstly, osteochondrogenitor cells differentiate into preosteoblasts through one or several steps in which Runx2 has a vital role. Then, the preosteoblasts differentiate into osteoblasts expressing marker genes such as OC. Osx is involved in at least the terminal process.

Osx contains a proline-rich region, outside of the zinc finger region, which has been identified as Smad interaction motifs[40]. Smad is a critical component of the BMP signal pathway. Osx also contains a domain binding to the polymorphic Sp1 binding site in the Col1α1 gene promoter[40]. Furthermore, there is an OSE2 element in Osx promoter which Runx2 may bind to. Thus, the structure basis is in part provided for Osx function in osteogenesis. The mechanism of action by Osx remains to be fully defined. Osx can transiently induce Notch 3 and Notch 4 genes which are involved in coordinating the osteoblast differentiation[39]. This indicates that Osx may also function indirectly by activating other signaling molecules and pathways that result in osteogenesis.

28.5. WNT/β-CATENIN: A PUTATIVE COMMON MECHANISM UNDERLYING OSTEOCHONDROGENITOR CELL FATE

Studies have shown that canonical Wnts signaling drives the differentiation of progenitor cells into osteoblasts. Various Wnts such as Wnt1, 3a, 4, 7a, 8c, 9a, 9b and 10b inhibit chondrocyte differentiation and promotes ossification[41-46]. Ectopic expression Wnt14, which acts through the β-catenin-mediated canonical Wnt pathway results in upregulation of Lef1, a direct transcription of β-catenin, and severely blocks chondrocyte differentiation[47].

In the canonical pathway, Wnts bind to the transmembrane receptor Frz family and the co-receptor LRP5/6. Activation of Frz recruits the cytoplasmic bridging molecule Dsh, so as to inhibit GSK3β. Inhibition of GSK3β stabilizes β-catenin levels. The stabilized β-catenin acts on the nucleus by activating Tcf/Lef-mediated transcription of target genes[48]. Components transducing the canonical Wnt signal upstream of β-catenin such as Frz, LRP5/6 and Dsh, all exhibit large degrees of functional redundancy. β-catenin is an obligatory and no redundant component. Several recent in vitro and in vivo studies regarding the mechanism of Wnt signaling function in osteoblast differentiation commitment focus on β-catenin. β-catenin protein upregulation precedes early Runx2 and Osx expressing osteoblast. Loss of β-catenin by using the Prx1-Cre line[49,50] or Dermo-Cre line[51] resulted in an early osteoblast differentiation arrest. No mineralized bone collar formed, and no mature osteoblasts were present in endochondral and membranous bones. Gene expression analysis reveals that osteoblastogenesis is arrested in long bones at the level of an osteochondrogenitor cell and that these cells differentiate into chondrocytes due to express chondrogenic markers such as Sox9 and Col2α1[50], indicating that β-catenin is required to suppress the chondrogenic potential of osteochondrogenitor cells. In skull, Osx expression is not detected while Runx2 is still present. In vitro deletion of β-catenin in primary osteoblast cultures further demonstrates that β-catenin activity is cell-autonomously required in osteochondrogenitor cells to suppress chondrogenesis. Stabilization of β-catenin suppresses chondrogenesis.

Interestingly, gain-of-function experiments in vivo show that stabilization of β-catenin does not result in a differentiation of mesenchymal cells into more osteoblasts, nor in long bones or in the skull, similar to the deletion of β-catenin[50]. It indicates, however, that β-catenin normally inhibits mesenchymal cells to enter osteochondro-progenitor cells in the early stage of bone formation.

Looking at these emerging studies simultaneously, β-catenin may act as a molecular switch that regulates lineage commitment between chondrocyte and osteoblast. Ectopic Wnt/β-catenin signaling inhibits chondrocyte differentiation and promotes ossification. Conversely, when Wnt/β-catenin signaling is genetically inactivated in the osteochondro-progenitors, osteoblast differentiation is replaced by ectopic chondrocyte formation regardless of the regional location or the ossification mechanism, whether it is through intramembranous or endochondral ossification.

28.6. RELATIONSHIP AMONGST SOX9, RUNX2 AND β-CATENIN

Little direct evidence is known about the relationship amongst these regulators vital osteochondroprogenitor cell fate determination. The reciprocal situation, regulation of Runx2 gene activity by Sox9, might also exist, given a number of evolutionarily conserved Sox-binding sites in the Runx2 promoters[52]. That Sox9 is downregulated by Runx2 is demonstrated by cDNA microarray and differential hybridization techniques[53]. Inactivation of Runx2 by Nkx3.2 binding to the promoter results in Sox9 expression upregulation[54].

Wnt/β-catenin signaling is upstream to the expression of the important bone matrix protein Col1 and to the two early transcription factors, Runx2 and Osx required for osteoblast differentiation. However, Runx2 expression is not activated when Wnt14 is ectopically expressed[46] or β-catenin synergizes with BMP2[55], suggesting that Runx2 is not immediately an early transcription target of Wnt/β-catenin signaling.

A physical and functional interaction exists between β-catenin and Sox9. Sox9 can inhibit β-catenin by competing with the binding site of Tcf/Lef within β-catenin and by promoting degradation of β-catenin by the ubiquitination/26s proteasome pathway, which can also cause degradation of Sox9[56]. This may explain, in part, that chondrocyte differentiation inhibition of β-catenin is analogous to the phenotype of Sox9 null mice.

28.7. CONCLUSIONS AND PROSPECTS

Osteochondrogenitor cells have the potential to enter either osteoblasts or chondrocytes terminally hypertrophic chondrocytes. The determination mechanism of lineage commitment is under the control of a complex network of factors which interact and cooperate (see Figure 28.1.). The emerging data summarized above indicate that Sox9, Runx2/Osx and β-catenin play key roles. β-catenin in the canonical Wnt pathway seems to act as a molecular switch. In brief, during intramembranous bone formation, high level β-catenin induces Sox9 and Runx2 dual expressing osteochondrogenitor cells into preosteoblasts by promoting Runx2 expression and inhibiting Sox9 expression. The preosteoblasts also have potential to chondrocytes and osteoblast. Following this, the expression of Osx further induces dual potential preosteoblasts into mature matrix-synthesizing osteoblasts. In endochondral bone formation, low level β-catenin suppresses Runx2 expression and increases Sox9 expression. In this case, chondrogenesis occurs and forms the cartilage. Later, Runx2 and Osx are upregulated by high level β-catenin in the perichondrium to form endochondral bone.

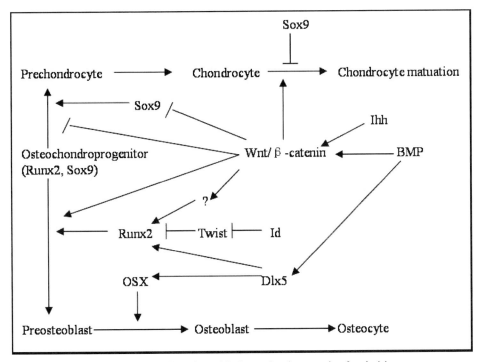

Figure 28.1. Paradigmatic model of osteochondroprogenitor fate decision

Due to the fact that other signaling pathways such as BMPs[38,57], FGF[58], IGF-1[38,59] and PTH[60,61] are involved in bone formation, how they synergize during bone formation remains to be answered. Wnt/β-catenin signaling may be controlled by more upstream events, which may also indicate other intrinsic differences between the two types of ossification mechanism. In vitro data show that β-catenin acts as either downstream or in parallel to BMP signaling in osteoblastogenesis. Continuous PTH can increase the levels of β-catenin, at least in part, via the cAMP-PKA pathway through the differential regulation of the receptor complex proteins (FZD-1/LRP5 or LRP6) and the antagonist (Dkk-1)[62].

In adult osteoblasts, Runx2 is expressed; however, Osx expression is below the level of detection. Although it remains to be determined whether loss of Osx is the result of partial de-differentiation in the in vitro culture conditions or whether it reflects the situation in aged bone, potential treatments that increase Osx expression by the gene delivery methods may be developed as an efficient therapeutic approach to repair bone damage. In addition, the bone marrow mesenchymal cell is regarded as a promising cell origin of tissue engineering due to its multilineage differentiation potential. How to enhance its osteogenesis or chondrogenesis is a crucial problem that needs to be solved. Direct increase of Runx2/Osx expression vital to osteogenesis or Sox9 expression vital to chondrogenesis by the gene delivery could enhance bone or cartilage repair. It is also possible to direct the cell differentiation by manipulating the β-catenin level. On the other hand, indirect increase of Runx2/Osx expression by optimization of culture condition in vitro by synergy of Wnt/β-catenin signaling and other signaling such as BMPs, IGF-1 may be as alternative method for bone repair.

Moreover, further studies of the interaction of those crucial factors, i.e. Sox9, Runx2/Osx and β-catenin and their upstream and downstream targets, will contribute to our understanding of molecular mechanism, regulating and controlling mesenchymal precursor differentiation direction. From a clinical point of view, this will also benefit bone repair, tissue engineering research and new drug discovery.

28.8. ACKNOWLEDGMENTS

This work is supported by Sino-Danish Scientific and Technological Cooperation Project between Chinese and Danish Governments (AM14:29NNP14) and Key International S&T Cooperation Project granted by Ministry of Science and Technology of the People's Republic of China (2005DFA30570). This financial support is greatly appreciated.

28.9. REFERENCES

1. J. Fang and B.K. Hall, Chondrogenic cell differentiation from membrane bone periostea, *Ana. Embryol.* **196**(5), 349-362(1997).
2. C.D. Toma, J.L. Schaffer, M.C. Meazzini, D. Zurakowski, H.D. Nah and L.C. Gerstenfeld, Developmental restriction of embryonic calvarial cell populations as characterized by their in vitro potential for chondrogenic differentiation, *J. Bone Miner. Res.* **12**(12), 2024-2039(1997).
3. T. Aberg, R. Rice, D. Rice, I. Thesleff and J. Waltimo-Siren, Chondrogenic potential of mouse calvarial mesenchyme, *J. Histochem. Cytochem.* **3**(5), 653-663(2005).

4. H. Akiyama, M.C. Chaboisser, J.F. Martin, A. Schedl and B. de Crombrugghe, The transcription factor Sox9 has essential roles in successive steps of the chondrocyte differentiation pathway and is required for expression of Sox5 and Sox6, *Genes Dev.* **16**(21), 2813-2828(2002).
5. Q. Zhao, H. Eberspaecher, V. Lefebvre and B. de Crombrugghe, Parallel expression of Sox9 and Col2a1 in cells undergoing chondrogenesis, *Dev. Dyn.* **209**(4), 377-386(1997).
6. V. Lefebvre, W. Huang, V.R. Harley, P.N. Goodfellow and B. de Crombrugghe, SOX9 is a potent activator of the chondrocyte-specific enhancer of the pro α1(II) collagen gene, *Mol. Cell Biol.* **17**(4), 2336-2346(1997).
7. L.C. Bridgewater, V. Lefebvre and B. de Crombrugghe, Chondrocyte-specific enhancer elements in the Col11a2 gene resemble the Col2a1 tissue-specific enhancer, *J. Biol. Chem.* **273**(24), 14998-15006(1998).
8. I. Sekiya, K. Tsuji, P. Koopman, H. Watanabe, Y. Yamada, K. Shinomiya, A. Nifuji and M. Noda, SOX9 enhances aggrecan gene promoter/enhancer activity and is up-regulated by retinoic acid in a cartilage-derived cell line, TC6, *J. Biol. Chem.* **275**(15), 10738-10744(2000).
9. P. Smits, P. Li, J. Mandel, Z. Zhang, J.M. Deng, R.R. Behringer, B. de Croumbrugghe and V. Lefebvre, The transcription factors L-Sox5 and Sox6 are essential for cartilage formation, *Dev. Cell* **1**(2), 277-290(2001).
10. V. Lefebvre, P. Li and B. de Crombrugghe, A new long form of Sox5 (L-Sox5), Sox6 and Sox9 are coexpressed in chondrogenesis and cooperatively activate the type II collagen gene, *EMBO J.* **17**(19), 5718-5733(1998).
11. J. Chimal-Monroy, J. Rodriguez-Leon, J.A. Montero, Y. Gañan, D. Macias, R. Merino R and J.M. Hurle, Analysis of the molecular cascade responsible for mesodermal limb chondrogenesis: sox genes and BMP signaling, *Dev. Biol.* **257**(2), 292-301(2003).
12. H. Tsuchiya, H. Kitoh, F. Sugiura and N. Ishiguro, Chondrogenesis enhanced by overexpression of sox9 gene in mouse bone marrow-derived mesenchymal stem cells, *Biochem. Biophys. Res. Commun.* **301**(2), 338-343(2003).
13. B.F. Eames, P.T. Sharpe and J.A. Helms, Hierarchy revealed in the specification of three skeletal fates by Sox9 and Runx2, *Dev. Biol.* **274**(1), 188-200(2004).
14. H. Akiyama, M.C. Chaboissier, J.F. Martin, A. Schedl and B. de Crombrugghe, The transcription factor Sox9 has essential roles in successive steps of the chondrocyte differentiation pathway and is required for expression of Sox5 and Sox6, *Genes. Dev.* **16**(21), 2813-2828(2002).
15. Y. Mori-Akiyama, H. Akiyama, D.H. Rowitch and B. de Crombrugghe, Sox9 is required for determination of the chondrogenic cell lineage in the cranial neural crest, *Proc. Natl. Acad. Sci. U.S.A.* **100**(16), 9360-9365(2003).
16. T. Komori, H. Yagi, S. Nomura, A.Yamaguchi, K. Sasaki, K. Deguchi, Y. Shimizu, R.T. Bronson, Y.H. Gao, M. Inada, M. Sato, R. Okamoto, Y. Kitamura, S. Yoshiki and T. Kishimoto, Targeted Disruption of Cbfa1 Results in a Complete Lack of Bone Formation owing to Maturational Arrest of Osteoblasts, *Cell* **89**(5), 755-764(1997).
17. P. Ducy, M. Starbuck, M. Priemel, J. Shen, G. Pinero, V. Geoffroy, M. Amling and G. Karsenty, A Cbfa1-dependent genetic pathway controls bone formation beyond embryonic development, *Genes Dev.* **13**(8),1025-36(1999).
18. H. Kobayashi, Y. Gao, C. Ueta, A. Yamaguchi and T. Komori, Multilineage differentiation of Cbfa1-deficient calvarial cells in vitro, *Biochem. Biophys. Res. Commun.* **273**(2), 630-636(2000).
19. W. Liu, S. Toyosawa, T. Furuichi, N. Kanatani, C. Yoshida, Y. Liu, M. Himeno, S. Narai, A. Yamaguchi and T. Komori, Overexpression of Cbfa1 in osteoblasts inhibits osteoblast maturation and causes osteopenia with multiple fractures, *J. Cell Biol.* **155**(1), 157-166(2001).
20. S. Stricker, R. Fundele, A. Vortkamp and S. Mundlos, Role of Runx genes in chondrocyte differentiation, *Dev. Biol.* **245**(1), 95-108(2002).
21. J.L. Frendo, G Xiao, S. Fuchs, R.T. Franceschi, G. Karsenty and P. Ducy, Functional hierarchy between two OSE2 elements in the control of osteocalcin gene expression in vivo, *J. Biol. Chem.* **273**(46), 30509-30516(1998).
22. B. Kern, J. Shen, M. Starbuck, G. Karsenty, Cbfa1 contributes to the osteoblast-specific expression of type I collagen genes, *J. Biol. Chem.* **276**(10), 7101–7107(2001).
23. M.A. Milona, J.E. Gough, A.J. Edgar, Expression of alternatively spliced isoforms of human Sp7 in osteoblast-like cells, *BMC Genomics* **4**(1),43-53(2003).
24. K.Y. Choi, S.W. Lee, M.H. Park, Y.C. Bae, H.I. Shin, S. Nam, Y.J. Kim, H.J. Kim and H.M. Ryoo, Spatio-temporal expression patterns of Runx2 isoforms in early skeletogenesis, *Exp. Mol. Med.* **34**(6), 426-433(2002).
25. M.H. Park, H.I. Shin, J.Y. Choi, S.H. Nam, Y.J. Kim, H.J. Kim and H.M. Ryoo, Differential expression patterns of Runx2 isoforms in cranial suture morphogenesis, *J .Bone. Miner. Res.* **16**(5), 885-892(2001).

26. C. Ueta, M. Iwamoto, N. Kanatani, C. Yoshida, Y. Liu, M. Enomoto-Iwamoto, T. Ohmori, H. Enomoto, K. Nakata, K. Takada, K. Kurisu and T. Komori, Skeletal malformations caused by overexpression of Cbfa1 or its dominant negative form in chondrocytes, *J.Cell. Biol.* **153**(1), 87-100(2001).
27. Z. Xiao, H.A. Awad, S. Liu, J. Mahlios, S. Zhang, F. Guilak, M.S. Mayo and L.D. Quarles, Selective Runx2-II deficiency leads to low turnover osteopenia in adult mice, *Dev. Biol.* **283**(2), 345-356(2005).
28. C.A. Yoshida, H. Yamamoto, T. Fujita, T. Furuichi, K. Ito, K. Inoue, K. Yamana, A. Zanma, K. Takada, Y. Ito and T. Komori, Runx2 and Runx3 are essential for chondrocyte maturation, and Runx2 regulates limb growth through induction of Indian hedgehog, *Genes Dev.* **18**(8), 952-963(2004).
29. N. Smith, Y. Dong, J.B. Lian, J. Pratap, P.D. Kingsley, A.J. van Wijnen, J.L. Stein, E.M. Schwarz, R.J. O'Keefe, G.S. Stein and M.H. Drissi, Overlapping expression of Runx1 (Cbfa2) and Runx2(Cbfa1) transcription factors supports cooperative induction of skeletal development, *J. Cell Physiol.* **203**(1), 133-143(2005).
30. M. Yousfi, F. Lasmoles and P.J. Marie, TWIST inactivation reduces CBFA1/RUNX2 expression and DNA binding to the osteocalcin promoter in osteoblasts, *Biochem. Biophys. Res. Commun.* **297**(3), 641-644(2002).
31. P. Bialek, B. Kern, X. Yang, M. Schrock, D. Sosic, N. Hong, H. Wu, K. Yu, D.M. Ornitz, E.N. Olson, M.J. Justice and G. Karsenty, A twist code determines the onset of osteoblast differentiation, *Dev. Cell* **6**(3), 423-435(2004).
32. H.M. Kronenberg, Twist genes regulate Runx2 and bone formation, *Dev. Cell* **6**(3), 317-318(2004).
33. I. Kazhdan, D. Rickard and P.S. Leboy, HLH transcription factor activity in osteogenic cells, *J. Cell Biochem.* **65**(1), 1-10(1997).
34. Y. Maeda, K. Tsuji, A. Nifuji and M. Noda, Inhibitory helix-loop-helix transcription factors Id1/Id3 promote bone formation in vivo, *J.Cell Biochem.* **93**(2), 337-344(2004).
35. K. Nakashima, X. Zhou, G. Kunkel, Z. Zhang, J.M. Deng, R.R. Behringer and B de Crombrugghe, The novel zinc finger-containing transcription factor osterix is required for osteoblast differentiation and bone formation, *Cell* **108**(1), 17-29(2002).
36. G. Tai, I. Christodoulou, A.E. Bishop and J.M. Polak, Use of green fluorescent fusion protein to track activation of the transcription factor osterix during early osteoblast differentiation, *Biochem .Biophys .Res. Commun.* **333**(4), 1116-1122(2005).
37. M.H. Lee, T.G. Kwon, H.S. Park, J.M. Wozney and H.M. Ryoo, BMP-2-induced Osterix expression is mediated by Dlx5 but is independent of Runx2, *Biochem. Biophys. Res .Commun.* **309**(3), 689-694(2003).
38. A.B. Celil and P.G. Campbell, BMP-2 and IGF-I mediate Osx expression in human mesenchymal stem cells via the MAPK and PKD signaling pathways, *J .Biol .Chem.* **280**(36), 31353-31359(2005).
39. G. Tai, J.M. Polak, A.E. Bishop, I. Christodoulou and L.D. Buttery, Differentiation of osteoblasts from murine embryonic stem cells by overexpression of the transcriptional factor osterix, *Tissue Eng.* **10**(9-10), 1456-1466(2004).
40. Y. Gao, A. Jheon, H. Nourkeyhani, H. Kobayashi and B. Ganss, Molecular cloning, structure, expression, and chromosomal localization of the human Osterix (SP7) gene, *Gene* **341**(1), 101-110(2004).
41. X. Guo, T.F. Day, X. Jiang, L. Garrett-Beal, L. Topol and Y. Yang, Wnt/beta-catenin signaling is sufficient and necessary for synovial joint formation, *Genes. Dev.* **18**(19), 2404-2417(2004).
42. C. Hartmann and C.J. Tabin, Wnt-14 plays a pivotal role in inducing synovial joint formation in the developing appendicular skeleton, *Cell* **104**(3), 341-351(2001).
43. J.A. Rudnicki, A.M. Brown, Inhibition of chondrogenesis by Wnt gene expression in vivo and in vitro, *Dev. Biol.* **185**(1), 104-118(1997).
44. N.S. Stott, T.X. Jiang and C.M. Chuong, Successive formative stages of precartilaginous mesenchymal condensations in vitro: modulation of cell adhesion by Wnt-7A and BMP-2, *J. Cell Physiol.* **180**(3), 314-324(1999).
45. G. Rawadi, B. Vayssiere, F. Dunn, R. Baron and S. Roman-Roman, BMP-2 controls alkaline phosphatase expression and osteoblast mineralization by a Wnt autocrine loop, *J. Bone Miner. Res.* **18**(10), 1842-1853(2003).
46. C.N. Bennett, K.A. Longo, W.S. Wright, L.J. Suva, T.F. Lane, K.D. Hankenson and O.A. MacDougald, Regulation of osteoblastogenesis and bone mass by Wnt10b, *Proc. Natl. Acad. Sci .U.S.A.* **102**(9), 3324-3329(2005).
47. T.F. Day, X. Guo, L. Garrett-Beal and Y. Yang, Wnt/beta-catenin signaling in mesenchymal progenitors controls osteoblast and chondrocyte differentiation during vertebrate skeletogenesis, *Dev. Cell* **8**(5), 739-750(2005).
48. J. Huelsken and W. Birchmeier, New aspects of Wnt signaling pathways in higher vertebrates, *Curr .Opin .Genet. Dev.* **11**(5), 547-553(2001).
49. M. Logan, J.F. Martin, A. Nagy, C. Lobe, E.N. Olson and C.J. Tabin, Expression of Cre Recombinase in the developing mouse limb bud driven by a Prxl enhancer, *Genesis* **33**(2), 77-80(2002).

50. T.P. Hill, D. Spater, M.M. Taketo, W. Birchmeier and C. Hartmann, Canonical Wnt/beta-catenin signaling prevents osteoblasts from differentiating into chondrocytes, *Dev. Cell* **8**(5), 727-738(2005).
51. H. Hu, M.J. Hilton, X. Tu, K. Yu, D.M. Ornitz and F. Long, Sequential roles of Hedgehog and Wnt signaling in osteoblast development, *Development* **132**(1), 49-60(2005).
52. J.H. Eggers, M. Stock, M. Fliegauf, B. Vonderstrass and F. Otto, Genomic characterization of the RUNX2 gene of Fugu rubripes, *Gene* **291**(1-2), 159-167(2002).
53. M. Stock, H. Schafer, M. Fliegauf, F. Otto, Identification of novel genes of the bone-specific transcription factor Runx2, *J .Bone Miner. Res.* **19**(6), 959-972(2004).
54. C.J. Lengner, M.Q. Hassan, R.W. Serra, C. Lepper, A.J. van Wijnen, J.L. Stein, J.B. Lian and G.S. Stein, Nkx3.2-mediated repression of Runx2 promotes chondrogenic differentiation, *J. Biol. Chem.* **280**(16), 15872-15879(2005).
55. G. Mbalaviele, S. Sheikh, J.P. Stains, V.S. Salazar, S.L. Cheng, D. Chen and R. Civitelli, Beta-catenin and BMP-2 synergize to promote osteoblast differentiation and new bone formation, *J. Cell Biochem.* **94**(2), 403-418(2005).
56. H. Akiyama, J.P. Lyons, Y. Mori-Akiyama, X. Yang, R. Zhang, Z. Zhang, J.M. Deng, M.M. Taketo, T. Nakamura, R.R. Behringer, P.D. McCrea and B. de Crombrugghe, Interactions between Sox9 and beta-catenin control chondrocyte differentiation, *Genes Dev.* **18**(9), 1072-1087(2004).
57. A.B. Celil, J.O. Hollinger and P.G. Campbell, Osx transcriptional regulation is mediated by additional pathways to BMP2/Smad signaling, *J. Cell Biochem.* **95**(3), 518-528(2005).
58. D.M. Ornitz, FGF signaling in the developing endochondral skeleton, *Cytokine Growth Factor Rev.* **16**(2), 205-213(2005).
59. M. Qiao, P. Shapiro, R. Kumar and A. Passaniti, Insulin-like growth factor-1 regulates endogenous RUNX2 activity in endothelial cells through a phosphatidylinositol 3-kinase/ERK-dependent and Akt-independent signaling pathway, *J .Biol .Chem.* **279**(41), 42709-42718(2004).
60. M. Sato, G.Q. Zeng and C.H. Turner, Biosynthetic human parathyroid hormone (1-34) effects on bone quality in aged ovariectomized rats, *Endocrinology* **138**(10), 4330-4337(1997).
61. C.P. Jerome, C.S. Johnson, H.T. Vafai, K.C. Kaplan, J. Bailey, B. Capwell, F. Fraser, L. Hansen, H. Ramsay, M. Shadoan, J.S. Thomsen and L. Mosekilde, Effect of treatment for 6 months with human parathyroid hormone (1-34) peptide in ovariectomized cynomolgus monkeys (Macaca fascicularis), *Bone* **25**(3), 301-309(1999).
62. N.H. Kulkarni, D.L. Halladay, R.R. Miles, L.M. Gilbert, C.A. Frolik, R.J. Galvin, T.J. Martin, M.T. Gillespie and J.E. Onyia, Effects of parathyroid hormone on Wnt signaling pathway in bone, *J. Cell Biochem.* **95**(6), 1178-1190(2005)

Author Index

Abberton, Keren, 403
Abousleiman, Rita I., 243
Ahmad, Shama, 125
Anseth, Kristi S., 135
Arkudas, Andreas, 311
Baatrup, Anette, 31
Bach, Alexander D., 311
Banas, Agnieszka, 3
Baroli, Biancamaria, 183
Benedict, J.J., 87
Blackband, Stephen J., 261
Blondeel, Phillip, 403
Blunk, Torsten, 379
Bos, P.K., 297
Brandl, Ferdinand, 413
Briest, A., 87, 393
Brune, Kay, 311
Buma, Pieter, 279
Bünger, Cody E., 31, 197, 209, 393, 431
Cai, N., 151
Cai, Shenshen, 125
Chan, V., 151
Chapel, Alain, 19
Chian, K.S., 151
Choi, Bangsil, 167
Chopp, Michael, 49
Constantinidis, Ioannis, 261
Daamen, Willeke F., 279
de Groot, Klaas, 327
Duch, Mogens, 31
Duflo, Suzy, 125
Eyrich, Daniela, 379
Faraj, Kaeuis A., 279
Feitz, Wout F., 279
Feng, Z., 151
Fisher, John P., 67
François, Agnès, 19
François, Sabine, 19
Frick, Johanna, 19

Fuchs, D., 115
Geutjes, Paul J., 279
Grant, Samuel C., 261
Gluhcheva, Y., 115
Göpferich, Achim, 379, 413
Greil, Peter, 311
Ha, Hyun Jung, 167
Habibovic, Pamela, 327
Hamdi, Moustapha, 403
Hellman, Kiki B., 363
Hess, Andreas, 311
Holtorf, Heidi L., 225
Horch, Raymund.E., 311
Huffer, W.E., 87
Hughes, Casey W., 125
Jansen, John A., 225
Khang, Gilson, 167
Kim, Moon Suk, 167
Kim, Soon Hee, 167
Kirker, Kelly R., 125
Kloxin, April M., 135
Kneser, Ulrich, 311
Kopp, Jürgen, 311
Labanaris, Apostolos, 311
Lee, Hai Bang, 167
Li, Haisheng, 31, 197, 209, 393, 431
Li, Yi, 49
Liao, K., 151
Lind, Martin, 31, 197, 209
Liu, Yanchun, 125
Long Jr., Robert C., 261
Lü, Nonghua, 431
Mhaisalka, P.S., 151
Mikos, Antonios G., 225
Mochida, Yoshiyuki, 101
Modin, Charlotte, 31
Morrison, Wayne, 403
Mouiseddine, Moubarak, 19
Mygind, Tina, 31, 197, 209, 431

Nuttelman, Charles R., 135
Ochiya, Takahiro, 3
Orlandi, Richard R., 125
Parisuthiman, Duenpim, 101
Park, Albert H., 125
Pedersen, Finn S., 31
Polykandriotis, Elias, 311
Prestwich, Glenn D., 125
Quinn, Gary, 3
Ratner, B.D., 151
Rettenmaier, R., 87
Rhee, John M., 167
Saché, Amandine, 19
Sambanis, Athanassios, 261
Sémont, Alexandra, 19
Shu, Xiao Zheng, 125
Sikavitsas, Vassilios I., 243
Simpson, Nicholas E., 261
Smith, Marshall E., 125
Sommer, Florian, 413
Springer, Marco, 393
Stiehler, Maik, 31

Stillaert, Filip, 403
Teratani, Takumi, 3
Thibeault, Susan L., 125
Thierry, Dominique, 19
Thompson, Erik, 403
Ulrich-Vinther, Michael, 31
van Blitterswijk, Clemens, 327
van Kuppevelt, Toin H., 279
van Osch, G.J.V.M., 297
Verhaar, J.A.N., 297
Walsh, Jennifer F., 125
Woodfield, Tim, 327
Yamamoto, Yusuke, 3
Yamauchi, Mitsuo, 101
Yang, Yoon Sun, 167
Yoon, Diana M., 67
Yoon, Sun Jung, 167
Yu, Bolan, 125
Zeng, Yuanlin, 431
Zvetkova, E., 115
Zou, Lijin, 197, 209, 431
Zou, Xuenong, 197, 209, 393, 431

Subject Index

A

$\alpha1\beta1$, 71
$\alpha2\beta1$, 71
$\alpha3\beta1$, 71
$\alpha5\beta1$, 71
$\alpha5\beta1$, 80
Accelerated endochondral bone formation, 91, 96
Acellular biomaterials, 249
Actin in cell adhesion, 162
Activin receptor-like kinase 1-6 (ALK1-6), 103
Adeno-associated virus (AAV) vector, 33
Adhesion contact, 152, 156
    area, 157–159
Adhesion energy, 160–161
Adhesion molecules and flow perfusion culture, 237
Adhesion prevention, 131
Adipoblasts, 406–407
Adipogenesis, 404–411
Adiponectin, 407
Adipose precursor cells, 406–407
Adipose stromal cells, 408
Adipose tissue, 12–13, 403–404
    induction, 403–411
    stromal-vascular fraction, 406–407, 411
    and vasculature, 409–410
Adipose tissue-derived stem cells (ADSCs), 4, 12–13
Age-related macular degeneration (ARMD), 414, 420
Aggrecan, 69, 75, 76, 80
    and epithelial growth factor, 77
Aggrecan genes, 432
Akp2, 108, 109, 111
Akt proteins, 80
Albumin, 5
Alginate, 81
    and fibrin, 387

Alginate encapsulating chondrocytes, 80
Alginate/poly-L-lysine/alginate (APA) beads, 263
ALK6, 108, 110, 111, 112
Alkaline phosphatase (ALP), 231
    activity, 38, 104–107, 111, 200, 253, 254–255, 300, 333
    and human mesenchymal stem cells, 139, 144
Allogeneic bone marrow stromal cells, 55–56
Allograft, 245, 247
Alpha-fetoprotein (AFP), 5
Alumina ceramics, 330
Amino terminal (MH1), 74
Amniotic membrane (AM), 416
    in retinal pigment epithelium transplantation, 422
Anabolic growth factors, 72
Angiogenesis, 282, 289, 319–320, 322, 414
    and brain repair, 57–58
Angiopoietins, 410
Animal models for cartilage tissue engineering
    load-bearing, 348
    non-load-bearing, 348
Annulus fibrosus (AF), 171, 174
Antagonists of extracellular signaling, 72
Anterior cruciate ligament, 247
Anterior lumbar interbody fusion (ALIF), 197–198
Anterograde degeneration, 58
Antibiotic delivery and fibrin, 383
Anti-cancer drugs and hydrogels, 130
Apatite glass ceramics, 330
Apligraf, 370
Apophysitis, 244
Apoptosis in brain injury, 57
Appositional growth, 244, 245
Aprotinin, 380–381, 385

Arginine-glycine-aspartic acid (RGD) sequences, 80, 249
ARPE-19 cells, 422
Arteriovenous vessel loop (AV Loop), 312–313
and vascular morphology, 317–319
Articular cartilage, 67, 245–246, 291, 298, 339–340, 342, 386
biology of, 69–70
L-ascorbic acid, 232
Astrocytes, 57, 58–59
Autocrine signaling, 72
Autograft, 197, 198, 245, 247
Autologous bone graft, 225
Autologous cells
in retinal pigment epithelium engineering, 421
transplantation, 250–251
Autologous fat transplantation, 405
Autologous limbal transplantation, 415

B

Basic fibroblast growth factor (bFGF), 57–59, 128, 130–131, 282, 285, 287, 289, 384, 414
BCP1150, 332, 333–335
BCP1300, 332, 333–335
bFGF. *See* Basic fibroblast growth factor (bFGF)
BGN-V5, 108, 110
Biglycan (BGN)
binding to ALK6, 108, 110, 111
binding to BMP-2, 105–106, 108, 110–112
and BMP-2 induced alkaline phosphatase activity, 107, 111
and BMP-2-induced Smad phosphorylation, 106–107
and expression of myogenic and osteogenic markers, 108, 111
and osteoblast differentiation, 101–112
recombinant, 103–104
Bioactive molecules in bone regeneration, 225
Biodegradable scaffolds, 175, 248, 404
Bioglass carriers, 99
Biologics license application, 368
Biomaterials
as a cell carrier, 416
in long-term hepatic functions, 13–14
surfaces and cell adhesion, 151–165

Bioreactors, 337
in autologous cell transplantation, 250–251
in cartilage tissue engineering, 347
for cell seeding, 234–235
and chondrogenesis, 344
electric and magnetic stimulation, 255
flow perfusion, 253
mechanical loading, 253–255
for musculoskeletal system, 243–255
rotating wall vessel, 252–253
for scaffolds in bone tissue engineering, 235–237
spinner flask, 252
static culture, 251–252
in vivo, 251
Bioscaffolds. *See* Scaffolds and specific types
Biosensors, 364
Biphasic calcium phosphate ceramics, 332, 333
Biphasic scaffolds, 341
Bladder augmentation with collagen scaffolds, 290–291
Blood vessel repair, 384–385
BMP-1, 75
BMP-2, 31–32, 36, 38, 75, 76, 102, 436
and alkaline phosphatase activity, 107
binding by BGN, 105–106, 108, 110–112
in bioreactor, 251
expression of, 38–39, 41–42, 45, 80
inducing osteoblast differentiation, 101–112
and myogenic and osteogenic markers, 108, 109, 111
and Smad phosphorylation, 106–107
BMP-3, 97
BMP-4, 75, 76, 102, 105, 106, 110
BMP-6, 102, 105, 106, 110
BMP-7, 75, 76, 80, 102, 105, 110
BMP-13, 97
BMPRII, 103
BMPs. *See* Bone morphogenetic proteins (BMPs)
Bonding osteogenesis, 331
Bone
components of, 229–230
induction, 168
properties and pathologies of, 244–245
structure of, 226–230
and use of fibrin, 386

SUBJECT INDEX

Bone cell culture systems, 329
Bone cells, 229
Bone defect models, 338–339
Bone defect repair, 131
Bone defects, 135
Bone formation
    ectopic, 33, 199, 202–206, 333
    by equine bone protein extract, 393–401
    induced by COLLOSS® and COLLOSS® E, 92–95, 96
    induced by GFm, 87, 88, 89–92, 96
    and osteochondroprogenitor fate, 431–438
    in vitro assays, 328–330
    in vivo, 230–231
Bone fractures, 245
    models, 338–339
Bone graft, 245
Bone graft substitutes
    cytotoxicity of, 330–331
    osteoconduction, 331–332
    osteoinduction, 332–335
    in vitro models, 330–337
    in vivo models for synthetic, 337–339
Bone-like tissue formation in vitro, 231–232
Bone marrow, 10–12, 21
    aspiration and isolation, 199
    hematopoietic stem cells derived, 10–11
    mesenchymal stem cells, 11–12
    non-fractioned, 10
Bone marrow-derived mesenchymal stem cells (BM-MSCs), 4
    and adipogenesis, 407
Bone marrow hematopoietic progenitors, 115–120
Bone marrow nucleated cells, 197–198
Bone marrow stromal cells (BMSCs)
    allogeneic, 55–56
    angiogenesis and brain repair, 57–58
    in autografting, 198–199
    gliogenesis and glial-axonal remodeling, 58–59
    immune priority of, 55–56
    intracerebral transplantation of, 51, 52
    neurogenesis, 59
    secretion of trophic and growth factors, 56–57
    synaptogenesis and synaptic modification, 58
    targeting to sites of cerebral damage, 56
    treatment of brain tumor, 54–55, 60
    treatment of CNS diseases, 49–60
    treatment of intracerebral hemorrhage, 52
    treatment of mechanism of action, 55–59
    treatment of multiple sclerosis, 54, 60
    treatment of Parkinson's disease, 53–54
    treatment of spinal cord injury, 52
    treatment of stroke, 50–51, 60
    treatment of traumatic brain injury, 52
Bone mass, 231
Bone morphogenetic proteins (BMPs), 50, 73, 75–76, 97–98, 101, 250, 333
    and β-catenin, 438
    in soft tissue models, 338
Bone regeneration, 225
    and hydrogel carriers, 135–136
Bone repair by synthetic extracellular matrix, 131
Bone sialoprotein, 433
Bone tissue engineering, scaffold materials for, 232–234
Bone volume fraction, 202, 204–205
Brain
    regeneration after injury, 49–50
    remodeling, 56–57
Brain-derived neurotrophic factor (BDNF), 50, 54, 57
Brain tumor, treatment by bone marrow stromal cells (BMSCs), 54–55, 60
Bromodeoxyuridine, 51, 59
Bruch's membrane (BM), 422–423
BSP, 108, 109, 111
Burn repair, 384

C

^{13}C in pancreatic constructs, 266–267
C2C12 cells, 333–335, 336
    alkaline phosphatase activity in, 107
    and bone formation, 333
    myogenic and osteogenic markers in, 108, 109, 111
    phosphorylation in, 106–107
Calcified chondromyxoid tissue, 92
Calcified hyaline cartilage, 92
Calcifying matrix vesicles, 91, 92
Calcium concentration in hydroxyapatite ceramics, 330–331, 335–336
Calcium-phosphate ceramics, 233, 331–332
Calcium phosphate co-precipitation of porcine mesenchymal stem cells, 34–36, 39, 43

Calcium polyphosphate, 167
Calvarial defect, 338
Cambium layer, 228
Canaliculi, 228
Cancellous bone, 92, 93, 96, 226
  and marrow, 89, 90, 92, 98
Cancer. *See* Tumor
Capillary-like tube formation, 58
Carboxylic acid groups and mineralization, 144–145
Carboxymethylcellulose (CMC) and ectopic bone formation, 393, 398–399, 401
Carboxy terminal (MH2), 74
Carbylan™-GSX, 129, 130, 131
Carbylan™-S, 129, 131
Carbylan™-SX, 129
Cardiovascular tissue engineering and fibrin, 385
Carotid artery, 51, 52
Carrier proteins, 5, 99
Carticel, 370
Cartilage, 67, 93–95. *See also* Articular cartilage
  age-related differences in wound healing, 297–307
  properties and pathologies of, 245–246
  and rotating wall vessel, 252
  and scaffolds, 249
  and tissue engineering, 291–292, 339–340
  and use of fibrin, 386–388
Cartilage tissue engineering
  cells and cell sources, 342–343
  scaffolds and matrices, 340–342
  in vitro models, 343–347
  in vivo models, 347–350
  limitations of in vitro models, 346–347
  limitations of in vivo models, 348–350
Catabolic growth factors, 72
Catabolic joint environment, 348
Cataracts, 424
β-catenin, 431, 432, 438
  and osteochondroprogenitor fate during bone formation, 435–436
  and Sox9, 436–437
Cationic liposome-mediated transfection, 35, 39, 43
Cbfa1/Runx2, 108, 109, 111
CCAAT/enhancer binding proteins, 408
CD44, 71, 344

CD34+ and neopterin, 115–120
Cell adhered rate, 200
Cell adhesion on biomaterial surfaces, 151–165
Cell expansion in chondrogenesis, 343
Cell fusion, 10
Cell growth and synthetic extracellular matrix, 127–128
Cell lines in bone graft substitutes, 336, 337
Cell morphology and viability of small intestine submucosa (SIS), 218
Cell proliferation rate in scaffolds, 171, 173–175, 179
Cells
  in cartilage tissue engineering, 342–343, 349–350
  in functional tissue engineering, 247–248
  scaffold interactions in chondrogenesis, 344
  stimulation of, 250
Cell seeding, 158–163, 205–206
  onto scaffolds, 234–235
Cell spreading during cell adhesion, 163–164
Cell surface receptors, 70
Cell survival theory, 405
Cellular differentiation, 409
Cellular signaling, principles of, 70
Cell viability in bioreactors, 269–270
Cement line, 228
Center for Biologics Evaluation and Research (CBER), 365
Center for Devices and Radiological Health (CDRH), 365
Center for Drug Evaluation and Research (CDER), 365
Central nervous system diseases
  brain tumor, 54–55, 60
  intracerebral hemorrhage, 52
  mechanism of action, 55–59
  multiple sclerosis, 54, 60
  Parkinson's disease, 53–54
  spinal cord injury, 52
  stroke, 50–51, 60
  traumatic brain injury, 52
  treatment by bone marrow stromal cells (BMSCs), 49–60
Centrifugation in retroviral gene transfer, 45, 47
CGTP Rule, 371–373

SUBJECT INDEX

Chemical vapor infiltration (CVI) process, 205
Chemotactic factors, 56
Chondrocytes, 69, 91, 92, 93–95, 244, 248, 249, 291
    in cartilage tissue engineering, 342–343
    and β-catenin, 436
    cell culture of, 299
    and cellular signaling, 70
    committed, 342
    death of, 299–300
    de-differentiation, 342, 343–345
    differentiation, 432–433
    encapsulation by polymers, 79–80
    and extracellular matrix in wound healing, 298
    and fibrin, 386–388
    in fibrin gel, 381
    and growth factors, 307
    and osteochondroprogenitor fate, 431–438
    and Runx2, 433–434
    transplantation of autologous, 251
    in wound healing, 301–302, 304
Chondrocyte signaling, 67, 72–79
    native effectors on, 70–71
    proteins involved in, 68–69
Chondrocyte-specific markers, 432
Chondrogenesis, 252, 307, 438
    and transcription factors, 432
    in vitro, 343–347
Chondroitin sulfate, 69, 285, 291
Chondroitin sulfate (CS)/dermatan sulfate (DS), 282
Chondroitin-6-sulfate, 80
Chondromxyoid tissue, 91
Chordin, 75
Choroidal layer, 420
Choroidal neovascularization, 420
Chronic wound repair, 130–131
Circumferential lamellae, 227, 228
CLONfectin reagent, 153, 154
Clot formation, 379, 380
c-met, 77
Co-culture of hepatic-like cells, 7
Col11α1, 432
CollA2, 108, 109, 111
Collage microsponges, 249
Collagen, 69–70, 281
    in cell adhesion, 160–162
    degeneration, 246
    in hepatic culture, 6
Collagen2α1, 432
Collagen gels, 249
    in scaffolds, 253
Collagenous scaffolds, 288–289
    bladder augmentation application, 290–291
Collagen type I, 139, 140, 146–147, 245, 433
Collage type II, 245
Collagraft, 197–198, 200, 202–206
COLLOSS®, 87, 88, 89
    and bone formation, 98–99
    and ectopic bone formation, 92–95
    and ectopic tissue, 95–97
COLLOSS® E, 87, 88, 89, 393–401
    and bone formation, 98–99
    and ectopic bone formation, 92–95
    and ectopic tissue, 95–97
    histology of, 398–399
    implant of, 384–395
    micro-CT images, 396–400
Colony forming units of fibroblasts (CFU-F), 11
CombiMag, 37
Combination products, regulation of, 366–367
Common Smads (Co-Smads), 74, 75
Complex moduli, 190–191
Complex viscosity, 190
Composite scaffolds, 249
Computed tomography (CT), 262
Confocal reflectance interference contrast microscopy (C-RICM), 151, 153, 155–157
Constructs. *See also* specific types
Constructs, implanted and vascularization, 314–324
Contact osteogenesis, 331
Contusion boundary zone, 52
Cord blood-derived mesenchymal stem cells, 4
Cornea, 414
    innervation of, 420
Corneal allograft transplantation, 415
Corneal endothelial regeneration, 419
Corneal endothelium
    culturing and transplantation, 419–420
Corneal epithelial cells (CEC), 419–420

Corneal epithelial stem cells, 415
Corneal epithelium, culturing and transplantation, 414–418
Corneal grafts, engineered, 425
Corneal stroma, culturing and transplantation, 418–419
Corneal tissue engineering, 414–420
Corrosion casting, 314–315
Cortical bone, 93, 226, 227
Corticosteroids, 386
Critical Path Initiative, 373
Critical Path Opportunities List, 373–374
Crosslinking
    density in hydrogels, 140–141
    of small intestine submucosa (SIS) sponge, 211
    in synthetic extracellular matrix, 126–127
Crypt cell proliferation, 24–28
Crystalline alumina ceramics, 330
CS-DTPH, 130–131
CS-DTPH-HP-DTPH-PEGDA, 127–128
Current Good Tissue Practice for Human Cell, Tissues, and Cellular- and Tissue-Based Product Establishments Rule, 371, 372
Cyclic stretching in scaffolds, 254
Cyclooxygenase-2 (COX2), 77
Cytochemical staining methods, 116–117
Cytokeratin, 9
Cytokines, 50
Cytoskeleton remodeling, 162
Cytospin, 116–117
Cytotoxic T lymphocyte response, 55

D

DAN, 75
DBP/PLGA scaffolds, 168
    characterization of, 172
    histological evaluation of, 175–179
    preparation of, 169–170
Degree of deformation, 160–161, 164
Demineralized bone matrix (DBM), 333, 399
Demineralized bone particle (DBP), 168
Demyelination, 54
De novo adipogenesis, 405
Dermagraft, 370
Dexamethasone, 7, 146, 232, 238
    in hydrogels, 136

Diabetic retinopathy (DR), 414
Diaphyseal fracture, 338
Differentiated intestinal epithelial cells, 20
Differentiation potential, hepatic, 4, 5
Differentiation stage factors, 6–7
Dilution effect in transgene expression, 44
Disc cells, density of, 175–176
3,3'-di(thiopropionyl)bishydrazide (DTPH), 127
Dlx5, 435
DNA extraction, 22
DNA/PolyMag complexes, 35
DNA quantification in scaffolds, 171, 173–175, 179
2,4-DNP, 268
Doublecortin (DCX), 59
DRAGON protein, 111
Drug discovery and hydrogels, 130
Dry eye, 420
Dsh, 435–436

E

Ectopic bone formation, 33, 88, 199, 202–206
    by equine bone protein extract, 393–401
    induced by COLLOSS® and COLLOSS E®, 92–95
    induced by GFm, 89–92
Ectopic tissue, 95–97
EDC
    crosslinking, 286
    crosslinking with SIS sponge, 211, 214, 216–217
Elastic cartilage, 245
Elastin, 281
    isolation of, 285
Electric stimulation of bioreactors, 255
Electroporation, 35, 39, 43
Embryoid bodies (EBs), 5
    differentiation of, 6–9
Embryonic stem cells, 4–9
    human, 9
    mouse, 5–9
    in vitro differentiation, 6–9
    in vivo differentiation, 5–6
Encapsulation of polyethylene hydrogels, 143–144
Endochondral bone formation, 91, 96, 244
Endocrine signaling, 72
Endogenous progenitor cells, 404

SUBJECT INDEX

Endothelial cells
  and adipogenesis, 409–410
  in corneal epithelium, 419
  in vascularization, 318
Endothelial denudation of endothelium, 322
Engineered tissues
  applications of, 363–364
  as biosensors, 364
  FDA approved, 370
  investigational studies, 367–368
  post-market surveillance, 369
  premarket submissions, 368
  product classification, 365–366
  product premarket submissions, 367–369, 369–371
  product regulatory process, 365–367
  regulation of, 364, 374–376
  special product designations and submissions, 368–369
  therapies, 363–364
Enhanced green fluorescent protein (eGFP), 31–32, 35, 36
  evaluation of expression, 37–39
  in MLV-based retroviral gene transfer, 41–42, 45
  in rAAV-mediated gene transfer, 40–41, 43
Episomal molecule, 44
Epithelial-cell sheet in corneal tissue engineering, 416
Epithelial growth factor (EGF), 77, 384
Epithelization in retinal pigment epithelium transplantation, 422
Equine bone protein extract inducing ectopic bone formation, 393–401
ERK1/2 pathway, 73
EROD enzyme activity, 130
1-ethyl-(3,3-dimethylaminopropyl) carbodiimide hydrochloride. See EDC
Experimental autoimmune encephalomyelitis, 54
Extracellular inducing signals, 408
Extracellular matrix (ECM), 69, 101, 168, 230, 404
  and cell attachment, 146–147
  and chondrocyte signaling, 70–71
  and chondrocytes in wound healing, 298
  deposition by cells, 247–248
  and flow perfusion culture, 237
  in retinal pigment epithelium transplantation, 423
  and scaffolds, 408–409
  and seeding, 249
Extracellular signaling molecules, 70, 72
Extracellular signal-related kinase (ERK), 75
Extrinsic vascularization, 311–324
Exudative age-related macular degeneration (ARMD), 420
Eye diseases, 414

F

Factor XIII, 381
Fat precursor cells, 409
Fat tissue graft, 405
FDA
  classification of products, 365–366
  legislative authority, 364–365
  mission and organization, 365
  regulation of combination products, 366–367
Federal Food, Drug, and Cosmetic (FD&C) Act, 364, 367
Fetal bovine serum (FBS), 231–232
Fetal calvarial cells, 231
Fetal tissues and stem cells, 13
Fibrillar collagen, 281
Fibrin
  as cell delivery vehicle, 382
  characteristics of, 381–383
  as culture bed, 384
  to engineer bone tissue, 386
  to engineer cartilage tissue, 386–388
  to engineer skin tissue, 384
  to engineer vascular tissue, 384–385
  and release of antibiotics, 383
  and release of growth factors, 382–383
  as scaffold material, 382
  in tissue engineering, 379–388
Fibrin glue, 380–381, 416
Fibrinogen, 379, 380–381
Fibrinolysis inhibitors, 382
Fibrin sealant, 380
Fibroblast growth factor-2 (FGF2), 304, 306–307
Fibroblast growth factors (FGFs), 6, 250, 343

Fibroblasts, 94–95, 246, 248, 254, 384
    in cell adhesion, 163–165
Fibrocartilage, 94–95, 96, 97, 245
Fibronectin, 71, 249, 344, 384
    in cell adhesion, 159–162
Fibrous tissue, 97
Fibrovascular core in bone formation, 89, 90, 96–97
Fibrovascular tissue in vascularization, 320–321
Flat flap transfer, 403
Flow cytometry, 37
Flow perfusion, 253
Fluid shear, 253
    and flow perfusion culture, 238
Fluorescence microscopy, 38
Fluorochrome markers, 339
Foaming in scaffolds, 340
Focal adhesion kinase (FAK), 70–71
Focal adhesions, 70
Free-form fabrication techniques to produce scaffolds, 342
Frz family, 435–436
Fumaryl acetoacetate hydrolase (Fah) gene, 10
Functional recovery, 50, 55, 60

G

Gastrointestinal tract damage, 20
Gel mass loss, 141–142
Gene delivery methods in porcine mesenchymal stem cells, 31–47
Gene expression of encapsulated human mesenchymal stem cells, 146–147
Gene transfer efficiency, 32, 43, 45
GFm
    bone formation, 98–99
    and ectopic tissue, 95–97
    inducing ectopic bone formation, 87, 89–92
Glaucoma, 414
Glial-axonal remodeling, 58–59
Gliogenesis, 58–59
9L-Gliosarcoma, 54
Global test, 50
Glucose concentration, 266
Glucose consumption, 268
Glucose consumption rate, 264–265

Glucose metabolism, 266–267
Glucose-6-phosphatase, 5
Glucose resonance, 269, 271
Gluthathione-s-transferase (GST), 103–104, 107
β-Glycerophosphate, 145, 232
Glycoproteins in extracellular matrix, 409
Glycosaminoglycans (GAGs), 69, 110, 282, 285, 287
    assessment of production, 300, 304
    response to collagenous scaffolds, 288–289
    in scaffolds, 279
    in synthetic extracellular matrices (sECMs), 125–131
Glycosylphosphatidylinositol (GPI)-anchoring protein, 111
Glypican-3 (GPC3), 111
Grafts, 413–414
    survival, 405
Granulocyte colonies, 117
Granulocyte-macrophageal colonies, 117
Green fluorescent protein (GFP)
    and embryonic stem cell differentiation, 5–6
Green fluorescent protein (GFP)-actin imaging, 157–160
Growth factors, 58, 72–77, 81, 101, 230, 282–283, 285, 349, 408
    anabolic, 72
    in brain injury, 56–57
    catabolic growth factors, 77–79
    as chemical stimulation of cells, 250
    in chondrogenesis, 343
    controlled release of, 128–129, 130
    epithelial growth factor, 78
    and fibrin, 382–383
    fibroblastic growth factor, 76–77
    hepatocyte growth factor, 78
    immunohistochemical staining for, 300
    insulin-like growth factor-I, 72–73
    platelet-derived growth factor, 76
    transforming growth factor-β super-family, 73–76
    vascular endothelial growth factor, 78
    in wound healing, 304, 306–307
GSK3β, 435–436
GST-BGN fusion protein, recombinant, 103–104, 105, 106, 107
GST-BGN protein, 108

SUBJECT INDEX

GST pull down assay, 104, 106, 110
Guanosine triphosphate (GTP), 116

H

HA-DTPH-Gelatin-DTPH-PEGDA, 127–128, 130
HA-DTPH-PEGDA, 127–128
Haversian canal, 228
Health Resources Services Administration (HRSA), 364
Helper genes, 44
Hematopoietic progenitors, 115
Hematopoietic cells, 231
Hematopoietic growth factor, 115–120
Hematopoietic marrow, 96
Hematopoietic stem cells
  bone marrow derived, 10–11
  and progenitor cells, 205
Heparan sulphate (HS), 285
Heparan sulphate(HS)/heparin, 282
Heparin and growth factor delivery, 383
Hepatic functions, long-term maintenance by biomaterials, 13–14
Hepatic induction factor cocktail (HIFC) differentiation system, 7, 8
Hepatic induction system, 6–9
Hepatic nuclear factor, 5
Hepatic transcription factors, 5
Hepatocyte growth factor (HGF), 6, 77
Hepatocyte nuclear factors, 7
Hepatocytes
  differentiation of, 8–9
  functional, 3
  generation of human, 4
HepG2 cells, 153, 154, 157–160
Heptide, 381
H80HrPE-6 cells, 424
Hippocampus-derived stem cells, 423
Histioinductive approaches to tissue engineering, 404–405
Histomorphometry, 202–206
Homeostasis, 380–381
Host replacement theory, 405
HP-DTPH, 130–131
Human 293 cells, 37
Human cellular- and tissue-based products (HCT/Ps)
  FDA approved, 370
  FDA regulation of, 371–373

Humanitarian Device Exemption (HDE), 368
Humanitarian Use Device (HUD), 368
Human mesenchymal stem cells
  analysis of, 139
  biochemical activity of encapsulated, 144
  and bone regeneration, 135–147
  culture and encapsulation, 21, 138
  DNA extraction and PCR analysis, 22
  encapsulation and proliferation, 143–144
  gene expression of, 139–140, 146–147
  histology, 22
  in NOD/SCID mouse model, 21
  mineralization of hydrogels by, 139, 144–145
Hyaline cartilage, 91, 93–95, 96, 97, 245
Hyaline nasal septal cartilage, 342
Hyaluronan, 125, 126
Hyaluronic acid (HA), 69, 81, 282
Hyaluronic acid (HA) gel, 197–198, 199, 206
  and nucleated cells, 200–202
Hyaluronic acid (HA) sponge, 14
Hydrazide derivatives, 127
Hydrogels, 379
  and bone regeneration, 135–147
  encapsulating chondrocytes, 80
  as scaffolds, 232
  in synthetic extracellular matrices (sECMs), 125–131
Hydrogen bonding in PEGDM-PLGA blends, 187, 192
Hydrolysis kinetic constant, 141–142
Hydroxyapatite ceramics, 330–332, 333
Hypoxia, 408
Hypoxia inducible factor I (HIF-1), 408

I

IGF-1, 72–73, 81, 304, 306, 343
IGFBP-3, 72
IGF-1R, 72
Immune privilege of bone marrow stromal cells, 55
Immunoprecipitation-Western blot analysis, 103
Immunosuppression, 119
India ink perfusion, 314
Indocyanin-green (ICG) uptake, 7
Indoleamine 2,3-dioxygenase (IDO), 119

Inflammation
  in scaffolds, 179
  in vascularization, 320–323
Infrared spectroscopy (IR), 185, 187–188
InFUSE bone graft, 370
Inhibitory Smads (I-Smads), 74, 75, 76
Injectability of PEGDM-PLGA blends, 191, 193
Inner cell mass (ICM), 4
Inner circumferential lamellae, 227–228
Insertional mutagenesis, 45
Insulin-like growth factor binding proteins (IGFBP), 72
Insulin-like growth factor-1 (IGF-1), 72–73, 81, 304, 306, 343
Insulin receptor substrates (IRS), 72–73
Insulin secretion, 265–266
Integrins, 70–71, 344
  and signaling, 80–81
Interbody fusion, 197, 198
Interleukin-1, 75, 76, 77–79
  associating protein, 78
Interleukin-6, 78, 79
Interleukin-8, 79
Interleukin-17, 79
Interleukin-18, 79
Interleukin-1β, 77–78
Interleukin-1 receptor I, 78
Interleukin-1 receptor II, 78
Interstitial growth, 244, 245
Interstitial lamella, 228
Intervertebral discs and tissue engineering, 167–180
Intestinal radiation injury and mesenchymal stem cells, 19–28
Intracellular signaling, 70, 408
Intracerebral hemorrhage, treatment by bone marrow stromal cells (BMSCs), 52
Intracerebral surgical transplantation, 51
Intracisternal cell injection, 51
Intramembranous ossification, 244
Intramuscular implantation in synthetic bone graft substitutes, 338
Intrinsic vascularization, 312–324
Intussusceptive angiogenesis, 322
Inverse terminal repeats (ITR), 33
Investigational Device Exemption (IDE) application, 367
Investigational New Drug (IND) application, 367

IRAK-1, 78
IRAK-2, 78
Ischemic boundary tissue, 49
Ischemic boundary zone, 51

J

Joint loading, 348

K

Keratan sulfate (KS), 282
Keratinocyte growth factor (KGF), 129
Keratinocytes, 384
Keratin sulfate, 69, 80
Keratocytes, 418
Kick-down factors, 372–373
Kinetic chain connectivity, 141–142
Knee replacements, 247

L

Lactate production, 268
Lamellae of osteons, 227, 228
Lamellar bone, 226–227
Laminin, 409
Large skeletal defects, 225
Lef1, 435
Lens regeneration, 424–425
Leptin, 407
Leukemia and possible induction by retroviral vectors, 45
Leukemia inhibitory factor (LIF), 5
Ligaments
  and bioreactors, 254
  properties and pathologies of, 246–247
Limbal allograft transplantation, 415
Limbal stem cells, 415
Limbus, 415
Lineage-uncommitted stromal cells, 406
LipofectAMINE™ transfection agent, 35
Liver
  target for stem cell therapy, 3
  tissue engineering of, 13–14
  transplantation, 3
Liver specific markers, 5, 7
Long-bone segmental defect, 338–339
L-Sox5, 431, 432–433

SUBJECT INDEX

M

Macro-monomers, 183
Magnetic force-based tissue engineering, 422
Magnetic resonance angiography, 315, 322
Magnetic resonance imaging (MRI) of tumor cells, 54–55
Magnetic stimulation of bioreactors, 255
Magnetofection™, 35–36, 37, 39, 43
MAPK pathway, 72–73, 78
MAPK signaling pathway, 79, 80
Marrow space, 202, 204–205
Marrow stimulation, 246
Marrow stromal cells, 231, 232–233
    growth and neopterin, 115–120
Mass culture technique in chondrogenesis, 343
Masson's trichrome staining, 176, 178–179
Mass swelling ratio, 140–141
Matrigel®, 404–405, 409, 411, 424
Matrix mineralization, 144
Matrix proteins, 6
MC3T3-E1 cell line, 333–335
Mean fluorescence intensity (MFI), 37, 40, 41, 43, 45
Mean pore diameter in scaffolds, 172, 176, 179
Mechanical loading, 253–255
Mechanical stimulation and chondrogenesis, 344
Mechano-chemical transduction, 152
Medical Device User Free and Modernization Act (2002), 366
Medium in bone graft substitutes, 335–337
MEK/Erk pathway, 57
Membrane-surface separation, 153
Membranous bone, 91, 92, 99
Me.PEG-PLA films, 233
Mesenchymal stem cells (MSCs), 11–12, 405
    and adipogenesis, 406
    engraftment in NOD/SCID mice, 23
    in functional tissue engineering, 248, 251, 254
    human, 21–22
    infusion on small intestine, 24–25
    isolation of porcine stem cells, 34
    supporting small intestine regeneration after radiation injury, 19–28
    viability in cartilage tissue engineering, 350
    viral and non-viral gene transfer methods, 31–47
Metalloproteases, 77–79, 81
Metalloproteinases, expression of, 80
Metals as scaffolds for bone tissue engineering, 233
1-methyl-4-phenyl-1,2,3,6-tetrahydropyridine (MPTP), 54
icrocontact printing, 421
Micro-CT scanning, 262, 397–398
Microencapsulation, 263
Microvessels in angiogenesis, 57–58
Middle cerebral artery (MCAo), 50–51
Mineral formation, 144
Mineralization, 96
    of bone, 230
    of hydrogels, 139, 144–145
Mitomycin-C containing synthetic extracellular matrix, 131
MMP1, 77
MMP3, 77
Modified neurological severity score (mNSS), 50
MOI 10, 40, 100, 40, 41, 43
Molecular markers, 59
Mouse bone marrow-derived cells (mBMCs), 116
Mouse embryonic stem cells, 5–9
Mucosa regeneration by mesenchymal stem cell infusion, 24–28
Mucosal epithelial cells in corneal transplant, 417–418
Multiple sclerosis, treatment by bone marrow stromal cells (BMSCs), 54, 60
Multipotent adult progenitor cells (MAPCs), 11
Multipotential mesenchymal stem cells, 12
Murine leukemia virus (MLV)-based retroviral system, 33, 36–37, 41–42
    application of, 46
    optimization of, 45
    safety issues, 45–46
Murine NIH3T3 cells, 37
Muscle derived stem cells, 407
Muscle xenograft, 406–407
Musculoskeletal disorders, statistics on, 243–244

Musculoskeletal system
  bioreactors and, 243–255
  properties and pathologies of, 244–247
MyD88, 78
Myelin proteolipid protein (PLP), 54
Myeloid stem cells, 115
Myocardial infarction, 20
Myod1, 108, 109, 111
Myofibroblasts, 385
Myogenesis, 407
Myogenic markers, 108, 109, 111

N

National Marrow Donor Program, 364
National Organ Transplant Program, 364
Neopterin as hematopoietic and stromal cell growth factor, 115–120
Neotissue, 244, 247
Neovascularization, 311, 404
Nerve growth factor (NGF), 7
Neural proteins, 51
Neural stem cells in retina regeneration, 423
Neurogenesis in brain injury, 59
Neuronal degeneration, 58
Neurotrophins, 50, 58
Neutrophilin-1, 77
NF-κB signaling pathway, 79
NG-2, 59
NIH-3T3 cell line, 37, 212, 217
Nitric oxide production, 73
NMR, 185, 188, 262–263
NOD/SCID mice and human mesenchymal stem cell engraftment, 21, 23
Noggin, 75
Non-exudative age-related macular degeneration (ARMD), 420
Noninvasive monitoring of constructs, 261–274
Non-load-bearing animal models, 348
Non-viral gene delivery methods, 32, 34–36, 39, 43, 46
  calcium phosphate co-precipitation, 34–35, 39
  cationic liposome-mediated transfection, 35, 39
  electroporation, 35, 39
  magnetofection™, 35–36, 39

Nuclear magnetic resonance spectroscopy (NMR), 185, 188, 262–263
Nucleated cells, 197–198
  in vitro assays of, 200–202
Nucleation, 144
Nucleofector™ programs, 35
Nucleus pulposus (NP), 171, 174

O

Ocular tissue engineering, 413–425
  corneal epithelium, 419–420
  corneal stroma, 418–419
  lens regeneration, 424–425
  retinal pigment epithelium engineering, 420–423
  retina regeneration, 423–424
Office of Combination Products (OCP), 365, 366
Office of Orphan Products (OOP), 365
Office of Regulatory Affairs (ORA), 365
Oligodendrocytes, 54, 59
Oligo[poly(ethylene glycol) fumarte] hydrogels, 232
Oncostatin M, 6
OP-1 implant, 370
OP-1 Putty, 370
Optical imaging, 262
Organ culture systems, 329–330
Orphan Drug Act (1982), 368
Orphan drugs, 368–369
Oscillatory experiments, 190–191
Ossicles, 89, 98
Ossification, 432, 433
Osteoarthritis, 70, 245, 246
Osteoblast differentiation
  induced by BMP-2, 101–112
  regulation by Osterix, 434–435
  regulation by Twist proteins, 434
  and Wnt/β-catenin, 435–436
Osteoblasts, 89, 90, 91, 93, 135, 136, 229, 230, 247–248
  in bone graft substitutes, 336, 337
  electric stimulation, 255
  and osteochondroprogenitor fate, 431–438
  and Runx2, 433–434
  in scaffolds, 254
  and Sox9, 433

SUBJECT INDEX

Osteocalcin, 231, 253, 332
Osteochondroprogenitor fate during bone formation, 431–438
   and Runx2, 435
   and Wnt/β-catenin, 435–436
Osteoclasts, 89, 90, 91, 93, 229
Osteoconduction, 331–332
Osteocytes, 229, 244
Osteogenesis, 438
   bonding, 331
   and Osterix, 434–435
   and Runx2, 433–434
   and transcription factors, 432
Osteogenesis imperfecta, 20
Osteogenic cells in bone regeneration, 226
Osteogenicity, 338
Osteogenic markers, 108, 109, 111, 333–334
Osteogenic proteins (OP), 75
Osteoinduction, 87–99, 332–335, 336
   by equine bone protein extract, 393–401
   and soft tissue models, 338
Osteonecrosis, 244–245
Osteonectin, 332
Osteopontin (OPN), 139, 140, 146–147, 231, 386, 433
Osteoprogenitor cells, 231–232
Osterix (Osx), 108, 109, 111, 432, 437, 438
   in osteogenesis, 434–435
OST (osteogenic differentiation) media, 144–147
Outer circumferential lamellae, 227–228

P

^{31}P in pancreatic constructs, 265–266
Packaging cells, 33, 45, 46
PAI-1, 408, 410
Pancreatic constructs
   cell organization, 264–265
   function of, 273–274
   integrity of, 263–264, 272–273
   in vivo experiments, 270–274
   metabolic activity of, 265–269
   noninvasive monitoring of, 263–274
   viable cell number, 269–272
Paracrine signaling, 72
Parallel elastic, 190–191
Parkinson's disease treatment by bone marrow stromal cells (BMSCs), 53–54
Partial oxygen pressure, 266, 268
Particle leaching in scaffolds, 340
Patellar tendon, 247
Patency, 317, 322
PCR analysis, 22
PDGF. *See* Platelet-derived growth factor (PDGF)
PDGF-α, 76
PDGF-β, 76
PDK1, 73
PDK2, 73
PEEK rings, 396–400
PEG4600-2Cap-DMA, encapsulation, 143–144
PEG4600DMA, 137, 139, 147
   biochemical activity of, 144
   encapsulation, 143–144
PEGDM-PLGA blends, 184–195
   characterization of, 185, 187–192
   non-polymerized, 186
   photopolymerized, 186, 192
   preparation of, 184–185
PEG4600-4Lac-DMA, 147
   biochemical activity of, 144
   encapsulation, 143–144
PEG4600-nCap-DMA, 137, 138
PEG4600-nLac-DMA, 137, 138, 139
   characterization of, 140–143
Pellet culture in chondrogenesis, 343, 346
Perfusion bioreactors, 235, 236–238
Perfusion in tissue engineering, 317, 322
Perichondrium, 342
Periosteum, 228, 342
Periostitis, 244
Peritoneal cavity, 270–271
Phase angle, 190
Phase contrast microscopy, 155
Phosphorus concentration in hydroxyapatite ceramics, 330–331, 335–336
Photopolymerizable systems, 183
Photopolymerization, 193–194
Photopolymerized poly(ethylene oxide) hydrogels, 81
Pigment epithelial (PE) cell line, 424
PI3K/Akt pathway, 57
PI3K signaling pathway, 72–73, 78, 80
PKC pathway, 73
Plasmids
   and fibrin, 383
   in rAAV-mediated gene transfer, 44

Platelet-derived growth factor (PDGF), 76, 307, 343
pLXSN transfer vector, 36, 38, 41–42
PMOA Proposed Rule, 366–367
Poly(α-hydroxy acid)s, 167
Polyethylene glycol diacrylate (PEGDA)-crosslinked HA-DTPH, 127
Poly(ethylene glycol)dimethyacrylate (PEGDM), 183–195
Poly(ethylene glycol) (PEG), 81
Poly(ethylene glycol) (PEG) hydrogels
 and bone regeneration, 136–147
 characterization of, 140–143
 mineralization of, 139
 in retinal pigment epithelium engineeing, 421–422
 synthesis of, 137–138
Poly(ethylene glycol)-terephthalate-poly(butylene terephthalate) (PEGT/PBT) polymer, 346
Polyethylene hydrogels, mineralization of, 144–145
Poly(glycolic acid) (PGA), 167
 meshes, 81
 scaffolds, 249
Poly(lactic acid) (PLA), 167
 blocks, 141–142
 in retinal pigment epithelium engineeing, 421–422
Poly(lactic-co-glycolic acid) (PLGA), 167–180
 photopolymerizable blends, 183–195
 in retinal pigment epithelium engineering, 421–422
Poly(lactic-co-glycolic acid) (PLGA) scaffolds
 characterization of, 172
 and fibrin, 386
 histological evaluation of, 175–179
 preparation of, 169–170
Poly(L-lactic acid) (PLLA), 248–249
Poly-L-lysine (PLL) layer, 263–264
Polymer films in retinal pigment epithelium engineering, 421–422
Polymerizing light, 183–184
Polymers, 13–14
 encapsulating chondrocytes, 79–80
 use in scaffolds, 232, 248–249, 341
Poly (propylene fumarate-co-ethylene glycol) hydrogels, 232

Poly(propylene fumarate) (PPF), 232
Polyurethane in tissue engineering, 13
Porcine mesenchymal stem cells, 31–47
 cell culture of, 34
 detection of replication-competent viruses (RCVs), 37
 evaluation of transgene expression, 37–39
 isolation of, 34
 non-viral gene delivery methods, 34–36, 39, 46
 viral gene delivery methods, 36–37, 40–42
Porcine small intestine submucosa (SIS), 209–220
Pore size
 of scaffold, 238
 of small intestine submucosa (SIS) sponge, 211, 215
Porogens, 340
Porosity
 of scaffolds, 172, 176, 179, 285–286, 340
 of small intestine submucosa (SIS) sponge, 211, 215
Porous tantalum trabecular metal, 197–206
 preparation of, 199–200
Positron emission tomography (PET), 262
Posterior capsule opacification, 424
Posterior cruciate ligament, 247
Preadipocytes, 405, 406–407, 408, 409
 and vasculature, 409–410
Pref-1, 406
Premarket Approval application, 368
Preosteoblasts, 437
 and Runx2, 435
Prevascularization, 311
Primary Mode of a Combination Product: Proposed Rule, 366–367
Primary porcine esophageal fibroblasts, 154–155, 163–165
Processed bovine cancellous bone (PBCB) matrices, 313
Processed-lipoaspirate (PLA), 405
Product development, 373–374
Product premarket submissions, 367–369, 369–371
Product regulatory process, 365–367
 of combination products, 366–367
Progenitor cells
 for adipose tissue, 406–407
 retinal, 423–424

SUBJECT INDEX

ProPak-X.36, 36
Prostaglandin E2 (PGE$_2$), 77
Prosthetic joint replacement, 245
Protein receptors, 69
Proteins
    in chondrocyte signaling, 68–69
    in damaged brains, 49
Proteoglycans, 69, 74, 76, 125
    in cartilage, 245
    small leucine-rich, 101
    synthesis, 80, 81
    in wound healing, 299, 301, 303
Pseudoperiochondrium, 387
PTH and β-catenin, 438
pXX2, 44
pXX6, 44

R

Radiation injury and mesenchymal stem cells, 19–28
Radiograph, 396
Radionuclide imaging, 262
Radiotherapy, 20
Rat bone marrow cells on calcium-phosphate ceramics, 331
Real-time quantitative reverse transcription polymerase chain reaction (RT-PCR), 38, 105, 139
Recombinant adeno-associated virus-enhanced green fluorescent protein (rAAV-eGFP) vector, 36, 38, 40
Recombinant adeno-associated virus(rAAV)-mediated gene delivery, 32, 36, 40–41, 43–44
    application of, 44
    gene transfer efficiency, 43
    safety of, 44
    temporal transgene expression, 43–44
Recombinant adeno-associated virus (rAAV) system, 33, 36, 40–41, 43–44, 46–47
Recombinant BGN, 103–104
Recombinant GST-BGN fusion protein, 103–104, 105, 106, 107, 110–111
Reflectance interference contrast microscopy (RICM), 152–153
Regenerative medicine, 3
Regular Smads (R-Smads), 74–76

Replication-competent viruses (RCVs)
    detection of, 37
    generation of, 46, 47
Request for Designation (RFD), 366
Retinal pigment epithelium (RPE)
    cell sheets, 421–423
    metabolism of, 422
    and tissue engineering, 420–423
Retinal progenitor cells, 423–424
Retina regeneration, 423–424
Retinitis pigmentosa, 423
Retinoid metabolism, 422
Retrograde degeneration, 58
Retroviral envelope, 45, 47
Retroviral gene delivery, 32
Retroviral gene transfer systems, 33
Retroviral transfer vector, 33
Retroviral vectors, 33
Retroviruses, 33
Reverse gel point, 142
Reverse transcription, 139–140
rhBMP-2, 104, 105, 107, 108, 111, 197, 200, 202–206
rhBMP-4, 104, 105
rhBMP-6, 104, 105
rhBMP-7, 104, 105
Rheological measurements of PEGDM-PLGA blends, 185, 188–192, 194
RIP, 54, 58
RNA
    integrity determination, 38
    transcription, 33
Rotating wall vessels in cell seeding, 234–235, 236, 252–253
Runx1, 434
Runx2, 432, 433, 438
    and chondrocyte maturation, 433–434
    isoforms, 433
    in osteogenesis, 433–434
    regulation of transcription, 434–435
    relationship with Sox9, 436
    Wnt/β-catenin signaling, 436
Runx3, 434
Runx2-I, 433–434
Runx2-II, 433–434

S

Safe Medical Device Act (1990), 366
Safranin O staining, 176, 178–179

Satellite cells, 407
Scaffolds, 13, 225–226
  applications of, 290–292
  architecture of in vivo models of cartilage tissue engineering, 349
  biodegradable, 175, 248, 404
  in bone tissue engineering, 232–234
  in cartilage tissue engineering, 291–292, 339–340
  and cell interactions in chondrogenesis, 344
  cell seeding onto, 234–235
  characterization of, 171, 286–288
  chemical stimulation of, 250
  and chondrogenesis, 343
  components of, 281–283
  crosslinking, 286–287
  and extracellular matrices, 408–409
  and fabrication techniques, 340–341
  foaming in, 340
  in functional tissue engineering, 248–249
  and hydrogels, 382, 1125–126
  mechanical stimulation of, 250, 252, 253
  nonbiodegradable, 248
  pore size of, 238
  porosity of, 344–345, 346–347
  porous tantalum trabecular metal as, 197–198, 202–206
  preparation of, 283–288
  purity of components, 283–285
  in retina regeneration, 424
  seeding techniques, 249
  surface modification of, 249
  synthetic, 81
  three-dimensional architecture of, 344–346
  for tissue engineered intervertebral discs, 167–180
  tissue response to, 288–289
  use of small intestine submucosa (SIS), 217–218
Scanning electron microscope, 211–212
SDS-PAGE, 283–285
Secondary forces in PEGDM-PLGA blends, 188
Seeding scaffolds, 234–235, 249, 251–255
  efficiencies of, 253
Semi-penetrating networks (semi-IPNs), 194

Shc pathway, 70–71
Shc proteins, 72–73
Shear stress, 322
Shear viscosity in PEGDM-PLGA blends, 188–190, 193
Sialoprotein, 231, 332
Signaling
  autocrine, 72
  of chondrocytes, 67–82
  endocrine, 72
  paracrine, 72
  pathways, 408–409
  pathways in bone formation, 438
  pathways of chondrocytes, 67
  regulated by tissue engineering, 79–81
  transduction, 152
Single-photo emission tomography (SPECT), 262
Sintering of ceramics, 331–332
SIS/DBP/PLGA scaffolds, 168
  characterization of, 172
  histological evaluation of, 175–179
  preparation of, 169–170
SIS/PLGA scaffolds, 168
  characterization of, 172
  histological evaluation of, 175–179
  preparation of, 169–170
Skeletal tissues, 95–97
Skin
  composite cultured, 370
  replacement therapies, 383
  tissue engineering of, 292–293
  and use of fibrin, 384
Smad-2, 75
Smad-3, 75
Smad-4, 75, 76
Smad-6, 75, 76
Smad-7, 75
Smad proteins, 74, 75
  assay, 104
  phosphorylation, 106–107
Small intestine
  atrophy, 26
  infusion by mesenchymal stem cells, 24–25
  regeneration after radiation injury using mesenchymal stem cells, 19–28
Small intestine submucosa (SIS), 168, 173–175, 290
  preparation of, 169

SUBJECT INDEX

Small intestine submucosa (SIS) sponge
　cell attachment to, 212
　measurement of, 211–212
　porosity and pore size of, 211
　preparation of, 170, 172, 176, 210–211, 213–214
　as a scaffold, 209–220
　structures of, 215
　water absorption of, 212, 216–217
　in wound healing, 212–213, 218–220
Small leucine-rich proteoglycans (SLRPs), 101
Soft tissue models for synthetic bone graft substitutes, 337–338
Solvent casting/salt leaching method, 169–170, 172, 176
Sox6, 431, 432–433
Sox9, 431, 432, 438
　and chondrogenic cell lineage, 432–433
　relationship with β-catenin, 436–437
　relationship with Runx2, 436
Spinal cord injury treatment by bone marrow stromal cells (BMSCs), 52
Spinal fusion, 205
Spinner flask, 234, 235–236, 252
　and chondrogenesis, 344
Sport injuries, 247
Sprouting angiogenesis, 319–320, 322
Static culture as seeding technique, 249, 251–252
Stem cells
　adult, 9–13
　adipose tissue, 12–13
　bone marrow, 10–12
　in fetal tissues, 13
　multipotent, 3, 10
　pluripotent, 3, 4
　transplantation, 3
Stretching in scaffolds, 253–254
Stroke
　and brain damage, 49–50
　treated by bone marrow stromal cells (BMSCs), 50–51
Stromal cell growth and neopterin, 115–120
Stromal cell progenitors, 115–120
Stromal cells, 231
Stromal/mesenchymal cell growth, 115–120
Stromal-vascular fraction of adipose tissue, 406–407, 411
Subcutaneous implantation, 348
　in synthetic bone graft substitutes, 338

Subgranular zone (SGZ), 52, 59
Subventricular zone (SVZ), 49, 52, 59
Surface wetting, 216
Surgery and use of fibrin glue, 380–381
Synapse formation, 58
Synaptogenesis and synaptic modification, 58
Synaptophysin, 58
Syngeneic bone marrow stromal cells, 55–56
Synthetic extracellular matrices (sECMs), 125–131
　applications of, 130–131
Synthetic scaffolds, 81

T

Tantalum ring, 197–198
TCA cycle, 266
βTC3 cells, 265–267
Tegaderm™, 218–220
Tendinopathies, 246
Tendinosis, 246
Tendonitis, 246
Tendons
　and bioreactors, 254
　properties and pathologies of, 246
Tenocytes, 246
Tensile strength, 246
Teratomas, production of, 5–6
TGF-β, 73–76, 101–102, 250, 343
TGF-β1, 73, 75, 80, 297–307
TGF-β2, 75
TGF-β3, 75
TGF-β/BMP receptors, 102, 103
TGF-β/BRII, 103
Thiols in synthetic extracellular matrix (sECM), 126–127
Thrombin, 379, 380–381
Tibial fracture, 338
Tissue constructs, 413
Tissue culture substrate, detachable, 422
Tissue defects in wound healing, 301–302, 305
Tissue-engineered devices, 115
Tissue engineering
　of articular cartilage, 339–340
　of cornea, 414–420
　of corneal endothelium, 419–420
　of corneal stroma, 418–419

functional, 247–250
and intervertebral discs, 167–180
magnetic force-based, 422
ocular, 413–425
of pancreatic constructs, 261–274
to regulate signaling, 79–81
retinal pigment epithelium, 420–423
strategies, 404–405
synthetic extracellular matrices for, 125–131
vascularization in, 311–324
Tissue growth, 244
Titanium fiber mesh as scaffold, 233, 237
T lymphocytes, 55
TNFα, 75, 79, 81, 384
TNF-R1, 73–74, 75, 79
TNF-R2, 73–74, 75, 79
Total choline resonance, 269–270, 271–272
Trabecular lamellae, 227, 228
TRAF protein, 79
Transcription factors during bone formation, 431, 432
Transcription of BMP-2 transgene, 38–39
Transdifferentiation, 11, 424
Transduction, 43–44
Transfection, cationic liposome-mediated, 35
Transfer vectors, 36
Transforming growth factor-β superfamily (TGF-β), 73–76, 101–102, 250, 343
bone morphogenetic protein, 75–76
transforming growth factor-β1, 74–75
Transforming growth factor β1 (TGFβ1), 74–75, 304, 306–307
Transgene expression
evaluation of, 37–39
temporal, 43–44
Transthyretin, 5
Traumatic brain injury treated by bone marrow stromal cells (BMSCs), 52
Trophic factors in brain injury, 56–57
Tropoelastin, 281
Tryptophan, 119
Tryptophan-2,3-dioxygenase, 5
Tumor cell lines and hydrogels, 130
Tumor necrosis factor-α, 75, 79, 81, 384
Twist-1, 434
Twist-2, 434
Twist proteins regulating Runx2, 434
Type I collagen, 70, 281, 283–284
in scaffolds, 291–292

Type II collagen, 69, 71, 76, 281, 285
and epithelial growth factor, 77
expression, 80
in scaffolds, 176, 178–179, 291 292
Type II receptor of transforming growth factor-β superfamily, 73–74, 75, 79
Type I receptor of transforming growth factor-β superfamily, 73–74, 75, 79
Type X collagen, 70
Tyrosine hydroxylase (TH), 54

U

Ultrasound, 255
Ultraviolet-visible spectroscopy (UV), 185, 187
Umbilical cord blood as source for stem cells, 13

V

Valve conduits, engineering of, 385
Vascular corrosion casts, 314–315
Vascular endothelial growth factor (VEGF), 49, 57–58, 77, 128–129, 282, 285, 408, 414
Vascularization
extrinsic, 311–324
intrinsic, 312–324
in tissue engineering, 311–324
Vascular tissue
and use of fibrin, 384–385
Vasculature, 404
and adipogenesis, 409–410
VEGF, 77, 384
VEGF-R1, 77
VEGF-RII, 77
Villus height affected by mesenchymal stem cell infusion, 24–26
Viral gene delivery methods, 36–37, 40–41, 43–46
murine leukemia virus (MLV)-based retroviral system, 36–37, 41–42, 45–46
recombinant adeno-associated virus (rAAV) system, 33, 36, 40–41, 43–44, 46–47
Viral load, effect of, 43
Viscosity in PEGDM-PLGA blends, 188–190, 193
Viscous moduli, 190–191

SUBJECT INDEX

Vitreous body, 425
Vitronectin, 344, 409

W

Water uptake, 216–217
Wnt14, 435, 436
Wnt/β-catenin, 435–436, 438
    and Runx2, 436
Wnt/β-catenin signal molecules, 431
Wound dressings, 126–127, 131

Wound healing, 380–381
    age-related differences in articular
        cartilage healing, 297–307
    histology of, 299–300
    use of small intestine submucosa (SIS)
        sponge, 212–213, 218–220
Woven bone, 226–227

X

Xenograft and hydrogels, 130